The Molecular and
Cellular Biology
of Wound Repair

The Molecular and Cellular Biology of Wound Repair

Edited by

R. A. F. Clark

and

P. M. Henson

National Jewish Center for Immunology and Respiratory Medicine
Denver, Colorado

PLENUM PRESS • NEW YORK AND LONDON

Library of Congress Cataloging in Publication Data

The Molecular and cellular biology of wound repair / edited by R. A. F. Clark and
P. M. Henson.
   p.   cm.
   Includes bibliographies and index.
   ISBN 0-306-42716-8
   1. Wound healing. I. Clark, R. A. F. (Richard A. F.) II. Henson, P. M. (Peter M.)
RD94.M65 1988
616'.1—dc 19   87-37683
                                                                          CIP

Cover illustration: Scanning electron micrograph of femoral artery
demonstrating fibrin strand formation and platelet deposition. (See Chapter 4,
Figure 11b.)

© 1988 Plenum Press, New York
A Division of Plenum Publishing Corporation
233 Spring Street, New York, N.Y. 10013

Printed in the United States of America

Contributors

Richard K. Assoian Department of Biochemistry and Molecular Biophysics, Center for Reproductive Sciences, College of Physicians and Surgeons, Columbia University, New York, New York 10032

Allen R. Banks Amgen, Inc., Thousand Oaks, California 91320

Robert A. Briggaman Department of Dermatology, University of North Carolina, Chapel Hill, North Carolina 27515

Richard A. F. Clark Department of Medicine, National Jewish Center for Immunology and Respiratory Medicine, Denver, Colorado 80206

John R. Couchman Connective Tissue Laboratory, Department of Medicine, B. R. Boshell Diabetes Hospital, University of Alabama in Birmingham, Birmingham, Alabama 35294

Louis DePalma Department of Pathology and Laboratory Medicine, Yale University School of Medicine, New Haven, Connecticut 06510

Harold F. Dvorak Department of Pathology, Beth Israel Hospital, Harvard Medical School, and the Charles A. Dana Research Institute, Boston, Massachusetts 02115

Gary M. Fox Amgen, Inc., Thousand Oaks, California 91320

Leo T. Furcht Department of Laboratory Medicine and Pathology, University of Minnesota, Minneapolis, Minnesota 55455

Heinz Furthmayr Department of Pathology, Yale University School of Medicine, New Haven, Connecticut 06510

Giulio Gabbiani Department of Pathology, University of Geneva, 1211 Geneva 4, Switzerland

Mark H. Ginsberg Department of Immunology, Scripps Clinic and Research Foundation, La Jolla, California 92037

Dean Handley   Division of Platelet Research, Sandoz, Inc., East Hanover, New Jersey 07936

Christopher Haslett   Department of Medicine, Royal Postgraduate Medical School, Hammersmith Hospital, London, W12 OHS, England

Ronald L. Heimark   Department of Pathology, University of Washington, Seattle, Washington 98195

Peter M. Henson   Department of Pediatrics, National Jewish Center for Immunology and Respiratory Medicine, Denver, Colorado 80206

Magnus Höök   Department of Biochemistry, Connective Tissue Laboratory, B. R. Boshell Diabetes Hospital, University of Alabama in Birmingham, Birmingham, Alabama 35294

Jung San Huang   E. A. Doisy Department of Biochemistry, St. Louis University School of Medicine, St. Louis, Missouri 63104

Shuan Shiang Huang   E. A. Doisy Department of Biochemistry, St. Louis University School of Medicine, St. Louis, Missouri 63104

Richard B. Johnston, Jr.   Department of Pediatrics, The University of Pennsylvania School of Medicine and The Children's Hospital of Philadelphia, Philadelphia, Pennsylvania 19104

Allen P. Kaplan   Division of Allergy, Rheumatology, and Clinical Immunology, Department of Medicine, The State University of New York at Stony Brook, Health Sciences Center, Stony Brook, New York 11794

Joseph A. Madri   Department of Pathology, Yale University School of Medicine, New Haven, Connecticut 06510

James B. McCarthy   Department of Laboratory Medicine and Pathology, University of Minnesota, Minneapolis, Minnesota 55455

John A. McDonald   Respiratory and Critical Care Division, Departments of Biochemistry and Medicine, Washington University School of Medicine, St. Louis, Missouri 63110

John M. McPherson   Connective Tissue Research Laboratories, Collagen Corporation, Palo Alto, California 94303

Paolo Mignatti   Department of Cell Biology and Kaplan Cancer Center, New York University School of Medicine, New York, New York 10016

Peter P. Nawroth   Department of Physiology and Cellular Biophysics, College of Physicians and Surgeons, Columbia University, New York, New York 10032

Thomas J. Olsen   E. A. Doisy Department of Biochemistry, St. Louis University School of Medicine, St. Louis, Missouri 63104

Karl A. Piez   Connective Tissue Research Laboratories, Collagen Corporation, Palo Alto, California 94303

Bruce M. Pratt   Department of Pathology, Yale University School of Medicine, New Haven, Connecticut 06510

David W.H. Riches   Department of Pediatrics, National Jewish Center for Immunology and Respiratory Medicine, Denver, Colorado 80206

Daniel B. Rifkin   Department of Cell Biology and Kaplan Cancer Center, New York University School of Medicine, New York, New York 10016

Daryl F. Sas   Department of Laboratory Medicine and Pathology, University of Minnesota, Minneapolis, Minnesota 55455; present address: Gastrointestinal Research Unit, Mayo Clinic, Rochester, Minnesota 55905.

Stephen M. Schwartz   Department of Pathology, University of Washington, Seattle, Washington 98195

Omar Skalli   Department of Pathology, University of Geneva, 1211 Geneva 4, Switzerland

Kurt S. Stenn   Department of Dermatology, Yale University School of Medicine, New Haven, Connecticut 06510

David M. Stern   Department of Physiology and Cellular Biophysics, College of Physicians and Surgeons, Columbia University, New York, New York 10032

Robert A. Terkeltaub   Veterans Administration Medical Center–UCSD, San Diego, California 92161

Marcia G. Tonnesen   Department of Pediatrics, National Jewish Center for Immunology and Respiratory Medicine, and Dermatology Service, Veterans' Administration Medical Center, Denver, Colorado 80206

Howard G. Welgus   Division of Dermatology, Department of Medicine, Jewish Hospital at Washington University Medical Center, St. Louis, Missouri 63110

Timothy J. Williams Section of Vascular Biology, MRC Clinical Research Centre, Harrow, Middlesex HA1 3UJ, England

David T. Woodley Department of Dermatology, University of North Carolina, Chapel Hill, North Carolina 27515

G. Scott Worthen Department of Medicine, National Jewish Center for Immunology and Respiratory Medicine, Denver, Colorado 80206

Preface

Editing a book of this nature was a simultaneously exhilarating and frightening experience. It was exhilarating to draw from cell biologists, biochemists, and molecular biologists, as well as those dermatologists, pathologists, and pulmonologists who are cell biologists at heart, to author chapters. At the same time, it was frightening to ask such busy investigators to devote their precious time to writing chapters that summarize not just their own endeavors but their entire area of expertise. However, the authors assuaged our fears by enthusiastically accepting the proposal to write on specific topics despite the time burden, and to update and willingly accept our editorial comments. In the editors' view, the authors have captured the important scientific data in their respective fields, have organized the data into an understandable outline, and have applied the information to elucidating wound repair processes.

The explosion of new, important discoveries in the field of wound repair and related areas as our book was developing has been very unsettling. This observation predicts obsolescence. In response to this possibility, the authors and the editors have attempted to build fundamental concepts upon existing data. Hopefully, these concepts will help provoke further experimentation to unravel the complex, interwoven processes of wound repair.

The book has been organized into three parts: Inflammation, Granulation Tissue Formation, and Extracellular Matrix Production and Remodeling. We believe that these parts comprehensively cover the molecular and cellular processes of wound repair that occurs when tissue damage has been sufficient to destroy tissue architecture and elicit a fibrotic response. What is not covered to any great extent are the processes that occur during tissue regeneration, that is, the repopulation of an injured area with tissue-specific parenchymal cells, as occurs when tissue damage has been insufficient to destroy the tissue architecture. In fact, the original intention of the editors was to have a fourth section entitled Tissue Regeneration, which would have drawn upon the expertise of investigators in the fields of lung, bone, liver, gastrointestinal, cardiovascular, nerve, and skin research. However, the length of the book became unwieldly and the only vestige of this plan lies in Chapter 23, which covers dermal–epidermal reepithelialization. Perhaps a future edition or, more likely, a second book, on the important topic of tissue regeneration will be generated.

This book is intended for all students of wound healing, who quest to understand the phenomenology of tissue repair at the level of molecular and cellular biology.

The editors would like to express their deep gratitude to the authors, without whom this book would have been only an idea and not a completed work. Special thanks goes to Pam Kirby, our managing editor, who organized the manuscripts into a book, corrected syntax, spelling, and punctuation, checked bibliographies against text references, and, finally, indexed the book. Thanks also go to our wives Marcia and Jan, our fellow workers, and the secretaries in the departments of Medicine and Pediatrics at the National Jewish Center for Immunology and Respiratory Medicine, who bore up under the immense pressure that overflowed from us onto them. Finally, our thanks to Plenum for patiently awaiting the final work.

Richard A. F. Clark
Peter M. Henson
Denver

Contents

Chapter 3

Potential Functions of the Clotting System in Wound Repair

Harold F. Dvorak, Allen P. Kaplan, and
Richard A. F. Clark

Chapter 4

Endothelial Cell Regulation of Coagulation

David M. Stern, Dean Handley, and Peter P. Nawroth

Chapter 5

**Factors That Affect Vessel Reactivity and Leukocyte
Emigration**

Timothy J. Williams

Chapter 6
Neutrophil Emigration, Activation, and Tissue Damage

Marcia G. Tonnesen, G. Scott Worthen, and
Richard B. Johnston, Jr.

Chapter 7
Resolution of Inflammation

Christopher Haslett and Peter M. Henson

Chapter 8
The Multiple Roles of Macrophages in Wound Healing
David W. H. Riches

PART II. GRANULATION TISSUE FORMATION

Chapter 9
The Role of Growth Factors in Tissue Repair I:
Platelet-Derived Growth Factor
Jung San Huang, Thomas J. Olsen, and
Shuan Shiang Huang

Chapter 10

The Role of Growth Factors in Tissue Repair II: Epidermal Growth Factor

Allen R. Banks

Chapter 11

The Role of Growth Factors in Tissue Repair III: Fibroblast Growth Factor

Gary M. Fox

Chapter 12

The Role of Growth Factors in Tissue Repair IV: Type β-Transforming Growth Factor and Stimulation of Fibrosis

Richard K. Assoian

Chapter 13
Mechanisms of Parenchymal Cell Migration into Wounds

James B. McCarthy, Daryl F. Sas, and Leo T. Furcht

Chapter 14
Re-epithelialization

Kurt S. Stenn and Louis DePalma

Chapter 15
Angiogenesis

Joseph A. Madri and Bruce M. Pratt

Chapter 16
The Role of Cell–Cell Interaction in the Regulation of Endothelial Cell Growth

Ronald L. Heimark and Stephen M. Schwartz

Chapter 17
The Biology of the Myofibroblast Relationship to Wound Contraction and Fibrocontractive Diseases

Omar Skalli and Giulio Gabbiani

PART III. EXTRACELLULAR MATRIX PRODUCTION AND REMODELING

Chapter 18
Fibronectin: A Primitive Matrix

John A. McDonald

Chapter 21
Role of Degradative Enzymes in Wound Healing

Paolo Mignatti, Howard G. Welgus, and Daniel B. Rifkin

Chapter 22
Basement Membranes

Heinz Furthmayr

Chapter 23
Re-formation of the Epidermal–Dermal Junction during Wound Healing

David T. Woodley and Robert A. Briggaman

Part I

Inflammation

Chapter 1

Overview and General Considerations of Wound Repair

RICHARD A. F. CLARK

1. Overview

During the past 20 years, an explosion of new knowledge has occurred in the fields of molecular and cellular biology. Application of this new knowledge to studies of tissue organization is having a major impact on our understanding of the molecular and cellular processes that interact to produce living tissue. Contributors have been selected to review topics of molecular and cellular biology that either provide new insights into or provoke important questions about the dynamic biologic processes of tissue repair. This introductory chapter attempts to outline the individual aspects of wound repair covered in the book and to arrange the extensive information into a continuum of events.

Although a time-scale compartmentalization of wound-repair phenomena risks oversimplification and inaccuracies, such modeling is useful in making a comprehensible outline of wound repair. For this purpose, tissue response to injury has been divided into three overlapping phases: inflammation, granulation tissue production, and matrix formation and remodeling (Fig. 1). To orient the reader, a brief overview of the three phases is presented; each phase is then discussed in more detail, with extensive referrals to the appropriate chapters in this book. Other chapters are organized according to the phases of wound repair they address.

During the early inflammatory phase, blood vessel disruption results in extravasation of blood constituents and concomitant platelet aggregation, blood coagulation, and generation of bradykinin and complement-derived anaphylatoxins. Activated platelets not only aggregate and trigger blood coagulation to effect hemostasis in disrupted blood vessels but also release a cadre of biologically active substances, including an array of molecules that promote cell migration and growth into the site of injury. Several intrinsic activities of the blood vessel endothelium limit the extent of platelet aggregation and blood coagulation to the wounded area.

RICHARD A. F. CLARK • Department of Medicine, National Jewish Center for Immunology and Respiratory Medicine, Denver, Colorado 80206.

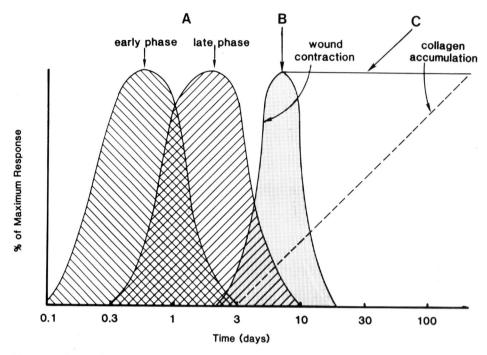

Figure 1. Phases of wound repair. Healing of a wound has been arbitrarily divided into three phases: (A) inflammation (early and late), (B) granulation tissue formation, and (C) matrix formation and remodeling. These phases overlap considerably with one another and are plotted along the abscissa as a logarithmic function of time. Inflammation is divided into early and late phases denoting neutrophil-rich and mononuclear cell-rich infiltrates, respectively. The magnitude of wound contraction parallels granulation tissue formation, as indicated. Collagen accumulation actually begins shortly after the onset of granulation tissue formation, continuing throughout the phase of matrix formation and remodeling.

Neutrophils are the first leukocyte observed to infiltrate an area of inflammation and injury; monocytes are seen shortly thereafter. Both cell types are attracted to sites of tissue injury by a variety of chemotactic factors. The major function of neutrophils during this early inflammatory phase of tissue injury is to rid the site of contaminating bacteria. By contrast, the influx of monocytes and their conversion to macrophages seem critical to the initiation of tissue repair. As the neutrophil infiltrate resolves and macrophage accumulation continues, an arbitrary division can be drawn between early and late inflammatory phases of wound repair. Macrophages, like neutrophils, phagocytose and digest pathogenic organisms; they also scavenge tissue debris, including effete neutrophils. In addition, macrophages release a plethora of biologically active substances. Although many of these substances facilitate the recruitment of additional inflammatory cells and aid the macrophage in tissue decontamination and debridement, growth factors and other substances are also released that are necessary for the initiation and propagation of granulation tissue. Thus, the macrophage plays a pivotal role in the transition between wound inflammation and the second phase of wound repair, the formation of granulation tissue.

Granulation tissue consists of a dense population of macrophages, fibroblasts, and neovasculature embedded in a loose matrix of collagen, fibronectin, and hyaluronic acid. Sometimes the fibroblast and neomatrix components of granulation tissue are referred to as fibroplasia. As fibroblasts proliferate and migrate into the wound space, they undergo an alteration of cell phenotype, permitting cell motility and concomitant deposition of the loose extracellular matrix (ECM). In addition, these cells align themselves and their newly deposited matrix along the radial axes of the wound, form cell–cell and cell–matrix links (fibronexus), and are thereby able to generate a concerted tension that results in wound contraction. Blood vessel growth (angiogenesis) into a wound occurs simultaneously with fibroplasia.

When the epithelium is disrupted at the time of tissue injury, re-epithelialization must occur as rapidly as possible in order to re-establish tissue integrity. This process begins within minutes to hours after injury by the movement of epithelial cells from the free edge of the tissue across the defect. Within a day or two, the epithelial cells remaining at the original edge of the wound begin to proliferate in order to generate an additional population of migrating cells. If the basement membrane is destroyed, the cells move over a provisional matrix of fibronectin and fibrin, gradually re-forming the basement membrane. If the basement membrane has not been destroyed then the hemidesmosomes are disrupted during re-epithelialization. In either case, the absence of tenacious binding at the epithelial–stromal interface is prerequisite to epithelial mobility. If large foreign objects or nonviable tissue lie within the wound space, the epithelium will dissect under these structures. Once re-epithelialization is complete, the cells revert to their normal phenotype and firmly reattach to the basement membrane through hemidesmosomes.

The third and final phase of wound healing is matrix remodeling. As with all of these time-scale compartmentalizations, this phase overlaps with the previous phase. In fact, matrix production and remodeling begins simultaneously with granulation tissue formation. Nevertheless, in the months following the dissolution of granulation tissue, the matrix is constantly altered, with the relatively rapid elimination of most fibronectin from the matrix and with the slow accumulation of large fibrous bundles of type I collagen that provide the residual scar with increasing tensile strength.

2. Inflammation

Blood vessel disruption during tissue injury leads to extravasation of blood constituents, with concomitant platelet aggregation (Chapter 2) and blood coagulation (Chapter 3). Nevertheless, several intrinsic activities of the blood vessel endothelium limit the extent of platelet aggregation and blood coagulation to the wounded area (Chapter 4). Clot formation occurs within vessel lumen to affect hemostasis, as well as in the surrounding connective tissue (Chapter 3); however, the interstitial fibrin gel is an important early component of wound repair, as judged by impaired wound healing in animals depleted of fibrinogen (Chapter 3). Mediators released by blood coagulation, complement pathways, and cell activation or death at the wound site induce the influx of inflammatory leukocytes and increase the permeability of undamaged vessels adjacent to the injured area resulting in more widespread leakage of plasma proteins (Chapter 5). The influx of neutrophils attempts to clear the area of foreign particles, especially bacteria but often further affects tissue damage (Chapter 6). If particle clearance is effective, no further generation of granulocyte chemoattractants occurs, and effete neutrophils at the site of injury are phagocytosed by macrophages (Chapter 7). Peripheral blood monocytes, however, continue to infiltrate the wounded site, probably in response to the generation of specific monocyte chemoattractants (Chapter 8). The monocytes are progressively activated, exhibiting the phenotype of macrophages. Macrophages, like platelets, produce growth factors that appear crucial to the initiation of granulation tissue formation (Chapters 9–12).

Platelet adhesion and aggregation are critical to hemostasis, stimulated by a number of components generated or expressed at the wound site, including thrombin (Detwiler and Feinman, 1973) and fibrillar collagens (Legrand et al., 1979; Barnes and MacIntyre, 1979). Platelets release ADP and facilitate the coagulation cascade, generating more thrombin. ADP and thrombin recruit additional platelets to the site of injury. In addition, several adhesive proteins are released when platelets discharge their α-granules, which include fibrinogen, fibronectin, thrombospondin, and von Willebrand factor VIII. The first three are important for proper platelet aggregation, and von Willebrand factor VIII mediates platelet adhesion to fibrillar collagens (see Chapter 2). Platelet adhesion to all four adhesive proteins is mediated through the platelet IIb/IIIa surface receptor. Cytoadhesins, receptors related to IIb/IIIa, were recently identified on a variety of cells (Plow et al., 1986). Platelet fibrinogen, once converted to fibrin by thrombin, adds to the fibrin clot, and both fibrin and fibronectin act as a provisional matrix for the influx of monocytes (see Chapter 3) and fibroblasts (see Chapter 13). Platelets also release growth factors concomitant with α-granule secretion that probably initially stimulates the formation of granulation tissue (Section 3) (see Chapters 9–12).

The leakage of plasma and formed blood elements from damaged blood vessels results in blood clotting by three major routes (Chapter 3):

1. Hageman factor (HF) activated by adsorption onto fibrillar collagen or other suitable surfaces along with its coactivators prekallikrein, and heavy-molecular-weight kininogen, induces the so-called intrinsic coagulation system (Kaplan, 1983).
2. Facior VII activated by tissue procoagulant factor found in the interstitium (Dvorak et al., 1985) and released from damaged cells (Maynard et al., 1975) induces the so-called extrinsic coagulation system (Josso and Prou-Wartelle, 1965; Marlar et al., 1982).

3. Platelets and endothelial cells activated by low levels of thrombin (see Chapters 2 and 4) and platelets activated by contact with fibrillar collagen (Barnes and MacIntyre, 1979) express coagulation factors (Sixma, 1978) and phospholipids (Bode et al., 1981) that greatly facilitate clotting (Chapter 4).

The inciting event in each route of clotting is the expression of a surface that promotes adsorption and activation of specific coagulation proenzymes (Chapter 3). Surface adsorption is prerequisite for proenzyme activation, since these proteins are otherwise literally afloat in a sea of enzyme inhibitors. Thus, although small amounts of proenzymes are activated under normal circumstances, once activated, the enzymes are almost immediately quenched by plasma protease inhibitors. When the proenzymes have been adsorbed on a surface in a microenvironment relatively free of protease inhibitors, however, minute amounts of spontaneous activation are quickly amplified into the physiologic response of blood clotting. Viewed from the standpoint of coagulation cessation, it follows that blood clotting automatically terminates when the stimuli for initiation dissipate. In addition, several intrinsic blood vessel activities limit the extent of platelet aggregation and clotting to the area proximate to the injury (Chapter 4). These activities include production of prostaglandin, which inhibits platelet aggregation (Moncada et al., 1976; Raz et al., 1977; Weksler et al., 1977); inactivation of thrombin (Lollar et al., 1980; Baker et al., 1980); generation of protein C, a potent enzyme that degrades coagulation factors V and VIII (Kisiel et al., 1977; Esmon and Owen, 1981); and release of plasminogen activator, which initiates clot lysis (Binder et al., 1979; Rijken et al., 1980; Loskutoff and Edgington, 1977).

Blood clotting can be considered a part of the inflammatory response, since HF activation leads to bradykinin generation (Kaplan & Austen, 1971; Habal et al., 1976) and to the initiation of the classic complement cascade (Ghebrehiwet et al., 1981) and perhaps generation of the anaphylatoxins, C3a and C5a (Craddock et al., 1977) (Chapter 3). The anaphylatoxins in turn not only increase blood vessel permeability directly and attract neutrophils and monocytes to sites of tissue injury (Fernandez et al., 1978) (Chapter 5) but also stimulate the release of vasoactive mediators, histamine (Hugli and Muller-Eberhard, 1978) and leukotriene C_4 and D_4 (Stimler et al., 1982) from mast cells, as well as the release of granule constituents and biologically active oxygen products from neutrophils (Hugli and Muller-Eberhard, 1978) and macrophages (McCarthy and Henson, 1979).

Neutrophils are considered the first leukocytes to infiltrate an area of inflammation and injury, but in fact monocytes probably begin to emigrate at the same time (Turk et al., 1976) (Chapter 7). Both cell types are attracted to sites of tissue injury by a variety of chemotactic factors, including kallikrein from the activated HF pathway (Kaplan et al., 1972; Gallin and Kaplan, 1974), fibrinopeptides generated during fibrin clot formation (Kay et al., 1974; Senior et al., 1986), fibrin degradation products (Stecher and Sorkin, 1972; McKenzie et al., 1975), C5a from complement activation (Fernandez et al., 1978; Snyderman et *al.,* 1972), leukotriene B4 released by activated neutrophils (Ford-Hutchinson *et al.,* 1980), bacteria-generated formyl methionyl peptides (Freer *et al.,* 1980), and platelet-released substances (Deuel *et al.,* 1981, 1982) (Chapter 5). The molecular mechanisms by which neutrophils adhere to blood vessel endothelium and diapedesis between adjacent endothelial cells and then through the blood vessel basement membrane are beginning to be elucidated, as discussed in Chapter 6. Neutrophils primarily function to destroy bacteria contaminating the wound site through phagocytosis and subsequent enzymatic and oxygen radical mechanisms (Chapter 6).

Neutrophil infiltration will cease after the first few days of tissue injury if no wound contamination has occurred, and effete neutrophils will be phagocytosed by tissue macrophages (Chapter 7). This marks the end of the early inflammatory phase of wound healing (Fig. 1). If wound contamination has occurred, however, the acute inflammatory phase will persist and interfere with the next phases of wound healing. Further inflammation and tissue destruction are side effects of the attempts to rid the injured area of bacteria or other foreign objects. These foreign substances initiate complement activity by providing a surface for alternative pathway activation. In a manner reminiscent of coagulation control, the proenzymes of the alternative pathway are continually undergoing slight activation; however, because they are surrounded by plasma protease inhibitors, any active complement enzymes are immediately inactivated. By contrast, an appropriate surface, such as bacteria (Fearon, 1978), or many other foreign objects (Fearon and Austen, 1977) that might contaminate a wound, provide a microenvironment on which the alternative pathway proenzymes can adsorb in the absence of their plasma inhibitors. Such surfaces continually activate the alternative pathway, resulting in opsonization of foreign surfaces with C3b and generation of C3a and C5a anaphylatoxins. Thus, additional neutrophils are attracted to the site of injury. In addition, the neutrophil may release lysosomal enzymes and toxic oxygen radicals, thereby extending the tissue damage (Chapter 6).

Regardless of whether the neutrophil infiltrate resolves or persists, macrophage accumulation continues, probably stimulated by selective chemoattractants, which include fragments of collagen (Postlethwaite and Kang, 1976), elastin (Senior *et al.,* 1980), and fibronectin (Norris *et al.,* 1982), as well as enzymatically active thombin (Bar-Shavit *et al.,* 1983). Macrophages, like neutrophils, phagocytose and digest pathogenic organisms; they also scavenge tissue debris, including effete neutrophils (Newman *et al.,* 1982) (Chapter 7). In addition, macrophages release a plethora of biologically active substances, such as vasoactive mediators (Humes *et al.,* 1977; Rouzer *et al.,* 1982), chemotactic and growth factors (Tsukamoto *et al.,* 1981; Lachman, 1983; Shimokado *et al.,* 1985; Sporn and Roberts, 1986), and enzymes (Schroff *et al.,* 1981), including proteases (Wahl *et al.,* 1977; Werb and Gordon, 1975a,b; van Furth, 1985). Although many of these substances facilitate the recruitment of additional inflammatory cells and aid the macrophage in tissue decontamination and debridement, growth factors and some chemotactic factors are necessary for the initiation and propagation of granulation tissue (Leibovich and Ross,

1975). Thus, the macrophage plays a pivotal role in the transition between wound inflammation and wound repair (see Chapter 8).

3. Granulation Tissue

The formation of granulation tissue occurs next on our time scale (Fig. 1). This process includes accumulation of macrophages, ingrowth of fibroblasts, deposition of loose connective tissue, and angiogenesis. The term granulation tissue derives from the granular appearance of such tissue when it is incised and visually examined. The numerous granules are in fact multiple newly formed blood vessels.

Macrophages, fibroblasts, and blood vessels have been observed to move into the wound space as a unit (Hunt, 1980), correlating well with the proposed biologic interdependence of these cells during tissue repair. Fibroplasia and angiogenesis are probably stimulated in part by a number of growth and chemotactic factors released by platelets and macrophages (Chapters 9–12). Fibroblasts respond to these stimuli by proliferation (Chapters 9–12), migration (Chapter 13), matrix deposition (Chapters 18–20), and wound contraction (Chapter 17). The connective tissue matrix formed by the fibroblasts provides a substrate on which macrophages, new blood vessels, and fibroblasts themselves can migrate into the wound (Chapters 13–15). Formation of a neovasculature provides the new tissue with the oxygen and nutrients needed for continued growth. Thus, macrophages, fibroblasts, and blood vessels are absolutely dependent on each other during granulation tissue generation.

Re-epithelialization of an epithelial defect begins within the first 24 hr after injury, several days before observable formation of granulation tissue. Nevertheless, the process of re-epithelialization is considered with granulation tissue development, since both represent new tissue generation and occur concomitantly. Rapid epithelial reformation (see Chapter 14) re-establishes the protective barrier of the organ, increasing the likelihood that the animal will survive the injury.

Signals for formation and re-epithelialization of granulation tissue are not well delineated but probably include biologically active substances such as chemotactic factors (Chapter 13), growth factors (Chapters 9–12), changes in structural molecules (Chapter 13 and 15), and loss of nearest-neighbor cells (Chapter 16). The net growth factor signal for cell proliferation depends on the kind and quantity of growth factors present and the type of target cell present (Sporn and Roberts, 1986) (Chapters 9–12). Although low levels of growth factor circulate in the plasma, upon aggregation and activation at a site of injury, platelets are the first cell component to release substantial amounts of preformed growth factors into the wounded areas. Growth factors stored in platelet granules include platelet-derived growth factor (PDGF), epidermal growth factor (EGF), transforming growth factor α (TGF-α), transforming growth factor β (TGF-β), and fibroblast growth factor-like (FGF) peptides (Sporn and Roberts, 1986). With the arrival of peripheral blood monocytes and their activation to inflammatory macrophages, a situation is established for the continual synthesis and release of growth factors. Macrophages produce PDGF (Shimokado et al., 1985; Martinet et al., 1986), TGF-α, TGF-β, and FGF-like peptides (Sporn and Roberts, 1986). In addition, it is possible that injured parenchymal cells begin to synthesize, secrete, and then respond to the same growth factors, a so-called autocrine process (Sporn and Roberts, 1986). Structural molecules of the ECM probably promote cell migration by providing a substratum for contact guidance (fibronectin and collagen) and a low-impedance matrix (hyaluronic acid) (Chapters 13 and 15).

3.1. Re-epithelialization

Re-epithelialization of a wound begins within hours after injury by the movement of epithelial cells from the free edge of the tissue across the defect. In the cutaneum, cells of the stratified epidermal sheet appear to move one over the other in a leapfrog fashion (Winter, 1962), while in the cornea, cells of the monolayer sheet appear to move in a single file with the lead cells remaining in front (Fujikawa et al., 1984) (Chapters 13 and 14). All epithelial cells undergo marked phenotypic alteration concomitant with their migration in a manner similar to the phenotypic modulation of fibroblasts that occurs during the formation of granulation tissue (see Section 3.2). The cellular metamorphosis of epithelial cells includes retraction of intracellular tonofilaments, dissolution of most intercellular desmosomes (structures that interlink epithelial cells and thereby provide tensile strength for epithelium), and formation of peripheral cytoplasmic actin filaments (Gabbiani et al., 1978). Similar phenotypic change in epidermal cells has been observed in vitro to occur rapidly (Hennings et al., 1980). The alteration of phenotype gives the cell mobility and the motor apparatus for motility. Thus, the epithelial cells at the wound edge tend to lose their apical–basal polarity and extend pseudopodia from their free basolateral side into the wound. The mechanism whereby epithelial sheets are able to move depends on whether the sheet is a monolayer or stratified layer of cells. Whether the driving force for epithelial cell movement is chemotactic factors, active contact guidance, or a loss of nearest-neighbor cells or a combination of these processes is unknown (Chapters 13 and 16); however, migration does not depend on cell proliferation (Winter, 1972).

Within 1 or 2 days, the epithelial cells at the original wound edge begin to proliferate, generating an additional population of migrating cells (Hall and Cruickshank, 1963; Krawczyk, 1971; Winter, 1972). The stimuli for epithelial proliferation during re-epithelization are unknown. Perhaps the absence of neighbor cells at the wound margin signals both epithelial migration and proliferation. This free edge effect has been postulated by Schwartz et al. (1982) to stimulate re-endothelialization of large blood vessels after intimal damage (see Chapter 16). Another possibility, not exclusive of the former, is local release of growth factors that directly induce epidermal proliferation. EGF is the leading candidate for this function (Cohen, 1965) (Chapter 10).

If the basement membrane is destroyed by injury or subsequent enzymatic degradation, epithelial cells migrate over a provisional matrix (see Chapters 13, 14, and 23). If the basement membrane is not destroyed, the hemidesmosomes that link epithelial cells and basement membrane are temporarily disrupted during cell migration (Krawczyk and Wilgram, 1973). In either situation, the absence of tenacious binding between epithelium and interstitium permits epithelial mobility. Once re-epithelialization is complete, epithelial cells revert to their normal phenotype and once again firmly attach to the basement membrane through hemidesmosomes. Hemidesmosomes reform very rapidly at least *in vitro* (Gipson et al., 1983).

3.2. Fibroplasia and Wound Contraction

The signals that induce fibroblast proliferation and migration into a wound space are unknown, although they probably include a number of fibroblast growth factors (Gospodarowicz, 1975; Zetter et al., 1976; Carpenter and Cohen, 1976; Glenn and Cunningham, 1979; Heldin et al., 1979; Adams et al., 1983; Ross et al., 1986; Sporn et al., 1986) and chemoattractants (Postlewaite et al., 1976, 1978, 1979, 1981, 1987; Gauss-Miller et al., 1980; Seppa et al., 1982). The various growth and chemotactic factors most likely act in concert to induce fibroblast migration and proliferation into wounds. The interplay of fibroblast growth and chemotactic factors in *in vitro* systems has been under intense investigation for a number of years (Oppenheimer et al., 1983; Assoian et al., 1984; Wrann et al., 1980; Stiles et al., 1979; Rozengurt et al., 1982; Clemmons et al., 1980; Grotendorst, 1984) (see Chapters 9–12). Combinations of growth factors have been added to wounds *in vivo* (Sporn et al., 1983; Lawrence et al., 1986; R. Ross, personal communication). These studies suggest that signals for fibroblast migration and proliferation are probably numerous, complex, and interrelated (see Chapters 12 and 20).

As fibroblasts migrate into the wound space, they deposit loose extracellular matrix initially composed of great quantities of fibronectin (Kurkinen et al., 1980; Grinnell et al., 1981). Since fibronectin has the capacity to bind connective tissue cells (Chapter 13) and extracellular matrix (Chapter 18) simultaneously and, since cells can rapidly adhere to and detach from fibronectin substratum, fibroblasts can use fibronectin matrix for movement over a surface (Hsieh and Chen, 1983) (Chapter 13). Recently the Arg-Gly-Asp-Ser tetrapeptide, occurring within the cell-binding domains of fibronectin and other ECM proteins, has been shown to be a critical ligand for the binding of these proteins to cell surface receptors (Ruoslahti and Pierschbacher, 1986). Cell receptors for fibronectin and other ECM proteins consist of related, but not identical, noncovalently associated α- and β-chains, called integrin receptors by Hynes (1987). The factors in a wound that regulate production of fibronectin by fibroblasts are unknown. However, *in vitro* thrombin can stimulate fibroblasts to proliferate (Glenn and Cunningham, 1979) and to synthesize and secrete fibronectin (Mosher and Vaheri, 1978). Additional candidates include

EGF, which not only promotes fibroblast proliferation (Carpenter and Cohen, 1976) but also increases fibronectin synthesis (Chen et al., 1977), and TGF-β, which does not promote cell proliferation but greatly enhances fibronectin synthesis by cultured human fibroblasts (Ignotz and Massangue, 1986).

Many, if not all, the fibroblasts that migrate into the wound space retract their endoplasmic reticula and Golgi apparati to perinuclear locations, forming large actin bundles that course through the peripheral cytoplasm oriented parallel to the long axes of the cells (Gabbiani et al., 1978) (Chapter 17). Thus, the phenotypically altered fibroblast or myofibroblast has gained motility and contractile capacity without relinquishing the ability to synthesize and secrete structural macromolecules, although the quantity and profile of macromolecules' synthesis is altered (Nusgens et al., 1984). The factor(s) that induce phenotype metamorphosis of fibroblasts are unknown but, since the phenotype alteration appears to occur in vivo when fibroblasts migrate and proliferate, the same factors may be involved in all three phenomena. An experimental situation that has impeded delineation of the factor(s) conducive to myofibroblast development is that resident tissue fibroblasts become phenotypically similar to myofibroblasts when cultured in plastic dishes (Abercrombie et al., 1971). Thus, classic tissue culture conditions may be the wrong in vitro system for the study of signals for phenotype modulation. The development of an in vitro system in which fibroblasts are grown in hydrated collagen gels (Bell et al., 1979, 1981, 1983) may remedy this problem, since these fibroblasts appear to be cytologically similar to resident skin fibroblast after 1 or 2 days (Bellows et al., 1982; Tomasek and Hay, 1984).

In recent years, wound contraction has been ascribed to actin-rich myofibroblasts, which are the most numerous cells in granulation tissue and which are aligned within the wound along the lines of contraction. By contrast, neither capillaries nor macrophages are aligned along wound contraction lines. Thus, myofibroblasts probably mediate the visible musclelike contraction observed in isolated strips of granulation tissue exposed to 5-hydroxytryptamine (5-HT), prostaglandin $F_{1\alpha}$ ($PGF_{1\alpha}$), angiotensin, vasopressin, bradykinin, epinephrine, or norepinephrine (Ryan et al., 1974; Gabbiani et al., 1972).

The unified contraction of granulation tissue observed when isolated strips of tissue are exposed to the mediators listed above necessitates molecular interconnections between myofibroblasts and between myofibroblasts and the surrounding extracellular matrix. In fact, several types of cell–cell and cell–stroma linkages are observed in granulation tissue by electron microscopy (Ryan et al., 1974; Gabbiani et al., 1978; Singer et al., 1984). It is postulated that the interconnections participate in the transmission of cellular contraction to other tissue components. Thus, the force of wound contraction is probably generated by actin bundles in the myofibroblasts and transmitted to the sides of the wound by cell–cell and cell–stroma links.

In a series of elegant transmission electron microscopic (TEM) studies, Singer (1979) delineated the co-linear assemblage of intracytoplasmic 5-nm microfilaments and extracellular matrix fibrils in human and hamster fibroblast monolayers, which he termed the fibronexus. Some of the chemical components comprising the fibronexus have been identified by immunoelectron microscopic investigations. Using indirect immunoferritin methods, fibronectin (Singer, 1979) and types I and III procollagen (Furcht *et al.*, 1980) were localized to the extracellular fibers of the fibronexus, while actin (Singer, 1979) and vinculin (Singer and Paradiso, 1981) were identified as the major cytoplasmic constituents of this assemblage. In addition, Singer *et al.* (1984) studied granulation tissue from 7- to 9-day open guinea pig skin wounds and found fibronectin fibers localized around the myofibroblasts' surface and along attenuated myofibroblast processes that extended some distance into the extracellular matrix of the granulation tissue. A large majority of these extracellular fibronectin fibrils were observed to be coincident with intracellular actin microfilaments. Singer and co-workers postulated that the fibronexus may function as the major cohesive complex that transmits the collective forces of contracting actin microfilaments across the wound space.

A functional *in vitro* model for wound contraction consists of fibroblasts dispersed within a hydrated collagen gel. During the first 24–48 hr after mixing, the fibroblasts contact the gel. The rate of contraction is proportional to the cell number and inversely proportional to the collagen concentration (Bell *et al.*, 1979). Collagen condensation results from a collection process executed by fibroblasts as they extended and withdrew pseudopodia attached to collagen fibers as judged by time-lapse photography. Thus, the fibers were drawn together toward the fibroblast cell body during the course of podial contraction (Bell *et al.*, 1981, 1983). The *in vitro* collagen gel system may ultimately help answer how the force of contracting microfilaments of myofibroblasts is transmitted over a collagen matrix and what the signals for contraction are.

3.3. Neovascularization

Neuvascularization of wounds occurs simultaneously with fibroplasia by capillary buds sprouting from blood vessels adjacent to the wound and extending into the wound space. The process of capillary formation (angiogenesis) has been studied morphologically in the usually avascular cornea, where capillary ingrowth can be induced by implantation of angiogenic factors (Ausprunk and Folkman, 1977). One or 2 days after implantation of angiogenic material into the cornea, basement membranes of parent venules in the adjacent limbus begin to fragment. Rifkin *et al.* (1982) observed that capillary endothelial cells grown *in vitro* release plasminogen activator and collagenase in response to angiogenic stimuli; these workers suggested that the early venule basement membrane fragmentation may represent local proteolysis secondary to endothelial cell enzyme release. In support of this hypothesis, Kalebic *et al.* (1983) found that endothelial cells migrating through a filter impregnated with radiolabeled basement membrane collagens degrade these collagens during their transit. Endothelial cells from the side of the venule closest to the angiogenic stimulus begin to migrate on the second day. Cytoplasmic pseudopods project through the fragmented basement membrane toward the stimulus. Subsequently, the entire endothelial cell migrates into the perivascular space, and other endothelial cells follow. Endothelial cells remaining in the parent vessel begin to proliferate by the second day, adding to the numbers of migrating cells. Although endothelial cells in the neovasculature ultimately proliferate, the cells at the capillary tip never undergo mitosis (Ausprunk and Folkman, 1977). The directional migration of capillary endothelial cells and subsequent capillary elongation continue temporarily even after all DNA synthesis has been blocked by X-irradiation (Sholley *et al.*, 1978). These findings imply that angiogenic stimuli may operate through chemotaxis and that endothelial replication may be a secondary event (Folkman, 1982). Capillary sprouts eventually branch at their tips and join to form capillary loops through which blood begins. New sprouts then extend from these loops to form a capillary plexus.

Angiogenesis is probably an extremely complex process that may depend on any or all of the following phenomena: (1) phenotype alteration, (2) stimulated migration, (3) mitogenic stimuli, (4) an appropriate extracellular matrix (Chapter 15), and (5) the free edge effect (i.e., absence of neighboring endothelial cells) (Schwartz *et al.*, 1982) (Chapter 16). Endothelial cell phenotype is modified during angiogenesis (Ausprunk and Folkman, 1977), but the ultrastructural changes are not as well delineated as the fibroblast and epidermal cell alterations described in Sections 3.1 and 3.2.

The soluble factors that stimulate angiogenesis in wound repair are unknown; however, many candidates exist from among numerous endothelial cell growth and chemotactic factors delineated by various *in vitro* systems as well as angiogenic substances demonstrated in corneal or chorioallantoic membrane *in situ* assays (Chapters 9–12). For example, activated macrophages induce vascular proliferation in the corneal angiogenesis assay (Polverini *et al.*, 1977), and a macrophage-derived growth factor stimulates cultured endothelial cell proliferation (Martin *et al.*, 1981). Several growth factors from a variety of tissues (Sidky and Auerbach, 1975; Brown *et al.*, 1980; D'Amore and Klagsbrun, 1984; Frederick *et al.*, 1984; Risan and Ekblom, 1986), including epidermis (Wolf and Harrison, 1973) and cutaneous wounds (Banda *et al.*, 1982) have angiogenic potential in the cornea system. The active molecular species in many of these extracts, however, may be fibroblast growth factor (see Chapter 11). In addition, low oxygen tension (Remensnyder and Majno, 1968), lactic acid (Imre, 1964), and biogenic amines (Zauberman *et al.*, 1969) are among factors occurring in wounds that appear to potentiate angiogenesis, possibly by injuring parenchymal cells and thereby causing the release of fibroblast growth factor which is otherwise not secreted.

Whether stimulation of cultured endothelial cells proliferation or migration relates to *in vivo* angiogenesis is undetermined. Furthermore, there is disagreement among investigators as to the proliferative response of cultured endothelial cells to various growth factors. For example, Haudenschild *et al.* (1976) found that confluent cultures of human endothelial cells failed to proliferate in the presence of growth factors. By contrast, other investigators found that cultured endothelial cells responded to platelet-derived serum factors (Gospodarowicz *et al.*, 1977; Clemmons *et al.*, 1983; King and Buchwald, 1984) and to non-platelet-derived serum factors (Wall *et al.*, 1978). Another area of controversy is whether the major endothelial cell mitogen from brain or pituitary extracts is identical to fibroblast growth factor (Gospodarowicz *et al.*, 1978, 1983) or a distinct molecular entity (Maciag *et al.*, 1982, 1984).

Folkman (1982) postulated that endothelial proliferation is an event secondary to migration. If this is true, endothelial cell chemotactic factors may be critical for angiogenesis. Adult tissue extracts and fibronectin stimulate endothelial cell migration across filters in chemotactic chambers (Glaser *et al.*, 1980; Bowersox and Sorgente, 1982), platelet-derived factors stimulate radial outgrowth from irradiated endothelial cell colonies (Wall *et al.*, 1978), and heparin as well as platelet factors stimulate phagokinetic migration of endothelial cells cultured on surfaces coated with colloidal gold particles (Azizkhan *et al.*, 1980; Bernstein *et al.*, 1982). On the other hand, Raju *et al.* (1984) suggested that angiogenesis is dependent on a mitogenic factor as well as an endothelial cell chemoattractant. Furthermore, Madri and Stenn (1982) demonstrated that cultured aortic endothelial cell migration depends on continued secretion of collagen, and Kinsella and Wight (1986) observed that migratory endothelial cells synthesized more proteoglycans, especially chondroitin sulfide and dermatan sulfate proteoglycans, compared with stationary endothelial cells. These observations support the hypothesis that angiogenesis depends not only on chemotactic and mitogenic factors but on an appropriate extracellular matrix for endothelial cell migration as well.

In studies of the microvasculature adjacent to and within wounds, Clark *et al.* (1982b) noted a transient increase in blood vessel wall fibronectin during endothelial cell proliferation. The proliferating blood vessels appeared to produce fibronectin *in situ* (Clark *et al.*, 1982c). Since cultured microvascular endothelial cells adhere avidly to fibronectin (Clark *et al.*, 1986), blood vessel fibronectin may act as a contact guidance system for endothelial cell movement at the tips of capillary buds. In addition, Ausprunk *et al.* (1981) showed that capillary buds have a homogeneous provisional substratum with altered proteoglycans instead of basement membranes. The homogeneous matrix surrounding capillary buds is reminiscent of the provisional matrix under migrating epithelia (Clark *et al.*, 1982a). That matrix alterations occur during angiogenesis is in concert with recent observation that extracellular matrix alterations *in vitro* have a profound effect on endothelial cell morphology and function (Chapter 15).

Endothelial cells in culture and *in vivo* grow as a single monolayer, making them an ideal cell for testing the concept of contact inhibition. Heimark and Schwartz (1985) showed that isolated endothelial cell membranes serve to inhibit proliferation of subconfluent endothelial cells in culture. This observation supports the concept of contact inhibition and also suggests that the absence of nearest-neighbor cells would release surrounding cells from the contact inhibition. Heimark and Schwartz termed the absence of nearest neighbors the free edge effect and speculated that this effect may be critical in repair of large vessel endothelium and possibly in angiogenesis.

In summary, evidence has accumulated that angiogenesis is a complex

process depending on at least five interrelated phenomena: phenotype alteration, chemoattractant-stimulated migration, mitogenic stimulation, an appropriate extracellular matrix, and the free edge effect. Within 1 or 2 days after
removal of angiogenic stimuli, capillaries undergo regression, as characterized
by mitochondrial swelling in the endothelial cells at the distal tips of the
capillaries, platelet adherance to degenerating endothelial cells, vascular stasis
and endothelial cell necrosis, and finally, ingestion of the effete capillaries by
macrophages (Ausprunk et al., 1978; Folkman, 1982).

4. Matrix Formation and Remodeling

The third phase of wound repair is matrix formation and remodeling. As
with all time-scale divisions, the third phase overlaps with the previous phase
(Fig. 1). In fact, matrix formation begins simultaneously with the formation of
granulation tissue as described in Section 3.2. Nevertheless, during the months
following dissolution of granulation tissue, the matrix is constantly altered,
with relatively rapid elimination of most fibronectin from the matrix and slow
accumulation of large fibrous bundles of type I collagen that provide the residual scar with increasing tensile strength.

Kinetically, the composition and structure of the extracellular matrix of
granulation tissue changes continuously from the time of its first deposition.
Spatially, extracellular matrix is deposited first at the wound margin along
with the initial development of granulation tissue and more centrally as the
granulation tissue grows into the wound space. At any given time, the extracellular matrix at the wound margin has different characteristics than that
situated centrally. Thus, the composition and structure of the extracellular
matrix of granulation tissue depends on both the time lapsed since tissue injury
and the distance from the wound margin. Recently, growth factors, especially
TGF-β, have been observed to have remarkable modulatory effects on fibroblast
synthesis of both fibronectin (Ignotz and Massague, 1986) and collagen (Roberts
et al., 1986). Thus, the ultimate matrix constituents probably depend not only
on the cells and enzymes present but on the growth factor profile impinging on
the cells as well (see Chapter 20).

Extracellular matrix components serve several critical functions for effective wound repair. First, during the formation of granulation tissue, fibronectin
provides a provisional substratum for the migration and ingrowth of cells (see
Chapter 13), a linkage for myofibroblasts to effect wound contraction (see Chapter 17), and a nidus for collagen fibrillogenesis (see Chapter 18). The presence
of large quantities of highly hydrated hyaluronic acid in granulation tissue
provides a matrix that is easily penetrated by ingrowing parenchymal cells (see
Chapter 19), and the early formation of types I, III, and V collagen fibrils
provides nascent tensile strength for the wound. As the matrix matures over the
ensuing weeks, (1) the fibronectin and hyaluronic acid disappear; (2) collagen
bundles grow in size, lending increased tensile strength to the wound site; and
(3) proteoglycans are deposited adding resilience to deformation of the tissue.

The next four subsections give an overview of these processes and the last subsection gives an overview of basement membrane re-formation.

4.1. Fibronectin

Initial extracellular matrix deposits contain considerable fibronectin (Chapter 18). In addition to its role in cell recruitment and wound contraction (Chapters 13 and 17), fibronectin may serve as a template for collagen deposition, as suggested by the observations that fibroblasts tend to be aligned in the same axis as fibronectin and that collagen is later oriented in the same pattern (see Chapter 18). In addition, fibronectin in cell culture matrix is closely associated with collagen and glycosaminoglycans (Bornstein and Ash, 1977; Vaheri et al., 1978; Hayman et al., 1982; Hedman et al., 1982). Several lines of indirect in vitro evidence demonstrate that collagen is deposited on a fibronectin matrix, and not vice versa. McDonald et al. (1982) noted that some fibrils in fibroblast cultures stain for fibronectin but not collagen. Fibroblasts grown in the absence of ascorbate produce little or no collagen but form a dense fibronectin matrix (Chen et al., 1978). Furthermore, collagenase releases collagen but not fibronectin from fibroblast matrices, while thrombin releases both fibronectin and collagen (Keski-Oja et al., 1981). It was suggested that the release of collagen by thrombin is unlikely to be a direct effect on the collagen, since thrombin does not digest native collagen but rather probably cleaves fibronectin or other glycoproteins that interact with collagen. In addition, an Fab' anti-fibronectin antibody that blocks collagen binding to fibronectin inhibited collagen accumulation in the extracellular matrix, as judged by immunofluorescence and [³H]hydroxyproline incorporation (McDonald et al., 1982). However, fibronectin deposition was also inhibited, which indicates that the fibronectin and collagen interaction is necessary for fibril formation. On the basis of their data, McDonald and co-workers suggest that "the deposition of fibrillar, extracellular fibronectin is essential for organization of types I and III collagen in vitro." Recent evidence has directly delineated fibronectin's role in matrix formation (McDonald et al., 1987) (Chapter 18).

The in vivo interrelationship of fibronectin and types I and III collagen deposition has been studied using cellulose sponge implants in rats (Kurkinen et al., 1980). Seven days after subcutaneous implantation, fibroblasts invaded 1–2 mm into the sponge, and argyrophilic reticulin fibers, which stained uniformly and strongly for fibronectin, appeared. Type III procollagen and some type I collagen were present but trailed behind the leading edge of fibroblasts. (Immunoelectron microscopy shows the fibronectin in wounds to be often associated with fine fibrils (Repesh et al., 1982) believed to be type III collagen and early forms of type I collagen that together form reticulin fibers.) By 3–5 weeks, the fibroblasts had reached the center of the sponge, where their numbers were now greatest, and the fibronectin and collagen distribution was as described in the sponge periphery at earlier times. The now more mature periphery contained birefringent collagen bundles that stained for type I collagen.

Fibronectin was diminished after 5 weeks as more mature birefringement collagen fibers were formed.

The sequence of fibronectin followed by interstitial collagen has also been observed in wounds of other mammals (Holund et al., 1982), including humans (Viljanto et al., 1981), in embryogenesis, and in certain pathologic processes. In each, fibronectin appears to be an early component, followed by type III collagen and then type I collagen. The initial fibronectin matrix can be easily degraded by either cell or plasma proteases (McDonald and Kelly, 1980; Vartio et al., 1981; Furie and Rifkin, 1980). The fibrillar collagens ultimately form fibrous bundles that greatly enhance the tissue tensile strength (see Section 4.4).

4.2. Hyaluronic Acid

Hyaluronic acid (HA), a linear polymer of repeating N-acetylglucosamine–glucuronic acid disaccharides (Chapter 19), also occurs in early granulation tissue. This molecule is in the general class of polysaccharides termed glycosaminoglycans (GAGs). Balazs and Holmgren (1950) first demonstrated that granulation tissue contains predominantly a nonsulfated GAG consistent with HA during the initial 4 days of healing but later consists mainly of sulfated polysaccharides. These workers proposed that HA has a critical role in the fibroblast proliferation of early granulation tissue and that later sulfated polysaccharides are essential for collagen production and maturation. Studying the GAG content of open cutaneous wounds, Bently (1967) found that HA content increased early, fell from day 5 to 10, and then remaining fairly constant, while the sulfated GAGs, chondroitin-4-sulfate and dermatan sulfate, increased from day 5 to 7. Similar matrix transitions from HA to sulfated GAGs have been observed in healing tendons (Dorner, 1967) and cornea (Anseth, 1961). In addition, during morphogenesis, hyaluronic acid appears at times of cell movement and mitosis and disappears at the onset of differentiation (Toole and Gross, 1971; Toole and Trelstad, 1971; Toole, 1972). Thus, Balazs and Holmgren's proposal that HA promotes cell movement is supported by the concomitant occurrence of HA and cell migration during both tissue repair and organ generation.

At least two possibilities exist, not necessarily mutually exclusive, for the role of HA in cell motility. First, HA may facilitate adhesion–disadhesion between the cell membrane and the matrix substratum during cell movement. Second, HA can become an extremely hydrated molecular structure, resulting in tissue swelling that would create additional space between collagen or cells and facilitate migration of more cells into these areas (Toole, 1981). The former possibility has been advanced by Culp and collageues (1979) on the basis of several elegant experiments (Lark et al., 1985; Rollins and Culp, 1979). These investigators proposed that interaction of cell-surface heparan sulfate, a sulfated GAG, and fibronectin mediates cell attachment to substratum and that accumulation of HA weakens this adhesion. Thus, precise regulation of cell-surface heparan sulfate and HA could result in waves of adhesion–disadhesion and cell movement.

In addition to evidence that HA may facilitate cell movement, several lines of investigation suggest that HA may promote cell division. HA production is greater during fibroblast proliferation *in vitro* than at confluency (Tomida *et al.*, 1974; Cohn *et al.*, 1976; Underhill and Keller, 1976; Hopwood and Dorfman, 1977). Furthermore, stimulated proliferation of cultured fibroblasts by serum (Tomida *et al.*, 1975), insulin (Moscatelli and Rubin, 1975), or EGF (Lembach, 1976) results in a marked increase in HA production. Thus, the presence of HA in the extracellular matrix may be important for cell division. The mechanistic reason may be similar to those proposed for cell motility.

As granulation tissue matures, HA is decreased through the action of tissue hyaluronidase, an enzyme that displays HA endoglycosidic activity (Bertolami and Donoff, 1982) (Chapter 21). The sulfated GAGs that replace HA are associated with a protein core (Hascall and Hascall, 1981) (Chapter 19). These substances, called proteoglycans, provide the tissue with more resilience than HA but accommodate cell movement and proliferation less well. Thus, early in the formation of granulation tissue, fibroblasts deposit a fibronectin and HA matrix conducive to cell migration and proliferation and later a collagen and proteoglycan matrix that increases tissue tensile strength and resilience.

4.3. Proteoglycans

Proteoglycans are the most complex structures in the GAG family. By definition, a proteoglycan contains a core protein to which at least one GAG chain is covalently bound (Chapter 19). However, many proteoglycans contain numerous GAG chains that may be of one or several types. A proteoglycan is named after the most prevalent GAG chain in its structure. Often proteoglycans form a noncovalent aggregate with HA. Thus, enormous molecular versatility permits proteoglycans to have many diverse structural and organizational functions in tissues.

Chondroitin-4-sulfate and dermatan sulfate increase during the second week of wound repair, as HA is on the wane (Bently, 1967). Since GAGs, other than HA, do not exist as free linear polysaccharides, the chondroitin 4-sulfate and dermatan sulfate found in maturing granulation tissue can be considered part of proteoglycan structures. Little is known of proteoglycan function *in vivo* except that these substances contribute substantially to tissue resilience (Hascall and Hascall, 1981). However, from several lines of *in vitro* and *in vivo* evidence, one can assume that proteoglycans may have the capacity to regulate collagen fibrillogenesis (Wood, 1960; Armitage and Chapman, 1971; Kischner and Shetlar, 1974; McPherson *et al.*, 1987). Chondroitin-4-sulfate has been shown to accelerate polymerization of monomer collagen *in vitro* (Wood, 1960). Since this GAG occurs at high levels in granulation tissue (Kirscher and

Shetlar, 1974) but not in mature scar (Shetlar *et al.*, 1972), it may facilitate collagen deposition during the matrix formation and remodeling phase of wound healing. That both collagen synthesis (Cohen *et al.*, 1971) and chondroitin-4-sulfate levels (Shetlar *et al.*, 1972) are elevated in hypertrophic scars supports this concept. In addition, proteoglycans may have the capacity to regulate cell function.

Heparan sulfate proteoglycan and fibronectin appear to mediate cell attachment to substratum, while HA weakens this bond (Culp *et al.*, 1979). Thus, the interplay of proteoglycans and HA at cell–substratum attachment sites determine the state of cell adhesion–disadhesion to surfaces, a critical phenomenon in cell motility. Likewise, as proliferating cells synthesize much more HA, they produce much less sulfated GAG proteoglycan (Tomida *et al.*, 1974; Cohn *et al.*, 1976; Underhill and Keller, 1976; Hopwood and Dorfman, 1977). In the case of cell-surface-associated heparan sulfate proteoglycan, specific shedding of this polysaccharide immediately precedes cell division (Kraemer and Tobey, 1972). In addition, heparan sulfate or heparin produced by confluent endothelial cells inhibits the growth of smooth muscle cells (Castellot *et al.*, 1981). From the combined data of these studies, one can speculate that heparan sulfate proteoglycan may serve to control cell proliferation. Many experiments suggest that cell shape and anchorage to a substratum may be a critical component of cell division. Inasmuch as GAGs may influence these parameters, they would also influence proliferation (Letourneau *et al.*, 1980).

Just as the interface between epithelium and mesenchyme is a critical site for the control of many morphogenetic sequences (Grobstein, 1967), it almost certainly plays a critical function during wound repair especially with regard to re-epithelialization (Chapter 14) and angiogenesis (Chapter 15). GAGs are recognized as a prominent component of this interface during both morphogenesis (Bernfield and Banerjee, 1972; Trelstad *et al.*, 1974; Hay and Meier, 1974) and wound healing (Ausprunk *et al.*, 1981). In an elegant set of studies, Bernfield and colleagues examined the role of GAG in branching morphogenesis of mouse epithelia (Bernfield and Banerjee, 1972; Bernfield *et al.*, 1972; Banerjee *et al.*, 1977; Cohn *et al.*, 1977; Gordon and Bernfield, 1980). That a similar phenomenon may occur during wound-healing neovascularization is suggested by Ausprunk's investigations (Ausprunk *et al.*, 1981). Proteoglycans, like fibronectin, HA and collagen, are probably remodeled continually during wound healing (Quintner *et al.*, 1982), especially at epithelial– and endothelial–stroma interfaces.

4.4. Collagen

Collagens are a family of closely related triple-chain glycoproteins found in the extracellular matrix (ECM) (see Chapter 20). At least three classes of collagen occur in connective tissue: (1) fibrillar collagens (types I, III, and V), which have uninterrupted triple helices; (2) basement membrane collagen (type IV), which has an interrupted triple helix and forms a meshwork in the laminia densa of membranes; and (3) other interstitial collagens with interrupted helices (types VI, VII, and VIII). Fibrillar collagens types II and XI and interrupted helical collagens types IX, X, and XII from cartilage are not discussed in this book. The principal characteristic of the fibrillar collagens is the ability of the monomeric collagen molecules to polymerize both side by side and end on end into long fibrillar aggregates (Trelstad and Silver, 1981). Type I collagen is thought to form the core of these aggregates, while types III and V collagen aggregate around the periphery of the fibril bundles limiting their size. These fibrillar bundles constitute the major structural collagens in all connective tissues. Type V collagen often occurs immediately adjacent to cells (Gay et al., 1981). Type IV procollagen fails to undergo proteolytic processing in the extracellular matrix and thus retains its large globular terminal domains which prevents fibrillar aggregation. Instead, these nonhelical domains interact resulting in a multimolecular collagen meshwork (Timpl et al., 1981). Type VI collagen is a major component of 100-nm periodic microfibrils that are clearly distinguishable from 67-nm periodic type I and III fibrils and are found around and between type I collagen fibrils in native tissue (Burns et al., 1986). Recently type VII collagen has been found to form the anchoring fibrils of epidermal basement membranes (Sakai et al., 1986). Type VIII collagen is produced by cultured endothelial cells, but its disposition in normal and wounded tissue is unknown (Benya and Padilla, 1986; Sage et al., 1983, 1984).

Most studies on the collagen content of healing wounds and artificially induced granulation tissue (sponge implants) have examined types I and III collagens, since these two collagens have been characterized for some time and their supramolecular structures are well defined. Bazin and Delauney (1964) first showed by biochemical techniques that granulation tissue contains a collagen distinct from the normal adult dermis and rather similar to that in embryonic skin. This collagen was later recognized as type III (Epstein, 1974; Chung and Miller, 1974), which does occur in small amounts in normal dermis but is greatly increased in granulation tissue (Gabbiani et al., 1976). Granulation tissue matrix deposition occurs in an ordered sequence of fibronectin, type III collagen, and type I collagen (see Section 4.1). Type V collagen was recently noted to increase during granulation tissue development in parallel with tissue vascularity, thus suggesting an association between capillary endothelial cells and type V collagen (Hering et al., 1983). The finding of abundant type V collagen in hypertrophic scars (Ehrlich and White, 1981) that have numerous capillaries provides additional support for this thesis.

Rigid helical collagen macromolecules aggregated into fibrillar bundles gradually provide the healing tissue with increasing stiffness and tensile strength (Trelstad and Silver, 1981; Levenson et al., 1965). After a 5-day lag, corresponding to early granulation tissue and a matrix composed largely of fibronectin and hyaluronic acid, an increase in wound breaking strength begins that coincides with collagen fibrogenesis. The rate at which wounds gain tensile strength thereafter, however, is slow. For example, wounds have gained only about 20% of their final strenth by the third week. In addition, wounded tissue fails to reattain the same breaking strength as uninjured skin. At maximum strength a scar is only 70% as strong as intact skin (Levenson et al., 1965).

The gradual gain in tensile strength is secondary not only to accruing collagen deposition but also to collagen remodeling with formation of larger collagen bundles (Kirscher and Shetlar, 1974) and an alteration of intermolecular crosslinks (Bailey et al., 1975). The high rate of collagen synthesis within a wound (Diegelmann et al., 1975) returns to normal tissue levels by 6–12 months (Barnes et al., 1975). Collagen remodeling during scar formation is dependent on both continued collagen synthesis and collagen catabolism. The degradation of wound collagen is controlled by a variety of collagenase enzymes from granulocytes (Lazarus et al., 1968; Robertson et al., 1972), macrophages (Wahl et al., 1977; Werb and Gordon, 1975a), epidermal cells (Donoff et al., 1971), and fibroblasts (Mainardi et al., 1986). These collagenase are specific for particular types of collagens, and most cells probably contain two or more of these enzymes (Hibbs et al., 1985; Hasty et al., 1986; Mainardi et al., 1986).

Besides providing structural support and strength to the new tissue, collagen can have a profound effect on the cells within and on its matrix. Collagen and collagen-derived peptides act as chemoattractants for fibroblasts in vitro (Postlethwaite et al., 1978) and may have a similar activity in vivo. In addition, collagen gels alter the phenotype and function of epithelial cell (Sugrue and Hay, 1981; J. B. Baskin and R. A. F. Clark, personal observation), endothelial cell (Madri et al., 1983) (Chapter 15) and fibroblasts (Bell et al., 1983; Nusgens et al., 1984). An interesting recent observation by Unemori and Werb (1986) suggests that a collagen gel matrix may provide fibroblasts with a signal to remodel the gel through the induction of fibroblast procollagenase. This phenomenon is a good example of how matrices may alter cells in a way that results in cellular modification of the matrix. Thus, during wound repair, matrix may induce cell phenotype changes that in turn induce matrix modification and so on in a chain reaction of events until the tissue stabilizes.

4.5. Basement Membranes

The constituents of basement membranes are reviewed in Chapter 22. During re-epithelialization or re-endothelialization of a wound in which the basement membrane zone has been disrupted, the migrating cells transit over a provisional matrix (see Chapters 14, 15, and 23). Basement membrane does not reform until after migration ceases (Stanley et al., 1981; Clark et al., 1982a) (Chapter 23). In both in vitro and in vivo studies, the re-formation of the epidermal basement membrane has been demonstrated to occur in stages. Bullous pemphigoid antigen is never absent during epidermal re-epithelialization and thus is present at the basal plasma membrane of all the migrating cells that juxtapose the extracellular matrix. As epithelial cells cease to migrate, type IV collagen and then laminin become detectable in the basement membrane zone.

The deposition of these two basement membrane proteins begins at the original wound margin and progresses inward simulating a zipper mechanism that interlocks the new epidermis to the neodermis (Chapter 23). A similar sequence of events probably occurs during angiogenesis (Chapter 15).

References

Abercrombie, M., Heaysman, J. E. M., and Pegrum, S. M., 1971, The locomotion of fibroblasts in culture. IV. Electron microscopy of the leading lamella, *Exp. Cell. Res.* **67**:359–367.

Adams, S. O., Nissley, S. P., Handwerger, S., Rechler, M. M., 1983, Developmental patterns of insulin-like growth Factor-I and -II synthesis and regulation in rat fibroblasts, *Nature (Lond.)* **302**:150–153.

Anseth, A., 1961, Glycosaminoglycans in corneal regeneration, *Exp. Eye Res.* **1**:122–127.

Armitage, P. M., and Chapman, J. A., 1971, New fibrous long spacing form of collagen, *Nature (New Biol.)* **229**:151–152.

Assoian, R. K., Frolik, C. A., Roberts, A. B., Miller, D. M., and Sporn, M. B., 1984, Transforming growth factor-B controls receptor levels for epidermal growth factor in NRK fibroblasts, *Cell* **36**:35–41.

Ausprunk, D. H., and Folkman, J., 1977, Migration and proliferation of endothelial cells in preformed and newly formed blood vessels during tumor angiogenesis, *Microvasc. Res.* **14**:53–65.

Ausprunk, D. H., Falterman, K., and Folkman, J., 1978, The sequence of events in the regression of corneal capillaries, *Lab. Invest.* **38**:284–294.

Ausprunk, D. H., Boudreau, C. L., and Nelson, D. A., 1981, Proteoglycans in the microvasculature. II. Histochemical localization in proliferating capillaries of the rabbit cornea, *Am. J. Pathol.* **103**:367–375.

Azizkhan, R. G., Azizkhan, J. C., Zetter, B. R., and Folkman, J., 1980, Mast cell heparin stimulates mirgration of capillary endothelial cells *in vitro*, *J. Exp. Med.* **152**:931–944.

Bailey, A. J., Bazin, S., Sims, T. J., LeLeus, M., Nicholetis, C., and Delaunay, A., 1975, Characterization of the collagen of human hypertrophic and normal scars, *Biochim. Biophys. Acta* **405**:412–421.

Baker, J. B., Low, D. A., Simmer, R. L., and Cunningham, D. D., 1980, Protease-nexin: A cellular component that links thrombin and plasminogen activator and mediates their binding to cells, *Cell* **21**:37–45.

Balazs, A., and Holmgren, H. J., 1950, The basic dye-uptake and the presence of growth inhibiting substance in the healing tissue of skin wounds, *Exp. Cell. Res.* **1**:206–216.

Banda, M. J., Knighton, D. R., Hunt, T. K., and Werb, Z., 1982, Isolation of a nonmitogenic angiogenesis factor from wound fluid, *Proc. Natl. Acad. Sci. USA* **79**:7773–777.

Banerjee, S. D., Cohn, R. H., and Bernfield, M. R., 1977, Basal lamina of embryonic salivary epithelial. Production by the epithelium and role in maintaining lobular morphology, *J. Cell Biol.* **73**:445–463.

Barnes, M. J., and MacIntyre, D. E., 1979, Collagen-induced platelet aggregation. The activity of basement membrane collagens relative to other collagen types, *Front. Matrix. Biol.* **7**:246–257.

Barnes, M. J., Morton, L. F., Bennett, R. C., and Bailey, A. J., 1975, Studies on collagen synthesis in the mature dermal scar in the guinea pig, *Biochem. Soc.* **3**:917–920.

Bar-Shavit, R., Kahn, A., Fenton, J. W., and Wilner, G. D., 1983, Chemotactic response of monocytes to thrombin, *J. Cell Biol.* **96**:282–285.

Bazin, S., and Delaunay, A., 1964, Biochimie de l'inflammation. VI. Fluctuations du taux de collagène et des proteines non fibrillaires dans differents types de foyers inflammatoires, *Am. Inst. Pasteur* **107**:163–172.

Bell, E., Ivarsson, B., and Merrill, C., 1979, Production of a tissue-like structure by contraction of collagen lattices by human fibroblasts of different proliferative potential *in vitro*, *Proc. Natl. Acad. Sci. USA* **76**:1274–1278.

Bell, E., Ehrlich, H. P., Buttle, D. J., and Nakatsuji, T., 1981, Living tissue formed in vitro and accepted as skin-equivalent tissue of full thickness, *Science* **211**:1052–1054.

Bell, E., Sher, S., Hull, B., Merrill, C., Rosen, S., Chamson, A., Asselineau, D., Dubertret, L., Coulomb, B., Lepiere, C., Nusgens, B., and Neveux, Y., 1983, The reconstitution of living skin, *J. Invest. Dermatol.* **81**(Suppl.):2S–10S.

Bellows, C. G., Melcher, A. H., Bargava, U., and Aubin, J. E., 1982, Fibroblasts contracting three-dimensional collagen gels exhibit ultrastructure consistent with either contraction or protein secretion, *J. Ultrastruct. Res.* **78**:178–192.

Bently, J. P., 1967, Rate of chondroitin sulfate formation in wound healing, *Ann. Surg.* **165**:186–191.

Benya, P. D., and Padilla, S. R., 1986, Isolation and characterization of type VIII collagen synthesized by cultured rabbit corneal endothelial cells. A conventional structure replaces the interrupted-helix model, *J. Biol. Chem.* **261**:4160–4169.

Bernfield, M. R., and Banerjee, S. D., 1972, Acid mucopolysaccharide (glycosaminoglycan) at the epithelial–mesenchymal interface of mouse embryo salivary glands, *J. Cell Biol.* **52**:664–673.

Bernfield, M. R., Banerjee, S. D., and Cohn, R. H., 1972, Dependence of salivary epithelial morphology and branching morphogenesis upon acid mucopolysaccharide-protein (proteoglycan) at the epithelial surface, *J. Cell Biol.* **52**:647–689.

Bernstein, L. R., Antoniades, H., and Zetter, B. R., 1982, Migration of cultured vascular cells in response to plasma and platelet-derived factors, *J. Cell. Sci.* **56**:71–82.

Bertolami, C. N., and Donoff, R. B., 1982, Identification characterization, and partial purification of mammalian skin wound hyaluronidase, *J. Invest. Dermatol.* **79**:417–421.

Binder, B. R., Spragg, J., and Austen, K. F., 1979, Purification and characterization of human vascular plasminogen activator derived from blood vessel perfusates, *J. Biol. Chem.* **254**:1998–2003.

Bode, A. P., Dombrose, F. A., Lentz, B. R., and Roberts, H. R., 1981, The platelet membrane as a catalytic surface in thrombin generation: Availability of platelet Factor I and platelet Factor 3, *Ann. NY Acad. Sci.* **370**:348–358.

Bornstein, P., and Ash, T. F., 1977, Cell surface-associated structural proteins in connective tissue cells, *Proc. Natl. Acad. Sci. USA* **74**:2480–2484.

Bowersox, J. C., and Sorgente, N., 1982, Chemotaxis of aortic endothelial cells in response to fibronectin, *Cancer Res.* **42**:2547–2551.

Brown, R. A., Weiss, J. B., and Tomlinson, I. W., 1980, Angiogenic factor from synovial fluid resembling that from tumors, *Lancet* **1**:682–685.

Bruns, R. R., Press, W., Engvall, E., Timpl, R., and Gross, J., 1986, Type VI collagen in extracellular, 100 nm periodic filaments and fibrils: Identification by immunoelectron microscopy, *J. Cell Biol.* **103**:393–404.

Carpenter, G., and Cohen, S., 1976, ^{125}I-labeled human epidermal growth factor (hEGF): Binding, internalization, and degradation in human fibroblasts, *J. Cell Biol.* **71**:159–171.

Castellot, J. J., Addonizio, M. L., Rosenberg, R., and Karnovosky, M. J., 1981, Vascular endothelial cells produce a heparin-like inhibitor of smooth muscle growth, *J. Cell Biol.* **90**:372–379.

Chen, L. B., Murray, A., Segal, R. A., Bushnell, A., and Walsh, M. L., 1978, Studies on intracellular LETS glycoprotein matrices, *Cell* **14**:377–391.

Chen, L. B., Gudor, R. C., Sun, T. T., Chen, A. B., and Mosesson, M., 1977, Control of a cell surface major glycoprotein by epidermal growth factor, *Science* **197**:776–778.

Chung, E., and Miller, E. J., 1974, Collagen polymorphism. Characterization of molecules with the chain composition $1(111)_3$, *Science* **183**:1200–1204.

Clark, R. A. F., Lanigan, J. M., DellaPelle, P., Manseau, E., Dvorak, H. F., and Colvin, R. B., 1982a, Fibronectin and fibrin provide a provisional matrix for epidermal cell migration during wound reepithelialization, *J. Invest. Dermatol.* **70**:264–269.

Clark, R. A. F., DellaPelle, P., Manseau, E., Lanigan, J. M., Dvorak, H. F., and Colvin, R. B., 1982b, Blood vessel fibronectic increases in conjunction with endothelial cell proliferation and capillary ingrowth during wound healing. *J. Invest. Dermatol.* **79**:269–276.

Clark, R. A. F., Quinn, J. H., Winn, H. J., Lanigan, J. M., DellaPelle, P., and Colvin, R. B., 1982c, Fibronectin is produced by blood vessels in response to injury, *J. Exp. Med.* **156**:646–651.

Clark, R. A. F., Folkvord, J. M., and Nielsen, L. D., 1986, Either exogenous or endogenous fibronectin can promote adherence of human endothelial cells, *J. Cell Sci.* **82**:263–280.

Clemmons, D. R., Van Wyk, J. J., and Pledger, W. J., 1980, Sequential addition of platelet factor and plasma to Balb/c 3T3 fibroblast cultures stimulates somatomedin-C binding early in cell cycle, *Proc. Natl. Acad. Sci. USA* **77**:6644–6648.

Clemmons, D. R., Isley, W. L., and Brown, M. T., 1983, Dialyzable factor in human serum of platelet origin stimulates endothelial cell replication and growth, *Proc. Natl. Acad. Sci. USA* **80**:1641–1645.

Cohen, I. K., Keiser, H. R., and Sjoerdsma, A., 1971, Collagen synthesis in human keloid and hypertrophic scar, *Surg. Forum* **22**:488–489.

Cohen, S., 1965, The stimulation of epidermal proliferation by a specific protein (EGF) *Dev. Biol.* **12**:394–407.

Cohn, R. H., Cassiman, J. J., and Bernfield, M. R., 1976, Relationship of transformation, cell density and growth control to cellular distribution of newly synthesized glycosaminoglycan, *J. Cell Biol.* **71**:280–294.

Cohn, R. H., Banerjee, S. D., and Bernfield, M. R., 1977, Basal laminia of embryonic salivary epithelia. Nature of glycosaminoglycan and organization of extracellular materials, *J. Cell Biol.* **73**:464–478.

Craddock, P., Fehr, J., Dalmasso, A.P., Brigham, K. L., and Jacob, H. S., 1977, Hemodialysis leukopenia: Pulmonary vascular leukostasis resulting from complement activation by dialyzer cellophane membrane, *J. Clin. Invest.* **59**:879–888.

Culp, L. A., Murray, B. A., and Rollins, B. J., 1979, Fibronectin and proteoglycans as determinants of cell-substratum adhesion, *J. Supramol. Struct.* **11**:401–427.

D'Amore, P., and Klagsbrun, M., 1984, Endothelial cell mitogens derived from the retina and hypothalamus: Biochemical and biological similarities, *J. Cell Biol.* **99**:1545–1549.

Detwiler, T. C., and Feinman, R. D., 1973, Kinetics of the thrombin-induced release of calcium by platelets, *Biochemistry* **12**:282–289.

Deuel, T. F., Senior, R. M., Chang, D., Griffin, G. L., Heinrikson, R. L., and Kaiser, E. T., 1981, Platelet factor 4 is chemotactic for neutrophils and monocytes, *Proc. Natl. Acad. Sci. USA* **78**:4584–4587.

Deuel, T. F., Senior, R. M., Huang, J. S., and Griffin, G. L., 1982, Chemotaxis of monocytes and neutrophils to platelet-derived growth factor, *J. Clin. Invest.* **69**:1046–1049.

Diegelmann, R. F., Rothkopf, L. C., and Cohen, I. K., 1975, Measurement of collagen biosynthesis during wound healing. *J. Surg. Res.* **19**:239–243.

Donoff, R. B., McLennan, J. E., and Grillo, H. C., 1971, Preparation and properties of collagenases from epithelium and mesenchyme of healing mammalian wounds, *Biochim. Biophys. Acta* **227**:639–653.

Dorner, R. W., 1967, Glycosaminoglycans of regenerating tendon, *Arthritis Rheum.* **10**:275–276.

Dvorak, H. F., Senger, D. R., Dvorak, A. M., Harvey, V. S., and McDonagh, J., 1985, Regulation of extravascular coagulation by microvascular permeability, *Science* **227**:1059–1061.

Ehrlich, H. P., and White, B. S., 1981, The identification of A and B collagen chains in hypertrophic scars, *Exp. Mol. Pathol.* **34**:1–8.

Epstein, E. H., 1974 [α1(III)]₃ human skin collagen. Release by pepsin digestion and preponderance in fetal life, *J. Biol. Chem.* **249**:3225–3231.

Esmon, C. T., and Owen, W. G., 1981, Identification of an endothelial cell cofactor for thrombin-catalyzed activation of Protein C, *Proc. Natl. Acad. Sci. USA* **78**:2249–2252.

Fearon, D. T., 1978, Activation of the alternative complement pathway by *E. coli*: Resistance of bound C3b to inactivation by C3b INA and IH, *J. Immunol.* **120**:1772.

Fearon, D. T., and Austen, K. F., 1977, Activation of the alternative complement pathway due to resistance of zymosan-bound amplification convertase to endogenous regulatory mechanisms, *Proc. Natl. Acad. Sci. USA* **74**:1683–1687.

Fernandez, H. N., Henson, P. M., Otani, A., and Hugli, T. E., 1978, Chemotactic response to human C3a and C5a anaphylatoxins. I. Evaluation of C3a and C5a leukotaxis *in vitro* and under simulated *in vivo* conditions, *J. Immunol.* **120**:109–115.

Folkman, J., 1982, Angiogenesis: initiation and control, *Ann. NY Acad. Sci.* **401**:212–227.

Ford-Hutchinson, A. W., Bray, M. A., Doig, M. V., Shipley, M. E., and Smith, M. J., 1980, Leuko-triene B, a potent chemokinetic and aggregating substance released from polymorphonuclear leukocytes, *Nature (Lond.)* **286:**264–265.

Frederick, J. L., Shimanuki, T., and DiZerega, G. S., 1984, Initiation of angiogenesis by human follicular fluid, *Science* **224:**389–390.

Freer, R. J., Day, A. R., Radding, J. A., Schiffmann, E., Aswanikumar, S., Showell, H. J., and Becker, E. L., 1980, Further studies on the structural requirement for synthetic peptide chemoattrac-tants, *Biochemistry* **19:**2404–2410.

Fujikawa, L. S., Footer, C. S., Gipson, I. K, and Colvin, R. B., 1984, Basement membrane com-ponents in healing rabbit corneal epithelial wounds: Immunofluorescence and ultrastructural studies, *J. Cell Biol.* **98:**128–138.

Furcht, L. T., Wendelschafer-Crabb, G., Mosher, D. F., and Foidart, J. M., 1980, An axial periodic fibrillar arrangement of antigenic determinants for fibronectin and procollagen on ascorbate treated human fibroblasts, *J. Supramol. Struct.* **13:**15–33.

Furie, M. B., and Rifkin, D. B., 1980, Proteolytically derived fragments of human plasma fibronectin and their localization within intact molecule, *J. Biol. Chem.* **365:**3134–3140.

Gabbiani, G., Lelous, M., Bailey, A. J., and Delauney, A., 1976, Collagen and myofibroblasts of granulation tissue. A chemical, ultrastructural and immunologic study, *Virchows Arch. [Cell Pathol]* **21:**133–145.

Gabbiani, G., Chapponnier, C., and Huttner, I., 1978, Cytoplasmic filaments and gap junctions in epithelial cells and myofibroblasts during wound healing, *J. Cell Biol.* **76:**561–568.

Gabbiani, G., Hirschel, B. J., Ryan, G. B., Statkov, P. R., and Majno, G., 1972, Granulation tissue as a contractile organ. A study of structure and function, *J. Exp. Med.* **135:**19–734.

Gallin, J. I., and Kaplan, A. P., 1974, Mononuclear cell chemotactic activity of kallikrein and plasminogen activator and its inhibition by C1 inhibitor and α_2-macroglubulin, *J. Immunol.* **113:**1928–1934.

Gauss-Muller, V., Kleinman, H. K., Martin, G. R., and Schiffman, E., 1980, Role of attachment factors and attractants in fibroblast chemotaxis, *J. Lab. Clin. Med.* **96:**1071–1080.

Gay, S., Rhodes, R. K., Gay, R. E., and Miller, E. J., 1981, Collagen molecules comprised of 1 (V)-chains (B chains): an apparent localization in the exocytoskeleton, *Cell. Res.* **1:**53–58.

Ghebrehiwet, B., Silverberg, M., and Kaplan, A. P., 1981, Activation of classic pathway of comple-ment by Hageman factor fragment, *J. Exp. Med.* **153:**665–676.

Gipson, I. K., Grill, S. M., Spun, S. J., and Brennan, S. J., 1983, Hemidesmosome formation *in vitro*, *J. Cell Biol.* **97:**849–857.

Glaser, B. M., D'Amore, P. A., Seppa, H., Seppa, S., and Schiffmann, E., 1980, Adult tissues contain chemoattractants for vascular endothelial cells, *Nature (Lond.)* **288:**483–484.

Glenn, K. C., and Cunningham, D. D., 1979, Thrombin-stimulated cell division involves proteolysis of its cell surface receptor, *Nature (Lond.)* **278:**711–714.

Gordon, J. R., and Bernfield, M. R., 1980, The basal lamina of the postnatal mammary epithelium contains glycosaminoglycans in a precise ultrastructural organization, *Dev. Biol.* **74:**118–135.

Gospodarowicz, D., 1975, Purification of fibroblast growth factor from bovine pituitary, *J. Biol. Chem.* **250:**2515–2520.

Gospodarowicz, D., Moran, J. S., and Braun, D. L., 1977, Control of proliferation of bovine vascular endothelial cells, *J. Cell Physiol.* **91:**377–386.

Gospodarowicz, D., Brown, K. D., Birdwell, C. R., and Zetter, B. R., 1978, Control of proliferation of human vascular endothelial cells. Characterization of the response of human umbilical vein endothelial cells to fibroblast growth factor, epidermal growth factor, and thrombin, *J. Cell Biol.* **77:**774–778.

Gospodarowicz, D., Cheng, J., and Lirette, M., 1983, Bovine brain and pituitary fibroblast growth factors: comparison of their abilities to support the proliferation of human and bovine vascular endothelial cells, *J. Cell Biol.* **97:**1677–1685.

Grinnell, F., Billingham, R. E., and Burgess, L., 1981, Distribution of fibronectin during wound healing *in vivo*, *J. Invest. Dermatol.* **76:**181–189.

Grobstein, C., 1967, Mechanisms of organogenetic tissue interaction, *Natl. Cancer Inst. Monog.* **26:**279–299.

Grotendorst, G. R., 1984, Alteration of the chemotactic response of NIH/3T3 cells to PDGF by growth factors, transformation and tumor promoters, *Cell* **36:**279–285.

Grobstein, C., 1967, Mechanisms of organogenetic tissue interaction, *Natl. Cancer Inst. Monog.* **26:**279–299.

Habal, F. M., Burrows, C. E., and Movat, H. Z., 1976, Generation of kinin by plasma kallikrein and plasmin, in: *Kinins, Pharmacodynamics and Biological Role* (F. Sicuteri, N. Black, and G. L. Haberland, eds.), pp. 23–36, Plenum, New York.

Hall, E., and Cruickshank, C. N. D., 1963, The effect of injury upon the uptake of ^{3}H thymidine by guinea pig epidermis, *Exp. Cell Res.* **31:**128–139.

Hascall, V. C., and Hascall, G. K., 1981, Proteoglycans, in: *Cell Biology of Extracellular Matrix* (E. G. Hay, ed.), pp. 39–63, Plenum, New York.

Hasty, K. A., Hibbs, M. S., Seyer, J. M., Mainardi, C. L., and Kang, A. H., 1986, Secreted forms of human neutrophil collagenase, *J. Biol. Chem.* **261:**5645–5650.

Haudenschild, C. C., Zahniser, D., Folkman, J., and Klagsbrun, D. M., 1969, Stimulation of neo-vascularization of the cornea by biogenic amines, *Exp. Eye Res.* **8:**77–83.

Haudenschild, C. C., Zahniser, D., Folkman, J., and Klagsbrun, M., 1976, Human vascular endo-thelial cells in culture. Lack of response to serum growth factors, *Exp. Cell Res.* **98:**175–183.

Hay, E. B., and Meier, S., 1974. Glycosaminoglycan synthesis by embryonic inductors: neural tube, notecord, and lens, *J. Cell Biol.* **62:**889–898.

Hayman, E. G., Oldburg, A., Martin, G. E., and Rouslahti, E., 1982, Codistribution of heparan sulfate proteoglycan, laminin, and fibronectin in the extracellular matrix of normal rat kidney cells, *J. Cell Biol.* **94:**28–35.

Hedman, K., Johansson, S., Vartio, T., Kjellen, L., Vaheri, A., and Hook, M., 1982, Structure of the pericellular matrix: Association of heparan and chondroitin sulfates with fibronectin-pro-collagen fibers, *Cell* **28:**663–671.

Heimark, R. L., and Schwartz, S. M., 1985, The role of membrane–membrane interactions in the regulation of endothelial cell growth, *J. Cell Biol.* **100:**1934–1940.

Heldin, C. H., Westermark, B., and Wasteson, A., 1979, Platelet-derived growth factor: Purification and partial characterization, *Proc. Natl. Acad. Sci. USA* **65:**3722–3726.

Hennings, H., Michael, D., Cheng, D., Steinert, P., Holbrook, K., and Yuspa, S. H., 1980, Calcuim regulation of growth and differentiation of mouse epidermal cells in culture, *Cell* **19:**245–254.

Herinmark, R. L., and Schwartz, S. M., 1985, The role of membrane–membrane interactions in the regulation of endothelial cell growth *J. Cell Biol.* **100:**1934–1940.

Hering, T. M., Marchant, R. E., Anderson, J. M., 1983, Type V collagen during granulation tissue development, *Exp. Mol. Pathol.* **39:**219–229.

Hibbs, M. S., Hasty, K. A., Seyer, J. M., Kang, A. H., and Mainardi, C. L., 1985, Biochemical and immunological characterization of the secreted forms of human neutrophil gelatinase, *J. Biol. Chem.* **260:**2493–2501.

Holund, B., Clemmensen, I., Junker, P., and Lyon, H., 1982, Fibronectin in experimental granula-tion tissue, *Acta Pathol. Microbiol. Immunol. Scand.* **90:**159–165.

Hopwood, J. J., and Dorfman, A., 1977, Glycosaminoglycan synthesis by cultured human skin fibroblasts after transformation with simian virus 40, *J. Biol. Chem.* **252:**4777–4785.

Hsieh, P., and Chen, L. B., 1983, Behavior of cells seeded on isolated fibronectin matrices, *J. Cell Biol.* **96:**1208–1217.

Hugli, T. E., and Muller-Eberhard, H. J., 1978, Anaphylatoxins, C3a and C5a, *Adv. Immunol.* **26:**1–53.

Humes, J. L., Bonney, R. J., Pelus, L., Dahlgren, M. E., Saelowski, S. J., Kuehl, F. A., Jr., and Davies, P., 1977, Macrophages synthesize and release prostaglandins in response to inflammatory stimuli, *Nature (Lond.)* **269:**149–151.

Hunt, T. K., 1980, *Wound Healing and Wound Infection: Theory and Surgical Practice,* Appleton-Century-Crofts, New York.

Hynes, R. O., 1987, Integrins: A family of cell surface receptors, *Cell* **48:**549–554.

Ignotz, R. A., and Massague, J., 1986, Transforming growth factor-β stimulates the expression of fibronectin and collagen and their incorporation into extracellular matrix, *J. Biol. Chem.* **261:**4337–4340.

Imre, G., 1964, Role of lactic acid, *Br. J. Ophthalmol.* **48:**75–82.

Josso, F., and Prou-Wartelle, O., 1965, Interaction of tissue factor and Factor VII at the earliest phase of coagulation, *Thromb. Diath. Haemorrh. (Suppl.)* **17:** 35–44.

Kalebic, T., Garbisa, S., Glaser, B., and Liotta, L. A., 1983, Basement membrane collagen: degradation by migrating endothelial cells, *Science* **221:**281–283.

Kaplan, A. P., 1983, Hageman factor-dependent pathways: Mechanism of initiation and bradykinin formation, *Fed. Proc.* **42:**3123–3127.

Kaplan, A. P., and Austen, K. F., 1971, A prealbumin activator of prekallikrein. II. Derivation of activators of prekallikreim from active Hageman factor with plasmin, *J. Exp. Med.* **133:**696–712.

Kaplan, A. P., Kay, A. B., and Austen, K. F., 1972, A prealbumin activator of prekallikrein. III. Appearance of chemotactic activity for human neutrophils by conversion of human prekallikreim to kallikrein, *J. Exp. Med.* **135:**81–97.

Kay, A. B., Pepper, D. S., and McKenzie, R., 1974, The identification of fibrinopeptide B as the chemotactic agent derived from human fibrinogen, *Br. J. Haematol.* **27:**669–677.

Keski-Oja, T., Todaro, G. J., and Vaheri, A., 1981, Thrombin affects fibronectin and procollagen in the pericellular matrix of cultured human fibroblasts, *Biochim. Biophys. Acta* **673:**323–331.

King, G. L., and Buchwald, S., 1984, Characterization and partial purification of an endothelial cell growth factor from human platelets, *J. Clin. Invest.* **73:**392–396.

Kinsella, M. G., and Wight, T. N., 1986, Modulation of sulfated proteoglycan synthesis by bovine aortic endothelial cells during migration, *J. Cell Biol.* **102:**679–687.

Kischer, C. W., and Shetlar, M. R., 1974, Collagen and mucopolysaccharides in the hypertrophic scar, *Connect. Tissue Res.* **3:**205–213.

Kisiel, W., Canfield, W. M., Ericsson, L. H., and Davie, E. W., 1977, Anticoagulant properties of bovine plasma protein C following activation by thrombin, *Biochemistry* **16:**5824–5831.

Kraemer, P. M., and Tobey, R. A., 1972, Cell-cycle dependent desquamation of heparan sulfate from the cell surface, *J. Cell Biol.* **55:**713–717.

Krawczyk, W. S., 1971, A pattern of epidermal cell migration during wound healing, *J. Cell Biol.* **49:**247–263.

Krawczyk, W. S., and Wilgram, G. F., 1973, Hemidesmosome and desmosome morphogenesis during epidermal wound healing, *J. Ultrastruct. Res.* **45:**93–101.

Kurkinen, M., Vaheri, A., Roberts, P. J., and Stenman, S., 1980, Sequential appearance of fibronectin and collagen in experimental granulation tissue, *Lab. Invest.* **43:**47–51.

Lachman, L. B., 1983, Human interleukin I: Purification and properties, *Fed. Proc.* **42:**2639–2645.

Lark, M. W., Laterra, J., and Culp, L. A., 1985, Close and focal contact adhesions of fibroblasts to fibronectin-containing matrix, *Fed. Proc.* **44:**394–403.

Lawrence, W. T., Sporn, M. B., Gorschbath, C., North, J. A., and Grotendorst, G., 1986, The reversal of an adriamycin induced healing impairment with chemoattractants and growth factors, *Ann. Surg.* **203:**142–147.

Lazarus, G. S., Brown, R. S., Daniels, J. R., and Fullmer, H. M., 1968, Degradation of collagen by a human granulocyte collagenolytic system, *J. Clin. Invest.* **47:**2622–2629.

Legrand, Y. J., Fauvel, F., and Caen, J. P., 1979, Adhesion of platelet to collagen, *Front. Matrix. Biol.* **7:**246–257.

Leibovich, S. J., and Ross, R., 1975, The role of the macrophage in wound repair: A study with hydrocortisone and antimacrophage serum, *Am. J. Pathol.* **78:**71–100.

Lembach, K. J., 1976, Enhanced synthesis and extracellular accumulation of hyaluronic acid during stimulation of quiescent human fibroblasts by mouse epidermal growth factor, *J. Cell. Physiol.* **89:**277–288.

Letourneau, P. C., Ray, P. N., and Bernfeld, M. R., 1980, The regulation of cell behavior by cell adhesion, in *Biological Regulation and Development*, Vol. 2 (R. Goldberger, ed.), pp. 339–376, Plenum, New York.

Levenson, S. M., Geever, E. F., Crowley, L. V., Oates, J. F. III, Berard, C. W., and Rosen, H., 1965, The healing of rat skin wounds, *Ann. Surg.* **161:**293–308.

Lollar, P., Hoak, J. C., and Owen, W. G., 1980, Binding of thrombin to cultured human endothelial cells. Nonequilibrium aspects, *J. Biol. Chem.* **255:**10279–10283.

Loskutoff, D. J., and Edgington, T. E., 1977, Synthesis of a fibrinolytic activator and inhibitor by endothelial cells, *Proc. Natl. Acad. Sci. USA* **74**:3903–3907.

Maciag, T., Hoover, G. A., and Weinstein, R., 1982, High and low molecular weight forms of endothelial cell growth factor, *J. Biol. Chem.* **257**:5333–5336.

Maciag, T., Mehlman, T., Friesal, R., and Schreiber, A. B., 1984, Heparin binds endothelial cell growth factor, the principal endothelial cell mitogen in bovine brain, *Science* **225**:932–935.

Madri, J. A., Williams, S. K., Wyatt, T., and Mezzio, C., 1983, Capillary endothelial cell cultures: phenotypic modulation by matrix components, *J. Cell Biol.* **97**:153–165.

Madri, J. A., and Stenn, K. S., 1982, Aortic endothelial cell migration. I. Matrix requirements and composition, *Am. J. Pathol.* **106**,180–186.

Mainardi, C. L., Hasty, K. A., and Hibbs, M. S., 1986, Type specific collagen degradation, *Adv. Inflam. Res.* **11**:135–144.

Majno, G., Gabbiani, G., Hirschel, B. J., Ryan, G. B., and Statkov, P. R., 1971, Contraction of granulation tissue *in vitro*: Similarity to smooth muscle, *Science* **173**:548–550.

Marlar, R., Kleiss, A., and Griffin, J. H., 1982, an alternative extrinsic pathway of human blood coagulation, *Blood* **60**:1353–1358.

Martin, B. M., Gimbrone, M. A., Jr., Unanue, E. R., and Cotran, R. S., 1981, Stimulation of non-lymphoid mesenchymal cell proliferation by a macrophage derived growth factor, *J. Immunol.* **126**:1510–1515.

Martinet, Y., Bitterman, P. B., Mornex, J., Grotendorst, G. R., Martin, G. R., and Crystal, R. G., 1986, Activated human monocytes express the c-sis proto-oncogene and release a mediator showing PDGF-like activity, *Nature (Lond.)* **319**:158–160.

Maynard, J. R., Heckman, C. A., Pitlick, F. A., and Nemerson, Y., 1975, Association of tissue factor activity with the surface of cultured cells, *J. Clin. Invest.* **55**:814–824.

McCarthy, K., and Henson, P. M., 1979, Induction of lysosomal enzyme secretion by macrophages in response to the purified complement fragments C5a and C5a des Arg, *J. Immunol.* **123**:2511–2517.

McDonald, J. A., and Kelley, D. G., 1980, Degradation of fibronectin by human leukocyte elastase, *J. Biol. Chem.* **255**:8848–8858.

McDonald, J. A., Kelley, D. G., and Broekelmann, T. J., 1982, Role of fibronectin in collagen deposition. Fab1 antibodies to the gelatin-binding domain of fibronectin inhibits both fibronectin and collagen organization in fibroblast extracellular matrix, *J. Cell Biol.* **92**:485–492.

McDonald, J. A., Quade, B. J., Broekelmann, T. J., LaChance, R., Forsman, K., Hasegawa, E., and Akiyama, S., 1987, Fibronectin's cell-adhesive domain and an amino-terminal matrix assembly domain participate in its assembly into fibroblast pericellular matrix, *J. Biol. Chem.* **262**:2957–2967.

McKenzie, R., Pepper, D. S., and Kay, A. B., 1975, The generation of chemotactic activity for human leukocytes by the action of plasmin on human fibrinogen, *Thromb. Res.* **6**:1–8.

McPherson, J. M., Sawamura, S., Condell, R. A., Rhee, W., and Wallace, D. G., 1987, The effects of heparin on the physicochemical properties of reconstituted collagen, *Cell. Relat. Res.*, in press.

Moncada, S., Gryglewski, R., Bunting, S., and Vance, J. R., 1976, An enzyme isolated from arteries transforms prostaglandin endoperoxidoses to an unstable substance that inhibits platelet aggregation, *Nature (Lond.)* **263**:663–665.

Moscatelli, D., and Rubin, H., 1975, Increased hyaluronic acid production on stimulation of DNA synthesis in chick embryo fibroblasts, *Nature (Lond.)* **254**:65–66.

Mosher, D. F., and Vaheri, A., 1978, Thrombin stimulates the production and release of a major surface-associated glycoprotein (fibronectin) in cultures of human fibroblasts, *Exp. Cell. Res.* **112**:323–334.

Newman, S. L., Henson, J. E., and Henson, P. M., 1982, Phagocytosis of senescent neutrophils by human monocyte derived macrophages and rabbit inflammatory macrophages, *J. Exp. Med.* **156**:430–442.

Norris, D. A., Clark, R. A. F., Swigart, L. M., Huff, J. C., Weston, W. L., and Howell, S. E., 1982, Fibronectin fragments are chemotactic for human peripheral blood monocytes, *J. Immunol.* **129**:1612–1618.

Nusgens, B., Merrill, C., Lapiere, C., and Bell, E., 1984, Collagen biosynthesis by cells in a tissue equivalent matrix *in vitro, Cell Relat. Res.* **4**:351–363.

Oppenheimer, C. L., Pessin, J. E., Massague, J., Gitomer, W., and Czech, M. P., 1983, Insulin action rapidly modulates the apparent affinity of the insulin-like growth factor II receptor, *J. Biol. Chem.* **258**:4824–4830.

Plow, E. F., Loftus, J. C., Levin, E. G., Fair, D. S., Dixon, D., Forsyth, and Ginsberg, M. H., 1986, Immunologic relationship between platelet membrane glycoprotein GPIIb/IIIa and cell molecules exposed by a variety of cells. *Proc. Natl. Acad. Sci. USA* **83**:6002–6006.

Polverini, P. J., Cotran, R. S., Gimbrone, M. A., Jr., and Unanue, E. R., 1977, Activated macrophages induce vascular proliferation, *Nature (Lond.)* **269**:804–806.

Postlethwaite, A. E., and Kang, A. H., 1976, Collagen and collagen peptide-induced chemotaxis of human blood monocytes, *J. Exp. Med.* **143**:1299–1307.

Postlethwaite, A. E., Snyderman, R., and Kang, A. H., 1976, Chemotactic attraction of human fibroblasts to a lymphocyte-derived factor, *J. Exp. Med.* **144**:1188–1203.

Postlethwaite, A. E., Seyer, J. M., and Kang, A. H., 1978, Chemotactic attraction of human fibroblasts to type I, II and III collagens and collagen-derived peptides, *Proc. Natl. Acad. Sci. USA* **75**:871–875.

Postlethwaite, A. E., Snyderman, R., and Kang, A. H., 1979, Generation of a fibroblast chemotactic factor in serum by activation of complement, *J. Clin Invest.* **64**:1379–1385.

Postlethwaite, A. E., Keski-Oja, J., Balian, G., and Kang, A., 1981, Induction of fibroblast chemotaxis by fibronectin. Localization of the chemotactic region to a 140,000 molecular weight non-gelatin binding fragment, *J. Exp. Med.* **153**:494–499.

Postlethwaite, A. E., Keski-Oja, J., Moses, H. L., and Kang, A. H., 1987, Stimulation of the chemotactic migration of human fibroblasts by transforming growth factor-β, *J. Exp. Med.* **165**:251–256.

Quintner, M. I., Kollar, E. J., and Rossomando, E. F., 1982, Proteoglycan modifications by granulation tissue in culture, *Exp. Cell. Biol.* **50**:222–228.

Raju, K. S., Alessandri, G., and Gullino, P. M., 1984, Characterization of a chemoattract for endothelium induced by angiogenesis effectors, *Cancer Res.* **44**:1579–1584.

Raz, A., Isakson, P. C., Minkes, M. S., and Needleman, P., 1977, Characterization of a novel metabolic pathway of arachidonate in coronary arteries which generates a potent endogenous coronary vasodilator, *J. Biol. Chem.* **252**:1123–1126.

Remensnyder, J. P., and Majno, G., 1968, Oxygen gradients in healing wounds, *Am. J. Pathol.* **52**:301–319.

Repesh, L. A., Fitzgerald, T. J., and Furcht, L. T., 1982, Fibronectin involvement in granulation tissue and wound healing in rabbits, *J. Histochem. Cytochem.* **30**:351–358.

Rifkin, D. B., Gross, J. L., Moscatelli, D., and Jaffe, E., 1982, Proteases and angiogenesis: Production of plasminogen activation and collagenase by endothelial cells, in: *Pathobiology of the Endothelial Cell* (H. L. Nossel and H. J. Vogel, eds.), pp. 191–197, Academic, New York.

Rijken, D., Wijngaards, G., and Welbergen, J., 1980, Relationship between tissue plasminogen activator and the activators in blood and vascular wall, *Thromb. Res.* **18**:815–830.

Risau, W., and Ekblom, P., 1986, Production of a heparin-binding angiogenesis factor by the embryonic kidney, *J. Cell Biol.* **103**:1101–1107.

Roberts, A. B., Spom, M. B., Assovan, R. K., Smith, J. M., Roche, M. S., Heine, U. F., Liottay, L., Falanga, V., Kehrl, J. H., and Fanci, A. S., 1986, Transforming growth factor beta: Rapid induction of fibrosis and angiogenesis *in vivo* and stimulation of collagen formation, *Proc. Natl. Acad. Sci. USA* **83**:4167–4171.

Robertson, P. B., Ryel, R. B., Taylor, R. E., Shyu, K. W., and Fullmer, H. M., 1972, Collagenase: Localization in polymorphonuclear leukocyte granules in the rabbit, *Science* **177**:64–65.

Rollins, B. J., and Culp, L. A., 1979, Glycosaminoglycans in the substrate adhesion sites of normal and virus-transformed murine cells, *Biochemistry* **18**:141–148.

Ross, R., Raines, E. W., and Bowen-Pospe, D. F., 1986, The biology of platelet-derived growth factor, *Cell* **46**:155–169.

Rouzer, C. A., Scott, W. A., Hamill, A. L., Liu, F. T., Katz, D. H., and Cohn, Z. A., 1982, Secretion of leukotriene C and other arachidonic acid metabolites by macrophages challenged with immunoglobulin E immune complexes, *J. Exp. Med.* **156**:1077–1086.

Rozengurt, E., Collins, M., Brown, K. D., and Pettican, P., 1982, Inhibition of epidermal growth factor binding to mouse cultured cells by fibroblast-derived growth factor, *J. Biol. Chem.* **257**:3680–3686.

Ruoslahti, E., and Pierschbacher, M. D., 1986, Arg-Gly-Asp: A versatile cell recognition signal, *Cell* **44**:517–518.

Ryan, G. B., Cliff, W. J., Gabbiani, G., Irle, C., Statkov, P. R., and Majno, G., 1974, Myofibroblasts in human granulation tissue, *Hum. Pathol.* **5**:55–67.

Sage, H., Trueb, B., and Bornstein, P., 1983, Biosynthetic and structural properties of endothelial cell type VIII collagen, *J. Biol. Chem.* **258**:13391–13401.

Sage, H., Balian, G., Vogel, A. M., and Bornstein, P., 1984, Type VIII collagen. Synthesis by normal and malignant cells in culture, *Lab Invest.* **50**:219–231.

Sakai, L., Keene, D. R., Morris, N. P., and Burgeson, R. E., 1986, Type VII collagen is a major structural component of anchoring fibrils, *J. Cell Biol.* **103**:1577–1586.

Schroff, G., Newman, C., and Song, C., 1981, Transglutaminase as a marker for subsets of murine macrophages, *Eur. J. Immunol.* **11**:637–642.

Schwartz, S. M., Gajdusek, C. M., and Owens, G. K., 1982, Vessel wall growth control in: *Pathobiology of the Endothelial Cell* (H. L. Nossel and H. J. Vogel, eds.), pp. 63–78, Academic, New York.

Senior, R. M., Griffin, G. L., and Mecham, R. P., 1980, Chemotactic activity of elastin-derived peptides, *J. Clin. Invest.* **66**:859–862.

Senior, R. M., Skogen, W. F., and Griffin, G. L., 1986, Effects of fibrinogen derivatives upon the inflammatory response, *J. Clin. Invest.* **77**:1014–1019.

Seppa, H. E. J., Grotendorst, G. R., Seppa, S. I., Schiffmann, E., and Martin, G. R., 1982, Platelet-derived growth factor is chemotactic for fibroblasts, *J. Cell Biol.* **92**:584–588.

Shetlar, M. R., Shetlar, C. L., Chien, S-F., Linares, H. A., Dobrokovsky, M., and Larson, D. L., 1972, The hypertrophic scar. Hexosamine containing components of burn scars, *Proc. Soc. Exp. Biol. Med.* **139**:544–547.

Shimokado, K., Raines, E. W., Madtes, D. K., Barrett, T. B., Benditt, E. P., and Ross, R., 1985, A significant part of macrophage-derived growth factor consists of two forms of PDGF, *Cell* **43**:277–286.

Sholley, M. M., Gimbrone, M. A., Jr., and Cotran, R. S., 1978, The effects of leukocyte depletion on corneal neovascularization, *Lab. Invest.* **38**:32–40.

Sidky, Y. A., and Auerbach, R., 1975, Lymphocyte-induced angiogenesis: A quantitative and sensitive assay of the graft-vs-host reaction, *J. Exp. Med.* **141**:1084–1100.

Singer, I. I., 1979, The fibronexus: a transmembrane association of fibronectin-containing fibers and bundles of 5 nm filaments in hamster and human fibroblasts, *Cell* **16**:675–685.

Singer, I. I., and Paradiso, P. R., 1981, A transmembrane relationship between fibronectin and vinculin (130 kd protein): Serum modulation in normal and transformed hamster fibroblasts, *Cell* **24**:481–492.

Singer, I. I., Kawka, D. W., Kazazis, D. M., and Clark, R. A. F., 1984, In vivo co-distribution of fibronectin and actin fibers in granulation tissue: Immunofluorescence and electron microscope studies of the fibronexus at the myofibroblast surface, *J. Cell Biol.* **98**:2091–2106.

Sixma, J. J., 1978, Platelet coagulant activities, *Thromb. Haemost.* **40**:163–167.

Smith, L. T., Holbrook, K. A., Sadai, L. Y., and Burgeson, R. E., 1987, The ontogeny of hemidesmosomes, anchoring fibrils and type VII collagen in human fetal skin, *Clin. Res.* **35**:252A.

Snyderman, R., Altman, L., Hausman, M. S., and Mergenhagen, S. E., 1972, Human mononuclear leukocyte chemotaxis: A quantitative assay for humoral and cellular chemotactic factors, *J. Immunol.* **108**:857–860.

Sporn, M. B., and Roberts, A. B., 1986, Peptide growth factors and inflammation, tissue repair, and cancer, *J. Clin. Invest.* **78**:329–332.

Sporn, M. B., Roberts, A. B., Shull, J. H., Smith, J. M., Ward, J. M., and Sodek, J., 1983, Polypeptide transforming growth factor isolated from bovine sources and used for wound healing *in vitro*, *Science* **219**:1329–1331.

Sporn, M. B., Roberts, A. B., Wakefield, L. M., and Assoian, R. K., 1986, Transforming growth factor-B: Biological function and chemical structure, *Science* **233**:532–534.

Stanley, J. R., Alvarez, O. M., Bere, E. W., Jr., Eaglstein, W. H., and Katz, S. I., 1981, Detection of basement membrane zone antigens during epidermal wound healing in pigs, *J. Invest. Dermatol.* **77**:240–243.

Stecher, V. J., and Sorkin, E., 1972, The chemotactic activity of fibrin lysis products, *Int. Arch. Allergy Appl. Immunol.* **43**:879–886.

Stiles, C. D., Capone, G., Scher, C. D., Antoniades, H. N., Van Wyk, J. J., and Pledger, W. J., 1979, Dual control of cell growth by somatomedins and platelet-derived growth factor, *Proc. Natl. Acad. Sci. USA* **76**:1279–1283.

Stimler, N. P., Bach, M. K., Bloor, C. M., and Hugli, T. E., 1982, Release of leukotrienes from guinea pig lung stimulated by C5a des arg anaphylatoxin, *J. Immunol.* **128**:2247–2257.

Sugrue, S. P., and Hay, E. D., 1981, Response of basal epithelial cell surface and cytoskeleton to solubilized extracellular matrix molecules, *J. Cell Biol.* **91**:45–54.

Timpl, R., Wiedemann, H., van Delden, V., Furthmayr, H., and Kuhn, K., 1981, A network model for the organization of type IV collagen molecules in basement membranes, *Eur. J. Biochem.* **120**:203–211.

Tomasek, J. J., and Hay, E. D., 1984, Analysis of the role of microfilaments and microtubules in acquisition of bipolarity and elongation of Rhoblasts in migrated collagen gels, *J. Cell Biol.* **99**:536–549.

Tomida, M., Koyama, H., and Ono, T., 1974, Hyaluronic acid synthetase in cultured mammalian cells producing hyaluronic acid. Oscillatory change during the growth phase and suppression by 5-bromodeoxyuridine, *Biochim. Biophys. Acta* **338**:352–363.

Tomida, M., Koyama, H., and Omo, T., 1975, Induction of hyaluronic acid synthetase activity in rat fibroblasts by medium change of confluent cultures, *J. Cell. Physiol.* **86**:121–130.

Toole, B. P., and Gross, J., 1971, The extracellular matrix of the regenerating newt limb: Synthesis and removal of hyaluronate prior to differentiation, *Dev. Biol.* **25**:57–77.

Toole, B. P., and Trelstad, R. L., 1971, Hyaluronate production and removal during corneal development in the chick, *Dev. Biol.* **26**:28–35.

Toole, B. P., 1972, Hyaluronate turnover during chondrogenesis in the developing chick limb and axial skeleton, *Dev. Biol.* **29**:321–329.

Toole, B. P., 1981, Glycosaminoglycans in morphogenesis, in: *Cell Biology of Extracellular Matrix* (E. B. Hay, ed.), pp. 259–294, Plenum, New York.

Trelstad, R. L., and Silver, F. H., 1981, Matrix assembly, in: *Cell Biology of Extracellular Matrix* (E. B. Hay, ed.), pp. 179–215, Plenum, New York.

Trelstad, R. L., Hayaski, K., and Toole, B. P., 1974, Epithelial collagen and glycosaminoglycans in the embryonic cornea. Macromolecular order and morphogenesis in the basement membranes, *J. Cell Biol.* **62**:815–830.

Tsukamoto, Y., Helsel, W. E., and Wahl, S. M., 1981, Macrophage production of fibronectin, a chemoattractant for fibroblasts, *J. Immunol.* **127**:673–678.

Turk, J. L., Heather, C. J., and Diengdoh, J. V., 1976, A histochemical analysis of mononuclear cell infiltrates of the skin with particular reference to delayed hypersensitivity in the guinea pig, *Int. Arch. Allergy Appl. Immunol.* **29**:278–289.

Underhill, C. B., and Keller, J. M., 1976, Density-dependent changes in the amount of sulfated glycosaminoglycans associated with mouse 3T3 cells, *J. Cell. Physiol.* **89**:53–63.

Unemori, E. N., and Werb, Z., 1986, Reorganization of polymerized actin: A possible trigger for induction of procollagenase in fibroblasts cultured in and on collagen gels, *J. Cell Biol.* **103**:1021–1031.

Vaheri, A., Kurkinen, M., Lehto, V. P., Linder, E., and Timpl, R., 1978, Codistribution of pericellular matrix proteins in cultured fibroblasts and loss in transformation: fibronectin and procollagen, *Proc. Natl. Acad. Sci. USA* **75**:4944–4948.

van Furth, R., 1985, Cellular biology of pulmonary macrophages, *Int. Arch. Allergy Appl. Immunol.* **76**(Suppl. 1):21–27.

Vartio, T., Seppa, H., and Vaheri, A., 1981, Susceptibility of soluble and matrix fibronectins to degradation by tissue proteinases, mast cell chymase and cathepsin G, *J. Biol. Chem.* **256**:471–477.

Viljanto, J., Penttinen, R., and Raekallio, J., 1981, Fibronectin in early phases of wound healing in children, *Acta Chir. Scand.* **147**:7–13.

Wahl, L. M., Olsen, C. E., Sandberg, A. L., and Mergenhagen, S. E., 1977, Prostaglandin regulation of macrophage collagenase production, *Proc. Natl. Acad. Sci. USA* **74**:4955–4958.

Wall, R. T., Harker, L. A., and Striker, G. E., 1978, Human endothelial cell migration. Stimulated by a released platelet factor, *Lab. Invest.* **39**:523–529.

Weksler, B. B., Marcus, A. J., and Jaffee, E. A., 1977, Synthesis of prostaglandin I_2 (prostacyclin) by cultured human and bovine endothelial cells, *Proc. Natl. Acad. Sci. USA* **74**:3922–3926.

Werb, A., and Gordon, S., 1975a, Secretion of a specific collagenase by stimulated macrophages, *J. Exp. Med.* **142**:346–360.

Werb, A., and Gordon, S., 1975b, Elastase secretion by stimulated macrophages, *J. Exp. Med.* **142**:361–377.

Winter, G. D., 1962, Formation of the scab and the rate of epithelialization of superficial wounds in the skin of the young domestic pig, *Nature (Lond.)* **193**:293–294.

Winter, G. D., 1972, Epidermal regeneration studied in the domestic pig, in: *Epidermal Wound Healing* (H. I. Maibach and D. T. Rovee, eds.), pp. 71–112, Year Book Medical, Chicago.

Wolf, J. E., and Harrison, R. G., 1973, Demonstration and characterization of an epidermal angiogenic factor, *J. Invest. Dermatol.* **61**:130–141.

Wood, G. C., 1960, The formation of fibrils from collagen solutions. Effect of chondroitin sulfate and other naturally occurring polyanions on the rate of formation, *Biochem. J.* **75**:605–612.

Wrann, M., Fox, C., and Ross, R., 1980, Modulation of epidermal growth factor receptors on 3T3 cells by platelet-derived growth factor, *Science* **210**:1363–1365.

Yamada, K., and Olden, K., 1978, Fibronectins—Adhesive glycoproteins of cell surface and blood, *Nature (Lond.)* **275**:179–184.

Zauberman, H., Michaelson, I. C., Bergmann, F., and Maurice, D. M., 1969, Stimulation of neovascularization of the cornea by biogenic amines, *Exp. Eye Res.* **8**:77–83.

Zetter, B. R., Chen, L. B., and Buchanan, J., 1976, Effects of protease treatment on growth, morphology, adhesion, and cell surface proteins of secondary chick embryo fibroblasts, *Cell* **7**:407–412.

Chapter 2

Platelets and Response to Injury

ROBERT A. TERKELTAUB and MARK H. GINSBERG

1. Introduction

Our understanding of the participatory role of platelets in biologic processes other than hemostasis and coagulation is rapidly evolving. Platelets are implicated in the maintenance of capillary integrity and wound healing. Platelets may also contribute to the acceleration of atherogenesis, as the activation of these cells promotes vascular injury and platelets promote cholesterol accumulation within smooth muscle cells and macrophages. This chapter addresses the structure, function, and modes of activation of platelets as they relate to the potential role of these cells in certain immunologically mediated and inflammatory diseases in which alterations of blood vessel function and integrity occur.

2. Morphology and Composition of Platelets as They Relate to Inflammatory Functions

Normal platelets are anucleate discoid fragments approximately 2 μm in diameter. They are derived from marrow megakaryocytes as fragments budding from the peripheral cytoplasm as reviewed in greater scope elsewhere (Pennington, 1981).

The cell contains at least three types of storage organelles:

1. The α-granule is a storage site of several platelet-specific proteins and adhesive glycoproteins (Kaplan, 1981).
2. The dense body, which is less numerous than the α-granule, is the main storage site for biogenic amines. The major biogenic amine in human platelets is serotonin, and virtually the entire blood content of serotonin is borne in platelet-dense bodies. Adenine nucleotides, calcium, and pyrophosphate are also stored in the dense bodies (da Prada et al., 1981).

ROBERT A. TERKELTAUB • Veterans Administration Medical Center-University of California San Diego, San Diego, California 92161. MARK H. GINSBERG • Department of Immunology, Scripps Clinic and Research Foundation, La Jolla, California 92037.

3. Lysosomes containing several neutral and acid hydrolases are also present (Gordon, 1975).

The normal platelet life-span is 7–10 days, with circulating cells being removed either by the reticuloendothelial system when senescent or by incorporation into hemostatic plugs. The cells have little or no ability to synthesize proteins.

The main function of platelets is to initiate hemostasis by forming and helping consolidate a cellular plug at sites of vascular injury (Born, 1980). Platelets adhere to exposed subendothelial collagen in blood vessels and, at these sites, stimulated, aggregated platelets release mediators that promote further aggregation and vasoconstruction to arrest hemorrhage; the platelet reaction is reviewed in detail by Skaer (1981). Platelets are thus recognized as specialized for adhesion, aggregation, and secretion (de Clerck et al., 1984).

Platelets also possess receptors for IgG Fc, as well as certain prostaglandins (Schafer et al., 1979) and complement proteins (Meuer et al., 1981). They interact directly with a number of particulate inflammatory agents, including microorganisms, and platelets may modulate clearance of some particles from the circulation (Gordon, 1975; Zucker-Franklin, 1981). Platelets also interact with other inflammatory cells; for example, they enhance monocyte adherence to certain surfaces (Musson and Henson, 1979). Therefore, platelets are well suited to participate in inflammatory vascular processes; several lines of evidence indicate that platelets participate in inflammation: (1) they contain and release, upon stimulation, mediators of inflammation; (2) they are stimulated by phlogistic agents, (3) they participate in the pathogenesis of animal models of inflammatory disease; and (4) there is evidence suggesting platelet localization and activation at sites of tissue injury in some human inflammatory diseases.

3. The Platelet as a Source of Mediators in Inflammation and Wound Repair

The inflammatory process that occurs in response to tissue injury is essential to healing. Complex signals mediated by humoral inflammatory mediator systems (Chapter 3) and inflammatory cells (Chapter 8) appear to direct orderly fibroplasia and new collagen synthesis, which begin within 24 hr of wounding and also to direct the angiogenesis, which follows during the first 48–72 hr. Platelets and the coagulation system respond directly to perturbations of vascular integrity and thus are held to be among the earliest factors in the production of inflammation in the wound-repair process. Moreover, in studies using a rabbit corneal system, the implantation of thrombin-stimulated antologous platelets (but not unactivated platelets) was sufficient to induce angiogenesis, fibroplasia, and new collagen synthesis. In addition, fibrin implantation elicited a cellular exudate from limbal vessels followed by angiogenesis and corneal opacification (Knighton et al., 1982).

Platelet production and modulation of inflammatory responses and wound healing result in a large part from the release of mediators of inflammation, which occurs in association with platelet activation and aggregation, similar in many respects to the release of mediators from neutrophils. The platelet mediators may be newly synthesized, as in the case of metabolites of arachidonic acid (Goetzl and Gorman, 1978; Vargaftig et al., 1981; Weksler and Goldstein, 1980), or preformed and concentrated in storage organelles. The materials released from stimulated platelets may contribute to the inflammatory process by modulating vascular tone and permeability, attracting more inflammatory cells, inducing tissue damage, and initiating repair by mitogenic effects on connective tissues. Many of the platelet mediators capable of these functions are listed in Table I. Some of the mediators, such as neutral proteinases in granules (Chesney et al., 1974; Henson et al., 1976; Legrand et al., 1977), are also present in other inflammatory cells. By contrast, the platelet has a uniquely well-developed capacity to generate vasoactive thromboxanes and 12-lipoxygenase products (Goetzl, 1981; Maclouf et al., 1982). Furthermore, the platelet is the major depot in the circulation of serotonin (da Prada et al., 1981; de Clerck et al., 1984), a potent vasoconstrictor that interacts with thromboxane A_2 to increase vascular permeability and that promotes fibroblast collagen synthesis. The potential role of serotonin in the human fibrotic disease, progressive systemic sclerosis, is discussed in Section 7.1.1.

Platelet α-granules contain three large adhesive glycoproteins (fibrinogen, von Willebrand factor, fibronectin), which are also found in plasma (Wencel-Drake et al., 1984, 1985). In addition, α-granules contain as their fourth adhesive protein, thrombospondin, a 450,000 M_r glycoprotein composed of three subunits of similar size. Many functions have been attributed to thrombospondin, including enhancement of aggregation of stimulated platelets (Leung, 1984), binding of fibrinogen and fibronectin (Leung and Nachman, 1982; Lahav et al., 1982), calcium-dependent binding to plasminogen and inhibition of plasmin generation in vitro (Silverstein et al., 1984). Thrombospondin is also synthesized by monocytes, fibroblasts, and endothelial cells in vitro (Jaffe et al., 1985) and is present at only very low concentrations in plasma. When platelets are stimulated sufficiently to extrude their α-granules, the adhesive proteins as well as the other granule constituents are released into the blood or the local tissue site.

The role of platelets and their constituents in hemostasis and in accelerating the coagulation system is reviewed by George et al. (1984). Importantly, the four large adhesive glycoproteins released from α-granules play a critical role in hemostasis via their ability to form contact interactions with platelet membrane proteins and vessel wall proteins and with each other. Platelet constituents are believed to modulate provisional matrix formation in areas of vascular damage in a variety of ways, including direction of cell attachment (e.g., endothelial cell spreading), facilitation of fibroblast growth competence by fibronectin (Bitterman et al., 1983), release of free sulfated glycosaminoglycans (which may regulate smooth muscle cell growth and movement) from cell-surface proteoglycans by platelet heparitinase (Castellot et al., 1982), and regulation of

smooth muscle replication and matrix deposition of smooth muscle cell-derived thrombospondin by platelet-derived growth factor (PDGF) (Majack et al.,
1985). In addition to thrombospondin, the platelet α-granule is the major
source of four other substances important in wound repair: (1) PDGF (Deuel
and Huang, 1984), a connective tissue mitogen (see Chapter 9, Section 1); (2)

Table I. Platelet-Derived Mediators of Inflammation

Class	Mediator	Actions
I: Cyclo-oxygenase dependent[a–c]	Thromboxane A_2	Vasoconstrictor, proaggregant, increases neutrophil adherence
	Thromboxane B_2	More stable thromboxane A_2 derivative
	Prostaglandins D_2, E_2, F_2	Vasoactive, modulates hemostasis and leukocyte function
	HHT	Chemotactic
II: Lipoxygenase dependent[d,e]	12-HPETE	Vasoconstrictor, cyclooxygenase
	LTB_4 synthesis	Inhibitor, stimulates leukocyte
	12-HETE	Chemotactic
III: Dense-body contents[f]	Serotonin	Vasoconstrictor, increases vascular permeability, fibrogenic
IV: α-Granule contents	Thrombospondin[g]	Endogenous platelet lectin, inhibits fibrinolysis, binds to matrix constituents
	Growth Factors: e.g. Platelet-derived growth factor (PDGF)[h]	Connective tissue mitogen, cell-transforming factor, chemotactic
	Platelet factor 4 (PF4)[i]	Proaggregant, chemotactic, inhibits neutral proteases, induces basophil histamine release
V: Granule contents	Cationic permeability factor release, chemotactic[j]	Stimulates mast cell histamine
	Serum-activating enzymes[k]	Generate C5a in serum
	Cathepsins A,C,D,E	Acid proteinases
	Elastase[l]	Neutral proteinase
	Collagenase[m]	Neutral proteinase
	α_1-Antitrypsin, α_2-macroglobin[n]	Proteinase inhibitors
	α_2-Antiplasmin	Primary plasmin inhibitor

[a]Vargaftig et al. (1981). [e]Maclouf et al. (1982). [i]Hiti-Harper et al. (1978). [m]Chesney et al. (1974).
[b]Weksler and Goldstein (1980). [f]daPrada et al. (1981). [j]Nachman et al. (1972). [n]Nachman and Harpel (1976).
[c]Goetzl and Gorman (1978). [g]Leung (1984). [k]Weksler and Coupal (1973).
[d]Goetzl (1981). [h]Deuel and Huang (1984). [l]Henson et al. (1976).

the transforming growth factor α family including epidermal growth factor (see Chapter 9, Section 2); (3) transforming growth factor β (see Chapter 9, Section 4); and (4) platelet factor 4, a protein that neutralizes heparin *in vitro* (Ginsberg *et al.*, 1980).

4. Platelet-Adhesive Mechanisms and Their Relationship to Endothelium

The capacity of circulating platelets to adhere to each other and to exposed tissue surfaces following vessel injury is crucial to their hemostatic function. When inappropriate platelet-adhesive aggregation occurs within the vasculature, the resulting vessel occlusion leads to tissue damage. Adhesive interactions are triggered by the activation of platelets by insoluble components of the subendothelial matrix, such as collagen or microfibrils (Fauvel *et al.*, 1984) as well as fluid-phase mediators generated locally such as thrombin, ADP, and certain arachidonate metabolites. This section briefly reviews some of the recent progress in our understanding of how platelets express these adhesive functions.

Current interest has focused on four large adhesive glycoproteins, fibrinogen, fibronectin, von Willebrand factor, and thrombospondin, which have the extracellular "glue" binding platelets both to other platelets and the constituents of the vessel wall. We recently extensively reviewed (Plow *et al.*, 1986*a*, Ginsberg *et al.*, 1985*b*) the means by which these glycoproteins function in platelet-adhesive reactions in depth and briefly summarize that information here. The function of fibrinogen and von Willebrand factor in hemostasis seems secure, since patients deficient in these proteins have bleeding disorders. By contrast, the evidence for the role of fibronectin in platelet function come primarily from *in vitro* studies (Houdijk *et al.*, 1985), as does the evidence for role of thrombospondin (Leung, 1984). Each of these proteins is a large (340,000-M_r) glycoprotein, which has intramolecular symmetry—that is, consisting of repeating subunits. The primary structure of fibrinogen has been known for some time (Doolittle, 1984), and recent studies (Kornblihtt *et al.*, 1985; Titani *et al.*, 1986; Lawler and Hynes, 1986) established the predicted primary amino acid sequence of fibronectin from fibroblasts as well as thrombospondin and von Willebrand factor from endothelial cells. Although these proteins share the above-noted gross structural and functional features, direct comparison of their primary sequences does not demonstrate strong evidence for a close evolutionary relationship. Fibronectin, fibrinogen, and von Willebrand factor are primarily plasma proteins; however, there are also intraplatelet pools (reviewed by Plow *et al.*, 1986*a*). The interactions of fibrinogen, fibronectin, and von Willebrand factor with intraplatelet pools have now been definitively localized to the platelet α-granule (Wencel-Drake *et al.*, 1985). Platelet von Willebrand factor is enriched in higher-molecular-weight multimers (Lopez-Fernandez *et al.*, 1982) and in rat platelet fibronectin appears to be enriched in the extra domain containing the variety typical of cellular fibronectin (Paul *et al.*, 1986). Circulating thrombospondin is primarily in platelet α-

granules (Wencel-Drake et al., 1985) but is also a biosynthetic product of endothelial cells (McPherson et al., 1981; Jaffe et al., 1983), smooth muscle cells,
and monocytes (Jaffe et al., 1985) in vitro. There have been no reported structural differences between platelet and endothelial cell thrombospondin. In
addition, thrombospondin, fibronectin, and von Willebrand factor are all incorporated into the endothelial cell matrix (Jaffe et al., 1983; Wagner et al., 1982).

In order to function in platelet adhesive responses, these proteins must
interact with the cell surface. One mechanism by which these proteins appear
on the cell surface is by externalization of their α-granule pools (Tollefsen and
Majerus, 1975; Courtois et al., 1986; Ginsberg et al., 1980; George and Onofre,
1982; Phillips et al., 1980). This process appears to be rapid and in part due to
direct expression of these proteins on the cell surface (Ginsberg et al., 1981;
Courtois et al., 1986) as well as by rebinding of released material. These proteins also interact with the surface of platelets, with the exception of thrombospondin (Wolff et al., 1986); this interaction appears to require an activation
event. These interactions, what is known of the receptors mediating the interactions, and the relationship of these receptors to the endothelial cell surface
forms the remainder of this discussion.

Fibrinogen, fibronectin, and von Willebrand factor bind to thrombin-acti-
vated platelets in saturable fashion consistent with a discrete receptor site
(Bennett and Vilaire, 1979; Marguerie et al., 1979; Plow and Ginsberg, 1981;
Fujimoto et al., 1982). The interactions of fibrinogen, fibronectin, and von
Willebrand factor with stimulated platelets share the requirement for divalent
cations and ADP dependence (reviewed by Plow et al., 1986a). In addition,
there is a reduction in these protein interactions with Glansmann's thrombasthenic platelets (Bennett and Vilaire, 1979; Ginsberg et al., 1983; Ruggeri et
al., 1982). Such platelets are selectively deficient in membrane glycoproteins
GPIIb/IIIa (Nurden and Caen, 1974). Moreover, monoclonal antibodies reactive
with GPIIb–IIIa that inhibit fibrinogen binding also inhibit the binding of fibronectin and von Willebrand factor (Plow et al., 1985a). All three of these adhesive proteins contain the Arg-Gly-Asp (RGD) sequence (Doolittle, 1984;
Pierschbacher et al., 1983; Sadler et al., 1986) originally identified by Pierschbacher and Ruoslahti (1984) as a potential common cell-adhesion signal. Peptides containing the RGD inhibit the binding of fibronectin, fibronectin, and
von Willebrand factor to activated platelets (Ginsberg et al., 1985a; Plow et al.,
1985b; Gartner and Bennett, 1985; Haverstick et al., 1985). Affinity chromatography of whole platelet extracts on immobilized RGD peptide matrix
results in the purification of GPIIb–IIIa (Pytela et al., 1986), as does affinity
chromatography on the 120,000-M_r fragment of Fibronectin (Gardner and
Hynes, 1985). Finally, purified GPIIb–IIIa incorporated into liposomes interacts with fibrinigen, fibronectin, and von Willebrand factor (Baldassare et
al., 1985; Parise and Phillips, 1985; Pytela et al., 1986). Thus, it appears quite
likely that platelet membrane glycoprotein IIb–IIIa is a constituent of a common membrane receptor for fibronectin, fibrinogen, and von Willebrand factor.
It is attractive to hypothesize that the shared RGD sequence among the otherwise structurally dissimilar proteins forms the common site recognized by
GPIIb–IIIa.

Peptides derived from the γ-chain of fibrinogen also inhibit the binding of fibrinogen (Kloczewiak et al., 1982) to platelets. They also inhibit the binding of fibronectin and von Willebrand factor (Plow et al., 1984). Surprisingly, fibronectin and von Willebrand factor contain no obvious homology to the γ-chain sequence of fibrinogen. Recent data have provided an explanation for this apparent paradox. Specifically, we found that γ-chain peptides could inhibit the binding of an RGD peptide to platelets with parameters consistent with those of competitive antagonism (Lam et al., 1987). Second, γ-chain peptides could elute GPIIb–IIIa bound to insolubilized RGD peptides, and conversely the RGD peptides can elute GPIIb–IIIa from insolubilized γ-chain peptides (Lam et al., 1987). These data indicate that the two peptide sets either bind to the same site or bind in a mutually exclusive manner to a GPIIb–IIIa-containing receptor. These findings may also explain the capacity of RGD peptides to inhibit binding to platelets of fibrinogen deficient in the RGD sequence of the α-chain (Plow et al., 1987).

The RGD sequence has been implicated in a variety of cell-adhesion events, and GPIIb–IIIa bears striking gross structurally relationship to a variety of cell-adhesion receptors (Pytela et al., 1986). Epitopes shared with platelet membrane GPIIb–IIIa have been found on a wide variety of cell types (Fitzgerald et al., 1985; Charo et al., 1986; Plow et al., 1986b; Burns et al., 1986; Thiagarajan et al., 1985) including endothelial cells. These related proteins are biosynthetic products of these cells (Thiagarajan et al., 1985; Fitzgerald et al., 1985; Charo et al., 1986; Plow et al., 1986b) and have similar subunit structure to GPIIb–IIIa. The antigenic, structural, and functional relationships have led to the proposal that there is a family of GPIIb–IIIa-related proteins in a variety of cells termed *cytoadhesins* (Plow et al., 1986b). Moreover, recent studies have directly demonstrated that GPIIIa is similar or identical to the β-subunit of another cytoadhesin, the vitronectin receptor. Although GPIIb is distinct from the α-subunit of the vitronectin receptor, it appears to be homologous to this protein and to the α-subunits of the leukocyte-adhesion receptors, LFA-1 and MAC-1 (Ginsberg et al., 1987; Charo et al., 1986). The GPIIb–IIIa-related heterodimers appear to share a common β-subunit and distinct but homologous α-subunits. The cytoadhesins appear to differ in ligand recognition specificity (Pytela et al., 1986); thus, it is tempting to speculate that ligand specificity is regulated by the α-subunit. The cytoadhesins also resemble the family of leukocyte-adhesion molecules (Sanchez-Madrid et al., 1983) as well as the very late lymphocyte activation antigen family beautifully described by Hemler et al. (1987) in having distinct α- and common β-subunits.

Note should be made of another well-documented adhesion receptor on human platelets, GPIb. Several recent reviews on the subject of the relationship of von Willebrand factor to BPIb appeared (Nurden et al., 1986; Ruggeri and Zimmerman, 1985; Ginsberg and Jaques, 1983). To summarize this important area of research, the adhesion of platelets at high shear rates is dependent on the presence of von Willebrand factor and GPIb on the platelet surface. GPIb has a nominal molecular weight of 170,000 in the unreduced state, consisting of disulfide-linked 143,000- and 22,000-M_r subunits. In addition, GPIb appears to be noncovalently associated with a 17,000-M_r GPIX on the external face of the plasma membrane and is associated with actin filaments and unactivated platelets via association with actin-binding proteins (Fox, 1985; Okita *et al.*, 1985).

The role of GPIb in von Willebrand factor-dependent adhesion and ristocetin-induced agglutination appears to be unequivocal based on the deficit in these reactions in platelets genetically or chemically deficient in GPIb, inhibition of the reactions by certain monoclonal antibodies against GPIb, and *in vitro* binding studies. Fujimura*et al.* (1986) recently identified an approximately 50,000-M_r domain of von Willebrand factor that interacts with GPIb. Similarly, a 38,000-M_r fragment of GPIb has been identified as a potential von Willebrand factor interaction site on the GPIb molecule (Handa *et al.*, 1986). Recently, a GPIb-related antigen was detected on endothelial cells. Perhaps the GPIb-like membrane protein plays a role in the adhesive reactions of endothelial cells as well.

5. Potential Activators of Platelets in Inflammatory Diseases

Platelets can clearly be activated by traditional hemostatic activators such as thrombin, ADP, arachidonate derivatives, and exposed subendothelial collagen at sites of vascular injury (see Chapter 3). A number of other agents stimulate platelets, and several of these materials may be involved in the initiation or propagation of inflammatory responses. Examples of such are agents listed in Table II. Activation of platelets may also be affected by several different types of immunologic reactions, as reviewed in greater scope elsewhere (Henson and Ginsberg, 1981). The presence or excessive expression of these factors at a site of traumatic injury may induce excessive platelet activation leading to either thrombosis or additional injury, or both.

Table II. Potential Activators of Platelets in Inflammatory Diseases

Types of activation	Activator
Hemostatic activation	Thrombin
Collagen	
ADP	
Prostaglandins, thromboxanes	
Immunologic activation	Platelet-activating factor (PAF)
Immune aggregates	
Antibodies to certain drugs (e.g., quinidine)	
Antiplatelet antibodies	
Nonimmunologic activation	Monosodium urate crystals
Microorganisms	
Double-stranded DNA	
Enhancers of activation	Complement
Single-stranded DNA	
Certain bacterial lipopolysaccharides	

5.1. Platelet-Activating Factor

Platelet-activating factor (PAF) is a well-characterized phospholipid mediator released from stimulated human mast cells, neutrophils, and macrophages.
Its biology is reviewed elsewhere in greater depth (O'Flaherty et al., 1983;
Vargaftig et al., 1981). PAF aggregates platelets at subnanomolar concentrations
and stimulates other cell types, including neutrophils. Injection of PAF into
animals induces thrombocytopenia, leukopenia, hypotension, and platelet-dependent bronchoconstriction.

5.2. Antibody-Mediated Platelet Activation

Immunoglobulin G (IgG)-containing immune complexes, aggregated γ-
globulin, and IgG-coated surfaces stimulate human platelets (Henson and
Ginsberg, 1981). Human platelets possess a receptor for Fc portion of IgG
(Pfueller et al., 1977) that has been suggested to be identical to membrane
glycoprotein IIIa by one group (Steiner and Luscher, 1986). A 40,000-M_r single-
chain platelet membrane protein, apparently identical to p40, a low-affinity
receptor on U937 cells for monomeric IgG, with the capacity to bind IgG aggregates or IgG-coated particles, has also been described, and monoclonal antibodies to p40 specifically block platelet aggregation induced by heat-aggregated IgG (Rosenfeld et al., 1985). Certain drug-induced thrombocytopenias are
probably mediated by immune-complex-mediated platelet sequestration and
lysis. Quinidine-induced purpura is the best studied of these (Christie et al.,
1985; Garty et al., 1985; Lerner et al. , 1985; Shulman, 1978), and both immunologically specific and nonspecific adsorption of drug–antibody complexes to
the platelet surface appear to be imporatnt in its pathogenesis. Such binding is
mediated by the platelet Fc receptor and by Fab domain-mediated binding.
Quinidine itself binds weakly to platelets when drug-dependent antibody is
absent.

Antibodies to antigens on the platelet surface may arise in autoimmune
states, such as systemic lupus erythematosus (SLE) or idiopathic thrombocytopenic purpura (ITP), or as a result of isoimmunization after transfusion
or pregnancy. In addition, antilymphocyte and antithymocyte globulins may
also possess antiplatelet activity (Csako et al., 1982). Antiplatelet antibodies
may either stimulate platelets or inhibit platelet function, and thrombocytopenia may be produced via increased reticuloendothelial clearance (Aster and
Jandl, 1964). In the case of alloantibodies, anti-Pla1 has been clearly shown to
react with a major cell-surface glycoprotein (Kunicki and Aster, 1979) and
antilymphocyte globulins in part with β_2-microglobulin on the cell surface
(Csako et al., 1982). In the case of autoantibodies, studies are just beginning to
characterize their antigens. The major platelet membrane glycoproteins GP IIb
and IIIa may be the major antigen in some patients with chronic ITP (Woods et
al., 1984; Beardsley et al., 1984). The mechanisms of antibody-mediated complement activation on the platelet surface and of platelet sequestration and

lysis on these disorders have been reviewed in greater depth previously (Henson and Ginsberg, 1981).

5.3. Collagen and Other Surfaces as Platelet Activators

Intact vascular endothelium normally prevents platelet adherence to the vessel wall. Upon damage, or removal of vessel-surface endothelium, platelets rapidly adhere to the exposed subendothelial surface and spread (reviewed by Packham and Mustard, 1986). Platelets adhere to collagen, microfibrils, and the basement membrane, but collagen appears to be the surface most able to activate platelets and promote the release of granule contents. von Willebrand factor may influence platelet–subendothelial interactions at high shear rates. Platelets appear most reactive to type I collagen from tendons. Type III collagen found in the media of muscular arteries also causes platelet aggregation, whereas type IV basement membrane collagen is a poor stimulator of the release reaction.

Platelets and monosodium urate crystals, the causative agent of gout, have the potential to interact at many intravascular and extravascular sites. The study of platelet–crystal interaction has proved useful as a model system for platelet activation by surfaces. Monosodium urate crystals have been shown to induce a selective secretion of dense-body constituents followed by platelet lysis in vitro (Ginsberg et al., 1977). More recent work suggests that four platelet-membrane glycoproteins (including GPIIb and IIIa) mediate platelet stimulation by urate crystals, as removal of these proteins by chymotryptic digestion, or incubation of platelets with F(ab')2 fragments of an antibody directed against these proteins specifically suppresses platelet secretory responses to urate crystals (Jaques and Ginsberg, 1982).

5.4. Effects of Complement, DNA, and LPS on Platelet Activation

Platelets interact with complement in a variety of ways (reviewed by Wiedmer et al., 1986). First, complement-dependent sequelae to the binding of antiplatelet antibodies occur and may modulate platelet lysis (reviewed by Henson and Ginsberg, 1981). Second, platelets may participate in the activation of complement via C5 cleavage by platelet-bound thrombin (Polley and Nachman, 1981). Third, platelets are directly activated by either classical or alternative pathway complement activation in platelet-rich plasma. Platelet membrane assembly of C5b-9 results in increased binding of coagulation factors Va and Xa to the membrane and a dramatic increase in platelet prothrombinase activity. Thrombin-mediated platelet activation and conversion of arachidonate to thromboxanes are also enhanced in the presence of certain complement proteins. Thus, it is believed that complement proteins may modulate enhanced procoagulant activity in some diseases associated with complement activation (e.g., SLE). Interestingly, prolonged bleeding times and impaired *in vitro* platelet aggregation are observed in some individuals genetically deficient in one of the proteins necessary for C5b-9 formation.

Free DNA has been described in serum and plasma in several conditions associated with tissue injury, including vasculitides and SLE. Single- and double-stranded (native) DNA both bind to platelets. Native DNA induces *in vitro* release of serotonin from platelets (Dorsch and Killmayer, 1983; Fiedel *et al.*, 1979). Single-stranded DNA, but not native DNA, enhances the platelet release reaction induced by heat-aggregated IgG (Dorsch and Killmayer, 1983).

The bacterial lipopolysaccharide (LPS) component of gram-negative bacteria may be responsible for a number of *in vitro* effects, including pryogenicity, toxicity, and lethality (Mathison and Ulevitch, 1983). LPS may also have several important immunologic actions, in part mediated by effects in Fc receptor-bearing cells such as macrophages and B cells (Chiller *et al.*, 1973). The lipid A region of LPS is responsible for many of these effects. Isolated lipid A and lipid A-rich LPS of certain strains have been found to enhance immune aggregate-induced platelet serotonin release approximately 50-fold and to enhance secretion of other platelet constituents as well (Ginsberg and Henson, 1978).

6. Platelets in Animal Models of Inflammatory Diseases and Wound Healing

Platelets are equipped with numerous mediators of inflammation and can be activated by a variety of means in inflammatory conditions. Numerous studies of animal models of human disease have thus assessed the effect of platelet depletion on tissue injury and have measured platelet deposition at sites of inflammatory tissue damage. Platelet deposition at sites of tissue injury has been detected quantitatively by the accumulation of ^{51}Cr-labeled platelets or by ultrastructural pathology in such animal models as sponge implantation (Bolam and Smith, 1977), reverse passive Arthus reaction in skin (Kravis and Henson, 1977), and IgE-mediated anaphylaxis (Pinckard, 1977). Protective effects of platelet depletion have been reported in models such as IgE anaphylaxis, the Shwartzman reaction, the Arthus reaction in the joint (Margarathen and McKay, 1971), and serum sickness nephritis (Kniker and Cochrane, 1968), where released platelet permeability factors may influence the deposition of immune complexes in blood vessel walls. In the case of the Arthus reaction and IgE-dependent skin reactions in the rabbit, platelet depletion does not prevent the lesions but may be associated with some lessening of the intensity of the reaction. This finding exemplifies the inherent redundancy of the inflammatory response. It should be pointed out that platelet deposition is without effect in various other animal models. It is thus important to study platelets in human disease directly, rather than with animal models, because of the known functional differences between human and nonprimate platelets.

7. Platelets in Human Disease and Wound Healing

7.1. Approaches to Document Platelet Localization and Activation in Inflammation and Wound Repair

Platelets are known to be the earliest circulating cell detected in areas of vascular injury; that is, platelets are sequestered rapidly in the microvasculature of burn wound tissue (Demling, 1985). This section reviews relevant approaches to, and knowledge of, the presence, activation, and potential roles of platelets in a variety of inflammatory diseases.

Light microscopic recognition of platelets in inflammatory lesions can be difficult. Ultrastructural techniques have demonstrated platelets in synovial fluids and platelet aggregation in glomerular capillaries (Duffy et al., 1970). More recently, the platelet-specific proteins platelet factor 4 and β-thromboglobulin (B-TG) have been demonstrated in rheumatoid synovial fluids (Ginsberg et al., 1978; Myers and Christine, 1982). There is suggestive evidence of platelet localization at sites of human immune injury, but newer investigation using immunolocalization techniques for platelet-specific antigens and ^{111}In-labeled platelets with external imaging (e.g., Henriksson et al., 1985) is anticipated in the future.

Measurement of platelet activation in human immunologic disease has dual significance. First, it implicates platelets in the disease. Second, it may provide a means of monitoring drug effects on platelet activation in a disease and an opportunity to elucidate the relationship between disease activity and platelet activation.

Approaches to date have included measurement of platelet turnover in patients with immunologic diseases. This test is inconvenient and does not measure activation per se, but rather the increased turnover that presumably accompanies platelet activation. Assays for detection of platelet activators in blood and tissue fluids of immunologic disease patients have been used as well (Ginsberg and O'Malley, 1977; Shapleigh et al., 1980). The presence of these activators also represents only an indirect indication of in vivo platelet activation. The availability of assays for detection of in vitro secretion of platelet-specific proteins (Kaplan and Owen, 1981) has provided a rapid and simple approach to measure the state of platelet activation in disease. Studies of several rheumatic diseases by these methods have provided evidence of platelet activation.

7.1.1. Platelets in Scleroderma and Raynaud's Phenomenon

Scleroderma is an inflammatory connective tissue disease characterized by fibrosis and degeneration of tissues in vasculature and tissues of the skin, musculoskeletal system, and a number of organs (Medsger, 1985). Tissue injury in this disease is believed to be initiated by ischemic and immunologic mechanisms; the excessive deposition of collagen at involved sites could be considered a form of exuberant tissue repair. Platelet interaction with small vessel subendothelium exposed by immune endothelial injury is a possible factor in the early pathogenesis of scleroderma. This process would be followed by release of platelet mediators, including PDGF and a distinct endothelial growth factor (King and Buchwald, 1984) and TGF-β (which could also be released by activated T lymphocytes (Chapter 9) in this disease). Smooth muscle cell migration and intimal proliferation with luminal narrowing and ultimate fibrosis would result. Serotonin is believed to be a modulator of episodic vasoconstriction (Raynaud's phenomenon) and systemic fibrogenesis in the disease (Seibold and Jageneau, 1984; Sternberg et al., 1980). Platelets of affected patients have a decreased content of serotonin compatible with enhanced release of this moiety (Zeller et al., 1983).

Other evidence of in vivo platelet participation in scleroderma includes the demonstration of elevated levels of circulating platelet aggregates and plasma concentrations of B-TG (Kahaleh et al., 1982), with reduction of these levels achieved in some patients treated with dipyridamole and aspirin. In vivo platelet adhesion to subendothelium was reported in a case study (Case Records of the Massachusetts General Hospital, 1978). Platelets from scleroderma patients also may have an enhanced ability to adhere to collagen in vitro (Kahaleh et al., 1985).

7.1.2. Platelets in Systemic Lupus Erythematosus and Glomerulonephritis

Defective platelet aggregation independent of therapy with aspirin or nonsteroidal anti-inflammatory agents is seen in a significant proportion of SLE patients (Dorsch and Meyerhoff, 1982; Weiss et al., 1980). Increased plasma levels of B-TG (Dorsch and Meyerhoff, 1980) and an acquired deficiency of platelet dense-body contents (storage pool deficiency) have been associated with this defect and suggest in vivo platelet activation. Potential platelet activators in SLE include immune complexes, antiplatelet antibodies, exposed subendothelial collagen (vasculitis), and thrombin, via activation of the clotting cascade (Hardin et al., 1978). Increased plasma levels of the free DNA are frequently observed in SLE. Single-stranded (ssDNA) and native DNA both bind to platelets, and both modulate platelet activation in vitro. Treatment of SLE platelet-rich plasma with deoxyribonuclease has been shown to restore defective aggregation to collagen in platelets of some SLE patients with an acquired storage pool deficiency, suggesting this abnormality to be possibly mediated by DNA (Dorsch and Meyerhoff, 1982).

Acute and chronic thrombocytopenias may be encountered in SLE. The course of chronic thrombocytopenia in SLE may be similar to that in chronic idopathic thrombocytopenic purpura (McMillan, 1981). In addition to antiplatelet antibodies, it has been suggested that antibodies to platelet-bound ssDNA may play a pathogenetic role in this condition (Dorsch, 1980).

7.1.3. Platelet Abnormalities in Rheumatoid Arthritis

Various studies have shown that sera and synovial fluids from rheumatoid arthritis patients can activate normal platelets (Zeller et al., 1983). Increased plasma concentrations of B-TG have been found in some rheumatoid arthritis patients (Myers *et al.*, 1980). The presence of increased amounts of platelet activating material in rheomatoid arthritis sera and synovial fluids may be of particular importance because of the frequent occurrence in rheumatoid arthritis of heightened platelet production and net thrombocytosis. The degree of thrombocytosis correlates directly with parameters of active disease and inversely with the hematocrit (Bennett, 1977). A relationship appears to exist between thrombocytosis and extraarticular manifestations of rheumatoid arthritis, particularly cutaneous vasculitis.

Degradation of articular cartilage is a consequence of synovial inflammation in rheumatoid arthritis. Proteolytic degradation of articular cartilage *in vitro* renders this tissue active as an adhesion site and aggregating factor for platelets (Zucker-Franklin and Rosenberg, 1977). The role of platelets in cartilage damage and repair remain to be elucidated in rheumatoid arthritis and other conditions.

8. Summary

Platelets have long been known to play an important role in thrombosis and hemostasis. The molecular mechanisms that mediate platelet–platelet aggregation and platelet–substratum adhesion are currently being delineated. In addition platelets are well equipped to function in inflammatory and wound-healing responses via release of numerous mediators that provoke increased vasculature permeability, leukocyte accumulation, fibroplasia, collagen synthesis, and angiogenesis.

References

Aster, R. H., and Jandl, J. H., 1964, Platelet sequestration in man. II. Immunological and clinical studies, *J. Clin. Invest.* **43:**856–869.

Baldassare, J. J., Kahn, R. A., Knipp, M. A., and Newman, P. J., 1985, Reconstruction of platelet proteins into phospholipid vesicles. Functional proteoliposomes, *J. Clin. Invest.* **75:**35–39.

Bennett, R. M., 1977, Hematological changes in rheumatoid disease, *Clin. Rheum. Dis.* **3:**433–465.

Bennett, J. S., and Vilaire, G., 1979, Exposure of platelet fibrinogen receptors by ADP and epinephrine, *J. Clin. Invest.* **64:**1393–1401.

Beardsley, D. S., Spiegel, J. E., Jacobs, M. M., Handin, R. I., and Lux, S. E. IV, 1984, Platelet membrane glycoprotein IIIa contains target antigens that bind anti-platelet antibodies in immune thrombocytopenas, *J. Clin. Invest.* **74:**1701–1707.

Bitterman, P. B., Rennard, S. I., Adelburg, S., and Crystal, R. G., 1983, Role of fibronectin as a growth factor for cells, *J. Cell Biol.* **97:**1925–1932.

Bolam, J. P., and Smith, M. J., 1977, Accumulation of platelets at acute inflammatory sites, *Br. J. Pharmacol.* **61:**158–159.

Born, G. U., 1980, Platelets in hemostasis and thrombosis, in: *Platelets: Cellular Response Mechanism and Their Biological Significance* (A. Rotman, ed.), pp. 3–17, Wiley (Interscience), New York.

Burns, G. F., Cosgrove, L., Triglia, T., Beall, J. A., Lopez, A. F., Werkmeister, J. A., Begley, C. G.,

Haddad, A. P., d'Apice, A. J. F., Vadas, M. A., and Cawley, J. C., 1986, The IIb–IIIa glycoprotein complex which mediates platelet aggregation is directly implicated in leukocyte adhesion, *Cell* **45**:269–280.

Case Records of the Massachusetts General Hospital, 1978, Case 34-1978, *N. Engl. J. Med.* **299**:466–474.

Castellot, J. J., Favreau, L. V., Karnovsky, M. J., and Rosenberg, R. D., 1982, Inhibition of vascular smooth muscle cell growth by endothelial cell-derived heparin: Possible role of a platelet endoglycosidase, *J. Biol. Chem.* **257**:11256–11260.

Charo, I. F., Fitzgerald, L. A., Steiner, B., Rall, S. C., Jr., Bekeart, L. S., and Phillips, D. R., 1986, Platelet glycoproteins IIb and IIIa: Evidence for a family of immunologically and structurally related glycoproteins in mammalian cells (adhesion/endothelial cells/leukocytes), *Proc. Natl, Acad. Sci. USA* **83**:8351–8356.

Chesney, C. M., Harper, E., and Colman, R. W., 1974, Human platelet collagenase, *J. Clin. Invest.* **53**:1647–1655.

Chiller, J. M., Skidmore, B. J., Morrison, D. C., and Weigle, W. O., 1973, Relationship of the structure of bacterial lipopolysaccharides to its function in mitogenesis and adjuvanticity, *Proc. Natl. Acad. Sci. USA* **70**:2129–2133.

Christie, D. J., Muller, P. C., and Aster, R. H., 1985, Fab-mediated binding of drug-dependent antibodies to platelets in quinidine- and quinine-induced thrombocytopenia, *J. Clin. Invest.* **75**:310–314.

Courtois, G., Ryckewaert, J. J., Woods, V. L., Woods, V. L., Jr., Plow, E. F., and Marguerie, G. A., 1986, Expression of intracellular fibrinogen on the surface of stimulated platelets, *Eur. J. Biochem.* **159**:61–67.

Csako, G., Suba, E. A., and Wistar, R., Jr., 1982, Activation of human platelets by antibodies to thymocytes and beta 2-microglobulin, *J. Clin. Lab. Immunol.* **7**:33–38.

da Prada, M., Richards, J. G., and Kettler, R., 1981, Amine storage organelles in platelets, in: *Platelets in Biology and Pathology*, Vol. 2 (J. L. Gordon, ed.), pp. 107–146, Elsevier/North-Holland, Amsterdam.

de Clerck, F., Somers, Y., and Van Gorp, L., 1984, Platelet-vessel wall interactions in hemostasis: implications of 5-hydroxytryptamine, *Agents Actions* **15**:627–635.

Demling, R. J., 1985, Burns, *N. Engl. J. Med.* **313**:1389–1398.

Deuel, T. F., and Huang, J. S., 1984, Platelet-derived growth factor: Structure, function and roles in normal and transformed cells, *J. Clin. Invest.* **74**:669–676.

Doolittle, R. F., 1984, Fibrinogen and fibrin, *Annu. Rev. Biochem* **53**:195–229.

Dorsch, C. A., 1980, Enhancement of binding of single-strand DNA to human platelets by aggregated IgG and ADP, *Arthritis Rheum.* **23**:666–667.

Dorsch, C. A., and Killmayer, J., 1983, The effect of native and single stranded DNA on the platelet release reaction, *Arthritis Rheum.* **26**:179–185.

Dorsch, C. A., and Meyerhoff, J., 1980, Elevated plasma beta-thromboglobulin levels in systemic lupus erythematosus, *Thromb. Res.* **20**:617–622.

Dorsch, C. A., and Meyerhoff, J., 1982, Mechanisms of abnormal platelet aggregation in systemic lupus erhythematosus, *Arthritis Rheum.* **25**:966–973.

Duffy, J. L., Cinquz, T., Grishman, E., and Churg, J., 1970, Intraglomerular fibrin, platelet aggregation, and subendothelial deposits in lipid nephrosis, *J. Clin. Invest.* **49**:251–258.

Fauvel, F., Campos, O. R., Leger, D., Pignaud, G., Rosenbaum, J., and Legrand, Y. J., 1984, Aortic endothelial cells in culture secrete glycoproteins reacting with blood platelets, *Biochem. Biophys. Res. Commun.* **123**:114–120.

Fiedel, B. A., Schoenberger, J. S., and Gewurz, H., 1979, Modulation of platelet activation by native DNA, *J. Immunol.* **123**:2479–2483.

Fitzgerald, L. A., Charo, I. F., and Phillips, D. R., 1985, Human and bovine endothelial cells synthesize membrane proteins similar to human platelet glycoproteins IIb and IIIa, *J. Biol. Chem.* **260**:10893–10896.

Fujimoto, T., Ohara, S., and Hawiger, J., 1982, Thrombin-induced exposure and prostacyclin inhibition of the receptor for factor VIII/von Willebrand factor on human platelets, *J. Clin. Invest.* **69**:1212–1222.

Fujimura, Y., Titani, K., Holland, L. Z., Russell, S. R., Roberts, J. R., Elder, J. H., Ruggeri, Z. M., and Zimmerman, T. S., 1986, von Willebrand Factor. A reduced and alkylated 52/48-kDa fragment beginning at amino acid residue 449 contains the domain interacting with platelet glycoprotein Ib, *J. Biol. Chem.* **261**:381–385.

Gardner, J. M., and Hynes, R. O., 1985, Interaction of fibronectin with its receptor on platelets, *Cell* **42**:439–448.

Gartner, T. K., and Bennett, J. S., 1985, The tetrapeptide analogue of the cell attachment site of fibronectin inhibits platelet aggregation and fibrinogen binding to activated platelets, *J. Biol. Chem.* **260**:11891–11894.

Garty, M., Ilfeld, D., and Kelton, J. G., 1985, Correlation of a quinidine-induced platelet-specific antibody with development of thrombocytopenia, *Am. J. Med.* **79**:253–255.

George, J. N., and Onofre, A. R., 1982, Human platelet surface binding of endogenous secreted factor VIII–von Willebrand factor and platelet factor 4, *Blood* **59**:194–197.

George, J. N., Nurden, A. T., and Phillips, D. R., 1984, Molecular defects in interactions of platelets with the vessel wall, *N. Engl. J. Med.* **311**:1084–1098.

Ginsberg, M. H., and Henson, P. M., 1978, Enhancement of platelet response to immune complexes and IgG aggregates by lipid A-rich bacterial lipopolysaccharides, *J. Exp. Med.* **147**:207–217.

Ginsberg, M. H., and Jaques, B. C., 1983, Platelet membrane proteins, in: *Measurements of Platelet Function* (L. A. Harker and T. S. Zimmerman, eds.), pp. 158–176, Churchill-Livingston, Edinburgh.

Ginsberg, M. H., and O'Malley, M., 1977, Serum factors releasing serotonin from normal platelets, *Ann. Intern. Med.* **87**:564–567.

Ginsberg, M. H., Kozin, F., O'Malley, M., and McCarty, D. J., 1977, Release of platelet constituents by monosodium urate crystals, *J. Clin. Invest.* **69**:999–1007.

Ginsberg, M. H., Breth, G., and Skosey, J. L., 1978, Platelets in the synovial space. (Letter.) *Arthritis Rheum.* **21**:994–995.

Ginsberg, M. H., Painter, R., Forsyth, J., Birdwell, C., and Plow, E., 1980, Thrombin increases expression of fibronectin antigen on the platelet surface, *Proc. Natl. Acad. Sci. USA* **77**:1049–1053.

Ginsberg, M. H., Plow, E. F., and Forsyth, J., 1981, Fibronectin expression on the platelet surface occurs in concert with secretion, *J. Supramol. Struct.* **17**:91–98.

Ginsberg, M. H., Forsyth, J., Lightsey, A., Chediak, J., and Plow, E. F., 1983, Reduced surface expression and binding of fibronectin by thrombin-stimulated thrombasthenic platelets, *J. Clin. Invest.* **71**:619–624.

Ginsberg, M., Pierschbacher, M. D., Ruoslahti, E., Marguerie, G., and Plow, E., 1985*a*, Inhibition of fibronectin binding to platelets by proteolytic fragments and synthetic peptides which support fibroblast adhesion, *J. Biol. Chem.* **260**:3931–3936.

Ginsberg, M. H., Plow, E. F., and Marguerie, G., 1985*b*, Platelet function, in: *Plasma Fibronectin Structure and Function*, Vol. 5 (J. McDonagh, ed.), pp. 149–174, Dekker, New York.

Ginsberg, M. H., Loftus, J. C., Ryckwaert, J.-J., Pierschbacher, M., Pytela, R., Ruoslahti, E., and Plow, E. F., 1987, Immunochemical and N-terminal sequence comparison of two cytoadhesins indicates they contain similar or identical beta subunits and distinct alpha subunits, *J. Biol. Chem.* **262**:5437–5440.

Goetzl, E. J., 1981, Oxygenation products of arachidonic acid as mediators of hypersensitivity and inflammation, *Med. Clin. North Am.* **65**:809–828.

Goetzl, E. J., and Gorman, R. R., 1978, Chemotactic and chemokinetic stimulation of human eosinophil and neutrophil polymorphonuclear leukocytes by HHT, *J. Immunol.* **120**:526–531.

Gordon, J. L., 1975, Blood platelet lysosomes and their contribution to the pathophysiological role of platelets, in: *Lyosomes in Biology and Pathology*, Vol. 4 (J. T. Dingle and R. T. Dean, eds.), pp. 3–31, Elsevier/North-Holland, Amsterdam.

Handa, M., Titani, K., Holland, L. Z., Roberts, J. R., and Ruggeri, Z. M., 1986, The von Willebrand factor-binding domain of platelet membrane glycoprotein Ib. Characterization by monoclonal antibodies and partial amino acid sequence analysis of proteolytic fragments, *J. Biol. Chem.* **261**:12579–12585.

Hardin, J. A., Cronlund, M., Haber, E., and Block, K., 1978, Activation of blood clotting in patients with systemic lupus erythematosus, *Am. J. Med.* **65**:430–436.

Haverstick, D. M., Cowan, J. F., Yamada, K. M., and Santoro, S. A., 1985, Inhibition of platelet adhesion to fibronectin, fibrinogen, and von Willebrand factor substrates by a synthetic tetrapeptide derived from the cell-binding domain of fibronectin, *Blood* **66**:946–952.

Henriksson, P., Edhag, O., Edlund, A., Junsson, B., Lantz, B., Nyquist, O., Sarby, B., and Wennmalm, A., 1985, A role for platelets in the process of infarct extension?, *N. Eng. J. Med.* **313**:1660–1661.

Henson, P. M., and Ginsberg, M. H., 1981, Immunological reactions of platelets, in: *Platelets in Biology and Pathology*, Vol. 2 (J. L. Gordon, ed.), pp. 265–308, Elsevier/North-Holland, Amsterdam.

Henson, P. M., Gould, D., and Becker, E. L., 1976, Activation of stimulus-specific serine esterases in the initiation of platelet secretion, *J. Exp. Med.* **144**:1657–1672.

Hiti-Harper, J., Wohl, H., and Harper, E., 1987, Platelet factor 4: An inhibitor of collagenase, *Science* **199**:991–992.

Houdijk, W. P. M., Sakariassen, K. S., Nievelstein, P. F. E. M., and Sizma, J. J., 1985, Role of factor VIII–von Willebrand factor and fibronectin in the interaction of platelets in flowing blood with monomeric and fibrillar human collagen Types I and III, *J. Clin. Invest.* **75**:531–540.

Jaques, B. C., and Ginsberg, M. H., 1982, The role of cell surface proteins in platelet stimulation by monosodium urate crystals, *Arthritis Rheum.* **25**:508–521.

Jaffe, E. A., and Mosher, D. F., 1978, Synthesis of fibronectin by cultured human endothelial cells, *J. Exp. Med.* **147**:1779–1791.

Jaffe, E. A., Ruggiero, J. T., Leung, L. L., Doyle, M. J., McKeown-Longo, P. J., and Mosher, D. F., 1983, Cultured human fibroblasts synthesize and secrete thrombospondin and incorporate it into extracellular matrix, *Proc. Natl. Acad. Sci. USA* **80**:998–1002.

Jaffe, E. A., Rugiero, J. T., and Falcone, D. J., 1985, Monocytes and macrophages synthesize and secrete thrombospondin, *Blood* **65**:79–84.

Kahaleh, M. B., Osborn, I., and Leroy, E. C., 1982, Elevated levels of circulating platelet aggregates and beta-thromboglobulin in scleroderma, *Ann. Intern. Med.* **96**:610–613.

Kahaleh, M. B., Scharstein, K., and LeRoy, E. C., 1985, Enhanced platelet adhesion to collagen in scleroderma, Effect of scleroderma plasma and scleroderma platelets, *J. Rheumatol.* **12**:468–471.

Kaplan, K. L., 1981, Platelet granule proteins: Localization and secretion, in: *Platelets in Biology and Pathology*, Vol. 2 (J. L. Gordon, ed.), pp. 77–90, Elsevier/North-Holland, Amsterdam.

Kaplan, K. L., and Owen, J., 1981, Plasma levels of beta-thromboglobulin and platelet factor 4 as indices of platelet activation *in vivo*, *Blood* **57**:199–202.

King, G. L., and Buchwald, S., 1984, Characterization and partial purification of an endothelial cell growth factor from human platelets, *J. Clin. Invest.* **73**:392–396.

Kloczewiak, M., Timmons, S., and Hawiger, J., 1982, Localization of a site interacting with human platelet receptor on carboxy-terminal segment of human fibrinogen gamma chain, *Biochem. Biophys. Res. Commun.* **107**:181–187.

Kornblihtt, A. R., Umezawa, K., Vibe-Pedersen, K., and Baralle, F. E., 1985, Primary structure of human fibronectin: Differential splicing may generate at least 10 polypeptides from a single gene, *EMBO J.* **4**:1755–1759.

Knighton, D. R., Hunt, T. K., Thakral, K. K., and Goodson, W. H., 1982, Role of platelets and fibrin in the healing sequence. An in vivo study of angiogenesis and collagen synthesis, *Ann. Surg.* **196**:379–387.

Kniker, W. T., and Cochrane, C. G., 1968, The localization of circulating immune complexes in experimental serum sickness, *J. Exp. Med.* **127**:119–136.

Kravis, T. C., and Henson, P. M., 1977, Accumulation of platelets at sites of antigen–antibody mediated injury, *J. Immunol.* **118**:1569–1580.

Kunicki, T. J., and Aster, R. H., 1979, Isolation and immunologic characterization of the human platelet alloantigen, P1AI, *Mol. Immunol.* **16**:353–360.

Lahav, J., Schwartz, M. A., and Haynes, R. O., 1982, Analysis of platelet adhesion with a radioactive chemical crosslinking reagent: Interaction of thrombospondin with fibronectin and collagen, *Cell* **31**:253–262.

Lam, S. C.-T., Plow, E. F., Smith, M. A., Andrieux, A., Ryckwaert, J.-J., Marguerie, G., and Ginsberg, M. H., 1987, Evidence that Arg-Gly-Asp and fibrinogen gamma chain peptides share a common binding site on platelets, *J. Biol. Chem.* **262**:947–950.

Lawler, J., and Hynes, R. O., 1986, The structure of human thrombospondin, an adhesive glycoprotein with multiple calcium-binding sites and homologies with several different peptides, *J. Cell Biol.* **103**:1635–1648.

Legrand, Y., Pignaud, G., and Caen, J. P., 1977, Human blood platelet elastase and proelastase, *Hemostatis* **6**:180–189.

Lerner, W., Caruso, R., Faig, D., and Karpatkin, S., 1985, Drug-dependent and non-drug-dependent anti-platelet antibody in drug-induced immunologic thrombocytopenic purpura, *Blood* **66**:306–311.

Leung, L. L., 1984, Role of thrombospondin in platelet aggregation, *J. Clin. Invest.* **74**:1764–1772.

Leung, L. L., and Nachman, R. L., 1982, Complex formation of platelet thrombospondin with fibrinogen, *J. Clin. Invest.* **70**:542–549.

Lopez-Fernandez, M., Ginsberg, M. H., Ruggeri, Z. M., Batlle, F. J., and Zimmerman, T. S., 1982, Multimeric structure of platelet factor VIII/von Willebrand factor: The presence of larger multimers and their reassociation with thrombin-stimulated platelets, *Blood* **60**:1132–1138.

Maclouf, J., de Laclos, B. F., and Borgeat, P., 1982, Stimulation of lekotriene biosynthesis in human blood leukocytes byd platelet-derived 12 HPETE, *Proc. Natl. Acad. Sci. USA* **79**:6042–6046.

Majack, R. A., Cook, S. C., and Bornstein, P., 1985, Platelet-derived growth factor and heparin-like glycosaminoglycans regulated thrombospondin synthesis and deposition in the matrix by smooth muscle cells, *J. Cell Biol.* **101**:1059–1070.

Margaretten, W., and McKay, D. G., 1971, The requirement for platelets in the active Arthus reaction, *Am. J. Pathol.* **64**:257–270.

Marguerie, G. A., Plow, E. F., and Edgington, T. S., 1979, Human platelets possess an inducible and saturable receptor specific for fibrinogen, *J. Biol. Chem.* **254**:5357–5363.

Mathison, J. C., and Ulevitch, R. J., 1983, Mediators involved in the expression of endotoxic activity, *Surv. Synth. Pathol. Res.* **1**:34–48.

McMillian, R., 1981, Chronic idiopathic thrombocytopenic purpura, *N. Engl. J. Med.* **304**:1135–1772.

McPherson, J., Sage, H., and Bornstein, P., 1981, Isolation and characterization of a glycoprotein secreted by aortic endothelial cells in culture. Apparent identity with platelet thrombospondin, *J. Biol. Chem.* **256**:11330–11336.

Medsger, T. A., Jr., 1985, Systemic sclerosis (scleroderma) eosinophilic fascitis, and calcinosis, in: *Arthritis and Allied Conditions*, 10th Ed. (D. J. McCarthy, ed.), pp. 994–1036, Lea & Febiger, Philadelphia.

Meuer, S., Ecker, U., Hudding, U., and Bitter-Suermann, D., 1981, Platelet–serotonin release by C3a C5a: Two independent pathways of activation, *J. Immunol.* **126**:1506–1509.

Mosher, D. F., Doyle, M. J., and Jaffe, E. A., 1982, Synthesis and secretion of thrombospondin by cultured human endothelial cells, *J. Cell Biol.* **93**:343–348.

Musson, R. A., and Henson, P. M., 1979, Humoral and formed elements of blood modulate the response of peripheral blood monocytes. I. Plasma and serum inhibit and placelets enhance monocyte adherence, *J. Immunol.* **122**:2026–2031.

Myers, S. L., and Christine, T. A., 1982, Measurement of beta-thromboglobulin connective tissue activating peptide–III platelet antigen concentrations in pathologic synovial fluids, *J. Rheumatol.* **9**:6–12.

Myers, S. L., Hossler, P. A., and Castor, C. W., 1980, Connective tissue activation. XIX. Plasma levels of CTAP-III platelet antigen in rheumatoid arthritis, *J. Rheumatol.* **7**:814–819.

Nachman, R. L., and Harpel, P. C., 1976, Platelet alpha 2-macroglobulin and alpha 1 antitrypsin, *J. Biol. Chem.* **251**:4512–4521.

Nachman, R. L., Weksler, B., and Ferris, B., 1972, Characterization of human platelet vascular permeability-enhancing activity, *J. Clin. Invest.* **51**:549–556.

Nurden, A. T., and Caen, J. P., 1974, An abnormal platelet glycoprotein pattern in three cases of Glanzmann's thrombasthenia, *Br. J. Haematol.* **28:**253–260.

O'Flaherty, J. T., and Wykle, R. L., 1983, Biology and biochemistry of platelet-activating factor, *Clin. Rev. Allergy* **1:**353–367.

Okita, J. R., Pidard, D., Newman, P. J., Montgomery, R. R., and Kunicki, T. J., 1985, On the association of glycoprotein Ib and actin-binding protein in human platelets, *J. Cell Biol.* **100:**317–321.

Packham, M. A., and Mustard, J. F., 1986, The role of platelets in the development and complications of atherosclerosis, *Semin. Hematol.* **23:**8–26.

Parise, L. V., and Phillips, D. R., 1985, Reconstitution of the purified platelet fibrinogen receptor fibrinogen binding properties of the glycoprotein IIb–IIIa complex, *J. Biol. Chem.* **260:**10698–10707.

Parise, L. V., and Phillips, D. R., 1986, Fibronectin-binding properties of the purified platelet glycoprotein IIb–IIIa complex, *J. Biol. Chem.* **261:**14011–14017.

Paul, J. I., Schwarzbauer, J. E., Tamkun, J. W., and Hynes, R. O., 1986, Cell-type-specific fibronectin subunits generated by alternative splicing, *J. Biol. Chem.* **261:**12258–12265.

Penington, D. G., 1981, Formation of platelets, in: *Platelets in Biology and Pathology,* Vol. 2 (J. L. Gordon, ed.), pp. 19–42. Elsevier/North-Holland, Amsterdam.

Pfueller, S. L., Jenkins, C. S., and Luscher, E. F., 1977, A comparative study of the effect of modification of the surface of human platelets on the receptors for aggregated immunoglobulins, *Biochim. Biophys. Acta* **465:**614–626.

Pierschbacher, M. D., and Ruoslahti, E., 1984, Cell attachment activity of fibronectin can be duplicated by small synthetic fragments of the molecule, *Nature (Lond.)* **309:**30–33.

Pierschbacher, M. D., Hayman, E. G., and Ruoslahti, E., 1983, Synthetic peptide with cell attachment activity of fibronectin (cell surface/cell culture/plastic surfaces/prosthetic materials), *Proc. Natl. Acad. Sci. USA* **80:**1224–1227.

Pinckard, R. N., Halonen, M., Palmer, J., Butler, C., Shaw, O., and Henson, P., 1977, Intravascular aggregation and pulmonary sequestration of platelets during IgE-induced systemic anaphylaxis in the rabbit, *J. Immunol.* **119:**2185–2194.

Plow, E. F., and Ginsberg, M. H., 1981, Specific and saturable binding of plasma fibronectin to thrombin-stimulated human platelets, *J. Biol. Chem.* **256:**9477–9482.

Plow, E. F., Srouji, A. H., Meyer, D., Marguerie, G., and Ginsberg, M. H., 1984, Evidence that three adhesive proteins interact with a common recognition site on activated platelets, *J. Biol. Chem.* **259:**5388–5391.

Plow, E. F., McEver, R. P., Coller, B. S., Woods, V. L., Jr., Marguerie, G. A., and Ginsberg, M. H., 1985a, Related binding mechanisms for fibrinogen, fibronectin, von Willebrand factor, and thrombospondin on thrombin-stimulated human platelets, *Blood* **66:**724–727.

Plow, E. F., Pierschbacher, M. D., Ruoslahti, E., Marguerie, G. A., and Ginsberg, M. H., 1985b, The effect of Arg-Gly-Asp-containing peptides on fibrinogen and von Willebrand factor binding to platelets (fibronectin/cell attachment/synthetic peptide/receptor), *Proc. Natl. Acad. Sci. USA* **82:**8057–8061.

Plow, E. F., Ginsberg, M. H., and Marguerie, G. A., 1986a, Expression and function of adhesive proteins on the platelet surface, in: *Biochemistry of Platelets* (D. R. Phillips and M. A. Shuman, eds.), pp. 226–256, Academic, New York.

Plow, E. F., Loftus, J., Levin, E., Fair, D., and Ginsberg, M. H., 1986b, Immunologic relationship between platelet membrane glycoprotein GPIIb/IIIa and cell surface molecules, *Proc. Natl. Acad. Sci. USA* **83:**6002–6006.

Polley, M. J., and Nachman, R. L., 1981, The human complement system in thrombin-mediated platelet function, in *Platelets in Biology and Pathology,* Vol. 2 (J. L. Gordon, ed.), pp. 309–319, Elsevier/North-Holland, Amsterdam.

Pytela, R., Pierschbacher, M. D., Ginsberg, M. H., Plow, E. F., and Ruoslahti, E., 1986, Plaetlet membrane glycoprotein IIb/IIIa: Member of a family of Arg-Gly-Asp-specific adhesion receptors, *Science* **231:**1559–1562.

Rosenfeld, S. I., Looney, R. J., Leedy, J. P., Phipps, D. C., Abraham, G. N., and Anderson, C. L., 1985, Human platelet Fc receptor for immunoglobulin G, *J. Clin. Invest.* **76:**2317–2322.

Ruggeri, Z. M., and Zimmerman, T. S., 1985, Platelets and von Willebrand disease, *Semin. Hematol.* **22**:203–218.

Ruggeri, Z. M., Bader, R., and DeMarco, L., 1982, Glanzman thrombasthenia: Deficient binding of von Willebrand factor to thrombin-stimulated platelets, *Proc. Natl. Acad. Sci. USA* **79**:6038–6041.

Sadler, J. E., Shelton-Inloes, B. B., Sorace, J. M., Harlan, J. M., Titani, K., and Davie, E. W., 1985, Cloning and characterization of two cDNAs coding for human von Willebrand factor, *Proc. Natl. Acad. Sci. USA* **82**:6394–6398.

Sanchez-Madrid, F., Nagy, J. A., Robbins, E., Simon, P., and Springer, T. A., 1983, A human leukocyte differentiation antigen family with distinct A-subunits and a common G-subunit: The lymphocyte function-associated antigen (LFA-1), the C3bi complement receptor (OKMl/Mac-1), and the p150,95 molecule, *J. Exp. Med.* **158**:1785–1803.

Schafer, A. I., Cooper, B., O'Hara, D., and Handin, R. I., 1979, Identification of platelet receptors for prostaglandin I$_2$ and D$_2$, *J. Biol. Chem.* **254**:2914–2917.

Schmaier, A. H., 1985, Platelet forms of plasma proteins: Plasma cofactors/substrates and inhibitors contained within platelets, *Semin. Hematol.* **22**:187–202.

Seibold, J. R., and Jageneau, A. H., 1984, Treatment of Raynaud's phenomenon with ketanserin, a selective antagonist of the serotinin 2 (5-HT$_2$) receptor, *Arthritis Rheum.* **27**:139–146.

Shadle, P. J., Ginsberg, M. H., Plow, E. F., and Barondes, S. H., 1984, Platelet–collagen adhesion: Inhibition by a monoclonal antibody that binds glycoprotein IIb, *J. Cell Biol.* **99**:2056–2060.

Shapleigh, C., Valone, F., Schur, P., Goetzl, E., and Austen, K., 1980, Platelet activity in synovial fluids of patients with rheumatoid arthritis, juvenile rheumatoid arthritis, gout, and noninflammatory arthropathies, *Arthritis Rheum.* **23**:800–807.

Shulman, N. R., 1958, Immunoreactions involving platelets, *J. Exp. Med.* **107**:665–690, 697–710, 711–729.

Silverstein, R. L., Leung, L. L., Harpel, P. C., and Nachman, R. L., 1984, Complex formation of platelet thrombospondin with plasminogen, *J. Clin. Invest.* **74**:1625–1633.

Skaer, R. J., 1981, Platelet degranulation, in: *Platelets in Biology and Pathology*, Vol. 2 (J. L. Gordon, ed.), pp. 321–348, Elsevier/North-Holland, Amsterdam.

Steiner, M., and Luscher, E., 1986, Identification of the immunoglobulin G receptor of human platelets, *J. Biol. Chem.* **261**:7230–7235.

Sternberg, E., Van Woert, M., Young, S., Magnussen, I., Baker, H., Gauthier, S., and Osterland, K., 1980, Development at a scleroderma-like illness during therapy with L-5-hydroxytrytophan and carbidopa, *N. Engl. J. Med.* **303**:782–787.

Thiagarajan, P., Shapiro, S. S., Levine, E., DeMarco, L., and Yalcin, A., 1985, A monoclonal antibody to human platelet glycoprotein IIIa detects a related protein in cultured human endothelial cells, *J. Clin. Invest.* **75**:896–901.

Titani, K., Kumar, S., Takio, K., Ericsson, L. H., Wade, R. D., Ashida, K., Walsh, K. A., Chopek, M. W., Sadler, J. E., and Fujikawa, K., 1986, Amino acid sequence of human von Willebrand factor, *Biochemistry* **24**:3171–3184.

Tollefsen, D. M., and Majerus, P. W., 1975, Inhibition of human platelet aggregation by monovalent and antifibrinogen antibody fragments, *J. Clin. Invest.* **55**:1259–1268.

Vargaftig, B. B., et al., 1981, Pharmacology of arachidonate metabolites and of platelet-activating factor, in: *Platelets in Biology and Pathology*, Vol. 2 (J. L. Gordon, ed.), pp. 373–406, Elsevier/North-Holland, Amsterdam.

Wagner, D. D., Olmsted, J. B., and Marder, V. J., 1982, Immunolocalization of von Willebrand protein in Weibel-Palade bodies of human endothelial cells, *J. Cell Biol.* **95**:355–360.

Weiss, H. J., Rosove, M. H., Lages, B. A., and Kaplan, K. L., 1980, Acquired storage pool deficiency with increased platelet-associated IgG, *Am. J. Med.* **69**:711–717.

Weksler, B. B., and Coupal, C. E., 1973, Platelet-dependent generation of chemotactic activity in serum, *J. Exp. Med.* **137**:1419–1430.

Weksler, B. B., and Goldstein, I. M., 1980, Prostaglandins: Interactions with platelets and polymorphonuclear leukocytes in hemostasis and inflammation, *Am. J. Med.* **68**:419–428.

Wencel-Drake, J. D., Plow, E. F., Zimmerman, T. S., Painter, R. G., and Ginsberg, M. H., 1984,

Immunofluorescent localization of adhesive glycoproteins in resting and thrombin-stimulated platelets, *Am. J. Pathol.* **115:**156–164.

Wencel-Drake, J. D., Painter, R. G., Zimmerman, T. S., and Ginsberg, M. H., 1985, Ultrastructural localization of human platelet thrombospondin, fibrinogen, fibronectin, and von Willebrand factor in frozen thin section, *Blood* **65:**929–938.

Wiedmer, T., Esmon, C. T., and Sims, P. J., 1986, On the mechanism by which complement proteins C5b-9 increase platelet prothombinase activity, *J. Biol. Chem.* **257:**11256–11260.

Wolff, R., Plow, E. F., and Ginsberg, M. H., 1986, Interaction of thrombospondin with resting and stimulated human platelets, *J. Biol. Chem.* **261:**6840–6846.

Woods, V. L., Oh, E. H., Mason, D., and McMillan, R., 1984, Autoantibodies against the platelet glycoprotein IIb/IIIa complex in patients with chronic ITP, *Blood:* 63:368–375.

Yaron, M., and Djaldetti, M., 1978, Platelets in synovial fluid, *Arthritis Rheum.* **21:**607.

Zeller, J., Weissbarth, E., Baruth, B., Mielke, H., and Deicher, 1983, Serotonin content of platelets in inflammatory rheumatic diseases, *Arthritis Rheum.* **26:**532–540.

Zucker-Franklin, D., 1981, Endocytosis by human platelets: Metabolic and freeze fracture studies, *J. Cell Biol.* **91:**706–715.

Zucker-Franklin, D., and Rosenberg, L., 1977, Platelet interaction with modified articular cartilage, *J. Clin. Invest.* **59:**641–651.

Chapter 3

Potential Functions of the Clotting System in Wound Repair

HAROLD F. DVORAK, ALLEN P. KAPLAN, and
RICHARD A. F. CLARK

1. Introduction

Injuries of many types and degrees, ranging from inflammation to frank blood vessel disruption, lead to plasma extravasation and extravascular fibrin clot formation. The clot is composed of crosslinked fibrin and fibronectin and platelets that together entrap plasma water, plasma proteins, and blood cells, primarily erythrocytes. This fibrin gel matrix not only halts bleeding but also establishes a provisional matrix for the influx of inflammatory cells and parenchymal cells into the injured tissue. With time, this surface clot dessicates to form the familiar scab, which in turn sloughs as wound healing proceeds from below.

Clots develop in the case of external or internal trauma and in a wide variety of disease processes. Clinical examples include entities affecting multiple organ systems and involving diverse etiologies, including inflammatory bowel disease, multiple sclerosis, and myocardial infarction (S. Robbins et al., 1984). Even malignant tumors regularly generate a local fibrin gel (Dvorak et al., 1983a). Injuries insufficient to induce hemorrhage also commonly generate an extravascular clot. For example, bee stings or intradermal injections of histamine raise a wheal; wheals represent local deposits of fibrin gel that bind water and feel indurated (Dvorak et al., 1985).

A characteristic common to all these examples is that the microvasculature has become leaky to plasma proteins, either secondary to trauma or in reaction to mediators such as histamine that transiently and reversibly increase local vascular permeability without causing endothelial or other cell damage. Majno et al. (1969) found that histamine and similar mediators act by causing post-

HAROLD F. DVORAK • Department of Pathology, Beth Israel Hospital, Harvard Medical School, and the Charles A. Dana Research Institute, Boston, Massachusetts 02115. ALLEN P. KAPLAN • Division of Allergy, Rheumatology, and Clinical Immunology, Department of Medicine, The State University of New York at Stony Brook, Health Sciences Center, Stony Brook, New York 11794. RICHARD A. F. CLARK • Department of Medicine, National Jewish Center for Immunology and Respiratory Medicine, Denver, Colorado 80206.

capillary venular endothelial cells to contract, pulling individual endothelial cells away from each other and thereby forming interendothelial cell gaps that permit escape of plasma water and proteins but not of platelets, erythrocytes, or leukocytes. Chapter 5 discusses vasopermeability mediators in depth.

After the extravasation of plasma constituents into the interstitial tissue, clotting is initiated through the interaction of plasma and tissue components. Although a direct demonstration of the steps by which fibrin is formed in this particular circumstance is lacking, several mechanisms are considered likely, including the extrinsic coagulation pathway, the intrinsic or Hageman factor (HF) pathway, and platelet activation. The extrinsic coagulation pathway is believed to be the primary source of clotting, while the intrinsic coagulation pathway is probably most important in producing bradykinin, a vasoactive mediator that increases vascular permeability. Platelet activation plays a major role when tissue injury is severe enough to disrupt blood vessels (see Chapter 2). All three mechanisms, regardless of how direct, generate prothrombinase, an enzyme complex that acts in the penultimate step of coagulation by catalyzing the conversion of prothrombin to thrombin. Thrombin in turn cleaves fibrinogen to fibrin, which polymerizes to form a clot.

Extravascular clotting is therefore a universal response of tissues to injury of even a mild degree. However, the mechanisms by which extravascular plasma clots form, and the role of such extravascular clotting in subsequent wound healing, are as yet rather poorly understood and represent an important and difficult problem that will require considerable effort to solve. Here we address three major questions that we hope will stimulate interest and additional investigation: (1) Why does extravasated plasma clot? (2) What regulates the extent of clotting? (3) What role does the resulting extravascular clot have in wound healing? While a good deal can be said in response to the first two questions, answers to the last are at best incomplete and speculative.

2. Extrinsic Coagulation Pathway

The extrinsic coagulation pathway is initiated by tissue thromboplastin, alternatively called tissue factor and procoagulant activity (Nemerson et al., 1980) (Fig. 1). This lipoprotein is expressed by fibroblasts, smooth muscle cells, and endothelial cells in injured tissue (Smariga and Maynard, 1982). In addition, endothelial cells express tissue factor when stimulated by endotoxin or interleukin-1 (IL-1) (Colucci et al., 1983; Bevilacqua et al., 1985). Tissue factor is also released and/or expressed on the surface of activated neutrophils (Niemetz, 1972), monocytes/macrophages (Edwards and Rickles, 1980), or tumor cells (Dvorak et al., 1983a,b). Thus endotoxin, IL-1, or other factors released at sites of sepsis or immunologic injury may induce extravascular clotting in sites where frank tissue destruction is not observed.

Tissue factor forms a 1 : 1 molecular complex with coagulation factor VII, and this complex converts factor X to factor Xa. As can be seen in Fig. 1, activation of factor X is the branch point of the intrinsic and extrinsic coagulation pathways. A positive feedback exists in which factor Xa cleaves factor VII

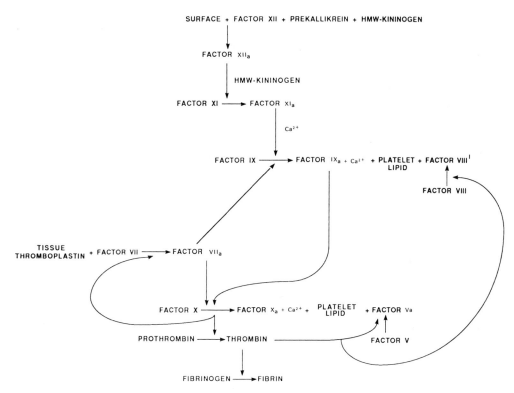

Figure 1. Coagulation pathways initiated by tissue injury. Plasma extravasation and blood vessel disruption, which follow tissue injury expose blood constituents to fibrillar collagen and tissue factor. Hageman factor (factor XII) becomes activated (XIIa) on the surface of fibrillar collagen, initiating the so-called intrinsic clotting cascade by activating factor XI (XIa). Tissue factor, present in the interstitium, activates factor VII (VIIa), the initiator of the so-called extrinsic pathway, which in turn activates factor IX–factor VIII and factor X–factor V complexes (IXa, VIIIa and Xa, Va, respectively). The IXa, VIIIa and Xa, Va complexes require phospholipids (PL) and calcium (Ca^{2+}) for their maximal activity. The Xa–Va complex generates thrombin from prothrombin. Thrombin then activates more factor VIII and factor V and generates fibrin monomer from fibrinogen. Fibrin monomer aggregates spontaneously to form fibrin polymers.

to factor VIIa, which has 50–200 times the activity of the factor VII zymogen. Nonetheless, native factor VII, or at least its complex with tissue factor, possesses functional activity (Broze and Majerus, 1980; Zur and Nemerson, 1979). However, factor IX of the intrinsic pathway can be activated by factor VIIa (Osterud and Rapaport, 1977) and at low tissue factor levels, activation of X by factor IXa rather than direct activation by factor VIIa may be significant (Marler et al., 1982a). In this circumstance, factor IX and the cofactor, factor VIII, would be part of the extrinsic coagulation pathway.

2.1. Monocyte/Macrophage Procoagulant Activities

The finding that fibrin deposits were a characteristic feature of delayed-type hypersensitivity reactions and the cause of reaction induration (Colvin et *al.*, 1979; Clark *et al.*, 1984) prompted a search for mechanisms of clotting that might occur in cellular immunity. The search focused primarily on cells of the immune response thought to participate in delayed reactions, namely, lymphocytes and monocytes/macrophages. It is now clear that macrophages are able to synthesize all coagulation factors of the extrinsic pathway, i.e., tissue factor, clotting Factors v, VII, and X, and prothrombin, and in addition provide a surface for generation of prothrombinase.

Edgington and co-workers (1985) have done much to clarify the mechanisms by which tissue factor activity is expressed by cells of the monocyte lineage. At least four distinct pathways may be involved in inducing tissue factor synthesis by monocytes, the first three of which are dependent on the activities of T lymphocytes:

1. The first pathway, which also gives the most rapid response, results from exposure of cultured monocytes and lymphocytes to lipopolysaccharide, its lipid A moiety, or to antigen–antibody complexes. Helper T lymphocytes are triggered over a 30-min period. Instruction of monocytes to produce tissue factor apparently involves close physical contact with lymphocytes, since soluble products capable of inducing procoagulant synthesis are not found in the culture medium. Monocyte instruction is quite rapid—15 min or less—after which lymphocytes are no longer necessary for continued development of monocyte tissue factor generation. The procoagulant products, fully expressed a few hours later, include not only tissue factor, but also prothrombinase activity as well as new synthesis of factor VII.

2. A somewhat slower expression of monocyte tissue factor results from a lymphokine produced in two-way mixed-lymphocyte cultures. The monocyte procoagulant inducing factor appears in culture fluids after about 72 hr. This unique 18,000-M_r protein, once formed, stimulates monocytes to express tissue factor at maximal levels in 4–6 hr.

3. A third and still slower pathway is driven by a specific antigen and is postulated to play an important role in cellular immunity. Monocytes must present soluble protein antigens to T lymphocytes in a step requiring cell–cell contact. T lymphocytes so triggered communicate with monocytes in a non-genetically restricted manner to induce the production of tissue factor. Although lymphokine production is not required, the lymphocyte to monocyte communication may also take place by way of soluble mediators, which Geczy and Hopper (1981) suggest is monocyte-inhibiting factor (MIF).

4. A fourth and as yet not well-defined pathway may also exist for generating expression of monocyte/macrophage tissue factor independent of T lymphocytes (Edwards and Rickles, 1978).

These four pathways demonstrate that macrophages can express tissue factor via different mechanisms over a prolonged length of time and thus may provide tissue factor at sites of injury not only during the acute inflammation but also during later phases of tissue repair. Macrophages also provide a surface for efficient prothrombinase assembly (Carr *et al.*, 1985). Prothrombinase assembly has been investigated by Tracy and Mann and their associates (1979,

1983) and involves formation of an enzyme complex of an active protease (factor Xa) with a nonenzymatic cofactor (factor Va) bound to an appropriate membrane surface in the presence of calcium ions. In addition to macrophages, platelets, some inflammatory cells, endothelial cells, and certain phospholipid vesicles of defined composition all provide an appropriate surface for pro-thrombinase complex assembly (see Chapter 4). In the absence of such a surface, the capacity of prothrombinase to cleave prothrombin to thrombin (hence fibrinogen to fibrin) falls nearly three orders of magnitude. Thus, provision of a suitable surface for prothrombinase activation, in addition to plasma clotting factors, is required for fibrin formation under any circumstances.

2.2. Tissue Factor-like Activity in Shed Membrane Vesicles

In addition to expressing these activities on their surfaces, macrophages were also found to shed ultramicroscopic vesicles from their surfaces, apparently without compromise of viability (Carr et al., 1985). These vesicles assumed functions analogous to those of intact cells, that is, expression of both tissue factor and prothrombinase-generating activity. If such shedding of plasma membrane fragments occurs in vivo, it would provide a mechanism for relatively wide dissemination of procoagulant activity, well removed from the cell doing the shedding.

Other normal nonmalignant cells (Maynard et al., 1975; Kadish et al., 1983; Carr et al., 1985) as well as tumor cells (Curatolo et al., 1979; Dvorak et al., 1981, 1983a,b) express tissue factor activity. Moreover, fibrin deposition in tumors is not confined to the immediate vicinity of malignant cells; for example, fibrin may be deposited in tumor stroma. Thus, procoagulants shed from the tumor cell surface may also have a role in tumor fibrin deposition. Apropos of the last observations, several groups have reported that tumor cells shed membrane-bound vesicles in tissue culture (Calafat et al., 1976; Black, 1980; Dvorak et al., 1981). Thus, cell-membrane shedding of vesicles is a mechanism by which clotting can be initiated in tissue stroma at a distance from cells under numerous circumstances, such as inflammation, tumor growth, and wound repair. In wound repair, shed vesicles may facilitate the deposition of a provisional matrix into which cells can then migrate (see Section 8.1.1.).

3. Intrinsic Coagulation Pathway

Hageman factor (factor XII), prekallikrein, and HMW-kininogen together comprise the initiating factors for the intrinsic coagulation cascade (see Fig. 1). The role of this pathway in hemostasis is unclear, since it is possible to be deficient in any of the above factors and not have a bleeding diathesis. However, as the cascade proceeds, the importance of each factor in terms of hemostasis becomes more evident, at least in regard to bleeding as a consequence of aberrant factor function. Once activated, HF converts factor XI to factor XIa;

factor XIa then activates factor IX in the presence of calcium ion (Fig. 1). Patients with deficiency of factor XI have a mild and often variable bleeding disorder while deficiency of either factor IX or factor VIII causes the severe forms of hemophilia. The explanation for these differences in clinical occurrence of bleeding (i.e., increasing severity when a more distal factor is missing) is not completely understood but may relate to the importance of factor IX in the extrinsic cascade (see Section 2.1).

In addition to initiating the intrinsic coagulation pathway, activated HF converts prekallikrein to kallikrein. Kallikrein then digests HMW-kininogen to liberate bradykinin, a potent vasoactive mediator that increases vascular permeability.

3.1. Hageman Factor

Hageman factor is an 80,000-M_r protein present in normal plasma at a mean concentration of about 35 µg/ml. The protein is a single-polypeptide chain that is glycosylated; some parts of the molecule have been sequenced (Fujikawa and McMullen, 1983). Although Hageman factor is the initiating protein of the cascade, it is readily cleaved by other proteases, the major one being kallikrein (Cochrane *et al.*, 1972). Thus, a reciprocal interaction exists whereby activated HF converts prekallikrein to kallikrein and kallikrein activates HF. When HF is activated by kallikrein, a single cleavage is initially made at an arginine residue located within a disulfide loop. The resulting molecule of activated Hageman factor (HFa) is thus a two-chain structure comprising a 50,000-M_r heavy chain and a 28,000-M_r light chain (Revak *et al.*, 1977). This molecule is a serine protease with the active site and catalytic mechanism located in the light chain. Enzymatic activity is readily demonstrated against its natural substrates, prekallikrein, or factor XI, and against low-molecular-weight synthetic substrates (Silverberg *et al.*, 1980). It is also inhibited by the classic serine protease inhibitor diisopropryl fluorophosphate (DFP), as well as by chloromethylketone derivatives of oligopeptides with suitable sequences (Dunn and Kaplan, 1982).

If digestion of HF by kallikrein continues, two further peptide bonds are cleaved. The new cleavage sites are located in the heavy chain, outside the disulfide bond that connects the two chains in HFa. The products are two forms of Hageman factor fragment (HFf) that make up the original light chain of HFa, with a small oligopeptide tail connected by a disulfide bond. It appears that the larger form of HFf (30,000 M_r) is formed first and that a subsequent cleavage trims the oligopeptide to produce the smaller form (28,500 M_r) (Dunn and Kaplan, 1982). Both forms remain enzymatically active, have very similar kinetics of hydrolysis of synthetic substrates to HFa (Silverberg *et al.*, 1980), and are efficient activators of prekallikrein (Kaplan and Austen, 1970; Revak *et al.*, 1977). However, whereas HFa is an efficient clotting factor, HFf is a very poor one (Kaplan and Austen, 1970, 1971). This difference may be ascribed to the surface requirements for factor XI activation, since HFf does not remain bound

(Revak and Cochrane, 1976). Thus, upon conversion of HFa to HFf, HFf leaves the surface and continues to activate the bradykinin-forming cascade at sites distant from the surface reaction, until it is inactivated by a plasma inhibitor.

3.2. Kallikrein

Prekallikrein is the precursor of the active serine protease, plasma kallikrein, and has two forms (85,000 and 88,000 M_r) in human plasma at a combined concentration of 25–50 µg/ml. Like Hageman factor, prekallikrein is a single-chain polypeptide that becomes cleaved within a disulfide-bonded loop upon activation; the active protein thus has a two-chain structure similar to that of HFa and like HFa, the active site is on the light chain (Mandle and Kaplan, 1977). Certain tissues are particularly rich in kallikreins (Orstavik et al., 1980), although many tissues possess cells containing kallikrein. A prokallikrein may exist within cells (Spragg, 1983), but tissue kallikrein appears already active when secreted.

The major activator of plasma prekallikrein in normal human plasma is activated Hageman factor. Once activated, kallikrein has a number of substrates. These include high-molecular-weight kininogen, which is cleaved extremely rapidly by kallikrein to liberate bradykinin (Habal et al., 1974; Thompson et al., 1978). This requires two cleavages, since the bradykinin sequence is located internally in the sequence of HMW-kininogen. Other substrates or potential substrates of plasma kallikrein include plasminogen (Colman, 1969; Mandle and Kaplan, 1977), plasma prorenin (Sealey et al., 1979) and complement components (DiScipio, 1982). Kallikrein may also have other effects in inflammatory reactions since it has chemotactic activity for neutrophils (Kaplan et al., 1972) and can cause neutrophil aggregation (Schapira et al., 1982) and enzyme secretion (Wachtfogel et al., 1983).

3.3. Kininogen

HMW-kininogen is a 120,000-M_r protein present in plasma at 80 µg/ml and contains within it the sequence of bradykinin. If this were its only function, deficiency of HMW-kininogen would not be expected to cause any change in coagulation parameters. In fact, however, plasmas deficient in HMW-kininogen show a very marked increase in their partial thromboplastin time (PTT), and studies with purified components show that the rates of activation of prekallikrein, HF and factor XI are all very much lower when HMW-kininogen is absent (Griffin and Cochrane, 1976; Meier et al., 1977). After the bradykinin has been liberated, the remainder of the molecule is in the form of a two-chain disulfide-linked protein. The isolated light chains can bind to prekallikrein and factor XI (Thompson et al., 1979) as well as to surfaces and therefore account for the cofactor (coagulant) activity of HMW-kininogen.

A more plentiful 50,000-M_r kininogen accounts for 85% of plasma kininogen, however. The heavy chains of the 50,000- and 120,000-M_r kininogen are known to be immunologically indistinguishable from each other (Thompson *et al.*, 1978), but the light chain of the low-molecular-weight form is much smaller and displays no coagulant activity (Kato *et al.*, 1976). Low-molecular-weight kininogen is cleaved only slowly by plasma kallikrein but is the primary substrate for tissue kallikrein. Thus, tissue kallikrein releases bradykinin from low-molecular-weight kininogen but generates no cofactor for coagulation.

3.4. Surface

The final component of the contact system to be considered is the surface. To date there is no unequivocal demonstration of a true physiologic surface that can support contact activation, although a number of substances are known, of both organic and nonorganic origin, that are functional. All these substances bear negative charges and are able to form either high-molecular-weight aggregates or are actually particulate. The classic inorganic substances, kaolin and celite, have been widely used both experimentally and as routine activators for PTT tests; another important inorganic activator is glass (or quartz).

Activation of the system can occur upon exposure of plasma or purified proteins to monosodium urate and pyrophosphate crystals (Ginsberg *et al.*, 1980; Kellermeyer and Breckenridge, 1965) and the lipid A portion of endotoxin (Morrison and Cochrane, 1974). These results raise the possibility that the contact system may be involved in several pathologic states, especially through the generation of bradykinin.

3.5. Initiation by Hageman Factor

The intrinsic coagulation pathway presents a dilemma, in that Hageman factor is clearly the initiating protein but it is present in zymogen form and appears to require cleavage to create the activated enzyme (Griffin and Beretta, 1979; Miller *et al.*, 1980; Revak *et al.*, 1977). Yet all the enzymes that might cleave it require activated HF for their formation. Thus, the process appears circular and the starting point is difficult to delineate.

It appears that surface-bound HF is more readily cleaved by other enzymes (Griffin, 1978); thus, an initiating surface appears to render Hageman factor a better substrate for proteases but does not form a new site within the uncleaved zymogen. The initiation of contact activation appears to be dependent on the ability of HF to autoactivate. Such activity was first suggested in studies of rabbit HF (Wiggins and Cochrane, 1979). A similar conclusion was suggested when human HF was examined (Miller *et al.*, 1980). It appeared that purified HF was slowly cleaved upon binding to surfaces, and such cleavage was not inhibited by agents known to inactivate possible HF activators (Miller *et al.*, 1980), such as kallikrein (Cochrane *et al.*, 1972), plasmin (Kaplan and Austen,

1971), or factor XIa (Meier *et al.*, 1977). Furthermore, the rate of HF cleavage appeared proportional to the percentage of cleaved (activated) enzyme in the starting material (Miller *et al.*, 1980). We have demonstrated that even the most highly purified preparations of HF possess a small amount of activity (Silverberg *et al.*, 1980). The source of HF enzyme for initiation of autoactivation is unclear. It could be due either to traces of activated (cleaved) HF that are always present in the circulation or to trace activity in the zymogen.

We estimate that if HF possesses any activity, it is not greater than ¼₀₀₀th the activity of HFa (Silverberg and Kaplan, 1982). Other reports (Heimark *et al.*, 1980; Kurachi *et al.*, 1980) estimate that the activity present in HF are far in excess of our estimates. We suspect that HFa generated from autoactivation are being measured.

Since the rate of HF digestion by kallikrein far exceeds that of the autoactivation reaction (Dunn *et al.*, 1982; Tankesley and Finlayson, 1984), the sequence in normal plasma appears to involve activation of prekallikrein by HFa, generated by autoactivation of surface bound HF, and then rapid cleavage of residual surface-bound HF by kallikrein. Once HFa is formed, cleavages occur external to the disulfide bond to form HFf.

3.6. Formation of Bradykinin in Plasma: A Product of the Intrinsic Coagulation Pathway

The formation of bradykinin in plasma is probably the most significant biologic event to result from initiation of the intrinsic coagulation pathway. Kinins are polypeptides that cause local peripheral vasodilatation and increase vascular permeability. This leads to extravasation of additional blood constituents in and around a site of tissue injury. Most studies have focused upon bradykinin, a 9-amino acid peptide with the sequence Arg-Pro-Pro-Gly-Phe-Ser-Pro-Phe-Arg. Bradykinin is derived from a plasma protein termed kininogen and its release requires cleavage at two sites (Lys-Arg and Arg-Ser) within kininogen. The enzymes that cleave kininogen to generate bradykinin are known as kallikreins (see Section 3.2). There are two general mechanisms by which bradykinin is generated in humans, and these involve plasma and tissue kallikreins, as well as the 50,000- and 120,000-M_r kininogens. Tissue kallikreins digest both forms of kininogen approximately equally; however, since 50,000-M_r kininogen is in far excess, most of the kinin formed by tissue kallikrein is derived from this form. The product is Lys-bradykinin or kallidin, a 10-amino acid peptide, rather than bradykinin (Webster and Pierce, 1963). An aminopeptidase in plasma can cleave at the N-terminal Lys-Arg group to convert it to bradykinin. The specificity of plasma kallikrein is much greater because it digests the 120,000-M_r kininogen selectively to form bradykinin. Studies of the amino acid sequence of high- and low-molecular-weight kininogens have demonstrated that they share a major portion of the molecule, from the N-terminal to just beyond the bradykinin moiety (Kitamura *et al.*, 1983; Thompson *et al.*, 1978) but that the residues subsequent to that point differ.

The level of bradykinin in plasma (and very likely other bodily fluids) is dependent on the rate of formation of bradykinin and its rate of destruction. The latter process is rapid and of considerable importance but renders the *in vivo* determination of bradykinin as a reflection of kininogen proteolysis difficult. Thus, assessment of the kinin-forming systems in human trauma and disease may require determination of kinin degradation products in addition to, or perhaps in place of, direct kinin assessment. There are two major pathways for *in vivo* bradykinin destruction. In plasma, a major enzyme known as carboxypeptidase N or kininase I (Erdos and Sloane, 1962; Plummer and Horwitz, 1978) removes the C-terminal arginine to leave an inactive octapeptide. This protein is identical to the anaphylatoxin inactivator (Bockisch and Muller-Eberhard, 1970), which similarly removes a C-terminal arginine from C3a, C4a, and C5a to cause loss of their contractile and permeability enhancing properties. The second enzyme is present in high concentration in the lung, where it rapidly degrades bradykinin in the pulmonary microcirculation. The products are a pentapeptide Arg-Pro-Pro-Gly-Phe, plus dipeptides Ser-Pro and Phe-Arg (Sheikh and Kaplan, 1985). This second enzyme is better known as the angiotensin converting enzyme (ACE) because it also converts angiotensin I to angiotensin II by removal of the dipeptide, His-Leu.

Recent studies of kinin metabolism in human plasma or serum reveal that these enzymes act on bradykinin sequentially. The carboxypeptidase acts first to remove the C-terminal arginine. The resultant octapeptide, des Arg^9 bradykinin, is then cleaved by ACE to yield Arg-Pro-Pro-Gly-Phe plus the tripeptide Ser-Pro-Phe (Sheikh and Kaplan, 1986). Finally the C-terminal Phe is removed from each peptide by enzymes with specificities suggesting carboxypeptidase A and prolyl carboxypeptidase, respectively (Sheikh and Kaplan, 1987). The initial rate of C-terminal Arg removal in serum is faster than plasma (Sheikh and Kaplan, 1987). Perhaps this is the result of another factor with carboxypeptidase B-like activity present in serum that is secreted by platelets or neutrophils. Radioimmunoassays (RIAs) are available for determination of plasma bradykinin (Scicli *et al.*, 1982; Talamo *et al.*, 1969). Normal levels appear to be as low at 25 pg/ml (Scicli *et al.*, 1982). An RIA for des Arg^9 bradykinin (the kininase I product) has also been reported (Odya *et al.*, 1983).

4. Platelet Role in Coagulation

Platelets interact with the coagulation cascade at the factor X activation step. Like the other vitamin K-dependent factors (factors VII and IX, and prothrombin), factor X contains glutamic acid residues within its amino-terminal domain, which possess an extra glutamic acid residue (γ-carboxyglutamic acid) (Stenflo *et al.*, 1974). Vitamin K acts as a cofactor for the carboxylase enzyme (Larson and Suttie, 1978) responsible for catalyzing the addition of these carboxyl groups as a post-translational modification (Munns *et al.*, 1976). The resultant γ-carboxyglutamic acid chelates calcium ion and binds to calcium-dependent sites on platelet membrane phospholipids (Esmon *et al.*, 1975).

Thus, factor X is bound to the platelet membrane and factor IX or IXa may be similarly bound. Like factor X, some prothrombin is bound to the platelet surface via γ-carboxyglutamic acid and calcium, and factor V is also weakly bound. Factor V, however, is a true metalloprotein and contains intrinsically bound cobalt (Greenquist and Colman, 1975), which is required for cofactor activity. As some factor Xa is formed, prothrombin is converted to thrombin and thrombin then cleaves and activates factor V. Factor V, like factor VIII and HMW-kininogen, acts as a cofactor when cleaved to facilitate specific enzyme and substrate reactions. A high-affinity binding site for factor Va exists at the platelet surface (Miletich et al., 1979) independent of γ-carboxyglutamic acid, and the bound factor Va acts as the factor Xa receptor (Kane et al., 1980). A binding site for factor Va also exists on one of the domains of prothrombin (Esmon and Jackson, 1974). Estimates of the ability of this platelet–factor Va–Xa complex to convert prothrombin to thrombin in the presence of calcium ion compared with factor Xa alone indicate an augmentation in reaction rate of as much as 300,000-fold (Kane et al., 1980).

Thrombin also activates factor VIII (Hultin, 1982), and it seems likely that the platelet, factor IXa, factor VIIIa, and factor X interact in the preceding step, in some analogous fashion. Coagulation factor VIII is known to be closely associated with plasma von Willebrand factor, and they circulate as a complex (Hoyer, 1981; Mikaelsson et al., 1983; Weinstein and Chute, 1984). von Willebrand factor is thought to be required for platelet–endothelial cell interactions, although the identification of the physiologic platelet receptor for von Willebrand factor is uncertain (Fujimoto et al., 1982; Schullek et al., 1984).

Thrombin is also a platelet activator, which has the following consequences on platelets: (1) the phospholipids that catalyze coagulation are exposed (Marcus, 1969); (2) platelets aggregate to form a hemostatic plug that may serve initially to limit bleeding (Marr et al., 1985); and (3) platelet granules, which contain clotting factors and mediators of the inflammatory process (see Chapter 2) and wound repair (see Chapters 9, Sections 1–4) are released. For example, one of the cationic proteins released appears capable of degranulating mast cells (Weiss, 1975). Thus, like the generation of bradykinin from the intrinsic coagulation pathway, this release of mast cell vasoactive mediators, such as histamine, PDG_2, as well leukotrienes C_4 and D_4, serves to facilitate the extravasation of blood constituents in and around a site of tissue injury. From the standpoint of blood coagulation, the ADP released from platelet granules serves to further sustain platelet aggregation (Marr et al., 1985); granule-derived serotonin acts as a small vessel vasoconstrictor that may facilitate the initial limitation of bleeding by the platelet plug; and the granule proteins fibrinogen, fibronectin, and thrombospondin (Gartner et al., 1978) serve to bind platelets together as a relatively stable mass (see Chapters 2 and 9).

Components of the contact activation system also appear to interact with platelets (Walsh, 1972). There are apparently separate platelet receptors for factors XI and XIa (Greengard et al., 1981; Sinha et al., 1984) and platelet-associated factor XI can be activated by both HF-dependent and -independent mechanisms (Walsh and Griffin, 1981). The cell membrane of activated platelets also appears to provide a surface upon which HF can be activated, a process dependent on prekallikrein and HMW-kininogen (Walsh and Griffin, 1981), activating bound factor XI. HMW-kininogen binds to platelets in a zinc-dependent reaction (Greengard and Griffin, 1984). Factor XI is also found as a platelet membrane constituent (Lipscomb and Walsh, 1979), and HMW kininogen has been shown to be present in the α-granules of platelets and becomes available during platelet activation (Schmair et al., 1983). Platelet-Derived factor XI differs from plasma factor XI in terms of size and charge but is reactive with antisera to factor XI. It is clear that platelets are not requisite for contact activation as they are for later steps in coagulation. Thus, contact activation proceeds unimpeded in platelet-poor plasma, and addition of platelets provides little augmentation. Nevertheless, platelet activation resulting from tissue injury and/or localized thrombosis may contribute to local contact activation and kinin formation.

5. Fibrin Formation

The last step in the blood coagulation pathway involves conversion of fibrinogen to form crosslinked fibrin. Again the enzyme thrombin is critical to these reactions. Thrombin cleaves two of the chains of fibrinogen in sequence to release fibrinopeptides A and B, respectively (Blomback et al., 1978). The resulting molecule (fibrin monomer) has exposed sites that result in lateral and end to end polymerization to form fibrin. The resultant clot, however, is friable, and stability is conferred on this structure by covalent crosslinking of the chains of adjacent fibrin stands. This is accomplished by a unique enzyme (the only nonserine protease in coagulation) known as factor XIIIa or fibrinoligase (Lorand, 1972). Like other coagulation factors, it circulates as a proenzyme that is converted to an active enzyme by thrombin (Takagi and Doolittle, 1974). Factor XIIIa crosslinks the γ-carboxyl group of glutamine to the ε-amino group of lysine residues to form a peptide bond thereby crosslinking the chains (Pisano et al., 1972). Cold insoluble globulin or plasma fibronectin (Mosesson and Umfleet, 1970) binds to fibrinogen (fibrin) and is also crosslinked to the fibrin matrix by factor XIIIa (Mosher, 1976). For a review of fibronectin structure and function in wound repair, see Chapter 15. Once fibrin is formed, the process for degradation of fibrin (i.e., fibrinolysis) is also set in motion. The plasma-derived protease plasmin degrades fibrin to a variety of intermediate products (Budzynski et al., 1974; Marder et al., 1982).

6. Fibrinolysis

Since the fibrin clot must ultimately be removed from the site of injury to permit repair to continue, the critical features of this pathway are briefly outlined. Various cells (tissues) contain an enzyme known as tissue plasminogen activator that rapidly converts plasminogen to plasmin. Like many coagulation factors (e.g., HF, prekallikrein, or factor X), a single cleavage in plasminogen at an Arg-Val bond within a disulfide bridge (Robbins et al., 1967) converts it from a 92,000-M_r single-chain to a two-chain molecule in which a 67,000-M_r heavy chain is disulfide linked to a 25,000-M_r light chain. The active site is in the light chain (Summaria et al., 1967).

The tissue plasminogen activator has been isolated from diverse sources, such as uterine tissue or pig heart (Cole and Bachman, 1977; Rijken et al., 1979), but the sources most relevant to this volume are probably from damaged endothelial cells (Allen and Pepper, 1981), previously called vascular plasminogen activator (Binder et al., 1979), or from activated neutrophils (Granelli-Piperno et al., 1977) or macrophages (Vassalli et al., 1976). Macrophages also secrete or express tissue factor activity (see Section 2.1); this may be important in coordinating local coagulation and fibrinolysis. Fibrin (but not fibrinogen) appears to possess a strong binding site for tissue plasminogen activator (Thorsen et al., 1972), so that this enzyme can localize at the surface of a clot. Plasminogen also contains a binding site for fibrin at its amino-terminal; thus, both enzyme and substrate are bound, and the resultant plasmin will degrade the fibrin.

Plasma also contains an intrinsic fibrinolytic cascade identical to the sequence of interactions described earlier for the formation of bradykinin. It appears that the main plasminogen activator is kallikrein (Colman, 1969; Mandle and Kaplan, 1977), but contributions are also made by factor XIa and HFa or HFf. This pathway, however, is many thousand-fold less effective than well-described plasminogen activators, such as urokinase or streptokinase (Goldsmith et al., 1978; Mandle and Kaplan, 1979), and the comparison with tissue plasminogen activator would be similar.

7. Control Mechanisms

One cannot really discuss coagulation and fibrinolytic mechanisms as they may relate to wound repair, without at least briefly considering control mechanisms. Clearly, once these cascades are set in motion, there must be a counterbalance so that reactions, once initiated, do not perpetually continue. In some pathologic circumstances, such as endotoxic shock and/or disseminated intravascular coagulation (DIC), coagulation continues until the underlying disorder is controlled. There are two general types of controls of all plasma proteolytic cascades: intrinsic ones in which one enzymatic reaction serves to limit another, and extrinsic controls in which protease inhibitors bind to plasma enzymes and inactivate them.

7.1. Intrinsic Controls

For the initiating step of contact activation, conversion of HFa to HFf by kallikrein can serve to limit coagulation, since factor XI is activated on the surface only by HFa (Bouma and Griffin, 1979; Ratnoff et al., 1961). HFf can continue kinin formation in plasma until extrinsic controls take effect. It is also well known that excessive digestion of HMW-kininogen by kallikrein leads to progressive destruction of the light chain (Chan et al., 1979) and loss of coagulant activity. A recent abstract suggests that factor XIa can also digest HMW-kininogen and, although its bradykinin-forming capability is minimal compared with kallikrein, it may digest the cleaved HMW-kininogen light chain and thereby limit its cofactor activity (Scott et al., 1984). Such mechanisms, i.e., destruction of coagulation cofactors to slow the reaction rates of their associated enzymes, occur in other steps of coagulation. Factors V and VIII are susceptible to proteolytic digestion and, after activation, further cleavage inactivates them. Multiple enzymes may function in this capacity. Thrombin itself can continue to digest factors V and VIII and inactivate them. A fifth relatively new vitamin K-dependent enzyme, however, may be the critical physiologic factor, called protein C (Stenflo, 1976). Protein C is activated by thrombin (Kisiel, 1979), and activated protein C cleaves and inactivates factors Va and VIIIa (Marler et al., 1982b). An endothelial cell cofactor (thrombomodulin) has also been described (Esmon and Owen, 1981), which binds to thrombin at the site of vascular injury and modifies the enzyme, so that it no longer activates platelets or clots fibrinogen but augments protein C activation 1000-fold. In some circumstances, factor Va can also serve as a thrombin cofactor for protein C activation (Salem et al., 1984). In fibrinolytic states, measurable quantities of plasmin circulate, often in addition to activated protein C. Together they can deplete factors V and VIII, as has been described in disorders associated with disseminated intravascular coagulation (see also Chapter 4).

Intrinsic controls also exist for the fibrinolytic cascade. At least one plasma protein, histidine-rich glycoprotein, binds to the site on plasminogen required for attachment to fibrinogen or fibrin (Lijen et al., 1980). This serves to limit plasminogen activation by tissue plasminogen activator. Recently, thrombospondin, the secreted platelet factor that has a role in platelet–platelet interactions, has been shown to bind fibrinogen and histidine-rich glycoprotein (Leung and Nachman, 1984).

7.2. Extrinsic Controls

The major plasma inhibitors of each enzyme of the coagulation cascade are summarized in Table I. The C1 inactivator (C1 INH), the enzyme initially described as the inhibitor of the activated first component of complement, is the main inhibitor of HFa or HFf in plasma (Forbes et al., 1970; Schreiber et al., 1972). The same protein is one of two inhibitors of plasma kallikrein (Gigli et al., 1970). Of particular interest is the disease hereditary angioedema, in which severe potentially fatal episodes of swelling occur due to absence of functional C1 INH. The swelling may be mediated by bradykinin (Fields et al., 1983), but further activation of the intrinsic coagulation cascade is not seen, presumably

Table I. Inhibitors of Proteases of the Coagulation,
Fibrinolytic, and Kinin-Forming Cascades

Enzyme	Main inhibitors
HFa, HFf	Cl⁻INH
Kallikrein	Cl⁻INH, α_2 macroglobulin
Factor XIa	α_1 Antitrypsin, Cl INH
Factor IXa	AT III
Factor Xa	AT III
Tissue factor-factor VII (factor VIIa)	Uncertain
Thrombin	AT III, heparin cofactor II
Plasmin	α_2 Antiplasmin, α_2 Macroglobulin

due to the effect of other inhibitors acting later in the cascade. The second kallikrein inhibitor in plasma is α_2-macroglobulin (Harpel, 1970). While C1 INH binds to the active site of enzymes and destroys their activity against any substrate, the effect of α_2-macroglobulin may be steric. Thus the kallikrein–β_2-macroglobulin complex can still hydrolyze low-molecular-weight synthetic substrates but retains only 1–2% proteolytic activity on protein substrates. Together C1 INH and α_2-macroglobulin account for more than 90% of plasma kallikrein inhibitory activity and are approximately equipotent. The main plasma inhibitor of factor XIa is α_1-antitrypsin (Heck and Kaplan, 1974; Scott et al., 1982); other inhibitors are C1 INH (Forbes et al., 1970) and antithrombin III (heparin cofactor) (Damas et al., 1973).

Most coagulation proteins, with the possible exception of factor VIIa, are inhibited by antithrombin III. ATIII, the major plasma inhibitor is activated by interaction with heparin; the heparin–ATIII complex interacts with coagulation factors to form a covalent bond at the active site serine residue and inactivates them. Thus, in the presence of heparin or similar substances, ATIII inactivates factors IXa and Xa and thrombin (Damas et al., 1973; Harpel and Rosenberg, 1976). For thrombin inactivation by ATIII, heparin has been shown to bind both to thrombin and antithrombin III affinity columns (Olson and Shore, 1982). Then, as the stable thrombin–ATIII complex forms, heparin is released (Pletcher and Nelsestuen, 1983), thereby recycling heparin. The in vivo heparin analogue may be heparan sulfate exposed at sites of connective tissue injury (Busch and Owen, 1982; Khoory et al., 1980). A second protein, termed heparin cofactor II, is also activatable by heparin or by dermatan sulfate but it is selective and seems to inhibit only thrombin (Tollefson et al., 1983).

Plasmin is inhibited first by α_2-antiplasmin (Collen, 1976; Moroi and Aoki, 1976; Mullertz and Clemmensen, 1976), which accounts for most of the rapid inhibitory activity of plasma, and then by α_2-macroglobulin. α_2-Antiplasmin binds to fibrin, as do plasminogen and tissue plasminogen activator. Thus, all the elements to form plasmin and to inactivate it seem to be confined locally.

Recently, a separate plasma inhibitor of tissue plasminogen activator was described (Kruithof et al., 1983; Verheijen et al., 1983).

8. Microvascular Permeability and Extravascular Fibrin Deposition

Under conditions of normal (i.e., low) vascular permeability to plasma proteins, levels of extravascular fibrinogen are negligible. Therefore, tissue fibrinogen levels, and probably levels of other plasma clotting factors as well, must be increased multifold if significant fibrin is to be deposited in the extravascular space. Such increased microvascular permeability is evident in tumors, at sites of inflammation, and in injury.

Although considerable attention in the literature has been devoted to cell-associated procoagulants that can initiate coagulation, changes in microvascular permeability may actually be the most important factor in initiating extravascular coagulation in most tissues. This fact stems from recent experiments that demonstrated that increased microvascular permeability alone led to maximal levels of local extravascular coagulation in several tissues, including the skin, subcutis, peritoneal wall, and eye (Dvorak et al., 1985). Injection of histamine or bradykinin into the skin of normal guinea pigs led to substantial, local, dose-dependent vascular leakage of plasma proteins including fibrinogen. Fibrin deposition could not be increased further by including tissue factor or even thrombin in the histamine injection (Dvorak et al., 1985). Nearly three-fourths of this extravasated fibrinogen was clotted and transglutaminated to crosslinked fibrin within a period of 20 min. Conclusive evidence for the crosslinked nature of the fibrin deposited was obtained from autoradiograms of sodium dodecyl sulfate-polyacrylamide gel electrophoresis (SDS-PAGE) gels run on tissue extracts; these revealed extensive γ-γ-dimers and α-chain polymerization, the characteristic signature of crosslinked fibrin. Similar results were obtained when a drop of histamine was placed in the eye, thereby avoiding even that minimal amount of trauma associated with an intradermal injection. Extravascular clotting in both the skin and eye could be largely inhibited either by local or systemic anticoagulation.

The extravascular localization of tissue fibrin as demonstrated by immunohistochemistry and electron microscopy was of particular interest. Fibrin was concentrated in localized deposits centered about individual fixed connective tissue cells, fibroblasts, and histiocytes; by electron microscopy, fibrin was found in intimate association with the surface of these cells. From this pericellular location, fibrin extended outward between collagen bundles of the connective tissue, forming a three-dimensional gel.

These data suggest that procoagulants are present in many normal tissues and in an active, or easily activated, form (see Section 2.1). Thus, they are available and ready for immediate action should vascular leakage or disruption (as in injury) occur. Apparently procoagulant is associated with the surfaces of tissue fibroblasts and histiocytes. The nature of the procoagulant(s) associated with these tissue cells has not been investigated; however, by analogy with tumor cells and macrophages, it is likely that the specific procoagulants represented include tissue factor and a surface for generating active prothrombinase. Taken together, these data argue strongly that increased microvascular permeability (see Chapter 5), rather than special or increased procoagulants, is the rate-limiting step in extravascular coagulation and that normal tissues contain more than sufficient amounts of procoagulants to clot extravasated fibrinogen.

8.1. Role of Extravascular Coagulation in Wound Healing

Extravascular fibrin deposits may have important biologic consequences. For example, by forming a water-trapping gel, extravascular fibrin deposits cause the induration characteristic of delayed hypersensitivity reactions and contribute importantly to the brain and spinal cord damage associated with autoimmune encephalomyelitis (Paterson, 1976). In addition, extravascular clotting and associated fibrinolysis have been implicated in depressing the immune response (Plow et al., 1976), in enhanced local blood vessel permeability (Gerdin and Saldeen, 1978), in chemotaxis (Richardson et al., 1976), and in tumor growth, angiogenesis (Clark et al., 1977), desmoplasia, and metastasis.

The fibrin gel is the substrate transformed over time into the vascular collagenous matrix that constitutes the healing wound. Transformation of a provisional fibrin matrix into mature stroma requires several sets of cellular events: (1) replication of adjacent fibroblasts and endothelial cells, mediated at least in part by platelet-secreted products (see Chapters 2 and 9); (2) cell migration into the fibrin gel including macrophages, fibroblasts, and blood vessels (see Chapters 8, 10, 12, and 14); (3) degradation of the provisional gel matrix (see Chapter 18); and (4) replacement of provisional matrix with newly synthesized stromal components such as collagen (see Chapters 17, 19, and 20). Cell invasion of the fibrin gel deserves further comment.

8.1.1. Cell Migratory Events

It is well known that neutrophils, macrophages, and later fibroblasts and endothelial cells migrate into the fibrin gel that fills the wound defect. Indeed, older studies indicate that fibrinogen degradation products are chemotactic for inflammatory cells (Stecher and Sorkin, 1972; Richardson et al., 1976), experiments that now need to be repeated in view of the fact that the fibrinogen employed in these studies was almost certainly contaminated with fibronectin and perhaps other proteins with potential chemotactic activities.

Recent studies of inflammatory cell migration in fibrin gels strongly support the view that fibrin provides a favorable substrate for inflammatory cell migration (Ciano et al., 1986). Cell migration has been extensively studied in vitro but almost entirely on artificial substrates. Neutrophils, macrophages, and fibroblasts migrate through nitrocellulose or other filters in Boyden chambers or other assay systems. Curiously, however, little attention has been paid to cell migration through the connective tissue matrices through which cells must move in the living organism if they are to arrive at sites of tissue injury. Recent experiments by Ciano et al. (1986) evaluated macrophage and neutrophil migration through fibrin gels of varying composition. Such experiments are particularly relevant because inflammatory cells must penetrate just such gels in zones of inflammation or tissue injury in vivo. Moreover, the biochemical nature of fibrin and its range of concentrations have been defined in two important pathologic processes: malignant tumors and delayed hypersensitivity reactions. Therefore, fibrin gels could be prepared in vitro that matched, at least to some extent, the gels deposited in vivo.

Fibrin gels γ-chain crosslinked and impregnated in nitrocellulose filters provided a superior matrix for macrophage migration as compared with filters alone. As fibrin concentrations were increased above 5 mg/ml, however, the migration advantage afforded at lower fibrin concentrations was progressively lost, and, above 7 mg/ml, fibrin provided a total barrier to macrophages. This barrier effect was attributable to the fibrin gel structure in that comparable amounts of soluble proteins actually enhanced cell migration. However, it must be remembered that the fibrin deposited in tissues in vivo demonstrates extensive α-chain polymerization in addition to γ-chain dimerization. In such gels, macrophage migration was inhibited at fibrin concentrations as low as 3 mg/ml and was totally stopped at concentrations of 5 mg/ml. Other properties of the fibrin gel, such as elasticity, solubility, and resistance to lysis, have been previously found to be more dependent on α-chain than on γ-chain crosslinking.

Thrombin concentration also played an important role in determining macrophage migration in fibrin gels. Independent of crosslinking, macrophage migration was optimal at thrombin concentrations of 1–3 U/ml and was significantly impeded at concentrations that were significantly lower or higher.

These data have obvious relevance to entry of neutrophils and macrophages into the fibrin gels found in wounds or sites of inflammation. In developing reactions of cellular immunity, fibrin concentrations of 0.25–3.0 mg/ml are typical. These concentrations consistently facilitate macrophage migration in the in vitro assay and therefore presumably facilitate the entry of macrophages in vivo. At later intervals and in more mature reactions, however, concentrations of fibrin may approach 7 mg/ml, approximately twice the plasma fibrinogen concentration; under these conditions, fibrin would be expected to impose an impenetrable barrier to macrophage migration.

That macrophages can migrate through any of the fibrin gels employed in these experiments is remarkable, given their small, highly uniform pore size

(0.3–2.8 μm) (Blomback and Okada, 1982). Guinea pig peritoneal macrophages (diameter approximately 15 μm) do not migrate effectively through cellulose nitrate filters of pore size below 5 μm (Senior *et al.*, 1980). How, then, do these cells migrate through the much smaller pores of fibrin gels? In addition to the radical changes in cell shape associated with macrophage migration through filters, two additional possibilities can be imagined. Macrophages could push apart relatively elastic fibrin gel fibrils, effectively increasing pore diameter to permit cell passage and/or dissolve the gel locally (Reich, 1975; Unkeless *et al.*, 1974; Danø *et al.*, 1985). Neither of these strategies would be available to macrophages migrating through untreated micropore filters composed of relatively rigid undigestable fibers. Gel pore size alone is clearly not the only determinant of macrophage migration in fibrin. Gels of comparable appearance by transmission electron microscopy (TEM), but prepared with 1 or 10 U/ml thrombin, permitted strikingly different amounts of macrophage migration. Physical properties of the fibrin gel (e.g., fiber diameter, elasticity, number of crosslinks) may be determinative under such conditions.

That fibrin gels of appropriate composition may not only permit, but even facilitate, macrophage migration is of considerable interest. Fibronectin content is apparently of lesser importance, since depletion of fibronectin did not affect migration (Ciano *et al.*, 1986). The mechanisms of fibrin facilitation are unknown but presumably reflect a positive interaction between the macrophage surface and the fibrin matrix. A fraction of guinea pig peritoneal exudate macrophages express surface receptors for fibrinogen/fibrin (Colvin and Dvorak, 1975; Gonda and Shainoff, 1982; Sherman and Lee, 1977). Macrophages exhibiting surface-associated fibrinogen/fibrin presumably have receptors that are partly or completely filled. It would be of considerable importance to know whether macrophages with free or filled fibrinogen/fibrin receptors migrate differently in micropore filters or in fibrin gels.

With regard to cell migration, a large number of protein factors has been identified that are potentially chemotactic for inflammatory and connective tissue cells in healing wounds (reviewed in Clark, 1983; Postlethwaite, 1983). These include components of the gel matrix itself, degradation fragments of that matrix, and products of tumor cells and lymphocytes. Thus, fibronectin is chemotactic for endothelium and its plasmin degradation products for several types of inflammatory cells. A surprisingly large number of factors are reportedly chemotactic for fibroblasts; including lymphokines, a complement fragment, native collagens of types I–V, fibronectin, and their respective proteolytic digestion fragments and PDGF. Further work will be needed to sort out the respective roles and relative importance of these several factors in stimulating and regulating cell migration and division. There are almost too many candidate mediators for comfort (also see Chapter 8).

Platelets play a major role in healing wounds, participating importantly in hemostasis and provisional matrix generation (see Chapter 1). Platelets may also be important at later stages of wound healing, since they contain potent mitogens and chemoattractants for fibroblasts (see Chapter 9).

8.1.2. Synthesis of New Stroma

Ingress of macrophages, fibroblasts, and capillaries transforms the fibrin–fibronectin provisional matrix deposited in wounds into a highly cellular, highly vascularized tissue called granulation tissue (Hunt, 1980). Granulation-like tissue acquires progressively more collagen, loses its cellularity and vascularity, and ultimately develops into scar tissue.

Recently, the structural proteins that accumulate in wound stroma were analyzed by immunohistochemistry (Clark *et al.*, 1982; Kurkinen *et al.*, 1980). Initially present in substantial amounts, fibrin stromal staining declined rapidly over a matter of days and was no longer detectable by 3 weeks in normally healing wounds induced in guinea pigs with a standard biopsy punch. Staining for fibronectin increased initially in early phases of wound healing but then declined precipitously. Loss of fibrin and fibronectin staining from wounds was accompanied by increasing deposits of type I and III collagen. In the few instances in which this has been studied in detail, relatively more type III collagen is deposited at earlier stages (granulation tissue), and relatively less is found in fully developed scar tissue (Bailey *et al.*, 1975; Kurkinen *et al.*, 1980). However, at all stages, type I collagen is more abundant than type III. It is generally agreed that the interstitial collagens of healing wounds are synthesized by fibroblasts that migrate into the fibrin–fibronectin stroma. In the case of tumors undergoing an analogous form of wound healing termed desmoplasia, collagen was often deposited initially in intimate association with fibrin strands (Harris *et al.*, 1982), and it would not be surprising if a similar association existed in normal wound healing. The reader is also referred to Chapters 15 and 20.

Epithelial cells synthesize type IV collagen and other basement membrane components required during the course of repair of epithelial defects. Fibrin (and fibronectin) may be deposited here as a provisional basement membrane that generally comes to be replaced by mature basement membrane components (Clark *et al.*, 1982; Repesh *et al.*, 1981) (see also Chapters 15 and 20).

8.1.3. Regulation of Mature Stroma Deposition

Little is known about the mechanisms that regulate the synthesis and deposition of mature stromal matrix or the subsequent remodeling events that lead finally to dense scar tissue in wounds. Recent experiments from our laboratory promise to shed important new light on these events as well as on the earlier events of cell migration (Dvorak *et al.*, 1987). Porous chambers, filled with fibrin or other contents, were implanted in the subcutaneous space of experimental animals. Chambers filled with crosslinked fibrin consistently induced brisk influx of macrophages, fibroblasts, and capillaries; chamber contents were progressively transformed into granulation tissue over the course of a few days. By contrast, chambers filled with agarose, with crosslinked fibrin supplemented with an angiogeneis inhibitor (Feinberg and Beebe, 1983), or with type I collagen elicited little or no angiogenic or fibroblastic response. Depletion of fibronectin did not affect the outcome. These data indicate that crosslinked fibrin itself, or perhaps certain of its degradation products, is critical to stroma generation, a finding with important implications for understanding the pathogenesis of wound healing. Of interest, platelets were not required for mature stroma generation in these chambers. Thus, platelets may be essential only at early stages of stroma formation, playing an important role in generating extravascular fibrin matrix. Thereafter, later steps of angiogenesis and fibroplasia are apparently able to proceed autonomously, independent of platelets.

9. Conclusions

Wound healing begins with an exudate of plasma fibrinogen, fibronectin, and other clotting proteins; platelets and other cellular elements that are normally confined to the vasculature may participate as well. Release of bradykinin by the intrinsic coagulation cascade is one of many important vasoactive mediators responsible for the extravasation of plasma products into an injured site. Extravasated fibrinogen is clotted and is crosslinked to itself and to fibronectin, inserting in the tissues an insoluble, water-binding gel. The conversion of fibrinogen to polymerized fibrin and clot deposition must be finely controlled, or tissue regeneration will not proceed properly. The extravascular fibrin–fibronectin clot serves as a provisional stroma, providing a matrix for macrophage, fibroblast, and new capillary migration. The fibrin–fibronectin gel is transformed to granulation tissue and eventually to dense relatively acellular collagen (scar tissue).

ACKNOWLEDGMENT. R.A.F. was supported by grant AM-31514 from the National Institutes of Health. H.F.D. was supported by grants CA-40624 and CA-28471 from the U.S. Public Health Service.

References

Allen, R. A., and Pepper, D. C., 1981, Isolation and properties of human vascular plasminogen activator, Thromb. Haemost. **45**:43–50.

Bailey, A., Sims, T., Le Lous, M., and Bazin, S., 1975, Collagen polymorphism in experimental granulation tissue, Biochem. Biophys. Res. Commun. **66**:1160–1165.

Bevilacqua, M. P., Pober, J. S., Wheeler, M. E., Cotran, R. S., and Gimbrone, M. A., Jr., 1985, Interleukin 1 activation of vascular endothelium. Effects on procoagulant activity and leukocyte adhesion, Am. J. Pathol. **121**:393–403.

Binder, B. R., Spragg, J., and Austen, K. F., 1979, Purification and characterization of human vascular plasminogen activator derived from blood vessel pertusates, J. Biol. Chem. **254**:1998–2003.

Black, P. H., 1980, Shedding from the cell surface of normal and cancer cells, Adv. Cancer Res. **32**:75–199.

Blomback, B., and Okada, M., 1982, Fibrin gel structure and clotting time, Thromb. Res. **25**:51–70.

Blomback, B., Hessel, B., Hagg, D., and Thirkildsen, L., 1978, A two-step fibrinogen fibrin transition in blood coagulation, Nature (Lond.) **275**:501–505.

Bock, P. E., and Shore, J. P., 1983, Protein interactions in contact activation of blood coagulation. Characterization of a fluorescein-labeled human high molecular weight kininogen light chain as a probe, *J. Biol. Chem.* **258**:15079–15083.

Bockisch, V. A., and Muller-Eberhard, H. J., 1970, Anaphylatoxin inactivator of human plasma: Its isolation and characterization as a carboxypeptidase, *J. Clin. Invest.* **49**:2427–2436.

Bouma, B. N., and Griffin, J. N., 1979, Human blood coagulation Factor XI. Purification, properties, and mechanism of activation by activated Factor XII, *J. Biol. Chem.* **252**:6432–6437.

Broze, G. J., Jr., and Majerus, P. W., 1980, Purification and properties of human coagulation Factor VII, *J. Biol. Chem.* **255**:1242–1247.

Budzynski, A. Z., Marder, V. J., and Schainoff, J. R., 1974, Structure of plasmic degradation products of human fibrinogen. Fibrinopeptide and polypeptide chain analysis, *J. Biol. Chem.* **249**:2294–2302.

Busch, C., and Owen, W. G., 1982, Identification *in vitro* of an endothelial cell surface cofactor for antithrombin. III. Parallel studies with isolated perfused rat hearts and microcarrier cultures of bovine endothelium, *J. Clin. Invest.* **69**:726–729.

Calafat, J., Hilgers, J., Van Blitterswijk, W. J., Verbeet, M., and Hageman, P. C., 1976, Antibody-induced modulation and shedding of mammary tumor virus antigens on the surfaces of GR ascites leukemia cells as compared with normal antigens, *J. Natl. Cancer Inst.* **56**:1019–1029.

Carr, J., Van De Water, L., Senger, D., Dvorak, A. M., and Dvorak, H. F., 1985, Macrophage procoagulants and microvascular permeability: Roles in the extravascular coagulation of cellular immunity, in: *Mononuclear Phagocytes: Characteristics, Physiology and Function* (R. van Furth, ed.), pp. 713–720, Martinus Nijhoff, Boston.

Chan, J. Y. C., Movat, H. Z., and Burrowes, C. E., 1979, High molecular weight kininogen: Its ability to correct the clotting of kininogen deficiency plasma after cleavage of bradykinin by plasma kallikrein, plasmin, or trypsin, *Thromb. Res.* **14**:817–824.

Ciano, P., Colvin, R., Dvorak, A., McDonagh, J., and Dvorak, H., 1986, Macrophage migration in fibrin gel matrices, *Lab. Invest.* **54**:62–129.

Clark, J. M., Altman, G., and Fromowitz, F. B., 1977, Basophil hypersensitivity response in rabbits, *Infect. Immun.* **15**:305–312.

Clark, R. A. F., 1983, Fibronectin in the skin, *J. Invest. Dermatol.* **81**:475–479.

Clark, R. A. F., Lanigan, J. M., DellaPelle, P., Manseau, E., Dvorak, H. F., and Colvin, R. B., 1982, Fibronectin and fibrin provide a provisional matrix for epidermal cell migration during wound reepithelialization, *J. Invest. Dermatol.* **79**:264–269.

Clark, R. A. F., Horsburgh, C. R., Hoffman, A. A., Dvorak, H. F., Mosesson, M. W., and Colvin, R. B., 1984, Fibronectin deposition in delayed-type hypersensitivity. Reactions of normals and a patient with afibrinogenemia, *J. Clin. Invest.* **74**:1011–1016.

Cochrane, C. G., Wuepper, K. D., Aiken, B. S., Revak, S. D., and Spiegelberg, H. L., 1972, The interaction of Hageman Factor and immune complexes, *J. Clin. Invest.* **51**:2736–2745.

Cole, E. R., and Bachmann, F. W., 1977, Purification of a plasminogen activator from pig heart, *J. Biol. Chem.* **252**:3729–3737.

Collen, D., 1976, Identification and some properties of a new fast-reacting plasmin inhibitor in human plasma, *Eur. J. Biochem.* **69**:209–216.

Colman, R. W., 1969, Activation of plasminogen by human plasma kallikrein, *Biochem. Biophys. Res. Commun.* **35**:273–279.

Colucci, M., Balconi, G., Lorenzet, R., Pietra, A., Locati, D., Donati, M. B., and Semeraro, N., 1983, Cultured human endothelial cells generate tissue factor in response to endotoxin, *J. Clin. Invest.* **71**:1893–1896.

Colvin, R. B., and Dvorak, H. F., 1975, Fibrinogen/fibrin on the surface of macrophages: Detection, distribution, binding requirements, and possible role in macrophage adherence phenomena, *J. Exp. Med.* **142**:1377–1390.

Colvin, R. B., Mosesson, M. W., and Dvorak, H. F., 1979, Delayed-type hypersensitivity skin reaction in congenital afibrinogenemia lack fibrin deposition and induration, *J. Clin. Invest.* **63**:1302–1306.

Curatolo, L., Colucci, M., Cambini, A. L., Poggi, A., Morasca, L., Donati, M. B., and Semeraro, N., 1979, Evidence that cells from experimental tumors can activate coagulation Factor X, *Br. J. Cancer* **40**:228–233.

Damas, P. S., Hicks, M., and Rosenberg, R. D., 1973, Anticoagulant activity of heparin, *Nature (Lond.)* **246**:355–357.

Danø, K., Andreasen, P. A., Grondahl-Hansen, J., Kristensen, P., Nielsen, L. S., and Skriver, L., 1985, Plasminogen activators, tissue degradation, and cancer, *Adv. Cancer Res.* **44**:139–266.

DiScipio, R. G., 1982, The activation of the alternative pathway C3 convertase by human plasma killikrein, *Immunology* **45**:587–595.

Dunn, J. T., and Kaplan, A. P., 1982, Formation and structure of human Hageman Factor fragments, *J. Clin. Invest.* **70**:627–631.

Dunn, J. T., Silverberg, M., and Kaplan, A. P., 1982, The cleavage and formation of activated Hageman factor by autodigestion and by kallikrein, *J. Biol. Chem.* **257**:1779–1784.

Dvorak, H. F., Harvey, S. V., Estrella, P., Brown, L. F., McDonagh, J., and Dvorak, A. M., 1987, Fibrin Containing Gels Induce Angiogenesis: Implications for Tumor Stroma Generation and Wound Healing, *Lab. Investig.* (in press).

Dvorak, H. F., Quay, S. C., Orenstein, N. S., Dvorak, A. M., Hahn, P., Bitzer, A. M., and Carvalho, A. C., 1981, Tumor shedding and coagulation, *Science* **212**:923–924.

Dvorak, H. F., Senger, D., and Dvorak, A., 1983a, Fibrin as a component of the tumor stroma: Origins and biological significance, *Cancer Metast. Rev.* **2**:41–73.

Dvorak, H. F., Van DeWater, L., Bitzer, A. M., Dvorak, A. M., Anderson, D., Harvey, V. S., Bach, R., Davis, G. L., DeWolf, W., Carvalho, A. C. A., 1983b, Procoagulant activity associated with plasma membrane vesicles shed by cultured tumor cells, *Cancer Res.* **43**:4434–4442.

Dvorak, H., Senger, D., Harvey, V., and McDonagh, J., 1985, Regulation of extravascular coagulation by microvascular permeability, *Science* **227**:1059–1061.

Edgington, T. S., Helin, H., Gregory, S. A., Levy, G., Fair, D. S., and Schwartz, B. S., 1985, Cellular pathways and signals for the induction of biosynthesis of initiators of the coagulation protease cascade by cells of the monocyte lineage, in: *Mononuclear Phagocytes: Characteristics, Physiology, and Functions* (R. Van Furth, ed.), pp. 687–696, Martinus Nijhoff, Boston.

Edwards, R. L., and Rickles, F. R., 1978, Delayed hypersensitivity in man: Effects of systemic anticoagulation, *Science* **200**:541–543.

Edwards, R. L., and Rickles, F. R., 1980, The role of human T cells (and T cell products) for monocyte tissue factor generation, *J. Immunol.* **125**:606–609.

Erdos, E. C., and Sloane, E. M., 1962, An enzyme in human plasma that inactivated bradykinin and kallidins, *Biochem. Pharmacol.* **11**:585–592.

Esmon, C. T., and Jackson, C. M., 1974, The conversion of prothrombin to thrombin IV. The function of the fragment 2 region during activation in the presence of Factor V, *J. Biol. Chem.* **249**:7791–7797.

Esmon, C. T., and Owen, W., 1981, Identification of an endothelial cell cofactor for thrombin-catalyzed activation of protein C, *Proc. Natl. Acad. Sci. USA* **78**:2249–2252.

Esmon, C. T., Suttie, J. W., and Jackson, C. M., 1975, The functional significance of vitamin K action. Difference in phospholipid binding between normal and abnormal prothrombin, *J. Biol. Chem.* **250**:4095–4099.

Feinberg, R., and Beebe, D., 1983, Hyaluronate in vasculogenesis, *Science* **220**:1177–1179.

Fields, T. R., Gerardi, E. N., Ghebrehiwet, B., Bennett, R. S., Lawley, T. J., Hall, R. P., Plotz, P., Karsh, J. R., Frank, M. M., and Hamburger, M. I., 1983, Reticuloendothelial system Fc receptor function in rheumatoid arthritis, *J. Rheumatol.* **10**:550–557.

Forbes, C. O., Pensky, J., and Ratnoff, O. D., 1970, Inhibition of activated Hageman factor and activated plasma thromboplastin antecedent by purified C inactivator, *J. Lab. Clin. Med.* **76**:809–815.

Fujikawa, K., and McMullen, B. A., 1983, Amino acid sequence of human Factor XIIa, *J. Biol. Chem.* **258**:10924–10933.

Fujimoto, T., O'Hara, S., and Hawiger, J., 1982, Thrombin-induced exposure and prostacyclin inhibition of the receptor for Factor VIII/Von Willebrand Factor on human platelets, *J. Clin. Invest.* **69**:1212–1222.

Gartner, T. K., Williams, D. C., Minion, F. C., and Phillips, D. R., 1978, Thombin-induced platelet aggregation is mediated by a platelet plasma membrane-bound lectin, *Science* **200**:1281–1283.

Geczy, C. L., and Hopper, K. E., 1981, A mechanism of migration inhibition in delayed-type hypersensitivity reactions. II. Lymphokines promote procoagulant activity of macrophages *in vitro*, *J. Immunol.* **126**:1059–1069.

Gerdin, B., and Saldeen, T., 1978, Effect of fibrin degradation products on microvascular permeability, *Thromb. Res.* **13**:995–1006.

Gigli, I., Mason, J. W., Colman, R. W., and Austen, K. F., 1970, Interaction of plasma kallikrein with the C1 inhibitor, *J. Immunol.* **104**:574–581.

Ginsberg, M. H., Jaques, B., Cochrane, C. G., and Griffin, J. H., 1980, Urate crystal dependent cleavage of Hageman factor in plasma and synovial fluid, *J. Lab. Clin. Med.* **45**:497–506.

Goldsmith, G., Saito, H., and Ratnoff, O., 1978, The activatin of plasminogen by Hageman Factor (Factor XII) and Hageman Factor fragments, *J. Clin. Invest.* **62**:54–60.

Gonda, S. R., and Shainoff, J. R., 1982, Adsorptive endocytosis of fibrin monomer by macrophages: Evidence of a receptor for the amino terminus of the fibrin alpha-chain, *Proc. Natl. Acad. Sci. USA* **79**:4565–4569.

Granelli-Piperno, P., Vassailli, J. D., and Reich, E., 1977, Secretion of plasminogen activation by human polymorphonuclear leukocytes: Modulation by glucocorticoids and other effectors, *J. Exp. Med.* **146**:1693–1706.

Greengard, J. S., and Griffin, J. H., 1984, Receptors for high molecular weight kininogen on stimulated washed human platelets, *Biochemistry* **23**:6863–6869.

Greengard, J. S., Heeb, M. J., Ersdal, E., Walsh, P. N., and Griffin, J. H., 1986, Binding of Factor XI to washed human platelets, *Biochemistry* **25**:3884–3890.

Greenquist, A. C., and Colman, R. W., 1975, Bovine Factor V: a calcium containing metalloprotein, *Blood* **46**:769–782.

Griffin, J. H., 1978, Role of surface in surface-dependent activation of Hageman factor (blood coagulation Factor XII), *Proc. Natl. Acad. Sci. USA* **75**:1998–2002.

Griffin, J. H., and Beretta, G., 1979, Molecular mechanisms of surface-dependent activation of Hageman Factor (Factor XII), *Adv. Exp. Med. Biol.* **120**:39–51.

Griffin, J. H., and Cochrane, C. G., 1976, Mechanism for the involvement of HMW-kininogen in surface-dependent reactions of Hageman factor, *Proc. Natl. Acad. Sci. USA* **73**:2559–2563.

Grinnell, F., Billingham, R. E., and Burgess, L., 1981, Distribution of fibronectin during wound healing *in vivo*, *J. Invest. Dermatol.* **76**:181–189.

Habal, F. M., Movat, H. Z., and Burrowes, C. E., 1974, Isolation of two functionally different kinonogens from human plasma: Separation from proteinase inhibitors and interaction with plasma kallikrein, *Biochem. Pharmacol.* **23**:2291–2302.

Harpel, P. C., 1970, Human plasma alpha$_2$-macroglobulin. An inhibitor of plasma kallikrein, *J. Exp. Med.* **132**:329–352.

Harpel, P. C., and Rosenberg, R. D., 1976, Alpha$_2$-macroglobulin and anti-thrombin–heparin cofactor: Modulators of hemostatic and inflammatory reactions, *Prog. Hemost. Thromb.* **3**:145–189.

Harris, N., Dvorak, A., Smith, J., and Dvorak, H., 1982, Fibrin deposits in Hodgkin's disease, *Am. J. Pathol.* **108**:119–129.

Heck, L. W., and Kaplan, A. P., 1974, Substrates of Hageman factor I. Isolation and characterization of human Factor XI (PTA) and inhibition of the activated enzyme by α_1 antitrypsin, *J. Exp. Med.* **140**:1615–1630.

Heimark, R. L., Kurachi, K., Fujikawa, K., and Davie, E. N., 1980, Surface activation of blood coagulation, fibrinolysis, and kinin formation, *Nature (Lond.)* **286**:456–460.

Hoyer, L. W., 1981, The Factor VIII complex: Structure and function, *Blood* **58**:1–11.

Hultin, M. B., 1982, Role of human Factor VIII in Factor X activation, *J. Clin. Invest.* **69**:950–958.

Hunt, T. K., 1980, *Wound Healing and Wound Infection*, Appleton-Century-Crofts, New York.

Kadish, J., Wenc, K., and Dvorak, H. F., 1983, Tissue factor activity of normal and neoplastic cells: Quantitation and species specificity, *J. Natl. Cancer Inst.* **70**:551–557.

Kane, W., Lindhout, M. J., Jackson, C. M., and Majerus, P. W., 1980, Factor Va dependent binding of Factor Xa to platelets, *J. Biol. Chem.* **255**:1170–1174.

Kaplan, A. P., and Austen, K. F., 1970, A prealbumin activator of prekallikrein, *J. Immunol.* **105**:802–811.

Kaplan, A. P., and Austen, K. F., 1971, A prealbumin activator of prekallikrein. II. Derivation of activators of prekallikrein from active Hageman factor by digestion with plasmin, *J. Exp. Med.* **133**:696–712.

Kaplan, A. P., Kay, A. P., and Austen, K. F., 1972, A prealbumin activator of kallikrein. III. Appearance of chemotactic activity in human neutrophils by the conversion of human prekallikrein to kallikrein, *J. Exp. Med.* **135**:81–97.

Kato, H., Han, Y. N., Iwanaga, S., Suzuki, T., and Komiya, M., 1976, Bovine plasma HMW and LMW kinonogens. Structural differences between heavy and light chains derived from the kinin-free proteins, *J. Biochem.* **80**:1299–1311.

Kellermeyer, R. W., and Breckenridge, R. T., 1965, The inflammatory process in acute gouty arthritis. I. Activation of Hageman factor by sodium urate crystals. *J. La. Clin. Med.* **65**:307–315.

Khoory, M. S., Nesheim, M. E., Bowie, E. J. W., and Mann, K. G., 1980, Circulating heparan sulfate proteoglycan anticoagulant from a patient with plasma cell disorder, *J. Clin. Invest.* **653**:666–674.

Kisiel, W., 1979, Human plasma protein C. Isolation, characlerization, and mechanism of activation by thrombin, *J. Clin. Invest.* **64**:761–769.

Kitamura, N., Takagaki, Y., Furoto, S., Tanaka, T., Nawa, H., and Nakanishi, S. A., 1983, A single gene for bovine high molecular weight and low molecular weight kininogens, *Nature (Lond.)* **305**:545–549.

Kruithof, E. K. O., Ransijn, A., Tren-Thang, C., and Bachmann, F., 1983, Characteristics of a fast-acting inhibitor of plasminogen activator in human plasma, *Thromb. Haemost.* **50**:193 (abst 592).

Kurkinen, M., Vaheri, A., Roberts, P. J., and Stenman, S., 1980, Sequential appearance of fibronectin and collagen in experimental granulation tissue, *Lab. Invest.* **43**:47–51.

Larson, A. E., and Suttie, J. W., 1978, Vitamin K-dependent carboxylase: Evidence for a hydroperoxide intermediate in the reaction, *Proc. Natl. Acad. Sci. USA* **75**:5413–5416.

Leung, L. L. K., and Nachman, R. L., 1984, Complex formation of platelet thrombospondin with fibrinogen, *J. Clin. Invest.* **73**:5–12.

Lijen, H. R., Hoylaerts, M., and Collen, D., 1980, Isolation and characterization of a human plasma protein with affinity for the lysine binding sites in plasminogen, *J. Biol. Chem.* **255**:10214–10222.

Lipscomb, M. S., and Walsh, P. N., 1979, Human platelets and Factor XI. Localization in platelet membranes of Factor XI-like activity and its functional distinction from plasma Factor XI, *J. Clin. Invest.* **63**:1006–1019.

Lorand, L., 1972, The fibrin-stabilizing factor system of blood plasma, *Ann. N.Y. Acad. Sci.* **202**:6–30.

Majno, G., Shea, S. M., and Leventhal, M., 1969, Endothelial contraction induced by histamine type mediators: An electron microscopic study, *J. Cell Biol.* **42**:647–672.

Mandle, R. J., Jr., and Kaplan, A. P., 1977, Hageman factor substrates: Human prekallikrein. Mechanisms of activation by Hageman Factor and participation in Hageman factor dependent fibrinolysis, *J. Biol. Chem.* **252**:6097–6104.

Mandle, R. J., Jr., and Kaplan, A. P., 1979, Hageman-factor dependent fibrinolysis: 18 generation of fibrinolytic activity by the interaction of human activated Factor XI and plasminogen, *Blood* **54**:850–862.

Mandle, R. J., Jr., Colman, R. W., and Kaplan, A. P., 1976, Identification of prekallikrein and HMW-kininogen as a circulating complex in human plasma, *Proc. Natl. Acad. Sci. USA* **73**:4179–4183.

Marcus, A. J., 1969, Platelet function, *N. Engl. J. Med.* **280**:1213–1220, 1278–1284, 1330–1335.

Marder, V. J., Budzynski, A. Z., and James, H. L., 1982, High molecular weight derivative of human fibrinogen produced by plasma. III. Their NH_2-terminal disulfide knot, *J. Biol. Chem.* **247**:4775–4781.

Marler, R. A., Kleiss, A. J., and Griffin, J. H., 1982a, An alternative extrinsic pathway of human blood coagulation, *Blood* **60**:1353–1358.

Marler, R. A., Kleiss, A. J., and Griffin, J. H., 1982b, Mechanism of action of human activated protein C, a thrombin dependent anticoagulation enzyme, *Blood* **59**:1067–1072.

Marr, J., Barboriak, J. J., and Johnson, S. A., 1985, Relationship of appearance of adenosine diphosphate, fibrin formation, and platelet aggregation in the haemostatic plug *in vivo*, *Nature (Lond.)* **205**:259–262.

Maynard, J. R., Heckman, C. A., Pitlick, F. A., and Namerson, Y. A., 1975, Association of tissue factor activity with the surface of cultured cells, *J. Clin. Invest.* **55**:814–824.

Meier, H. L., Pierce, J. V., Colman, R. W., and Kaplan, A. P., 1977, Activation and function of human Hageman factor; the role of HMW-kininogen and prekallikrein, *J. Clin. Invest.* **60**:18–31.

Meier, H. L., Thompson, R. E., and Kaplan, A. P., 1977, Activation of Hageman factor by factor XIa-HMW-kininogen, *Thromb. Haemost.* **38**:14 (abst).

Mikaelsson, M. E., Forsman, N., and Oswaldsson, D. M., 1983, Human Factor VIII: A calcium-linked protein complex, *Blood* **62**:1006–1015.

Miletich, J. P., Kane, W. H., Hofmann, S. L., Stanford, N., and Majerus, P. W., 1979, Deficiency of Factor Xa–Factor Va binding sites on the platelets of a patient with a bleeding disorder, *Blood* **54**:1015–1022.

Miller, G., Silverberg, M., and Kaplan, A. P., 1980, Autoactivatability of human Hageman factor (Factor XII), *Biochem. Biophys. Res. Commun.* **92**:803–810.

Moroi, M., and Aoki, N., 1976, Isolation and characterization of α_2 plasmin inhibitor from human plasma. A novel proteinase inhibitor which inhibits activator-induced clot lysis, *J. Biol. Chem.* **251**:5956–5965.

Morrison, D. C., and Cochrane, C. G., 1974, Direct evidence for Hageman factor (Factor XII) activation by bacterial lipopolysaccharides (endotoxins), *J. Exp. Med.* **140**:797–811.

Mosesson, M. W., and Umfleet, R., 1970, The cold insoluble globulin of human plasma. I. Purification, primary characterization, and relationship to fibrinogen and other cold insoluble fraction components, *J. Biol. Chem.* **245**:5726–5736.

Mosher, D. F., 1976, Action of fibrin-stabilizing factor on cold-insoluble globulin and α_2-macroglobulin in clotting plasma, *J. Biol. Chem.* **251**:1639–1645.

Mullertz, S., and Clemmensen, I., 1976, The primary inhibitor of plasmin in human plasma, *Biochem. J.* **159**:545–553.

Munns, T. W., Johnston, M. F. M., Liszewski, M. K., and Olson, R. E., 1976, Vitamin K-dependent synthesis and modification of precursor prothrombin in cultured H-35 hepatoma cells, *Proc. Natl. Acad. Sci. USA* **73**:2803–2807.

Nemerson, Y., Zur, M., Bach, R., and Gentry, R., 1980, The mechanisms of action of tissue factor: A provisional model, in: *The Regulation of Coagulation* (K. G. Mann and F. B. Taylor, eds.), pp. 193–203, Elsevier/North-Holland, New York.

Niemetz, J., 1972, Coagulant activity of leukocytes. Tissue factor activity. *J. Clin. Invest.* **5**:307–313.

Odya, C. E., Moreland, P., Stewart, J. M., Barabe, J., and Regoli, D. C., 1983, Development of a radioimmunoassay for (Des-Arg 9)-bradykinin, *Biochem. Pharmacol.* **32**:337–342.

Olson, S. T., and Shore, J. D., 1982, Demonstration of a two step reaction mechanism for inhibition of alpha thrombin by antithrombin III and identification of the step affected by heparin, *J. Biol. Chem.* **257**:14891–14895.

Orstavik, T. B., Brandtzaeg, P., Nustad, K., and Pierce, J. V., 1980, Immunohistochemical localization of kallikrein in human pancreas and salivary glands, *J. Histochem. Cytochem.* **28**:557–567.

Osterud, B., and Rapaport, S. I., 1977, Activation of Factor IX by the reaction product of tissue factor and Factor VII: Additional pathway for initiating blood coagulation, *Proc. Natl. Acad. Sci. USA* **74**:5260–5264.

Paterson, P. Y., 1976, Experimental allergic encephalomyelitis: Role of fibrin deposition in immunopathogenesis of inflammation in rats, *Fed. Proc.* **35**:2428–2434.

Pisano, J. J., Bronzert, T. J., and Peyton, M. P., 1972, ϵ(γ-glutamyl)lysine cross-links: Determination in fibrin from normals and Factor XIII-deficient individuals, *Ann. NY Acad. Sci.* **202**:98–113.

Pletcher, C. H., and Nelsestuen, G. L., 1983, Two substrate reaction models for the heparin-catalyzed bovine antithrombin/protease reaction, *J. Biol. Chem.* **258**:1086–1091.

Plow, E. F., Freaney, D., and Edgington, T. S., 1976, Chemotaxis for human monocytes by fibrinogen-derived peptides, *Br. J. Haematol.* **32**:507–513.

Plummer, T. H., Jr., and Horwitz, M. Y., 1978, Human plasma carboxypeptidase N. Isolation and characterization, *J. Biol. Chem.* **253**:3907–3912.

Postlethwaite, A., 1983, Cell–cell interaction in collagen biosynthesis and fibroblast migration, *Adv. Inflamm. Res.* **5**:27–55.

Ratnoff, O. D., Davie, E. W., and Mallett, D. L., 1961, Studies on the action of Hageman factor. Evidence that activated Hageman factor in turn activates plasma thromboplastin antecedent, *J. Clin. Invest.* **40**:803–819.

Reich, E., 1975, Plasminogen activator: Secretion by neoplastic cells and macrophages, in: *Proteins and Biological Control* (E. Reich, D. B. Rifkin, and E. Shaw, eds.), pp. 333–341, Cold Spring Harbor Laboratory, New York.

Repesh, L. A., Furcht, L. T., and Smith, D., 1981, Immunocytochemical localization of fibronectin in limb tissues of the adult newt, Notophthalmus viridescens, *J. Histochem. Cytochem.* **29**:937–945.

Revak, S. D., and Cochrane, C. G., 1976, The relationship of structure and function in human Hageman factor. The association of enzymatic and binding activities with separate regions of the molecule, *J. Clin. Invest.* **57**:852–860.

Revak, S. D., Cochrane, C. G., and Griffin, J. H., 1977, The binding and cleavage characteristics of human Hageman factor during contact activation, *J. Clin. Invest.* **59**:1167–1175.

Richardson, D. L., Pepper, D. S., and Kay, A.B., 1976, Chemotaxis for human monocytes by fibrinogen-derived peptides, *Br. J. Haematol.* **32**:507–513.

Rijken, D. C., Wijngaards, G., Zaal-de Jong, M., and Wolbergen, 1979, Purification and partial characterization of plasminogen activator from human uterus tissue, *Biochim. Biophys. Acta* **580**:140–153.

Robbins, K. C., Summaria, L., Hseih, B., and Shah, R., 1967, The peptide chains of human plasmin. Mechanism of activation of human plasminogen to plasmin, *J. Biol. Chem.* **242**:2333–2342.

Robbins, S., Cotran, R., and Kumar, V., 1984, *Pathologic Basis of Disease*, 3rd ed., WB Saunders, Philadelphia.

Salem, H. H., Esmon, N. L., Esmon, C. T., and Majerus, P. W., 1984, Effects of thrombomodalin and coagulation factor Va light chain on protein C activation in vitro, *J. Clin. Invest.* **73**:968–972.

Schmair, A. H., Zuckerberg, A., Silverman, C., Kuchibhotlea, J., Tuszynski, G. P., and Colman, R. W., 1983, High molecular weight kininogen. A secreted platelet protein, *J. Clin. Invest.* **71**:1477–1489.

Schreiber, A. D., and Frank, M. M., 1972, The role of antibody and complement in the clearance and destruction of erythrocytes. I. *In vivo* effects of IgG and IgM complement fixing sites, *J. Clin. Invest.* **51**:575–582.

Schullek, J., Jordan, J., and Montgomery, R. R., 1984, Interaction of Von Willebrand Factor with human platelets in the plasma milieu, *J. Clin. Invest.* **73**:421–428.

Scicli, A. G., Mindroiu, T., Scicli, G., and Carretero, O. A., 1982, Blood kinins; their concentration in normal subjects and in patients with congenital deficiency in plasma prekallikrein and kininogen, *J. Lab. Clin. Med.* **100**:81–93.

Scott, C. F., Chapira, M., James, H. L., Cohen, A. B., and Colman, R. W., 1982, Inactivation of factor XIa by plasma protease inhibitors. Predominant role of α_1-protease inhibitor and protective effect of high molecular weight kininogen, *J. Clin. Invest.* **69**:844–852.

Scott, C. F., Silver, L. D., Purdon, A. D., and Colman, R. W., 1984, Plasma Factor XIa regulates contact-activated coagulation, *Fed. Proc.* **43**:775 (abst).

Sealey, J. E., Atlas, S. A., Laragh, J. H., Silverberg, M., and Kaplan, A. P., 1979, Initiation of plasma prorenin activation by Hageman factor-dependent conversion of plasma prekallikrein to kallikrein, *Proc. Natl. Acad. Sci. USA* **76**:5914–5918.

Senior, R. M., Griffin, G. L., and Mecham, R. P., 1980, Chemotactic activity of elastin derived peptides, *J. Clin. Invest.* **66**:859–862.

Sheikh, I., and Kaplan, A. P., 1985, Assessment of histamine release and kinin formation in man: Identification of kinin degradation products and characterization of a lymphocyte independent histamine releasing factor, *Int. Arch. Allergy Appl. Immunol.* **77**:64–68.

Sheikh, I. A., and Kaplan, A. P., 1986. Studies of the digestion of bradykinin, Lys-bradykinin, and des-Arg⁹ bradykinin by angiotensin converting enzyme, *Biochem. Pharmacol.* **35**:1951–1956.

Sheikh, I. A., and Kaplan, A. P., 1987, Evidence of carboxypeptidase A and B like activities on the degradation of kinins in human plasma and serum, *J. Biol. Chem.*, in press.

Sherman, L. A., and Lee, J., 1977, Specific binding of soluble fibrin to macrophages, *J. Exp. Med.* **145**:76–85.

Silverberg, M., and Kaplan, A. P., 1982, Enzymatic activities of activated and zymogen form of human Hageman factor (Factor XII), *Blood* **60**:64–70.

Silverberg, M., Dunn, J. T., Garen, L., and Kaplan, A. P., 1980, Autoactivation of human Hageman factor. Demonstration utilizing a synthetic substrate, *J. Biol. Chem.* **255**:7281–7286.

Sinha, D., Seaman, F. S., Koshy, A., Knight, L. C., and Walsh, P. N., 1984, Blood coagulation Factor XI$_A$ binds specifically to a site on activated platelets distinct from that for Factor XI, *J. Clin. Invest.* **73**:1550–1556.

Smariga, P. E., and Marnard, J. R., 1982, Platelet effects on tissue factor and fibrinolytic inhibition of cultured human fibroblasts and vascular cells, *Blood* **60**:140–147.

Spragg, J., 1983, Characterization of purified human latent kallikrein, in: *Kinins III.* (Advances in Experimental Medicine and Biology Series), Vol. 156A (H. Fritz, N. Back, G. Dietz, and G. L. Haberland, eds.), pp. 393–398, Plenum, New York.

Stecher, V. J., and Sorkin, E., 1972, The chemotactic activity of fibrin lysis products, *Int. Arch. Allergy* **43**:879–886.

Stenflo, J., Fernlund, P., Egan, W., and Roepstorff, P., 1974, Vitamin K-dependent modifications of glutamic acid residues in prothrombin, *Proc. Natl. Acad. Sci. USA* **71**:2730–2733.

Stenflo, J., 1976, A new vitamin K-dependent protein. Purification from bovine plasma and preliminary characterization, *J. Biol. Chem.* **251**:355–363.

Summaria, L., Hsieh, B., Groskopf, W. R., and Robbins, K. C., 1967, The isolation and characterization of the S-carboxymethyl (light) chain derivative of human plasmin. The location of the active site on the (light) chain, *J. Biol. Chem.* **242**:5046–5052.

Summaria, L., Arzadon, L., Bernabe, P., and Robbins, K. C., 1975, The activation of plasminogen by urokinase in the presence of the plasmin inhibitor trasylol. The preparation of plasmin with the same NH$_2$-terminal heavy (A) chain sequence as the parent zymogen, *J. Biol. Chem.* **250**:3486–3995.

Takagi, T., and Doolittle, R. F., 1974, Amino acid sequence studies on Factor XIII and the peptide released during its activation by thrombin, *Biochemistry* **13**:750–756.

Talamo, R. C., Haber, E., and Austen, K. F., 1969, A radioimmunoassay for bradykinin in plasma and synovial fluid, *J. Lab. Clin. Med.* **74**:816–827.

Tankersley, D. L., and Finlayson, J., 1984, Kinetics of activation and autoactivation of human Factor XII, *Biochemistry* **23**:273–279.

Thompson, R. E., Mandle, R., Jr., and Kaplan, A. P., 1977, Association of Factor XI and high molecular weight kininogen in human plasma, *J. Clin. Invest.* **60**:1376–1380.

Thompson, R. E., Mandle, R., Jr., and Kaplan, A. P., 1978, Characterization of human HMW-kininogen. Procoagulant activity associated with the light of chain kinin-free HMW kininogen, *J. Exp. Med.* **147**:488–499.

Thompson, R. E., Mandle, R., Jr., and Kaplan, A. P., 1979, Studies of the binding of prekallikrein and Factor XI to high molecular weight kininogen and its light chain, *Proc. Natl. Acad. Sci. USA* **76**:4862–4866.

Thorsen, S., Glas-Greenwalt, P., and Astrup, T., 1972, Difference in the binding to fibrin of urokinase and tissue plasminogen activator, *Thromb. Pathol. Haemorrh.* **28**:65–74.

Tollefson, D. M., Pestka, C. A., and Monafo, W. J., 1983, Activation of heparin cofactor II by dermatan sulfate, *J. Biol. Chem.* **258**:6713–6716.

Tracy, P. B., Peterson, J. M., Nesheim, M. E., McDuffie, F. C., and Mann, K. G., 1979, Interaction of coagulation Factor V and Factor Va with platelets, *J. Biol. Chem.* **254**:10354–10361.

Tracy, P. B., Rohrbach, M. S., and Mann, K. G., 1983, Functional prothrombinase complex assembly on isolated monocytes and lymphocytes, *J. Biol. Chem.* **258**:7264–7267.

Unkeless, J. C., Gordon, S., and Reich, E., 1974, Secretion of plasminogen activator by stimulated macrophages, *J. Exp. Med.* **139**:834–850.

Vassalli, J. D., Hamilton, J., and Reich, E., 1976, Macrophage plasminogen activator modulation of enzyme production by anti-inflammatory steroids, mitotic inhibitors, and cyclic nucleotides, *Cell* **8**:271–281.

Verheijen, J. H., Chang, G. I. C., and Mullaart, E., 1983, Inhibition of extrinsic (tissue-type) plasminogen activator by human plasma: Evidence for the occurrence of a fast-acting inhibitor, *Thromb. Haemost.* **50**:294 (abst 930).

Wachtfogel, Y. T., Kucich, U., James, U. L., Scott, C. H., Schapira, M., Zimmerman, M., Cohen, A. B., and Colman, R. W., 1983, Human plasma kallikrein releases neutrophil elastase during blood coagulation, *J. Clin. Invest.* **72:**1672–1677.

Walsh, P. N., 1972, The role of platelets in the contact phase of blood coagulation, *Br. J. Haematol.* **22:**237–254.

Walsh, P. N., and Griffin, J. H., 1981, Contributions of human platelets to the proteolytic activation of blood coagulation Factor XII and XI, *Blood* **57:**106–118.

Webster, M. E., and Pierce, J. V., 1963, The nature of the kallidins released from human

Weinstein, M. J., and Chute, L. E., 1984, Two distinct forms of Factor VIII coagulant protein in human plasma. Cleavage by thrombin and differences in coagulant activity and association with von Willebrand factor, *J. Clin. Invest.* **73:**307–316.

Weiss, H. J., 1975, Platelet physiology and abnormalities of platelet function (first of two parts), *N. Engl. J. Med.* **293:**531–541.

Wiggins, R. C., and Cochrane, C. G., 1979, The autoactivation of rabbit Hageman factor, *J. Exp. Med.* **150:**1122–1133.

Zur, M., and Nemerson, Y., 1979, The esterase activity of coagulation Factor VII. Evidence for intrinsic activity of the zymogen, *J. Biol. Chem.* **253:**2203–2209.

Chapter 4

Endothelial Cell Regulation of Coagulation

DAVID M. STERN, DEAN HANDLEY, and
PETER P. NAWROTH

1. Introduction

The cessation of hemorrhage around wounded tissue and isolation of pathologic processes, such as an infection or solid neoplasias, are mediated in part by
thrombus formation and occlusion of blood vessel lumina. The clinical outcome of blood vessel occlusion may be quite devastating in certain processes,
such as myocardial infarction or vasculitis. Nevertheless, thrombotic phenomena are ubiquitous and closely linked to the body's response to injury
(Dvoarak, 1980, 1984, 1985). The limitation of clot formation to inflamed or
injured tissue suggests that the coagulation is under local regulation and therefore involves more than plasma protein–protein interactions. Thus, local cell
mediators may play a central role in the regulation of procoagulant events. The
ideal characteristics of these mediators would include high efficiency when
inducing intravascular coagulation following stimulation, balanced by little or
no activity in the quiescent state.

   The study of coagulation reactions in solution has flourished since the
original description of the cascade or waterfall theory (Davie and Ratnoff, 1964;
MacFarlane, 1964). Subsequent studies have provided a basic outline of the
coagulation mechanism and defined kinetic parameters of individual reactions.
Factors regulating the initiation and propagation of coagulant reactions in vivo,
however, have remained elusive. Although coagulation factors are the essential
building blocks of the clotting mechanism, coagulation is ultimately controlled
by cellular mediators which are responsive to local pathologic processes. These
considerations lead to the prediction that, although infusion of pharmacologic
amounts of procoagulant enzymes could force the coagulation pathway along
the lines defined by in vitro studies, the actual generation of physiologic concentrations of procoagulants would be under cellular control. Thus, infusion of
large amounts of activated factors VII and IX leads to intravascular coagulation,

DAVID M. STERN and PETER P. NAWROTH • Department of Physiology and Cellular Biophysics, College of Physicians and Surgeons, Columbia University, New York, New York 10032.
DEAN HANDLEY • Division of Platelet Research, Sandoz Inc., East Hanover, New Jersey 07936.

while infusion of low concentrations of procoagulant enzymes does not (Hedner and Kisiel, 1983; Gurewich *et al.*, 1979). As additional examples, low-dose thrombin infusion primes the protein C pathway, leading to anticoagulation rather than intravascular coagulation (Comp *et al.*, 1982), and low concentrations of infused factor Xa are promptly removed from the circulation and/or inactivated (Fuchs and Pizzo, 1983). Therefore, in the unperturbed endothelium of animals, anticoagulant mechanisms predominate, ensuring the normal flow of blood.

As the cells forming the luminal vascular surface, endothelial cells are strategically located to play an important role in the regulation of coagulation. In addition to their well-known role in anticoagulant reactions, the endothelium is also the first line of defense in vascular injury, promoting and stabilizing procoagulant activities. Thus, in the perturbed state, the endothelium requires a unidirectional shift in its coagulant properties whereby anticoagulant effects are downregulated and procoagulant activities are enhanced. For example, the monokine interleukin-1 (IL-1) (Mizel, 1982; Unanue, 1981; Oppenheim and Gery, 1982), released from cells at sites of inflammation, would be an appropriate mediator of the shift from an anticoagulant to procoagulant phenotype of the endothelial cell surface. Thus, signals from multiple cells may converge on the endothelial cell, leading to a basic change in the balance of anticoagulant and procoagulant mechanisms operative on the vessel surface.

Recent studies have indicated that endothelial cells can play an active role in coagulation reactions (Nawroth and Stern, 1985; Stern *et al.*, 1985c; Rodgers and Shuman, 1983b; Colucci *et al.*, 1983; Lyberg *et al.*, 1983; Cerveny *et al.*, 1984). Perturbed endothelium can promote an entire pathway of coagulation, leading to the localized deposition of fibrin (Stern *et al.*, 1985c). The sequence of coagulation reactions depends on specific endothelial cell binding sites for coagulation factors, which also function as cofactors, promoting the activity of the bound enzymes. Although these phenomena suggest a passive template-like function for the endothelial cell, this is not the case. Coagulation proteases generated on the endothelial cell surface play an active role not only in blood clotting, but in influencing the physiology of endothelium as well. For example, factor Xa formed on the endothelial cell surface leads to the release of mitogenic activity, including platelet-derived growth factor (PDGF) -like molecules (Gajdusek *et al.*, 1987). Other compounds of the endothelial cell response to factor Xa include elevation of cytosolic calcium levels (Sternberg *et al.*, 1985) and clearance of factor Xa from the cell surface by receptor-mediated endocytosis (Nawroth *et al.*, 1985a). Another example of endothelium activity is thrombin-induced synthesis and elaboration of IL-1 by endothelium (Stern *et al.*, 1985b). IL-1, a regulator of inflammation, induces a procoagulant cofactor, tissue factor, on the endothelial cell surface. Recent studies have also shown that interleukin 1 can decrease endothelial cell cofactor activity for the protein C pathway (Nawroth *et al.*, 1986). Thus coagulation enzymes, such as thrombin and factor Xa, generated in response to injury can also function as hormones by modulating endothelial cell physiology and altering the coagulant phenotype of the vessel surface.

This chapter covers a cellular approach to coagulation prompted by the hypothesis that important hemostatic reactions occur on the endothelial cell surface and that the outcome of these reactions plays a critical role in the coagulant response to injury. IL-1 elaborated by inflammatory cells can lead to activation of coagulation by inducing procoagulant activity in the vessel wall. By contrast, generation of the central coagulation enzyme thrombin can lead to endothelial cell elaboration of IL-1, thereby allowing for self-regulation of procoagulant events on the vessel surface. The goal of this chapter is to delineate the multiple levels of endothelial cell–coagulation factor interactions and to demonstrate how these interactions influence both endothelial cell physiology and the regulation of coagulation.

2. Initiation of Coagulation by Endothelium: Tissue Factor and Interleukin-1

Tissue factor is a cellular cofactor promoting factor VIIa-mediated activation of factors IX and X (Nemerson and Bach, 1982). The role of tissue factor in coagulation has been studied *in vitro* by employing high concentrations of tissue factor inserted into phospholipid vesicles. Under these conditions, factor VIIa–tissue factor-mediated activation of factor X is considerably more effective than the activation of factor IX (Jesty and Silverberg, 1979; Zur and Nemerson, 1980). These data, along with the normal prothrombin time observed with plasmas deficient in factor VIII or IX (Rizza, 1972), suggest that factors VIII and IX may have an ancillary role in coagulation. However, factors VIII and IX are not ancillary. They have a central role in normal hemostasis. In fact, deficiency of either factor VIII or IX leads to hemophilia, the most frequently inherited severe bleeding diathesis (Rizza, 1972). When vessels rupture, patients deficient in factors VIII and IX hemorrhage, although subendothelial layers of the vessel wall theoretically contain sufficient quantities of tissue factor to initiate coagulation. The continuing dichotomy between *in vitro* predictions and clinical observations indicates that enzymatic studies on phospholipid vesicles alone are insufficient to explain mechanisms involved in the pathogenesis of coagulopathies and the maintenance of normal hemostasis. In this context, mechanisms responsible for the initiation and localization of thrombotic events are poorly understood elements of coagulation.

The interaction of coagulation factors with formed elements of the blood, such as platelets and monocytes, has enriched the model of coagulation by indicating that major coagulation reactions, such as assembly of the prothrombinase complex, can occur on physiologic surfaces (Miletich *et al.*, 1977; Tracy *et al.*, 1981; Dahlback and Stenflo, 1978; Broze, 1982; Edwards *et al.*, 1979; Osterud and Eskeland, 1982; Prydz and Allison, 1978; Tracy *et al.*, 1985). The surface of formed elements can propagate activation of coagulation and, in the case of monocytes, even initiate coagulation by expressing tissue factor after stimulation (Edwards *et al.*, 1979; Osterud and Eskeland, 1982; Prydz and Allison, 1978). However, despite potent procoagulant activities, the role of formed elements in the localization of thrombotic events is not clear.

Several problems are related to the procoagulant activities of monocyte and platelet surfaces. First, platelets have to be stimulated by thrombin or other agents to actively and efficiently propagate coagulation; that is, unstimulated platelets do not express factor V, nor do they support the factor $IX_a VIII$-dependent activation of factor X (Miletich *et al.*, 1977; Tracy *et al.*, 1981; Dahlback and Stenflo, 1978; Hultin, 1982; Rosing *et al.*, 1985). A cellular surface central to the pathogenesis of a localized thrombotic event theoretically should not depend on stimulation by thrombin formed elsewhere, but rather should be capable of initiating and propagating thrombin formation. Second, such a cellular surface should have diverse and powerful tools capable of controlling thrombin formation. Our understanding of the pathogenesis of localized thrombus formation would then depend on the elucidation of factors affecting a delicate balance of cell-surface-dependent coagulant activities promoting and inhibiting clot formation. Furthermore, since the generalized thrombin formation that occurs in disseminated intravascular coagulation (DIC) is quite distinct from the localized thrombotic process, probably additional factors, perhaps on the vessel wall, play a critical role in clot localization.

There are two general models, both of which involve the vessel wall, used to explain the initiation and localization of thrombotic events. Factors promoting the binding of platelets and monocytes to discrete loci on the vessel may be the crucial element in localized coagulation. In support of this view, adherence and activation of platelets to exposed subendothelium in areas of the vessel wall denuded of endothelium has been observed and is assumed to be an important factor in fibrin formation (Kaplan, 1982). Thus, the platelets probably play an important role when traumatic vessel wall rupture exposes hemostatic components to subendothelium. By contrast, the pathogenesis of localized coagulation in more chronic disorders, such as atheroslcerosis, is probably quite different. Although endothelial denudation and fibrin deposition on subendothelium are observed in advanced lesions, there is not strong evidence that endothelial cell denudation is an early event in lesion formation (Schwartz and Gajdusek, 1982). In addition, studies of small injuries to vessels (Schwartz *et al.*, 1981; Reidy and Schwartz, 1981) have shown that endothelium can cover denuded areas rapidly, possibly even maintaining the continuity of the monolayer despite moderate cell loss. Thus, in the absence of subendothelium exposure, the endothelium itself may play a direct role in the initiation of clot formation.

If the regulation of localized thrombus formation involves the endothelium, synthesis and expression of tissue factor is a plausible mechanism for initiating the activation of coagulation. However, unperturbed endothelial cells express little tissue factor (Maynard *et al.*, 1977). Previous studies have confirmed that quiescent endothelial cells do not initiate coagulation via either the tissue factor-dependent extrinsic or intrinsic pathway. Nevertheless, by analogy with the monocyte, it could be hypothesized that perturbation of endo-thelium would lead to increased expression of tissue factor. Endotoxin is a reasonable candidate for a perturbing agent because of its association with coagulopathies in vivo.

Lyberg and colleagues (1983) demonstrated that treatment of human um-bilical vein endothelial cells with endotoxin, phorbol myristate acetate (PMA), and phytohemagglutinin (PHA) leads to the induction of tissue factor activity. In our own studies employing bovine aortic endothelial cells (Nawroth et al., 1985b), we observed a time- and dose-dependent acquisition of tissue factor activity after exposing endothelial cells to endotoxin lipopolysaccharide. The procoagulant activity was characterized as tissue factor based on (1) the ability of the procoagulant to activate factor X, but only in the presence of factor VIIA (Kisiel and Davie, 1975), and (2) the inability of the procoagulant to induce factor Xa formation when anti-tissue factor antibodies were added (Bach et al., 1981). Induction of tissue factor was dependent on RNA and protein synthesis, as indicated by the inhibitory effects of actinomycin D and cycloheximide. Endotoxin is thus one agent that can stimulate the transcription and translation of the tissue factor gene product.

The discovery that endothelial cells can be stimulated to synthesize and express tissue factor raises two major issues. First, what are physiologic agents capable of inducing tissue factor in endothelium, and second, what is the consequence of tissue factor expressed on the endothelial cell surface in terms of thrombotic phenomena? Although exposure of endothelium to lipopolysac-charide may occur in certain clinical circumstances, such as sepsis with gram-negative organisms, endothelial cells do not generally interact with endotoxin. A more likely physiologic mediator of endothelial cell tissue factor activity was revealed in a recent study by Bevilacqua and colleagues (1984). In this study, purified human monocyte-derived IL-1 was shown to induce synthesis and expression of tissue factor in human umbilical vein endothelial cells. The induction of endothelial cell tissue factor by interleukin 1, a mediator of the inflammatory response, allows endothelium to initiate an entire pathway of coagulation (Stern et al., 1985c). The release of interleukin 1 by monocytic cells in an inflamed area could result in localized coagulation through the induc-tion of endothelial cell tissue factor.

Classically, the endothelium was believed to play a passive role in hemo-static and inflammatory phenomena. Clinical and laboratory observations, however, have suggested that the endothelium actively participates in the in-flammatory and coagulation systems and forms a link between these systems. One agent probably involved in these endothelial activities is IL-1, a potent mediator of inflammatory and immunologic events. IL-1 appears to have multi-ple affects on a variety of cells ranging from tissue factor induction to the elaboration of interleukin 2 (Mizel, 1982; Unanue 1981; Oppenheim and Gery, 1982), and these cellular responses to IL-1 may act in concert as a unified response to injurious stimuli.

In addition to responding to interleukin 1, endothelial cells synthesize and elaborate IL-1 (Windt and Rosenwasser, 1984; Shanah and Korn, 1984). Thus, endothelial cell IL-1 may promote local inflammation while simultaneously inducing procoagulant activity in the vessel wall. Recent results from our laboratory suggest that this hypothesis may be correct. Cultured human umbilical vein endothelial cells treated with endotoxin lipopolysaccharide synthesize and elaborate enhanced amount of IL-1 (Stern *et al.*, 1985b). In addition, the coagulation enzyme thrombin, a vessel wall perturbant generated by the activated coagulation system, induced comparable amounts of IL-1 activity. Only the enzyme form of thrombin induced endothelial cell expression of interleukin. Inactivation of thrombin by antithrombin III (Rosenberg and Damus, 1973) or diisopropylfluorophosphate (Fenton *et al.*, 1977) rendered it ineffective. Endothelial cell IL-1 elaboration induced by thrombin was dependent on the concentration of enzyme added and the incubation time (Fig. 1). Although the amount of thrombin causing optimal IL-1 elaboration is relatively high, IL-1 is generated at lower concentrations, which may occur as prothrombin is generated on the endothelial cell surface.

These results indicate that a potent procoagulant enzyme, thrombin, can induce IL-1 expression in a highly specific manner. Since IL-1 is known to induce tissue factor activity in cultured endothelial cells, amplification of procoagulant events on the endothelial cell surface is possible. To test this hypothesis, IL-1-containing supernatants from endothelial cells treated with thrombin were incubated with fresh cultures, after the residual thrombin was inactivated, and induction of tissue factor activity was tested (Fig. 2). Procoagulant activity characterized as tissue factor, based on the factor VIIa dependence of factor X activation (Nemerson and Bach, 1982), was induced in endothelium. Similar inducion of tissue factor activity was observed when cultures were incubated with exogenous IL-1 (Fig. 2). Thus, in contrast to the multiple known inhibitory mechanisms that block thrombin procoagulant activity, these data suggest an amplification pathway in which thrombin induces endothelial cell IL-1, a mediator of endothelial cell procoagulant activity. The generation of IL-1 by perturbed endothelium indicates a new mechanism by which the systems involved in coagulation and inflammation can influence each other via the endothelium (Fig. 3).

Perturbed endothelium expressing tissue factor is an attractive nidus of localized procoagulant events on the vessel surface. Induction of tissue factor activity by IL-1, coupled with the elaboration of IL-1 by endothelium, allows for the self-regulation of procoagulant events on the endothelial cell surface.

3. Assembly of Procoagulant and Anticoagulant Complexes on the Endothelial Cell Surface

Endothelium has been called the only true blood-compatible surface. This statement would appear to be true, since blood does not form clots continuously as it passes over the vessel surface. However, what are the details of the interactions between coagulation factors in the blood and endothelium? At the outset, we would like to propose the hypothesis that the apparent inertness of the endothelium in hemostatic reactions actually masks a delicate balance of anticoagulant and procoagulant mechanisms operating at the endothelial surface. A bridge from these hypothetical considerations to clinical thrombosis is provided by observations in the Wessler stasis model of thrombosis (Wessler et al., 1959; Gitel et al., 1977). The Wessler model does not require endothelial cell denudation, but instead involves the injection of a procoagulant enzyme in a rabbit ear vein followed by ligation of the contralateral jugular vein. Following a ten minute period of stasis, the ipsilateral jugular vein is opened and thrombus formation evaluated. Using the Wessler model, Gurewich and colleagues (1979) showed that infusion of factor IXa into rabbits shortens the

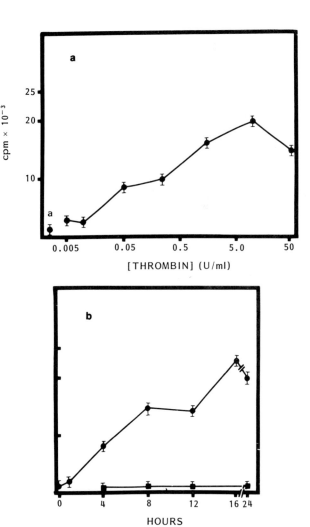

Figure 1. Elaboration of interleukin-1 (IL-1) activity by endothelial cells treated with α-thrombin. (a) Dependence on dose of α-thrombin. Endothelial cell monolayers were incubated for 16 hr at 37°C with medium 199 (1 ml) containing 0.5% bovine serum albumin (BSA), polymyxin B (1 μg/ml), and the indicated concentrations of thrombin. A hundredfold molar excess of bovine antithrombin III was then added to each culture dish for 10 min at 37°C; supernatants were assayed in the thymocyte proliferation assay. The direct effect of thrombin (50 U/ml) in the thymocyte assay is shown at a. (b) Time course of α-thrombin-induced elaboration of IL-1. Endothelial cell monolayers were incubated for the indicated times at 37°C with medium 199 (1 ml) containing 0.5% BSA—fatty acid free and polymyxin B (1 μg/ml) in the presence (●) or absence (■) of thrombin (5 U/ml). Antithrombin III (0.8 mM) was added for 10 min; supernatants were then assayed in the thymocyte proliferation assay. Mean ±1 SD.

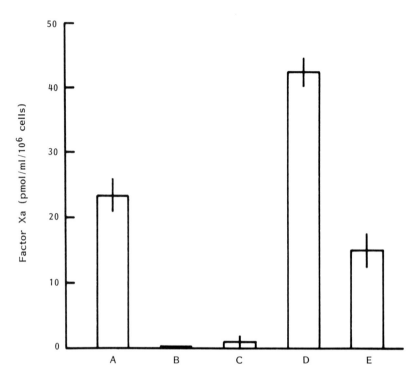

Figure 2. Effect of culture supernatants from thrombin-treated endothelial cells on the pro-coagulant activity of fresh endothelial cell cultures. Human endothelial cell monolayers were treated with α-thrombin (10 U/ml) in medium 199 containing bovine serum albumin (BSA) (0.5%) and polymyxin B (1 μg/ml) for 8 hr at 37°C. After this incubation period, the supernatant (endothelial cell-conditioned medium) was incubated with antithrombin III (2 μM) (10 min at 37°C) to inactivate residual thrombin, filtered (0.22 μm) and added to fresh endothelial cells for 6 hr. Monolayers were washed, after which 1 ml 10 mM HEPES (pH 7.4) containing 137 mM NaCl, 4 mM KCl, 11 mM glucose, 2.5 mil $CaCl_2$, 2 mg/ml BSA, along with human factor VIIa (0.5 nM) and/or factor X (300 nM) was added for 7 min at 23°C. The reaction mixture was assayed for factor Xa admidolytic activity, using the synthetic peptide substrate Bz-Ile-Glu-Gly-Arg-p-nitroanilide (0.5 mM). The amount of factor Xa formed after 7 min (mean ±SEM) is shown. (a) Endothelial cell-conditioned medium was incubated with the cells and factor Xa formation was assessed in the presence of factors VIIa and X. (b) Endothelial cell-conditioned medium was incubated with the cells, and factor Xa formation was assessed in the presence of factor X alone. (c) Medium 199 containing thrombin (10 U/ml) was incubated for 8 hr in a glass tube, and antithrombin III (2 μM) was added to inactivate the thrombin. This medium (1 ml) was then incubated with the cells for 6 hr at 37°C, and factor Xa formation was assessed in the presence of factors VIIa and X. (d,e) Medium 199 containing purified exogenous IL-1 [(D) 5 U/ml; (E) 1 U/ml] was incubated with endothelial cells, and factor Xa formation was assessed in the presence of factors VIIa and X. The mean and SEM of triplicates are shown.

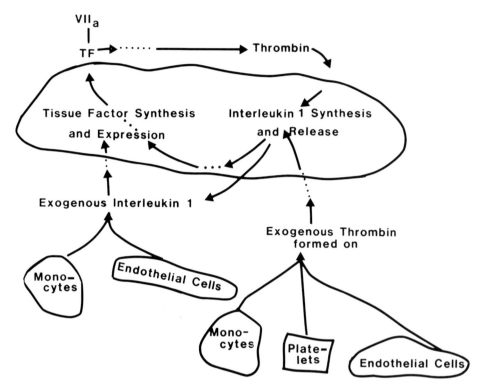

Figure 3. Schematic depiction of regulation of procoagulant events on the endothelial cell surface by Interleukin-1. VIIa, activated factor VII; TF, tissue factor.

partial thromboplastin time and results in local thrombus formation; however, disseminated intravascular coagulation was not observed. In contrast, infusion of tissue factor, factor Xa, or thrombin did not lead to localized thrombus formation, but rather prolongation of the partial thromboplastin time, fibrin monomer formation, and defibrination.

Further evidence suggesting the possibility of factor IXa–vessel wall interaction comes from *in vivo* factor IX clearance studies showing a biphasic clearance with an initial rapid phase (Aggeler, 1961; Tompson *et al.*, 1980; Fuchs *et al.*, 1984). When the clearance of radiolabeled factor IX is studied after the infusion of an excess of unlabeled factor IX, the initial rapid clearance phase is prevented. These observations indicate the possibility of intravascular binding sites. Prompted by these findings, we began studies of procoagulant reactions on the endothelial cell surface by examining the interaction of factor IX with endothelium.

3.1. Interaction of Factors IX/IXa with Endothelial Cells

Although factor IX, along with factor VIII, plays a central role in the hemostatic mechanism by linking the intrinsic and extrinsic coagulation pathways to the final common pathway, a cellular surface localizing this coagulation protein has not been previously described. Furthermore, a cellular surface selectively binding the enzyme factor IXa would provide a powerful focus of procoagulant reactions. Thus, as an initial step in our studies of mechanisms responsible for the localization of procoagulant activity on the vessel wall, our laboratory and others (Heimark and Schwartz, 1983; Stern et al., 1983) examined the specific binding of factor IX/IXa to endothelial cells. When radiolabeled factor IX or IXa was incubated with cultured bovine aortic endothelial cells, reversible and time-dependent binding was observed. Factor IX binding to endothelial cells was saturable with half-maximal binding occurring at a free factor IX concentration of approximately 2 nM. Two nM is considerably lower than the plasma concentration of factor IX (70–100 nM), suggesting that these sites are saturated under normal conditions. Consistent with this hypothesis, experiments employing bovine aortic vessel segments have shown that endogenously bound factor IX can be eluted with calcium-free buffer (Stern et al., 1984b). Furthermore, once the endogenously bound material was eluted, radiolabeled factor IX showed binding comparable to that observed in studies employing cultured endothelial cells. Thus, factor IX binds to, and can be eluted from, the native endothelium of bovine aortic vessel segments. Although factor IX receptor sites are saturated at normal plasma levels of factor IX, and even in mild deficiency states decreased occupancy of these sites probably occur in patients with severe factor IX deficiency who have a serious bleeding diathesis.

Competitive binding studies (Stern et al., 1983) have shown that other coagulation factors, including the vitamin K-dependent coagulation factors VII and X, prothrombin, and protein C, did not inhibit factor IX–endothelial cell interaction. Although expected, since endogenously bound factor IX was eluted from aortic segments, the high degree of specificity for the factor IX molecule raises the possibility that factor IX–vessel wall interaction is not simply secondary to phospholipid binding. Thus, even though initially it seemed likely that the factor IX/IXa binding to endothelium might represent the binding of a vitamin K-dependent coagulation factor to acid phospholipids, the specificity of factor IX binding and the nanomolar affinity constant (a dissociation constant of 2 μM has been reported using synthetic phospholipids) (Nelsestuen, 1978) suggest that a specific receptor may be involved. This hypothesis is supported by preliminary experiments demonstrating loss of specific factor IX binding sites after gentle treatment of endothelial cells with trypsin (1.0 μg/ml for 5 min at room temperature) (unpublished observations).

The endothelial binding of the zymogen factor IX and of the enzyme factor IXa was quite similar; they had equal affinity and competed for the same class of binding sites (Stern et al., 1983), in contrast to most cells which often bind only the enzyme form of coagulation factors. For example, the binding of activated factor X to the platelet in the presence of factor Va and calcium is highly specific for the enzyme form of factor X (Miletich et al., 1977; Tracy et al., 1981; Dahlback and Stenflo, 1978). Since only small amounts of factor IX and X are activated in the plasma during clot formation, in order for factor IXa and Xa to interact with a cellular receptor, a site specific for the enzyme form should exist. If not, all the sites would be occupied by the zymogen. One could argue, then, that activation of cell-bound factor IX would lead to its dissociation, since binding is reversible, thus protecting the body from unnecessary coagulation. These considerations have prompted the hypothesis that there is a factor IXa–vessel wall interaction, which is specific for the enzyme. In order to demonstrate a specific endothelial cell factor IXa-binding site, it was necessary to correlate the results of kinetic studies of factor Xa formation with factor IXa-binding studies.

Since our principal question in these studies of factor IX/IXa endothelial cell interaction concerned the effect of cell-surface binding on the coagulant properties of the coagulation proteins, functional studies were performed. Factor IXa, bound to native or cultured aortic endothelium, promoted the activation of factor X in the presence of factor VIII; no exogenous source of phospholipid such as the platelet was required (Stern et al., 1984a,b). The effective activation of factor X over endothelial cell monolayers incubated with factors IXa and VIII is shown by the data presented in Fig. 4. Half-maximal rates of endothelial cell-dependent factor IXa-VIII-mediated activation of factor X occurred at a factor IXa concentration of 0.15 nM, in contrast with the previously mentioned binding studies, in which factor IX/IXa binding was half-maximal at 2 nM. The solution to the apparent paradox is that in the presence of all components of the factor X activation mixture, factors IXa, VIII, and X, there is a selective factor IXa–endothelial cell interaction. The factor IXa site is rela-

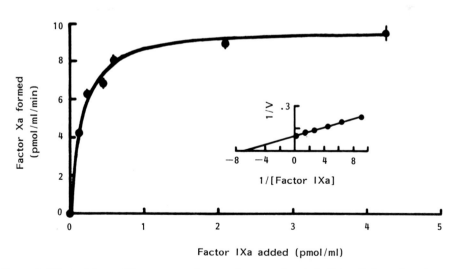

Figure 4. Effect of factor IXa concentration on the rate of endothelial cell-dependent factor X activation. Factor VIII (2.4 U/ml), factor X (300 pmole/ml), and the indicated concentrations of factor IXa were mixed and incubated over endothelial cell monolayers at 23°C, and samples for factor Xa assay were obtained. Inset (- - -) calculated using nonlinear regression analysis applied to the Michaelis–Menten equation.

tively specific for the enzyme form and requires the presence of both the cofactor, factor VIII, and the substrate, factor X.

The results indicate that endothelial cells have a binding site shared by factors IX and IXa. There is also a specific factor IXa-binding site, which may represent a modification of the shared site in the presence of factors VIII and X. When the enzyme, cofactor, and substrate are all present, a complex leading to the activation of factor X assembles on the endothelial cell binding site for factor IXa. These findings suggest that activation of cell-bound factor IX results in the assembly of an effective procoagulant complex on the endothelial cell surface. Once formed, factor IXa remains tightly bound to the cell surface in the factor IXa–VIII–X complex. Thus, from this site factor IXa may function as a vessel-localized focal point for the activation of the coagulation system. It is interesting to speculate whether this is an isolated procoagulant reaction on the endothelial cell surface or part of an entire endothelial cell-dependent pathway of coagulation. Further the study of the interaction of factor Xa with endothelium and its role in thrombin formation may answer such questions.

3.2. The Prothrombinase Complex and Recruitment of Platelets by Endothelial Cell Coagulation Pathway

In order to propagate the whole sequence of coagulation starting with factor IXa, endothelial cells must also interact with factor Xa, leading to assemblage of the prothrombinase complex. The parameters and conditions of factor Xa binding to endothelium differ from those described for the formation of the prothrombinase complex on the surface of stimulated platelets (Stern *et al.*, 1984b; Rodgers and Shuman, 1983a). In this context, it is reasonable to ask what cofactor activity the endothelial cell provides for factor Xa-mediated prothrombin activation.

When factor Xa and prothrombin are incubated with the native endothelium of bovine aortic vessel segments, thrombin formation occurs, as first observed by Rodgers and Shuman (1983b) using nonconfluent cultured endothelial cell. These investigators observed that as the cells approached confluence, their ability to promote factor Xa-mediated thrombin formation decreased. Although thrombin formation does decrease at confluence, it is observed even on native endothelium. Since effective factor Xa-catalyzed prothrombin activation *in vitro* depends on the presence of factor V/Va, in addition to calcium ions and phospholipids (Miletich *et al.*, 1977; Tracy *et al.*, 1981; Dahlback and Stenflo, 1978), endothelial cells might be providing two cofactor activities for prothrombin activation: a factor V-like and a phospholipid cofactor. Although initially it seemed likely that the source of factor V/Va was the fetal calf serum in the growth medium, subsequent studies have shown that factor V-like cofactor activity persists even when endothelial cells are grown in serum-free medium (Rodgers and Shuman, 1983b). Furthermore, synthesis of factor V by cultured bovine aortic endothelium was shown by immunoprecipitation in a study by Cerveny *et al.* (1984).

Factor Xa binds at least two distinct classes of surface sites (Stern, 1984b). A rapid phase of reversible binding (K_d = 1 nM) is followed by a slower phase of irreversible binding involving the formation of covalent bond between factor Xa and a cell-associated protein. Factor Xa irreversibly bound to the endothelial cell surface has no coagulant activity. These protease nexinlike sites (Baker *et al.*, 1980) were abundant on the surface of native endothelium. Thus, in addition to promoting prothrombin activation, the endothelium can inactivate factor Xa (see also Section 4.1).

The results presented thus far indicate that endothelial cells can play a role in the activation of factor X by the cell-surface factor IXa–VIII–X complex and in thrombin formation mediated by factor Xa. The next question then is: Can these reactions be linked? or, more generally, Can endothelial cells assemble an entire pathway of coagulation?

Cultured bovine aortic endothelial cells in the presence of factors XIa, VIII, IX, and X, prothrombin, and fibrinogen can promote a cell-dependent procoagulant pathway leading to fibrin clot formation and release of fibrinopeptide A. In these experiments, the coagulation, initiated by the addition of factor XIa, required the presence of factors VIII, IX, and X, prothrombin, and fibrinogen to go to completion with release of fibrinopeptide A. The interaction of coagulation proteins with cellular binding sites on the endothelium was essential, since no fibrinogen cleavage resulted in the absence of endothelial cells. When endothelial monolayers were preincubated with antibody to bovine factor V (Tracy *et al.*, 1979), subsequent fibrinopeptide A generation was blocked by greater than 90%. Thus, endothelial cells provided a factor V-like activity required for assembly of the prothrombinase complex. No exogenous source of phospholipid, such as the platelet, was necessary for factor X and prothrombin activation. Perturbed endothelial cells not only promoted procoagulant reactions but also activated coagulation via the interaction of factor VII/VIIa with cell-surface tissue factor (Fig. 5).

The endothelial cell-dependent procoagulant pathway is more than bal-

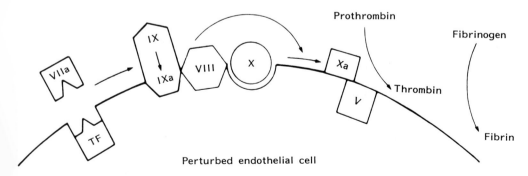

Figure 5. Schematic depiction of the endothelial cell procoagulant pathway on the surface of a perturbed endothelial cell. TF, tissue factor.

anced by multiple anticoagulant mechanisms usually operative on the vessel surface (see Sections 3.3 and 3.4). The crucial issue is the existence of augmentation mechanisms of the procoagulant response. One possibility was to examine the interaction between coagulation events on the endothelial cell surface and platelets. Our first experiments (Stern, 1985c) in this context were carried out by adding unstimulated human platelets to endothelial cell monolayers (Fig. 6). For these experiments, bovine endothelial cells were incubated with Factors IXa and VIII, washed, and factor X and prothrombin were then added in the presence of human platelets. Platelets increased thrombin formation by about 15-fold; similar results were observed with bovine platelets. The inhibition of thrombin formation by an antibody to human factor V (Hartubise, 1979) indicates that the platelet effect was due in large part to release of their endogenous factor V, which, after activation, promotes rapid factor Xa-mediated thrombin formation. In the absence of platelets, anti-human factor V antibodies decreased thrombin formation by bovine endothelial cells only minimally. The anti-factor V antibody appeared to block the activity of human factor V/Va from platelets more efficiently than did endothelial cell bovine factor V/Va (Cer-

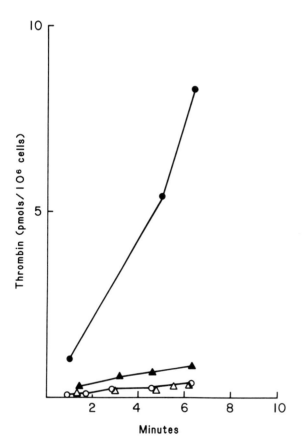

Figure 6. Effect of platelets of the thrombin formation by endothelial cells. Monolayers of bovine aortic endothelial cells in 1 ml of buffer were incubated with factors IXa (0.9 nM), VIII (1.2 U/ml), X (175 nM), and prothrombin (1.5 μM) in the presence ($\bullet$) or absence ($\bigcirc$) of 1.1 $\times$ 10^8 platelets/ml. Another set of monolayers was incubated with the same coagulation proteins and anti-human factor V IgG (100 μg/ml) in the presence ($\blacktriangle$) or absence ($\triangle$) of platelets. Addition of normal human IgG (100 μg/ml) had no effect on prothrombin activation in the presence or absence of platelets. Addition of human anti-factor V IgG (100 μg/ml) did not effect factor X activation in the presence or absence of platelets in contrast to its effect on thrombin formation in the presence of platelets ($\blacktriangle$). In each case, aliquots of 0.1 ml were removed at the indicated times and assayed in the chromogenic substrate assay. The mean of duplicates is plotted.

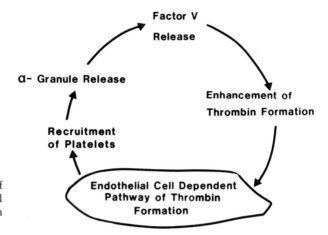

Figure 7. Schematic depiction of the interaction of the endothelial cell-dependent coagulation pathway and platelets.

veny, 1984). The source of factor Xa in these experiments was probably the endothelial cell-dependent pathway, since unstimulated platelets, in the absence of endothelial cells, did not promote significant factor IXa-VIII catalyzed factor X activation. Thus, endothelial cells can initiate a procoagulant pathway that results via thrombin formation in platelet activation, recruiting them to augment the procoagulant response (Fig. 7).

3.3. Interaction of Antithrombin III with Anticoagulantly Active Heparin-like Molecules Associated with the Vessel Wall

Since blood does not form clots continuously as it passes over the endothelium, a central issue concerning the endothelial cell procoagulant pathway concerns its regulation. The next two sections examine the antithrombin III–heparin system and the protein C pathway as regulators of coagulation reactions on the endothelial cell surface.

Our initial studies of endothelial cell-dependent factor Xa-mediated thrombin formation indicated that considerably more thrombin activity was found in the supernatant of cultured bovine aortic endothelial cells than with the native endothelium of bovine aortic vessel segments. When radiolabeled prothrombin was added to the reaction mixtures, it became evident that prothrombin cleavage on native and cultured endothelial cells was comparable, but a high-molecular-weight peak comigrating with a thrombin–antithrombin III complex standard was observed on sodium dodecyl sulfate polyacrylamide gel electrophoresis of medium from native endothelium. Subsequent studies showed that formation of this high-molecular-weight material could be blocked by a specific antibody to antithrombin III resulting in the appearance of a thrombin peak on the gels. Since no antithrombin III was added to these reaction mixtures, the source of antithrombin III must have been a pool of inhibitor associated with the vessel wall (Stern et al., 1985a). The functional significance of this vessel-associated antithrombin III, in terms of the amount of thrombin activity found in the supernatants of aortic segments incubated with factor Xa antithrombin III and prothrombin, is observed from the results of experiments carried out with antibody to antithrombin III. In the presence of antibody to antithrombin III, 20–50-fold greater amounts of thrombin activity are found in the reaction mixture supernatant. By complexing with antithrombin III, the antibody prevents formation of factor Xa and thrombin–antithrombin III complex, thereby augmenting the amount of thrombin found in culture supernatants (Stern et al., 1984b).

Since antithrombin III associated with the endothelial cell surface is clearly an important regulator of thrombin formation on the cell surface, antithrombin III–vessel wall interaction was examined (Stern et al., 1985a). After the vessel segments were washed to remove endogenously bound antithrombin III, incubation of native endothelium with radiolabeled antithrombin III resulted in specific, time-dependent, and saturable binding. Antithrombin III binding sites were half-maximally occupied at a concentration of 11 nM and completely occupied by 1 μM (Fig. 8). Thus, it is highly probable that these binding sites are occupied at the plasma concentration of antithrombin III (2.5 μM). Competitive binding studies demonstrated inhibition of [^{125}I]antithrombin III–vessel wall binding in the presence of unlabeled platelet factor 4. Since platelet factor 4 inhibits antithrombin III interactions with heparin, the experiment raised the possibility that heparin-like molecules were involved in the vessel wall–antithrombin III-binding site. Chemical modification of antithrombin III lysine and tryptophan residues, which blocks its heparin cofactor activity (Rosenberg and Damus, 1973; Heimark and Schwartz, 1983), prevented subsequent antithrombin III–vessel wall binding. Similarly, purified flavobacterium heparinase treatment of vessel segments precluded antithrombin III binding to these vessels. Thus, heparin-like molecules appear instrumental for antithrombin III binding to vessel segments. This concept is supported by the observed enhancement of antithrombin III anticoagulant activity in the presence of endothelium which can be prevented by treating the vessel segment with heparinase. Furthermore, both heparin and heparin-like glycosaminoglycans with anticoagulant activity have been isolated from calf vessel preparations and appear to be localized to the intima (Marcum and Rosenberg, 1984; Marcum et al., 1983, 1984).

The study of factor Xa-mediated prothrombin activation on native endothelium thus led to an understanding of vessel-bound antithrombin III as a regulator of prothrombin activation. Under steady-state conditions, the pool of endothelial cell-bound antithrombin III may effectively downregulate coagulant reactions on the endothelium, during activation of coagulation. However, when platelets undergo the release reaction, high local concentrations of platelet factor 4 may be achieved, thus preventing antithrombin III-endothelial cell interaction. Furthermore, platelets contain an endoglucuronidase that can degrade heparin-like molecules (Oosta et al., 1982), and potentially destroy the endothelial cell–antithrombin III binding site. In vivo modulation of the anti-

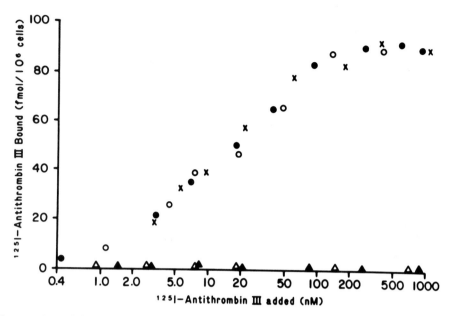

Figure 8. Saturability of [125I]antithrombin III is plotted against the concentration of added tracer. Aortic segments were washed to remove endogenously bound antithrombin III, a binding assay was then carried out (●). Wells were washed and then preincubated with heparinase (5 U/ml) (△), chondroitinase ABC (0.5 U/ml) (○), chondroitinase AC (0.5 U/ml) (X), or [125I]antithrombin III modified by treatment with O-methylisourea was used in place of untreated antithrombin III (▲).

thrombin III–endothelial cell axis may play an important role in the regulation of procoagulant reactions on the vessel surface such as factor Xa-mediated prothrombin activation.

3.4. The Protein C Pathway and Endothelium

An alternative mechanism of regulation of procoagulant reactions involves inactivation of the cofactors, factors Va and VIIIa by the protein C pathway. Protein C is a vitamin K-dependent plasma protein which has anticoagulant properties after its activation to a serine protease by thrombin (Esmon, 1984). The role of protein C as an effective anticoagulant was not appreciated until recently, since only minimal protein C activation occurs when blood clots *in vitro*. Nevertheless, studies employing native and cultured endothelium demonstrated that a cofactor on the cell surface promoted effective thrombin-mediated protein C activation (Esmon, 1983, 1984; Esmon et al., 1982). The endothelial cell cofactor for protein C activation, a cell-surface protein, has been isolated and named thrombomodulin (Esmon et al., 1982). As its name implies, thrombomodulin modulates the coagulant properties of thrombin: the procoagulant properties such as fibrinogen cleavage and factor V activation are attenuated, while activation of the anticoagulant, protein C, is enhanced. The current view of protein C activation as it occurs *in vivo* involves formation of a reversible complex between thrombin and cell-surface thrombomodulin, which cleaves protein C to its active form. The mechanism is responsive to low concentrations of thrombin and can effectively block thrombin-mediated activation of platelets. *In vivo* experiments have demonstrated that infusion of low levels of thrombin into dogs results in anticoagulation via the formation of activated protein C rather than via the activation of the coagulation pathway.

Once activated protein C is formed, it inhibits coagulation by inactivating the cofactors V and VIII (Esmon, 1983, 1984). Activated protein C requires the presence of negatively charged phospholipid surfaces and protein S for optimal anticoagulant activity (Walker, 1980, 1981, 1984). Protein S has been shown to function as a nonenzymatic cofactor for the binding of activated protein C to phospholipid surfaces by forming an enzyme complex that has enhanced affinity for membrane surfaces. The clinical importance of the protein C pathway is demonstrated by the thrombotic diathesis observed in kindreds deficient in either protein C or protein S (Griffin et al., 1981; Bertina et al., 1982; Broekmans et al., 1983; Seligsonn et al., 1984; Comp et al., 1984a; 1984b). Since endothelium effectively promotes the activation of protein C, these findings prompted us (Stern et al., 1986) to examine the vessel surface as a template for assembly of the activated protein C–protein S complex, thereby promoting the anticoagulant function of activated protein C (Fig. 9).

When endothelial cells were incubated with activated protein C and Factor Va, effective inactivation of factor Va was dependent on the presence of protein S. Kinetic studies indicated that the rate of factor Va inactivation was half-maximal at a protein S concentration of 0.2 nM and an activated protein C concentration of 0.05 nM. Binding of ^{125}I-activated protein C to endothelial cell monolayers was absolutely dependent on the presence of protein S. At saturating levels of protein S, activated protein C binding was saturable with K_d = 0.04 nM. By contrast, specific time-dependent and saturable binding of [125I]protein S to endothelium occurred in the absence of activated protein C. Addition of activated protein C increased the affinity of protein S from K_d = 11 nM to 0.2 nM but did not change the number of molecules bound per cell at saturation (85,000 molecules/cell). These studies suggest that activated protein

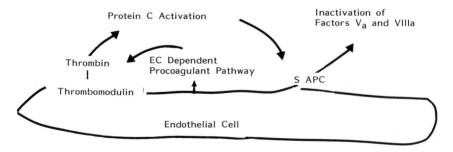

Figure 9. Schematic depiction of protein C pathway on the endothelial cell surface. APC, activated protein C; S, protein S; TM, thrombomodulin.

C increases the affinity of protein S for pre-existing sites on the endothelial cell surface. The close correlation between the parameters of protein S-activated protein C binding to endothelium and factor Va inactivation supports the concept that bound protein S and activated protein C are the active species. Formation of functional activated protein C–protein S complexes thus occurs effectively on the endothelial cell surface and represents a new addition to the list of vessel wall anticoagulant properties. Particularly in the microcirculation, where a high surface to volume ratio exists, the vessel wall protein S–activated protein C mechanism should provide an effective clearance pathway for circulating factor Va and perhaps factor VIIIa.

Clinical studies have demonstrated the existence of steady-state levels of both thrombin and fibrinopeptide A (Nossel et al., 1974; Shuman and Majerus, 1976; Teitel et al., 1982), and the capacity of low levels of thrombin to result in anticoagulation through activation of the protein C pathway (Comp, 1984). In summary, the endothelial cell surface is a powerful regulator of coagulation, since it promotes the generation of thrombin via the procoagulant pathway, and simultaneously primes the protein C pathway, protecting from excess thrombin formation.

4. Endothelial Cell Responses to Cell-Surface Coagulant Events

4.1. Endocytosis of Factors X and Xa

Cell processing is an important determinant of the coagulant activity of cell-associated coagulation proteins. If an enzyme remains localized on the cell surface, its activity can be modulated by the cells while it remains in contact with its substrates and inhibitors in the plasma. In addition, cellular binding can initiate clearance via endocytosis and degradation. Since factor X/Xa-endothelial cell integration forms a vital link between assembly of the factor IXa–VIII–X complex and the prothrombinase complex on the vessel surface, we examined the cellular processing of factor X/Xa. Coagulation factor X and its activated form, Factor Xa, bind specifically to distinct sites on the endothelial cell surface (Stern et al., 1984a,b; Rodgers and Shuman, 1983a). Following surface binding, both factors X and Xa are endocytosed. The factor Xa–binding site complex then dissociates in acidic prelysosomal compartments, allowing factor Xa to enter lysosomes, where degradation occurs. Factor Xa cellular processing is thus analogous to that described for low-density lipoprotein (LDLs) (Basu, 1978), asialoglycoproteins (Ashwell and Morell, 1974), and a variety of other ligands (Ciechanover et al., 1985). By contrast, factor X is slowly internalized and principally shuttled back to the cell surface in a manner similar to that for the transferrin pathway (reviewed in Ciechanover et al., 1985). Thus, cellular processing of cell-bound coagulation factors once again indicates that the endothelial cell surface is not a passive template for the assembly of coagulation factor complexes, but is a dynamic surface with its own regulatory mechanisms (Fig. 10).

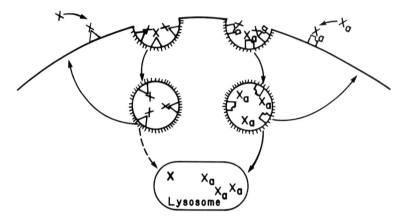

Figure 10. Schematic depiction of the cellular processing of factors X and Xa by cultured endothelium. X, factor X; Xa, Factor Xa.

Several mechanisms have been described by which endothelial cells can regulate the coagulant activity of serine proteases. In each case, these mechanisms are distinct from internalization involving specific binding sites for factors X and Xa. Protease nexins, for example, are a class of serine protease inhibitors synthesized by fibroblasts and other anchorage-dependent cells (Scott *et al.*, 1985; Kraver *et al.*, 1983). Enzyme–protease nexin complexes bind to the cell surface and are subsequently internalized and degraded (Scott *et al.*, 1985; Kraver *et al.*, 1983). Although protease nexin reacts rapidly with thrombin, complex formation with Factor Xa is quite slow.

When factor Xa is added to cultured endothelial cells, only a small fraction, 1–8%, binds to the monolayers, suggesting that factor Xa generated in the fluid phase would predominantly remain in the supernatant, even in the presence of endothelial cells. Mechanisms such as the heparin–antithrombin III system may be the principal inactivators under these conditions. However, when the surface/volume ratio is increased, altering the *in vitro* model to more closely simulate the microvasculature, mechanisms involving clearance of cell-associated factor Xa may become important.

When factor Xa is formed on the cell surface, it can associate with endothelial cell factor V promoting activation of prothrombin (see Section 3.2), or it can be removed from the cell surface by endocytosis. Thus, endocytosis and degradation of cell-bound factor Xa, the physiologic prothrombin activator, provides another pathway for regulation of procoagulant events on the vessel surface.

4.2. Factor Xa as a Hormonal Agent

Another facet of endothelial cell–coagulation factor interaction concerns the effect of coagulation enzymes on endothelial cell physiology. One example is thrombin induction of interleukin 1 elaboration by endothelium (discussed in Section 2). Two other examples concern the effect of factor Xa on the release of endothelial cell mitogenic activity and the elevation of cytosolic calcium.

Recently, endothelial cells have been shown to elaborate growth factors, which led us to examine the effect of coagulation reactions on the cell surface as regulators of mitogen release. In initial studies, we have found that factor Xa enhances the release of endothelial cell mitogens (Gajdusek et al., 1986). Mitogenic activity generated by cultured bovine aortic endothelial cells in response to Factor Xa included platelet-derived growth factor-like molecule(s) based on a radioreceptor assay. Release of mitogenic activity occurred as factor X was activated on the endothelial cell surface. Other studies have shown that thrombin (Harlan et al., 1986) can also induce the release of platelet-derived growth factor-like molecules. These data suggest a new mechanism by which the coagulation system can locally regulate endothelial cell function via interaction with factor Xa and thrombin.

To better understand the mechanism by which factor Xa influences endothelial cell functions, its effect on cellular calcium was examined. Preliminary results (Steinberg et al., 1985) indicated that factor Xa can elevate cytosolic calcium in a dose-dependent manner. Thus, factor Xa may regulate endothelial cell physiology, such as mitogen release, by inducing a change in cytosolic calcium.

5. Induction of a Unidirectional Shift in the Coagulant Phenotype of Endothelial Cells: A Model for the Thrombotic State

The clinical importance of endothelial cell participation in the regulation of coagulation is emphasized by the thrombotic diathesis observed in kindreds deficient in protein C or S (see Section 3.4), since function of the protein C anticoagulant pathway depends on cofactors present on the endothelial cell surface (Esmon et al., 1982; Stern et al., 1986). In addition to these anticoagulant properties, endothelial cells propagate a whole sequence of procoagulant reactions, starting with the expression of Tissue Factor and culminating in the formation of fibrin (see Fig. 5) (see Sections 3.1 and 3.2). It is our hypothesis that mechanisms preventing fibrin formation predominate on the surface of quiescent endothelial cells, but perturbed endothelial cells can promote clot formation.

The coagulant properties of quiescent endothelial cells result from both a lack of procoagulant activity and the presence of potent anticoagulant mechanisms. Tissue factor is not normally expressed on the surface of endothelial cells (Maynard et al., 1977) but can be induced in cultured endothelium in response to a variety of agents, including IL-1. By contrast, anticoagulant properties, such as endothelial cell cofactor activity for the protein C pathway (Esmon et al., 1982; Stern et al., 1986), are readily accessible. Since endothelium has potent anticoagulant mechanisms, induction of procoagulant activity may not be sufficient for the vessel surface to promote development of a prethrombotic state. This led us to examine the effect of IL-1 infusion on anti-

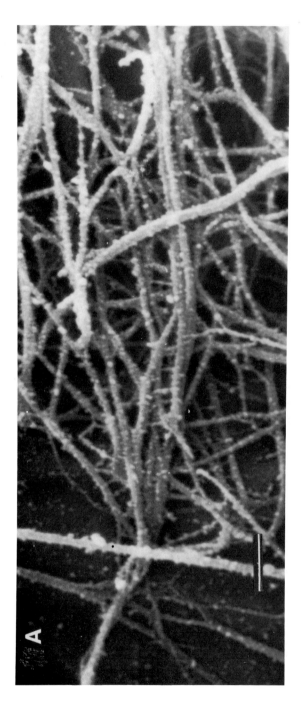

Figure 11. The association of fibrin with the endothelium of rabbits treated with interleukin-1 (IL-1). Rabbits were infused with IL-1 (100 ng/kg), 8 hr later, subjected to whole-body beating heart perfusion fixation, and major arteries were examined by scanning electron microscopy (SEM). (a) SEM of carotid artery in which fibrin is seen as an interlocking strand network in direct apposition to the luminal surface of the vascular endothelium. Marker bar represents 1 μm. (b) SEM of femoral artery demonstrating fibrin strand formation and platelet deposition. Platelets (P) exhibit an activated state, as indicated by pseudopodial projections in direct association with the fibrin strands. Also evident are white cells (W) and associated red blood cells (R). Fibrin strands have an apparent direct association with the endothelial cell surface (marker points). Marker bar represents 5 μm. In each case, the endothelial cells demonstrate a confluent morphology, and no evidence of exposure of the internal elastic lamina was observed.

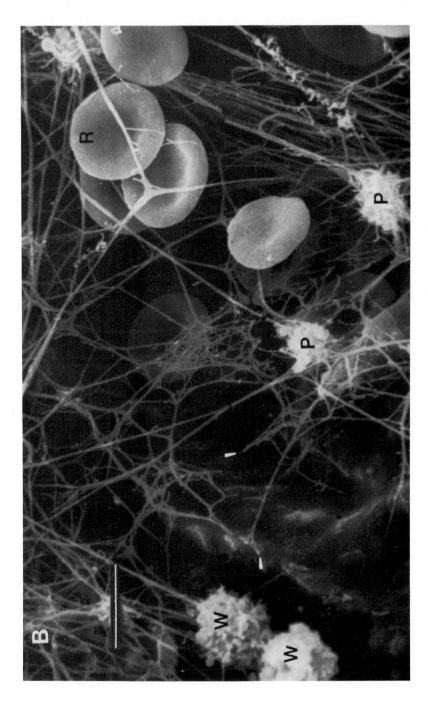

Figure 11. (Continued)

coagulant properties of endothelium. We chose to monitor the protein C pathway, since endothelium supplies both a cell-surface protein promoting thrombin-mediated protein C activation, thrombomodulin (Esmon et al., 1982), and cofactor activity allowing formation of functional activated protein C–protein S complex (Stern et al., 1986). IL-1 infusion resulted in a time-dependent decrease in thrombin-mediated protein C activation on the endothelial cell surface. Furthermore, activated protein C-protein S-mediated factor Va inactivation on aortic endothelium was attenuated following IL-1 infusion.

In addition to monitoring specific endothelial cell anticoagulant and procoagulant properties, the rabbit arterial bed was examined for evidence of fibrin deposition after the interleukin 1 infusion. Fibrin strands closely opposed to the endothelial cell surface (Fig. 11a), often with associated platelets (Fig. 11b), were observed in the vasculature with a predilection for arterial bifurcations. These studies demonstrate that *in vivo* infusion of IL-1 can modulate endothelial cell hemostatic properties and result in fibrin formation. Quiescent endothelial cells from untreated animals exhibited very little tissue factor activity and promoted both the formation and anticoagulant function of activated protein C. Perturbed endothelial cells from interleukin 1-treated animals, in contrast, had considerably enhanced tissue factor activity and did not supply cofactor activity for the protein C pathway effectively. These results indicate that the balance of anticoagulant and procoagulant activities on the endothelial cell surface can be shifted from the quiescent state, in which inhibitory mechanisms predominate, to the perturbed state, in which fibrin formation is promoted. The unidirectional shift in the balance of endothelial cell anticoagulant and procoagulant properties may explain the enhanced thrombotic tendency in inflammatory disease and provides a model of thrombus formation in which endothelial cells are active participants.

6. Summary

Endothelial cells are uniquely positioned to play an important role in vessel wall biology. To function effectively in this role, endothelium must be capable of responding to a variety of stimuli, ranging from mediators of inflammation, such as IL-1, and products of the activated coagulation system, such as factor Xa and thrombin, to products of the anticoagulation system, such as protein C and protein S. The response to these stimuli is equally varied, reflecting the regulatory role of endothelium. IL-1 of monocyte origin, or elaborated by endothelium in response to thrombin, can induce tissue factor in endothelium while concomitantly decreasing cofactor activity for the protein C pathway. The result is a unidirectional shift in the balance of endothelial cell anticoagulant and procoagulant activities, favoring the activation of coagulation on the vessel surface. Factor Xa and thrombin can induce the release of mitogenic activity from endothelium, including PDGF-like molecules. Furthermore, factor Xa can affect endothelial cell function globally by elevating cytosolic calcium. The endothelial cell in turn provides binding sites for factor Xa, which can promote its procoagulant activity or, alternatively, result in its clearance from the cell surface by receptor-mediated endocytosis. These data indicate that endothelium cannot be regarded as an inert surface insulating hemostatic components from extravascular tissues. Rather, endothelium is a dynamic modulator of vessel wall physiology.

ACKNOWLEDGMENTS. DMS completed this work during the tenure of a Clinician Scientist Award from the American Heart Association with funds contributed in part by the Oklahoma affiliate. This work was supported by a Young Investigator Award from the Oklahoma affiliate of the American Heart Association and by grant HL-34625 from the National Institutes of Health.

References

Aggeler, P., 1961, Physiological basis for transfusion therapy in hemorrhagic disorders, *Transfusion* **1**:71–86.

Ashwell, G., and Morell, A. G., 1974, The role of surface carbohydrates in the hepatic recognition of circulating glycoproteins, *Adv. Enzymol.* **41**:99–143.

Bach, R., Nemerson, Y., and Konigsberg, W., 1981, Purification and characterization of bovine Tissue Factor, *J. Biol. Chem.* **256**:8324–8331.

Baker, J. B., Low, D. A., Simmer, R. L., and Cunningham, D. D., 1980, Protease-nexin: A cellular component that links thrombin and plasminogen activator and mediates their binding to cells, *Cell* **21**:37–45.

Basu, S. K., Goldstein, J. L., and Brown, M. S., 1978, Characterization of the low density lipoprotein receptor in membranes prepared from human fibroblasts, *J. Biol. Chem.* **253**:3852–3861.

Bertina, R. M., Broekmans, A. W., van der Linden, I. K., and Mertens, K., 1982, Protein C deficiency in a Dutch family with thrombotic disease, *Thromb. Haemost.* **48**:1–5.

Bevilacqua, M. P., Pober, J. S., Majeau, G. R., Cotran, R. S., and Gimbrone, M. A., 1984, Interleukin 1 induces biosynthesis and cell surface expression of procoagulant activity in human vascular endothelial cells, *J. Exp. Med.* **160**:618–621.

Broekmans, A. W., Veltkamp, J. J., and Bertina, R. M., 1983, Congenital protein C deficiency and venous thromboembolism. A study of three Dutch families, *N. Engl. J. Med.* **309**:340–344.

Broze, G., 1982, Binding of human Factor VII and VIIa to monocytes, *J. Clin. Invest.* **70**:526–535.

Cerveny, T., Fass, D., and Mann, K., 1984, Synthesis of Factor V by cultured bovine endothelial cells, *Blood* **63**:1476–1484.

Ciechanover, A., Schwartz, A. L., and Lodish, H. I., 1985, Sorting and recycling of cell surface receptors and endocytosed ligands. The asialoglycoprotein and transferin receptors, *J. Cell Biochem.* **23**:107–122.

Colucci, M., Balconi, G., Lorenzet, R., Pietra, A., Locati, D., Donati, M. D., and Semerano, M., 1983, Cultured human endothelial cells generate Tissue Factor in response to endotoxin, *J. Clin. Invest.* **71**:1893–1896.

Comp, P. C., 1984, Animal studies of protein C physiology, *Semin. Thromb. Hemost.* **10**:149–153.

Comp, P. C., Nixon, R. R., Cooper, R. M., and Esmon, C. T., 1984a, Familial protein S deficiency is associated with recurrent thrombosis, *J. Clin. Invest.* **74**:2082–2088.

Comp, P. C., Nixon, R. R., and Esmon, C.T., 1984b, Determination of protein C, an antithrombotic protein, using thrombin–thrombomodulin complex, *Blood* **63**:14–21.

Dahlback, B., and Stenflo, J., 1978, Binding of bovine coagulation Factor Xa to platelets, *Biochem. J.* **23**:4938–4945.

Davie, E. W., and Ratnoff, O. D., 1964, Waterfall sequence for intrinsic blood clotting, *Science* **145**:1310–1311.

Dvorak, H. F., Galli, S. J., and Dvorak, A. M., 1980, Expression of cell-mediated hypersensitivity *in vivo*—Recent advances, *Int. Rev. Exp. Pathol.* **21:**119–194.

Dvorak, H. F., Harvey, V. S., and McDonagh, J., 1984, Quantification of fibrinogen influx and fibrin deposition and turnover in line 1 and line 10 guinea pig carcinoma, *Cancer Res.* **44:**3348–3354.

Dvorak, H. F., Senger, D. R., Dvorak, A. M., Harvey, V. S., and McDonagh, J., 1985, Regulation of extravascular coagulation by microvascular permeability, *Science* **229:**1059–1061.

Esmon, C. T., 1983, Protein C: biochemistry, physiology and clinical implications, *Blood* **62:**455–1158.

Esmon, C. T., 1984, Protein C, *Prog. Hemost. Thromb.* **7:**25–54.

Esmon, N. L., Owen, W. G., and Esmon, C. T., 1982, Isolation of a membrane-bound cofactor for thrombin-catalyzed activation of protein C, *J. Biol. Chem.* **257:**859–864.

Estes, D., and Christian, C. L., 1971, The natural history of systemic lupus erythematosus by prospective analysis, *Medicine (Baltimore)* **50:**85–103.

Fenton, J. W., II, Fascow, M. J., Stackrow, A. B., Aronson, D. L., Young, A. M., and Finlayson, J. S., 1977, Human thrombin, *J. Biol. Chem.* **252:**3587–3598.

Fuchs, H. E., and Pizzo, S. V., 1983, Regulation of Factor Xa *in vitro* in human and mouse plasma and *in vivo* in mouse, Role of the endothelium and plasma proteinase inhibitors, *J. Clin. Invest.* **72:**2041–2049.

Fuchs, H., Trap, H., Griffith, M., Roberts, H., and Pizzo, S., 1984, Regulation of Factor IXa *in vivo* in human and mouse plasma and *in vivo* in the mouse, *J. Clin. Invest.* **73:**1696–1703.

Gajdusek, C. M., Carbon, S., Ross, R., Nawroth, P., and Stern, D., 1986, Activation of coagulation releases endothelial cell mitogens, *J. Cell Biol.* **103:**419–428.

Gitel, S. N., Stephenson, R. C., and Wessler, S., 1977, *In vitro* and *in vivo* correlation of clotting protease activity: Effect of heparin, *Proc. Natl. Acad. Sci. USA* **74:**3028–3032.

Griffin, J. H., Evatt, B., Zimmerman, T. S., Kleiss, A. J., and Wideman, C., 1981, Deficiency of protein C in congenital thrombotic disease, *J. Clin. Invest.* **68:**1370–1373.

Gurewich, V., Nunn, T., and Lipinski, B., 1979, Activation of extrinsic or intrinsic blood coagulation in experimental venous thrombosis and disseminated intravascular coagulation: Pathogenic differences, *Thromb. Res.* **14:**931–940.

Harlan, J. M., D. F., Thompson, P. J., Ross, R. R., and Bowen-Pope, 1986, Alpha-thrombin induces release of platelet-derived growth factor-like molecule(s) by cultured human endothelial cells, *J. Cell Biol.* **103:**1129–1133.

Hartubise, P., Coots, M., Jacob, D., Mahleman, A., and Glueck, H., 1979, Monoclonal IgG$_4$ with Factor V inhibitory activity, *J. Immunol.* **122:**2119–2121.

Hedner, A., and Kisiel, W., 1983, Use of human Factor VIIa in the treatment of two hemophilia A patients with high-titer inhibitor, *J. Clin. Invest.* **71:**1836–1841.

Heimark, R. L., and Schwartz, S., 1983, Binding of coagulation Factors IX and X to the endothelial cell surface, *Biochem. Biophys. Res. Commun.* **111:**723–731.

Hultin, M. B., 1982, Role of human Factor VIII in Factor X activation, *J. Clin. Invest.* **69:**950–958.

Jesty, J., and Silverberg, S. A., 1979, Kinetics of the Tissue Factor-dependent activation of coagulation Factors IX and X in a bovine plasma system, *J. Biol. Chem.* **254:**12337–12345.

Kaplan, K. L., 1982, Interactions of platelets with endothelial cells, in: *Pathobiology of the Endothelial Cell* (H. I. Nossel and H. J. Vogel, eds.), pp. 337–349, Academic, New York.

Kisiel, W., and Davie, E. W., 1975, Isolation and characterization of bovine Factor VII, *Biochemistry* **14:**4928–4934.

Kraver, D. J., Thompson, J. A., and Cunningham, D. D., 1983, Protease nexus: Cell-secreted proteins that mediate the binding, internalization, and degradation of regulatory serine protease, *J. Cell Physiol.* **117:**385–394.

Lyberg, T., Galdal, K. S., Evensen, S. A., and Prydz, H., 1983, Cellular cooperation in endothelial thromboplastin synthesis, *Br. J. Haematol.* **53:**85–95.

MacFarlane, R. G., 1964, An enzyme cascade in the blood clotting mechanism, and its function as a biochemical amplifier, *Nature (Lond.)* **202:**498–499.

Marcum, J., and Rosenberg, R., 1984, Anticoagulantly active heparin-like molecules from vascular tissue, *Biochemistry* **23:**1730–1737.

Marcum, J., Fritze, L., Galli, S., Karp, G., and Rosenberg, R., 1983, Microvascular heparin-like species with anticoagulant activity, *Am. J. Physiol.* **245:**725–733.

Marcum, J., McKenney, J., and Rosenberg, R., 1984, The acceleration of thrombin–antithrombin III complex formation in rat hind quarters via heparin-like molecules bound to endothelium, *J. Clin. Invest.* **74**:341–350.

Maynard, J. R., Dryer, B. E., Stemerman, M. E., and Pitlick, F. A., 1977, Tissue Factor coagulant activity of cultured human endothelial and smooth muscle cells and fibroblasts, *Blood* **50**:387–396.

Miletich, J. C., Jackson, C., Majerus, P., 1977, Interaction of coagulation Factor Xa with human platelets, *Proc. Natl. Acad. Sci. USA* **74**:4033–4036.

Mizel, S. B., 1982, The interleukins: Regulation of lymphocyte differentiation, proliferation and functional activation, in: *Biological Responses in Cancer* (E. Mirich, ed.), pp. 89–119, Plenum, New York.

Nawroth, P. P., and Stern, D. M., 1985, A pathway of coagulation on endothelial cells, *J. Cell Biochem.* **28**:253–264.

Nawroth, P. P., McCarthy, D., Kisiel, W., Handley, D., Stern, D. M., 1985a, Cellular processing of bovine Factor X and Xa by cultured bovine aortic endothelial cells, *J. Exp. Med.* **162**:559–572.

Nawroth, P. P., Stern, D. M., Kisiel, W., and Bach, R., 1985b, Cellular requirements for Tissue Factor generation by bovine aortic endothelial cells in culture, *Thromb. Res.* **40**:677–691.

Nawroth, P. P., Handley, D., Esmon, C. T., and Stern, D. M., 1986, Interleukin 1 induces endothelial cell procoagulant while suppressing cell surface anticoagulant activity, *Proc. Natl. Acad. Sci. USA* **83**:3460–3464.

Nelsestuen, G. L., Kisiel, W., and DiScipio, R. G., 1978, Interaction of vitamin K-dependent proteins with membranes, *Biochemistry* **17**:2134–2138.

Nemerson, Y., and Bach, R., 1982, Tissue Factor revisited, *Prog. Hemost. Thromb.* **6**:237–261.

Nossel, H. L., Yudelman, I., Canfield, R. E., Butler, V. P., Spanondis, K., Wilner, G. D., and Qureshi, G. D., 1974, Measurement of fibrinopeptide A in human blood, *J. Clin. Invest.* **54**:43–53.

Oosta, G. M., Favreau, L. V., Beeler, D. L., and Rosenberg, R. D., 1982, Purification and properties of human platelet heparitinase, *J. Biol. Chem.* **257**:11249–11255.

Oppenheim, J. J., and Gery, I., 1982, Interleukin is more than an interleukin, *Immunol. Today* **3**:113–132.

Osterud, B., and Eskeland, T., 1982, The mandatory role of complement in the endotoxin-induced synthesis of tissue thromboplastin in blood monocytes, *FEBS Lett.* **149**:75–79.

Prydz, H., and Allison, A. C., 1978, Tissue thromboplastin activity of isolated human monocytes, *Thromb. Haemost.* **39**:582–591.

Ratnoff, O. D., and Colopy, J. E., 1955, A familial hemorrhagic trait associated with a deficiency of a clot promoting fraction of plasma, *J. Clin. Invest.* **34**:602–613.

Reidy, M. A., and Schwartz, S. M., 1981, Endothelial regeneration. III. Time course of minimal changes after small defined injury to rat aortic endothelium, *Lab. Invest.* **44**:301–308.

Rizza, C. R., 1972, The clinical features of clotting factor deficiencies, in: *Human Blood Coagulation, Haemostasis and Thrombosis* (R. Biggs, ed.), pp. 210–224, Blackwell Scientific, Oxford, England.

Rodgers, G. M., and Shuman, M. A., 1983a, Characterization of a novel receptor for Factor Xa on bovine aortic endothelial cells, *Blood* **62**(Suppl. II):308 (abst).

Rodgers, G. M., and Shuman, M. A., 1984b, Prothrombin is activated on vascular endothelial cells by Factor Xa and calcium, *Proc. Natl. Acad. Sci. USA* **80**:7001–7005.

Rosenberg, R., and Damus, P., 1973, The purification and mechanism of action of human antithrombin-heparin cofactor, *J. Biol. Chem.* **248**:6490–6503.

Rosing, J., Van Rijn, J. L. M. L., Bevers, E. M., van Dieijen, G., Comfurius, P., and Zwall, R. F. A., 1985, The role of activated human platelets in prothrombin and Factor X activation, *Blood* **65**:319–332.

Schwartz, S. M., and Gajdusek, C. M., 1982, Growth factors and the vessel wall, *Prog. Hemost. Thromb.* **6**:85–112.

Schwartz, S. M., Gajdusek, C. M., Selden, S. C., 1981, Vascular wall growth control: The role of endothelium, *Arteriosclerosis* **1**:107–161.

Scott, R. W., Bergman, B. L., Bajpai, A., Herxh, R. T., Rodriquez, H., Jones, B. N., Baneda, C., Watts, S., and Baker, J., 1985, Protease nexin, *J. Biol. Chem.* **260**:7029–7304.

Seligsonn, U., Berger, A., Abend, M., Rubin, L., Attias, D., Zivelin, A., and Rappaport, S. I., 1984,

Homozygous protein C deficiency manifested by massive venous thrombosis in the newborn, *N. Engl. J. Med.* **310:**559–562.

Shanah, W., and Korn, J., 1984, Endothelial cells express IL-1-like activity as assessed by enhancement of fibroblast PGE synthesis, *Clin. Res.* **32:**666 (abst).

Shuman, M., and Majerus, P., 1976, The measurement of thrombin in clotting blood by radioimmunoassay, *J. Clin. Invest.* **58:**1249–1258.

Steinberg, S., Stern, D. M., Nawroth, P. P., and Bielizikian, J., 1985, Factor Xa elevates cytosolic calcium in cultured endothelial cells, *Thromb. Haemost.* **54:**994 (abst).

Stern, D. M., Drillings, M., Nossel, H. L., Hurlet-Jensen, A., La Gamma, K., and Owen, J., 1983, Binding of Factors IX and IXa to cultured vascular endothelial cells, *Proc. Natl. Acad. Sci. USA* **80:**4119–4123.

Stern, D. M., Drillings, M., Kisiel, W., Nawroth, P., Nossel, H. L., and La Gamma, K. S., 1984a, Activation of Factor IX bound to cultured bovine aortic endothelial cells, *Proc. Natl. Acad. Sci. USA* **81:**913–917.

Stern, D. M., Nawroth, P. P., Kisiel, W., Handley, D., Drillings, M., and Bartos, J., 1984b, A coagulation pathway on bovine aortic segments leading to generation of Factor Xa and thrombin, *J. Clin. Invest.* **74:**1910–1921.

Stern, D. M., Nawroth, P. P., Marcum, J., Handley, D., Kisiel, D., Rosenberg, R., and Stern, K., 1985a, Interaction of antithrombin III with bovine aortic segments, *J. Clin. Invest.* **75:**272–279.

Stern, D. M., Bank, I., Nawroth, P. P., Cassimeris, J., Kisiel, W., Fenton II, J. W., Dinarello, C., Chess, L., and Jaffe, E. A., 1985b, Self-regulation of procoagulant events on the endothelial surface, *J. Exp. Med.* **162:**1223–1235.

Stern, D. M., Nawroth, P. P., Handley, D., and Kisiel, W., 1985c, An endothelial cell-dependent pathway of coagulation, *Proc. Natl. Acad. Sci. USA* **82:**2523–2527.

Stern, D. M., Nawroth, P. P., Harris, K., and Esmon, C. T., 1986, Cultured bovine aortic endothelial cells promote activated protein C protein S-mediated inactivation of Factor Va, *J. Biol. Chem.* **261:**713–718.

Teitel, J. M., Bauer, K. A., Lau, H. K., and Rosenberg, R. D., 1982, Studies of the prothrombin activation pathway utilizing radioimmunoassays for the F_1/F_{1+2} fragment and thrombin-antithrombin complex, *Blood* **59:**1086–1087.

Thompson, A., Forney, A., Gentry, P., Smith, K., and Harker, L., 1980, Human Factor IX in animals: Kinetics from isolated radiolabeled protein and platelet destruction following crude concentrate infusions, *Br. J. Haematol.* **45:**329–342.

Tracy, P. B., Petersen, J., Nesheim, M., McDuffie, F., and Mann, K. G., 1979, Interaction of coagulation Factor V and Factor Va with platelets, *J. Biol. Chem.* **254:**10354–10361.

Tracy, P. B., Nesheim, M. E., and Mann, K. G., 1981, Coordinate binding of factor Va and Xa to the unstimulated platelet, *J. Biol. Chem.* **256:**743–751.

Tracy, P. B., Eide, L. L., and Mann, K. G., 1985, Human prothrombinase complex assembly and function on isolated blood cell populations, *J. Biol. Chem.* **260:**2119–2124.

Unanue, E. R., 1981, The regulatory role of macrophages in antigenic stimulation. Part II. Symbiotic relationship between lymphocytes and macrophages, *Adv. Immunol.* **31:**1–43.

Walker, F. J., 1980, Regulation of activated protein C by a new protein, *J. Biol. Chem.* **255:**5521–5524.

Walker, F. J., 1981, Regulation of protein C by protein S, the role of phospholipid in Factor Va inactivation, *J. Biol. Chem.* **256:**11128–11131.

Walker, F. J., 1984, Protein S and the regulation of activated protein C, *Semin. Thromb. Hemost.* **10:**131–138.

Wessler, S., Reimber, S. M., and Sheps, M. C., 1959, Biologic assay of a thrombosis inducing activity in human serum, *J. Appl. Physiol.* **14:**943–946.

Windt, M. R., and Rosenwasser, L. J., 1984, Human vascular endothelial cells produce interleukin 1, *Lymphokine Res.* **3:**175 (abst).

Zur, M., and Nemerson, Y., 1980, Kinetics of Factor IX activation via the extrinsic pathway, *J. Biol. Chem.* **255:**5703–5710.

Chapter 5

Factors That Affect Vessel Reactivity and Leukocyte Emigration

TIMOTHY J. WILLIAMS

1. Introduction

The first phase of wound healing consists of an inflammatory response. It was the study of wounds that first led to the proposal that the visual manifestations of inflammation are caused by changes in blood vessels: dilatation underlying redness and plasma extravasation underlying tissue swelling (Hunter, 1794). Inflammation is important in wound healing because the associated micro-vascular changes result in the transfer of blood constituents from the vessels to the tissues. Thus, intradermal injection of autologous blood into rat skin, 2 days before an incision was found to result in accelerated healing (Myers and Rightor, 1978).

The event initiating wound healing may be tissue injury induced by, for example, a mechanical or thermal stimulus. Local infection, if sufficiently severe, can also lead to tissue injury and as the infective agent and necrotic host tissue are being eliminated by leukocyte phagocytosis, suppuration or shedding, the process of wound healing either restores the tissue to its normal function or produces fibrosis.

It is the purpose of this chapter to discuss the changes that occur in the microvascular bed in inflammation and the factors that bring about these changes. Many different chemicals are involved in this process, with considerable duplication of functions. The plethora of mediators probably is a consequence of the vital role of inflammation in host defense. The redundancy of mediator function minimizes the possibility of chemical interference by products emanating from foreign organisms.

The microvascular bed distributes the blood supply to a tissue to provide it with oxygen and nutrients and to remove metabolic waste products. This general function of microvessels is supplemented by the specialized functions of particular organs. Physiologic mechanisms exist to regulate local blood flow for

TIMOTHY J. WILLIAMS • Section of Vascular Biology, MRC Clinical Research Centre, Harrow, Middlesex HA1 3UJ, England.

three reasons: (1) blood vessels must adjust to widely varying requirements of an individual tissue, i.e., tissue metabolism changes; (2) the tissue blood vessels need to compensate for changes in arterial blood pressure to maintain local blood supply (autoregulation); and (3) arterial blood pressure is regulated in part by controlling peripheral resistance in certain areas (e.g., splanchnic-induced vasconstriction to compensate for increased blood flow in skeletal muscle during exercise).

In the face of these changes in local flow, it is essential to have a state of dynamic fluid equilibrium between the tissue and its blood supply. This is maintained by a balance between the hydraulic pressure tending to move fluid out of blood microvessels and an osmotic pressure tending to move fluid in the reverse direction. Lymphatic clearance compensates for a small excess outward movement. Proper equilibrium depends on a low conductivity of blood microvessels to plasma proteins across the vessel wall, which constitutes an important function of the lining endothelial cells.

The equilibrium existing in a tissue can change radically following a local inflammatory stimulus. Depending on the nature of stimulus, local blood flow can cease altogether or rise dramatically, overriding the previously physiologic needs of the tissue. Furthermore, the low conductivity of the endothelial cell barrier to macromolecules is lost, and fluid with a high protein concentration leaks from microvessels resulting in tissue swelling. Subsequently, the tissue becomes host to high numbers of blood cells normally largely confined to the vascular compartment.

2. Direct Injury to Blood Vessels

The changes in vessel tone and permeability seen in inflammatory reactions can result from exogenous or endogenous factors. These changes may occur separately or simultaneously in such a manner that it is often difficult to distinguish them. The changes in vessel tone may occur by direct action of the inflammatory stimulus on the blood vessel wall or, as discussed in subsequent sections, by the effects of endogenous chemical mediators released by the stimulus. In some cases, the direct effect of the stimulus is clear (e.g., a cut destroys the permeability barrier). Other examples of direct injury to the vessel are thermal injury, radiation injury, and exogenous chemical injury, where the damage to the microvascular smooth muscle cells and/or endothelial cells results in changes in vessel tone and permeability (Arthurson, 1979).

In many tissues, increased permeability occurs specifically in small venules in response to chemical mediators (see Section 6). Thus, direct injury may sometimes be distinguished from endogenous chemically mediated changes in the microvasculature by a loss of regional specialization. In addition, direct injury will be confined to the area of tissue exposed to the stimulus, whereas chemically mediated effects will extend beyond the area of damage. This effect can be demonstrated by observation of vasodilatation in skin at the edges of a masked area exposed to different wavelengths of ultraviolet (UV) light.

3. Concept and Classification of Inflammatory Mediators

The concept of endogenous chemical mediators of inflammation was first proposed by Ebbecke (1923), who postulated that erythema in the skin was caused by the irritated epithelium producing chemicals that diffused to the capillaries and arterioles in the cutis and induced dilatation. The first such mediator to be identified was histamine. Dale and Laidlaw (1910) found that intravenous injection of histamine caused peripheral vasodilatation and lowered arterial blood pressure in animals. Subsequently, Dale (1913) and Schultz (1910) postulated that histamine was the mediator of anaphylactic reactions.

Lewis and Grant (1924) first attempted to correlate observations of the skin response to histamine with the theory of chemical mediators proposed by Ebbecke (1923). Lewis and Grant, on the advice of Dale, studied the wheal and flare response induced in the skin by histamine and concluded that histamine, or a histamine-like substance, was liberated in the tissue in response to a mild mechanical or thermal injury. This use of mimicry as a criterion for the identification of endogenous mediators remains an important part of current research. Lewis and Grant were unable to detect histamine in trauma-induced wheal fluid, using the isolated guinea pig uterus as an assay tissue. They were therefore careful not to state categorically that the endogenous mediator was histamine.

The first challenge to the histamine theory of Lewis and Grant developed from a different approach adopted by Menkin (1938a,b). Menkin collected exudates induced in rabbits and dogs by turpentine, croton oil, *Staphylococcus aureus*, and thermal injury and partially purified a dialyzable factor that induced vasodilatation and increased microvascular permeability when injected into rabbit skin. He found that the factor also had the important property of inducing leukocyte accumulation, calling it leukotaxine. Menkin concluded that this factor was not histamine, as it failed to contract the isolated guinea pig ileum and also the skin reactions to the factor and histamine were characteristically different. The doubts about the universal importance of histamine as an inflammatory mediator were confirmed following the development of effective receptor antagonists, which failed to suppress completely the inflammatory response to chemical mediators (Halpern, 1942). A combination of the three approaches to mediators described in this section using mimicry, exudate analysis, and specific antagonists or inhibitors, forms the basis of modern research into inflammatory mediators.

In subsequent sections, mediators are classified according to their actions. Mediators can be further subclassified according to their (1) chemical nature (e.g., lipid, phospholipid, amino acid metabolite, polypeptide), (2) their source (i.e., tissue fluid, tissue cell, or inflammatory cell), and (3) whether they are stored and released or synthesized *de novo* on stimulation of a cell.

4. Mediators Affecting Vessel Tone

4.1. Physiologic Control of Vessel Tone

Normally the tone of blood microvessels is controlled by local factors, gas tensions, and metabolites, with arteriolar diameter largely governing tissue blood flow in most tissues. Superimposed on this control are the effects of transmitters, released from nerve endings, and the effects of circulating hormones. A major determinant of vascular smooth muscle tone is norepinephrine, released from sympathetic nerve endings. In most vascular smooth muscle, norepineprhine acts on α_1-receptors to induce vasoconstriction, although in coronary and lung vessels there are also β_2-receptors and dilatation usually predominates. The effect of circulating epinephrine varies according to the tissue, that is, dilatation of arterioles in skeletal muscle and liver by an effect on β_2-receptors, vasoconstriction in other abdominal viscera. Blood vessels of some tissues receive a parasympathetic cholinergic innervation, and acetylcholine (ACh) acts on muscarinic receptors to induce vasodilatation.

This is a brief description of the normal control of vessel tone. In response to an inflammatory stimulus, these control systems are overridden by the local release of chemical mediators.

4.2. Direct-Action and Endothelium-Dependent Vasodilator Mechanisms

Interest in vasodilators has been considerably increased by the recent discovery that the responses to some agents are dependent on the release of a factor from endothelial cells. Before the work of Furchgott and Zawadzki (1980), the engima had persisted that ACh induced arteriolar and arterial vasodilatation *in vivo* but contraction of isolated strips of circular artery *in vitro*. Furchgott and Zawadzki (1980) discovered that, if care was taken to prevent damage to the endothelium when preparing strips of rabbit aorta and tone was induced with norepinephrine, ACh induced relaxation. This phenomenon can be induced in the presence of prostaglandin synthesis inhibitors and has now been demonstrated for a variety of vasodilators. The factor generated by endothelial cells has been termed endothelium-derived relaxing factor, EDRF (Cherry *et al.*, 1982). The precise chemical nature of EDRF has not been determined because the substance is very unstable (having a half-life ($t\frac{1}{2}$) of 6 sec) (Griffith *et al.*, 1984).

Although the chemical structure of EDRF is unknown, its discovery is beginning to show an interesting parallel with the original discovery of ACh itself and more recently endorphins. The discovery of acetylcholine and endorphins was preceded by the finding that plant-derived substances (nicotine, muscarine, and morphine) had potent effects in animals. Acetylcholine, which is chemically related to nicotine and muscarine, and endorphins, which are chemically related to morphine, were subsequently identified as endogenous substances. In a similar manner, EDRF may be related to the nitrate vasodilators, such as glyceryl trinitrate. Nitric oxide itself, and substances such as glyceryl trinitrate and sodium nitroprusside, which probably have their effects after conversion to nitric oxide (NO), appears to stimulate guanylate cyclase in vascular smooth muscle (Katsuki et al., 1977). It is then proposed that relaxation is produced as a result of cyclic guanosine monophosphate (cGMP)-dependent phosphorylation of myosin light chain (Rapoport et al., 1983). Nitric oxide and nitrodilators stimulate cGMP in tissue homogenates (Kimura et al., 1975), and this is blocked by hemoglobin, myoglobin, and Methylene Blue (Miki et al., 1977; Greutter et al., 1979). Interestingly, these agents also block the relaxation and cGMP elevation induced by EDRF (Holzmann, 1982; Ignarro et al., 1984; Martin et al., 1984). These observations suggest that NO, derived from vasodilator nitrates, acts on the EDRF receptor of vascular smooth muscle cells.

In spite of all these interesting observations on arteries in vitro, it is still not clear whether arteriolar dilatation induced by neural transmitters released extravascularly is dependent on EDRF release.

4.3. Histamine-Induced Vasodilatation

Histamine (β-imidazolylethylamine) is widely distributed in mammalian tissues and at a particularly high concentration in the human epidermis, lungs, gastrointestinal (GI) mucosa, and central nervous system (CNS). Some of these tissues have a high turnover of histamine; it has been postulated that histamine plays a role in the physiologic control of vascular tone (Schayer, 1965). Except in the context of the control of gastric acid secretion, the strictly physiologic roles of histamine are controversial; the discussion here is limited to the established role of histamine in inflammatory reactions.

Histamine is synthesized from the amino acid L-histidine by the action of histidine decarboxylase and is stored in high concentrations in tissue mast cells, circulating basophil leukocytes, and platelets of some species. Histamine can be released from these cells by a wide variety of inflammatory stimuli, as well as by certain other inflammatory mediators. Thus, histamine may be a primary or secondary mediator in different reactions. Mast cells and basophils have immunoglobulin E (IgE), and in some species IgG, antibody receptors, and Ca^{2+}-dependent histamine secretion occurs on contact with antigen. Other stimuli inducing release are mechanical, thermal, and chemical (e.g., a side effect of certain drugs, such as tubocurarine). Histamine release can be induced by basic polypeptides and proteins and some of these may be generated by infiltrating leukocytes and injured tissues. Among the inflammatory mediators acting partly via histamine release are the polypeptides C3a, C5a, and substance P. Their other effects are discussed separately in subsequent sections.

One of the first actions of histamine to be discovered was a lowering of arterial blood pressure upon intravenous injection in animals (Section 3). This effect, which occurs in all mammalian species except the rabbit, is caused by peripheral arteriolar vasodilatation. With the advent of the first antihistamines, studies on histamine receptors in the vasculature could be undertaken (Folkow et al., 1948). Responses to large doses of histamine could not be antagonized, however, indicating the presence of a second type of histamine receptor. Other actions of histamine, such as stimulation of gastric acid secretion, were found to be entirely unaffected by the available antihistamines; hence Ash and Schild (1966) defined two types of receptors: H_1 (blocked by classic antihistamines) and H_2 (not blocked). Histamine antagonists acting on the H_2-receptor, were subsequently developed by Black et al. (1972). H_1- and H_2-agonists and antagonists have now been employed to characterize the receptors involved in particular vascular responses (Levi et al., 1982).

The tone of arteries and arterioles is controlled by both H_1- and H_2-receptors (Black et al., 1972, 1975; Boyce and Wareham, 1980), as suggested in early studies (Folkow et al., 1948). In humans, cats, and dogs, both H_1- and H_2-receptor-mediated effects are dilator. However, in the rabbit H_1 effects are constrictor, while the H_2 effects are dilator. It was shown in experiments in humans that a temporal difference exists between the effects of histamine on H_1- and H_2-receptors (Chipman and Glover, 1976). When an infusion of histamine was given intra-arterially to the forearm, the initial increase in blood flow was more effectively suppressed by an H_1-antagonist (mepyramine), whereas the later increase was more effectively suppressed by an H_2-antagonist (metiamide). Interestingly, it has been reported recently that H_1-receptor-mediated relaxation of rat aorta by histamine in vitro is endothelial cell dependent (Van de Corde and Leusen, 1983). Thus, it is possible that in humans the H_2-receptors are located predominantly on vascular smooth muscle, while H_1-receptors are located predominantly on endothelial cells, with both types of receptor mediating vasodilatation, but by different mechanisms. A different situation exists in the pulmonary circulation where, in all species studied, H_1-receptors mediate vasoconstriction, while H_2-receptors mediate vasodilatation, thus resembling the rabbit peripheral circulation (Levi et al., 1982).

Intradermal injection of histamine in human skin induces a wheal with local reddening and a surrounding red flare. The wheal is caused by an increase in microvascular permeability and local reddening by the vasodilator activity of histamine. The surrounding flare is caused by an axon reflex mechanism; impulses from skin pain receptors pass along branches of afferent nerves (c fibers) and release a vasodilator substance peripheral to the site of histamine injection. These responses are difficult to quantify. However, all the features of the response appear to be partly suppressed by combined H_1- and H_2-antagonists.

Since it was discovered before other inflammatory agents, histamine has probably been accredited with too large a role in pathophysiology. It is probable that histamine is important in certain acute inflammatory reactions, or in the acute phases of more protracted responses. However, it is intriguing that high numbers of mast cells are seen in association with forming vessels during wound healing. In addition, the histamine forming capacity of healing tissue is markedly elevated (Kahlson and Rosengren, 1971). Whether histamine has a role in the persistent vasodilatation seen in such tissue is open to question.

4.4. 5-Hydroxytryptamine and Vessel Tone

It was discovered during the last century that a stable vasoconstrictor substance is generated during blood clotting named vasotonin or serotonin. It was found empirically that this substance could be removed by perfusing serum through the vasculature of the lungs. The activity was attributable to 3-(β-aminoethyl)-5-hydroxyindole) (5-HT) synthesized in the body from the amino acid tryptophan (Rapport, 1948). Subsequently, it was discovered that the same substance, originally termed enteramine, was also present in the gut. 5-HT is found in enterochromaffin cells of the gut, the CNS, and in blood platelets. In certain species, rodents and cattle, 5-HT is also found together with histamine, in tissue mast cells.

5-Hydroxytryptamine has a broad spectrum of biologic activities and is thought to be a neurotransmitter, but its other functions remain unclear. Local release of 5-HT from platelets during clotting can contribute to hemostasis, although 5-HT can induce vasodilatation in skeletal muscle and erythema when injected into human skin. The latter involves stasis because of venous constriction, which is characteristic of 5-HT. These direct actions of 5-HT can be complicated by secondary reflex actions since the amine has potent effects on nerves. The role of 5-HT in inflammation is obscure, except in rodents where it is potent in increasing microvascular permeability.

4.5. Kinin-Induced Vasodilatation

Early experiments demonstrated that intravenous injection of urine in humans and animals resulted in a hypotensive response (Abelous and Bradier, 1909; Frey and Kraut, 1928). Large amounts of the hypotensive substance (termed kallikrein) were then found in the pancreas (Kraut and Werle, 1930). Subsequently, it was found that a substance (kallidin) that contracted the isolated guinea pig ileum was generated on incubation of urinary kallikrein with plasma (Werle et al., 1937). Similarly, incubation of certain snake venoms or trypsin with plasma globulins was found to generate a hypotensive substance that contracted guinea pig ileum; this substance was called bradykinin because of the slow contraction induced (Roche e Silva et al., 1949).

The kinin-generating system in plasma and extravascular tissue fluid is intimately involved with the clotting and fibrinolytic systems. Factor XII (Hageman factor) can be activated by particulate matter, bacterial lipopolysaccharides, collagen, crystals, damaged tissues or plasmin, etc. Activated factor XII then transforms, by direct and indirect mechanisms, prekallikrein to kallikrein, which is the enzyme that cleaves the plasma protein kininogen to form kinin. Two kininogens have been recognized—a high- and low-molecular-weight form. In addition to plasma kallikrein there are also glandular and leukocyte kallikreins. (For a detailed review of the kinin–kallikrein system, see Chapter 3.) Two kinins have been mainly studied, bradykinin (H-Arg-Pro-Pro-Gly-Phe-Ser-Pro-Phe-Arg-OH) and kallidin, which has an extra lysine at the N-terminal. They have a similar spectrum of activity and kallidin is converted to bradykinin by aminopeptidases *in vivo*.

Synthetic kallidin and bradykinin are potent vasodepressors when injected intravenously. Intradermal injections induce arteriolar dilation. These observations suggest that kinins may be involved in inflammation and shock, although no successful therapeutic agent has been found as a result of this suggestion. Of particular interest are the mechanisms involved in bradykinin-induced vasodilatation. The peptide is potent in inducing prostaglandin production (Terragno *et al.*, 1972) which may contribute to its dilator activity. In addition, bradykinin induces relaxation of the precontracted isolated artery strips by an endothelium-dependent mechanism (see Section 4.2).

Recent work has revealed the heterogeneity of bradykinin receptors (Regoli *et al.*, 1977; Regoli and Barabe, 1980). Plasma carboxypeptidase N (kininase I) rapidly removes C-terminal arginine from bradykinin, leaving des Arg^9-bradykinin. Originally, it was thought inactive; however, Regoli *et al.* (1977) found des Arg^9-bradykinin to be more active than bradykinin when tested on the isolated rabbit aorta but less active than bradykinin when tested on isolated rabbit jugular. The receptor present on the rabbit aorta was designated B_1 (responding to des Arg^9-bradykinin but less well to bradykinin) and the receptor on the rabbit jugular B_2 (responding to bradykinin but not to des Arg^9-bradykinin). Other tissues having B_1-receptors are the rabbit renal artery, pulmonary artery, carotid artery, portal vein, anterior mesenteric vein, jejunum, cat aorta, and carotid artery. B_2-receptors are found on the rat uterus, guinea pig ileum, and dog carotid. Other tissues have both types of receptor (e.g., rabbit posterior vena cava and renal vein).

Of considerable interest in the context of injury is the finding that the synthesis of B_1-receptors can be induced (Regoli *et al.*, 1978). A progressive increase in the sensitivity of the rabbit anterior mesenteric vein to des Arg^9-bradykinin (and bradykinin) has been observed with increasing time following isolation of the tissue. Increased sensitivity correlates with increased binding of tritiated des Arg^9-bradykinin. This phenomenon, which is not seen with other agonists such as substance P, is not affected by inhibition of prostaglandin synthesis using indomethacin, but is suppressed by protein synthesis inhibition using cycloheximide and actinomycin D. It has been concluded that there may be low numbers of B_1-receptors *in vivo* but that their synthesis may increase in response to noxious stimuli (Regoli and Barabe, 1980). In support of this, it has been found that intravenous des Arg^9-bradykinin induces no response in normal rabbits, but a marked depressor response in rabbits 5 hours after intravenous endotoxin. This depressor response is blocked by B_1-receptor antagonists. Blood vessels (e.g., the anterior mesenteric vein) taken from rabbits given endotoxin are sensitized to des Arg[9]-bradykinin without further incubation *in vitro*. Thus, blood vessels may become sensitized to des Arg[9]-bradykinin (and the less stable bradykinin itself) in inflammatory reactions, a situation that may gradually revert to normal during wound healing. These concepts may be applicable to receptors for other mediators.

4.6. Prostaglandins, Thromboxane A_2, and Vessel Tone

The potent vascular activities of the prostaglandins were discovered some time after the initial discovery of uterine spasmogenic activity in human semen (Kurzrok and Lieb, 1930). The vasodepressor activity in semen was found by Goldblatt (1935) and von Euler (1936), the latter coining the term *prostaglandin*. There is an immense literature on the chemistry and biologic activities of the prostaglandins (for review, see Moncada, 1983). This section is limited to their actions on blood vessels; effects relating to other aspects of inflammation are discussed in later sections.

Many inflammatory stimuli activate cell phospholipases and liberate arachidonic acid. Arachidonic acid is then converted to unstable endoperoxides (PGG_2 and PGH_2) by cyclo-oxygenase. Depending on the cells involved, the endoperoxides are then converted to different prostaglandins or thromboxane A_2. The unstable thromboxane A_2 is released by stimulated platelets (Hamberg *et al.*, 1975). Thromboxane A_2 induces platelet aggregation and vasoconstriction, and thus is thought to have a role in hemostasis (see Chapter 2). The local vasodilator effects of prostaglandins were first observed on injection into human skin using E-type prostaglandins (Bergstrom *et al.*, 1959). The responses in skin are characterized by an intense local erythrema that persists for 1½–2 hr (Juhlin and Michaelsson, 1969). Some persons also exhibit a wheal and surrounding flare, possibly due to histamine release (Sondergaard and Greaves, 1971). The more recently discovered unstable prostaglandin, prostacyclin (PGI_2) is a potent inhibitor of platelet aggregation and has been shown to induce a vasodepressor response upon intravenous injection (Armstrong *et al.*, 1978). Intradermally injected prostacyclin induces increased blood flow when tested in rabbit skin using ^{133}Xe clearance, and the potency of this prostaglandin is similar to that of PGE_2 (Peck and Williams, 1978; Williams, 1979). When tested in the same system, PGD_2 and $PGF_{2\alpha}$ are much less potent (Williams, 1979), although the relative potencies of the prostaglandins vary between tissues and species. Prostaglandins exert a direct relaxant effect on vascular smooth muscle cells, independent of endothelial cells. There is a clear evidence of prostaglandin-induced vasodilation in certain acute models of inflammation (Williams and Peck, 1977) but the contribution of these substances to vascular changes in chronic inflammation is a matter of contention.

Prostaglandin E_2 has been detected in wound fluid of rat skin 5 days after injury. However, a locally applied inhibitor of prostaglandin synthesis, indomethacin, reduced PGE_2 levels by 98% but had no detectable effect on blood flow (Lundberg and Gerdin, 1984). This suggests that other factors govern blood flow at this stage of healing in this particular model, although the importance of prostaglandins in wound healing in general is unknown.

4.7. Leukotrienes and Vascular Tone

The slow-acting spasmogenic activity, slow-reacting substance (SRS), released from venom-stimulated or anaphylatic guinea pig lung *in vitro* (Feldberg and Kellaway, 1938; Brocklehurst, 1960), is derived from metabolites of arachidonic acid produced by the 5-lipoxygenase pathway, an enzymatic pathway distinct from cyclo-oxygenase (Murphy *et al.*, 1979; Morris *et al.*, 1980). Aspirin and related compounds do not inhibit this pathway. However, corticosteroids can alter the availability of arachidonic acid. The 5-lipoxygenase products are generated in the lung by leukocytes and by vessel walls. Biosynthesis was first determined in rabbit leukocytes, hence the coining of leukotrienes for these metabolites. Although much attention has been given to the bronchoconstrictor activity of leukotrienes in the lung, with reference to asthma, the peptidoleukotrienes, C_4 and D_4, also have activities relevant to vascular changes in inflammation. Biosynthetic leukotriene D_4, from anaphylactic guinea pig lung (SRS-A), was shown to have potent vasoconstrictor activity in guinea pig skin using ^{133}Xe clearance (Williams and Piper, 1980). Chemically synthesized leukotriene C_4 was also shown to display this vasoconstrictor activity (Drazen *et al.*, 1980), and a comparative study of D_4 and C_4 showed leukotriene C_4 to be more active in guinea pig skin (Peck *et al.*, 1981). The vasoconstrictor activity has since been shown in many other tissues, including the coronary circulation (for review, see Feuerstein, 1984). In human skin these leukotrienes induce erythema (Bisgaard *et al.*, 1982), which may be due to the release of secondary mediators.

The chemistry of the leukotrienes has only recently been elucidated. (A discussion of their activity as chemoattractants and permeability-increasing mediators will be found in Sections 5.3 and 6.) The contribution of these substances to inflammation and wound healing remains to be determined.

4.8. Platelet-Activating Factor and Vessel Tone

Platelet-activating factor (PAF), originally discovered as a platelet-aggregating substance released from IgE-sensitized rabbit basophils stimulated with antigen (Benveniste *et al.*, 1972), is now known to possess a broad spectrum of biologic activities (for review, see Pinckard *et al.*, 1982). The structure of PAF, which is identical to a kidney-derived antihypertensive agent (Blank *et al.*, 1979), is 1-0-hexadecyl-2-acetyl-*sn*-glyceryl-3-phosphorylcholine or AGEPC (Benvensite *et al.*, 1979; Demopoulos *et al.*, 1979).

Intravenous administration of PAF induces systemic hypotension in rabbits (Halonen *et al.*, 1980) and baboons (McManus *et al.*, 1981). However, when applied locally to the hamster cheek pouch, PAF induces vasoconstriction

(Bjork and Smedegard, 1983). This may reflect a species difference, although there is some evidence that the effects of intravascular PAF may involve platelets. (A further discussion of PAF in the context of increased microvascular permeability may be found in Section 6.1).

4.9. Neuropeptides and Vessel Tone

Several neuropeptides are known to have potent effects on blood vessels. This brief discussion is limited to three vasodilators that are of particular interest: substance P, vasoactive intestinal polypeptide (VIP), and calcitonin gene-related polypeptide (CGRP).

Substance P was originally discovered as an activity in extracts of gut and brain (for review, see von Euler and Pernow, 1977), and much later purified, characterized, and synthesized as an 11-amino acid polypeptide (Tregear et al., 1971). Vasoactive intestinal polypeptide (VIP), a 28-amino acid polypeptide, was discovered as a vasodepressor activity extracted from the small intestine (Said and Mutt, 1970). Both substance P and VIP are found in the brain and in certain peripheral nerves (for review, see Bloom and Polak, 1983). The effects of these peptides in lowering arterial blood pressure on intravenous injection are well established. In humans, intradermally injected substance P induces a wheal-and-flare reaction (Hagermark, 1978), which is thought to involve the release of mast cell histamine (Foreman et al., 1983). In the rabbit, substance P is a weak vasodilator when injected intradermally. By contrast, VIP is potent, exceeding the potency of the vasodilator prostaglandins PGE_2 and PGI_2 (Williams, 1982). The result of an experiment that demonstrates increased local blood flow in skin induced by VIP in comparison with PGE_2 is shown in Fig. 1. Intradermal injection of VIP in humans induces a wheal-and-flare reaction that

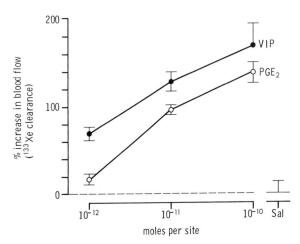

Figure 1. Comparison of the blood flow-increasing activity of vasoactive intestinal polypeptide (VIP, 28-amino acids) and prostaglandin E_2 (PGE_2) in rabbit skin. Agents were mixed with ^{133}Xe and injected intradermally in 0.1-ml volumes. After 20 min, the animal was killed and injection sites punched out for counting in a gamma counter, together with samples of injection fluid. The ordinate represents the increase in blood flow obtained by comparing isotope washout in agent- and saline-injected sites. The abscissa represents the doses of VIP and PGE_2 injected. Results are expressed as mean $\pm$SEM for $N = 6$ sites. (Based on Williams, 1982.)

may, like responses to substance P, involve histamine released (Anand *et al.*, 1983).

Recently, it was found that the gene encoding the hormone calcitonin in the rat thyroid also encodes flanking peptides (Amara *et al.*, 1982; Rosenfeld *et al.*, 1983), including a 37-amino acid polypeptide called calcitonin gene-related peptide (CGRP). CGRP is thought to be a neuropeptide in the CNS, based on immunocytochemical studies (Rosenfeld *et al.*, 1983; Fisher *et al.*, 1983). In the peripheral nervous system, immunoreactive CGRP was detected in beaded fibers associated with vascular smooth muscle (Rosenfeld *et al.*, 1983). The sequence of human CGRP (differing from rat CGRP in four residues) has been determined (Morris *et al.*, 1984). CGRP is a potent arteriolar dilator as assessed using ^{133}Xe clearance in rabbit skin and microscopically in the hamster cheek pouch (Brain *et al.*, 1985). In human skin, CGRP induces intense local erythema with little wheal or surrounding flare, except at high doses (Brain *et al.*, 1985). The local erythema is induced by doses as low as 15 fmoles; with higher doses, responses last 10–12 hr.

As with ACh, relaxation of strips of aorta *in vitro* induced by substance P (Furchgott, 1981), VIP (Davies and Williams, 1984), and CGRP (Brain *et al.*, 1985), is endothelium dependent (see Section 4.2 for a discussion on EDRF). It is not known, however, whether EDRF is involved in arteriolar vasodilatation induced by extravascular peptides, i.e., when intradermally injected or released from nerves supplying arterioles (Brain *et al.*, 1985).

Stimulation of the appropriate sensory nerves at the dorsal roots results in vasodilatation of the hindlimbs (Bayliss, 1901). Thomas Lewis first suggested that these antidromic impulses may account for the flare surrounding responses to histamine or mild injury in the skin (Lewis, 1927). Impulses are thought to travel up pain C fibers from cutaneous receptors, and branches of these fibers supplying peripheral arterioles are believed to release a vasodilator (see Section 4.3). The endogenous dilator is widely thought to be substance P (Foreman *et al.*, 1983), although CGRP has recently been proposed for this role (Brain *et al.*, 1985). Further examples of neurogenic inflammation are given later within the context of increased microvascular permeability (see Section 6.1). The contribution of neuropeptides to hyperemia during wound healing remains to be established.

5. Leukocyte Chemoattractants

Injured cells, foreign materials, or infectious organisms in a tissue stimulate the release of chemical signals that bring about the accumulation of defensive cells from the blood. These cells are essential both for the removal of the stimulating agent and apparently for subsequent wound healing. This process is complex: different cell types predominate both in response to different stimuli and in the phases of a given response, implying that different chemical signals are generated for different types of leukocytes. This discussion is limited to the neutrophilic polymorphonuclear leukocyte, which generally predominates in the acute phase of inflammation and about which most is known. The reader is referred to Chapter 8 for a discussion of monocyte/macrophage attractants and to Chapter 10 for a discussion of connective tissue cell migration.

Neutrophil chemoattractants owe their discovery to chemotactic and chemokinetic activity in test systems *in vitro* (for a review of the techniques, see Gallin and Quie, 1978). The relationship between these activities and the process of neutrophil emigration from blood vessels *in vivo* is controversial (for review, see Wilkinson, 1982). A fundamental question which remains open is whether the vessel wall plays an active role in the process. (The essential points are mentioned here briefly; a more detailed discussion will be found in Chapter 6.)

The first stage in neutrophil accumulation is leukocyte adherence to endothelial cells. In most tissues, adherence takes place in venules (in the lung, capillaries are involved). This selectivity of adherence site implies either an active change in the surface of specialized endothelial cells induced by the chemoattractant, or a favored site for the adherence of activated neutrophils. The surface of endothelial cells can be made more adhesive by direct injury; neutrophils adhere only to that side of the vessel that has received such an injury (Clark and Clark, 1935). However, it is not clear whether such a change in the endothelial cell surface can occur in response to chemoattractants. Some experiments have suggested that cultured endothelial cell monolayers show increased adhesive properties in response to chemoattractants (Hoover *et al.*, 1980, 1984). However, other experiments show no such effect (Tonnesen *et al.*, 1984). As these cultured cells are from major rather than microvessels, these experiments may not reflect the conditions *in vivo*. Neutrophils adhere to each other and to artificial surfaces when stimulated with chemoattractants *in vitro*. Thus, the most economical theory is that chemoattractants generated extravascularly diffuse into the lumen of microvessels and act on neutrophils, possibly during their passage along capillaries when the area of contact between neutrophil membrane and vessel wall is maximal. It is not clear what change takes place in the neutrophil membrane which results in increased adherence, although chemoattractants are known to decrease cell surface charge (Gallin *et al.*, 1980) and stimulate the presentation of an adhesive-promoting glycoprotein (Mo-1 or Mac-1) on the cell surface (Arnout *et al.*, 1983; Springer *et al.*, 1985). The stimulated neutrophils may then adhere downstream (in the venules in most tissues); the region of vessel where adherence takes place is governed either by differences in endothelial cell surfaces or rheological factors (i.e., low shear rate).

To answer whether the endothelial cell actually participates in this process will depend on experiments on the intact microvascular bed. One recent report of *in vivo* experiments does suggest such an active involvement. It was reported that skin sites in the rabbit could be specifically desensitized to particular chemoattractants by a previous intradermal injection of the chemoattractant

(Colditz and Movat, 1984*a* and *b*). These experiments, using radiolabeled leukocytes, offer the intriguing possibility that receptors for chemoattractants may be present upon endothelial cells or adjacent tissue cells.

Following adherence, neutrophils pass through junctions between adjacent endothelial cells (diapedesis), remain for some time flattened between endothelial cells and perivascular basement membrane and then penetrate the basement membrane. The mechanisms involved in the different stages of emigration are unknown. Whether the vessel wall plays an active role in the adherence and diapedesis of neutrophils is an important question in the understanding of the mechanisms involved in the modulation of both neutrophil accumulation (see Section 5.4) and neutrophil function (see Section 6.3) *in vivo*.

The chemoattractant activities of C5a, the formyl peptides, and LTB_4 are most studied, but there are many other substances with chemoattractant activity. Two of these are produced by neutrophils and as neutrophil recruiting factors, may have a role similar to that of LTB_4. These are PAF (Humphrey *et al.*, 1982) and a glycoprotein (8400 M_r) released by neutrophils stimulated with urate crystals (Spilberg and Mehta, 1979).

5.1. C5a

Systemic administration of complement-activated serum induces a shock reaction resembling anaphylaxis (Freideberger, 1910). The active substances involved, cleavage products of the third and fifth complement components, C3a and C5a, release mast cell histamine, which contributes to the shock reaction (Hahn and Oberdorf, 1950). The potent chemoattractant activity of complement-activated rabbit serum *in vitro* was discovered by Boyden (1962) and later shown to be due to C5a (Snyderman *et al.*, 1970). The amino acid sequence of human C5a (74 amino acid-glycosylated polypeptide) has now been determined (Fernandez and Hugli, 1978). In addition to its well-documented effects on neutrophils *in vitro*, namely, stimulation of chemotaxis, chemokinesis, aggregation, enzyme release, and the respiratory burst, C5a has been shown to cause neutrophil accumulation in the guinea pig pleural cavity (Damerau *et al.*, 1976) and in the hamster cheek pouch (Björk *et al.*, 1983). C5a rapidly loses carboxyl-terminal arginine in tissue field because of the action of carboxypeptidase N to produce C5a des Arg. Human C5a des Arg is active as a chemoattractant (with one-tenth the activity of C5a) but has little histamine-releasing activity (Gerard and Hugli, 1981). In some *in vitro* test systems, C5a des Arg requires the addition of a plasma cofactor, an anionic peptide, in order to express chemoattractant activity (Perez *et al.*, 1980); however, it is unclear whether this cofactor is required *in vivo*. In recent studies, a specific radioimmunoassay (RIA) has been used to detect C5a in inflammatory exudates. Levels of up to 800 ng/ml have been measured in rabbit peritoneal exudate fluid induced by injection of zymosan and significant levels were induced in Arthus reactions (Jose *et al.*, 1983).

Because of its potency as a chemoattractant, and because the complement system can be activated by many stimuli (e.g., immune complexes, microbial cell walls, endotoxin, and damage host tissue), C5a probably has a major role in mediating local neutrophil accumulation *in vivo* (see Section 6.3).

5.2. Formyl Peptides

Schiffmann *et al.*, (1975) showed that synthetic formyl peptides, resembling chemotactic substances in bacterial cultures, were chemotactic for neutrophils. Formyl-methionyl-leucyl-phenylalanine (FMLP) was found to be the most potent (Showell *et al.*, 1976). These peptides, now known to be present in bacterial cultures (Marasco *et al.*, 1984), have the same wide spectrum of effects that C5a has on neutrophils, but they act on a different receptor. FMLP has been shown to induce neutrophil accumulation in the lung (Desai *et al.*, 1979) and in rabbit skin (Colditz and Movat, 1984b).

Bacteria use a formyl-blocked N-terminal during protein synthesis, which is subsequently cleaved. Thus, mammals appear to have developed receptors in order to facilitate the recognition of bacterial products. Whether these peptides fall strictly within the definition of inflammatory mediators is a semantic question, but they may well contribute in inducing neutrophil accumulation in infected tissues *in vivo*.

5.3. Leukotriene B_4

The background to the discovery of the leukotrienes was given in Section 4.7. In an early study, it was shown that the platelet-derived monohydroxy arachidonic acid metabolite, 12-L-hydroxy-5,8,10,14-eicostetraenoic acid (12-HETE), is chemotactic for neutrophils (Turner *et al.*, 1975) and subsequently that 5-HETE is more active (Goetzl *et al.*, 1980). A much more powerful chemoattractant was found in a dihydroxy acid, leukotriene B_4 (5,12-dihydroxy-6,8,10,14-eicosatetraenoic acid) (Ford-Hutchinson *et al.*, 1980). LTB_4 may mediate leukocyte accumulation in particular inflammatory reactions. In experiments in animal models in which this has been tested, inhibition of 5-lipoxygenase has had only a partial effect on neutrophil accumulation (Higgs *et al.*, 1980).

5.4. Modulation of Leukocyte Accumulation

Neutrophil accumulation can be initiated in a tissue by the local extravascular generation of chemoattractants, which in turn can be influenced by the generation of nonchemotactic mediators in the tissue. Much of the published work in this area of leukocyte accumulation concerns the effects of prostaglandins. Experimental observations of prostaglandin activity are, in some ways, parallel with the longer-established effects of prostaglandins on edema formation, discussed in Section 6.2.

E-type prostaglandins have been shown to increase neutrophil accumulation when given intradermally, together with complement-activated plasma (as a source of C5a des Arg), in the rabbit (Issekutz and Movat, 1979). This effect is thought to result from vasodilatation increasing the supply of neutrophils to the skin. Blood flow may be a limiting factor in determining the rate of neutrophil accumulation in a tissue with low basal flow, such as skin. Whether nonprostaglandin vasodilators have the same effect has not been determined. The effect of prostaglandins on neutrophil accumulation in other tissues may not be the same. In tissues with high basal flow rates, vasodilators may have less effect on neutrophil accumulation. In fact, a high flow could reduce accumulation by increasing the shear force on neutrophils attached to the vessel wall (Atherton and Born, 1973).

Leukocyte emigration in the skin takes place in the postcapillary venules to which blood supply is regulated by arteriolar tone. However, arterioles do not control capillary blood supply in the same way in the lung; therefore, the mechanism of prostaglandin enhancement of neutrophil emigration in the lung is not clear (Henson et al., 1982). Evidence of an effect of prostaglandins on neutrophil emigration has also been obtained in a major vessel (Tonnesen et al., 1982). It was shown that PGE_2, applied to the outside of a rabbit carotid along with C5 fragments, had a marked enhancing effect on neutrophil migration into the vessel wall, an effect independent of changes in blood flow. The situation is complicated further by the fact that prostaglandins can inhibit neutrophil function by elevating intracellular cyclic adenosine monophosphate (cAMP) (Boxer et al., 1980). Thus, some experiments have shown that PGI_2 can inhibit neutrophil adherence to venular walls (Jones and Hurley, 1984).

With these different effects of prostaglandins on neutrophil accumulation, it is not surprising that the effects of prostaglandin synthesis inhibition are complex. Some nonsteroid anti-inflammatory drugs (NSAIDs) appear to interfere with chemoattractant binding to receptors on neutrophils; for example, FMLP binding is inhibited by phenylbutazone, sulfinpyrazone (Dahinden and Fehr, 1980), and indomethacin (Coste et al., 1981). NSAIDs also appear to be able to inhibit neutrophil function in vitro by an unknown mechanism (MacGregor et al., 1974; Brown and Collins, 1977; Matzner et al., 1984; Kaplan et al., 1984; Pham Huy et al., 1985). NSAIDs have also been shown to inhibit neutrophil accumulation in inflammatory reactions in vivo (Issekutz and Bhimji, 1982; Higgs, 1984), although it is not clear whether this is secondary to inhibition of blood flow, inhibition of chemotactic factor generation, or an effect on the neutrophil itself. Of particular interest is ibuprofen, which suppresses experimentally induced myocardial infarct size by an effect on neutrophils (Flynn et al., 1984; Maderazo et al., 1984; Rampart and Williams, 1986).

As NSAIDs can suppress plasma leakage from microvessels (see Section 6.2), they can also suppress the supply of C5 and thus indirectly inhibit the extravascular generation of C5a (Lo et al., 1984). Other NSAIDs (e.g., BW755C) can inhibit the generation of the chemoattractant LTB_4 as well as that of prostaglandins (see Higgs et al., 1979).

Clearly, prostaglandins can have multiple effects on neutrophil accumulation. In experimental injury of rat skin (Lundberg and Gerdin, 1984), PGE_2

applied locally 5 days after the injury increased blood flow but did not affect neutrophil accumulation. This suggests that blood flow did not limit neutrophil traffic at 5 days. Levels of endogenous PGE_2 were elevated in the wound fluid at this time, but indomethacin treatment failed to decrease neutrophil accumulation. In fact, indomethacin had a small enhancing effect on neutrophil accumulation, possible because of inhibition of a negative feedback system involving PGI_2 production by endothelial cells. These data only give information on the mediators present and their effect on neutrophil accumulation in one time frame of wound repair. The factors present and their effect on neutrophil accumulation are likely to vary considerably in the different stages of wound healing.

6. Mediators Increasing Microvascular Permeability

This discussion covers mediator effects on the microvessels' permeability to macromolecules, leading to tissue edema and extravascular clotting, the two hallmarks of the inflammation phase of wound repair (see Chapter 3). In the later phases of a healing wound, assessment of mediator effects on microvascular permeability is complicated by the observation that new vessels are abnormally leaky to proteins (Schoefl, 1963). New vessels appear unresponsive to mediators, which might further increase permeability, such as histamine (Hurley et al., 1970). The reader is referred to Section 4 for the chemical nature and source of mediators.

6.1. Mediators Increasing Permeability by a Direct Action on the Vessel Wall

Thomas Lewis (1927) described the wheal produced by intradermally injected histamine as the result of an increase in capillary permeability to plasma proteins. The leakage of plasma proteins was demonstrated in early animal studies of inflammatory reactions in animal skin, using intravascular protein-bound dye (Ramsdell, 1928). Much later, Majno et al. (1961) revealed in their classic studies that histamine acts on the small postcapillary venules to increase permeability. Rats were given an intravenous injection of a suspension of carbon (India ink) or mercuric sulfide, followed by application of histamine to the cremaster muscle. The carbon leaked from the endothelial cell barrier and became trapped under the perivascular basement membrane, leaving leaky vessels labeled. Electron microscopic studies revealed open junctions between adjacent endothelial cells (Majno and Palade, 1961). Subsequently, evidence was presented that the junctions resulted from contraction of endothelial cells (Majno et al., 1969; Joris et al., 1972). Endothelial cells do contain contractile filaments, but the detailed mechanics of how contraction leads to opening of junctions or whether other changes are concomitant (e.g., a change in the nature of the junctional regions) remains to be determined.

Majno and colleagues also showed that 5-HT acted on postcapillary venules; it has since been shown that all known permeability-increasing mediators act in the same area (although some mediators may affect larger venules as well (see Section 6.3). Use of histamine–ferritin conjugates has revealed high-affinity binding sites located on venular endothelial cells (Heltianu et al., 1982). Other mediators thought to act directly on venules to increase permeability include bradykinin via B_2-receptors (Regoli and Barabe, 1980); leukotrienes LTC_4; LTD_4 (Drazen et al., 1980; Williams and Piper, 1980; Peck et al., 1981; Dahlen et al., 1981); substance P (Lembeck and Holzer, 1979); PAF (Vargaftig and Ferreira, 1981; Wedmore and Williams, 1981a; Pinckard et al., 1982); and certain fibrin-derived peptides (Saldeen, 1983).

In most animal models, H_1-antagonists abolish histamine-induced plasma protein leakage. However, in human skin it has been suggested that a combination of H_1- and H_2-antagonists may be necessary (Levi et al., 1982). The use of histamine antagonists has shown that some mediators act, at least in part, by the release of histamine from mast cells. The anaphylatoxins, C3a and C5a, release mast cell histamine (Hahn and Oberdorf, 1950). Both polypeptides rapidly lose carboxy-terminal arginine by the action of carboxypeptidase N; in some species, the resulting des Arg forms of the molecules are poor histamine releasers (Huey et al., 1983). For example, removal of the carboxy-terminal arginine from human C5a, which is glycosylated, almost abolishes histamine release activity; however, removal of the carboxyhydrate group restores some of this activity (Gerard and Hugli, 1981). Other species (e.g., hog C5a has been studied intensively) have no carboxyhydrate group on C5a and the des Arg form is an active histamine releaser (Gerard and Hugli, 1981).

Substance P also has histamine-releasing activity (Foreman et al., 1983) but can act directly to increase permeability (Foreman et al., 1983). Substance P has been implicated as the endogenous mediator of vasodilation (see Section 4.9) and increased microvascular permeability induced by antidromic electrical stimulation of sensory nerve fibers (Lembeck and Holzer, 1979). This is supported by the observation that substance P antagonists inhibit the effects of antidromic stimulation of sensory nerve fibers (Holmdahl et al., 1981; Lembeck et al., 1982; Lundberg et al., 1983). Inflammatory reactions with neurogenic components have now been demonstrated in many tissues (Lundberg and Saria; 1983; Saria and Lundberg, 1985). Two other neuropeptides related to substance P may also contribute to local increased microvascular permeability: neurokinins A and B (Kangawa et al., 1983; Nawa et al., 1984; Saria and Lundberg, 1985).

By implication, venular endothelial cells appear to be equipped with a wide variety of receptors that respond to mediators derived from different cell types and from different enzyme systems in tissue fluid. The situation is complicated by the fact that some mediators may act, at least partly, by releasing other endogenous mediators. For instance, the anaphylatoxins may release prostaglandins or leukotrienes, as well as histamine in some situations (Pavek and Smedegard, 1979; Stimler et al., 1982). Histamine can initiate the release of substance P and vice versa (Foreman et al., 1983) and PAF may release leukotrienes (Voelkel et al., 1982; Lin et al., 1982). Further complexities include marked species and tissue differences in the responses to different mediators. Thus, 5-HT increases microvascular permeability in rodents, but not in other species, while peptidoleukotrienes increase permeability in guinea pig skin and human skin, but not in rabbit skin.

Clearly, many factors may increase the permeability of microvessels during wound healing; these factors will vary with the animal and organ involved, as well as the phase of the healing process. After the initial inflammation stage of wound repair, the high permeability of new vessels within the wound to plasma proteins (Schoefl, 1963) may be an intrinsic property, independent of the mediators described above. In one study, there was no evidence for an involvement of histamine and 5-HT when antagonists were tested in a 5-day-old wound in rat skin (Lundberg and Gerdin, 1984). The availability of antagonists to other mediators may provide more information about the endogenous substances involved in controlling vessel permeability throughout the healing process.

6.2. Modulation of Plasma Protein Extravasation

Thomas Lewis proposed that once increased permeability is established, the rate of plasma protein leakage from microvessels depends on blood flow (Lewis, 1927). This phenomenon is not obvious when observing the effect of a single mediator, such as histamine, which acts both to dilate arterioles and to increase the permeability of venules. However, when mediators that have specific effects on the microvascular bed are used in combination dramatic synergism can be observed. For instance, synergism was seen in guinea pig skin where E-type prostaglandins caused little edema given alone, but markedly potentiated edema induced by histamine and bradykinin (Williams and Morley, 1973). A similar phenomenon was observed in the rat (Moncada et al., 1973). A good correlation was found between the vasodilator activity of different prostaglandins and their ability to potentiate edema in the rabbit (Williams, 1976; Johnston et al., 1976). Evidence was obtained that two types of mediators, one vasodilator and one predominantly permeability increasing, were generated together in response to an intradermal injection of a bacterial suspension (Williams and Peck, 1977). More recently, the potent edema-potentiating activities of PGI_2 (Williams, 1979), VIP (Williams, 1982), and CGRP (Brain and Williams, 1985) have been observed. Other substances that potentiate edema include adenosine (Williams and Peck, 1977; Sugio and Daly, 1984), ATP (Chahl, 1977), and isoproterenol (Williams and Peck, 1977). An example of edema induced by synergism between vasodilator and permeability-increasing mediators in the skin is shown in Fig. 2.

The mechanism of synergism in these experiments has been interpreted as arteriolar dilatation inducing an increased hydrostatic pressure downstream within the venule lumen, thereby increasing plasma protein leakage. In tissues with a low blood flow, such as the skin, the effect of prostaglandins on the formation of inflammatory edema can be marked. For example, inhibition of

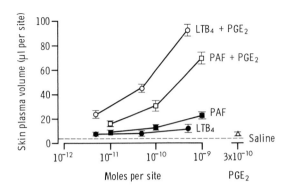

Figure 2. Comparison of edema formation induced by leukotriene B_4 (LTB$_4$) and platelet-activating factor (PAF) in rabbit skin, showing the potentiating effect of prostaglandin E_2 (PGE$_2$). The rabbit was given an intravenous injection of [^{125}I]albumin, followed by intradermal injections (0.1 ml) of LTB$_4$ or PAF, with or without the addition of PGE$_2$ (3×10^{-10} moles per site). The animal was killed after 30 min, the skin was removed, and the injection sites punched out for counting together with plasma samples, in a gamma counter. The ordinate represents albumin leakage, expressed in terms of volumes of plasma per skin site. The small values obtained with saline alone (– – – – –) or PGE$_2$ alone are included for comparison. Results are expressed as mean ±SEM for $N = 6$ sites.

prostaglandin synthesis in the acute response to zymosan in rabbit skin has been shown to reduce edema by approximately 80% (Williams and Jose, 1981). In tissues in which the basal blood flow is high, the effect of a vasodilator on edema formation would be expected to be less substantial. In accord with this, inhibition of prostaglandin synthesis in the acute response to zymosan in the rabbit peritoneal cavity has been shown to reduce edema by a maximum of only approximately 20% (Forrest et al., 1986).

These observations suggest that prostaglandins do not have a major effect in potentiating leakage by an action on the venule itself (e.g., sensitization of receptors to permeability-increasing mediators). However, there is some evidence that this can occur in other situations. For instance, it has been observed that the leakage response to bradykinin can be enhanced by prostaglandins in the cat forelimb perfused at a constant rate by a pump (Ameland et al., 1981). Potentiation of leakage by prostaglandins has also been observed in the lung (Henson et al., 1982), where arteriolar tone does not govern downstream hydrostatic pressure. Thus, prostaglandins may affect leakage by mechanisms additional to those dependent on vasodilatation.

Synergism between prostaglandins and other mediators has so far been observed only in models of acute inflammation. This would presumably hold true for the acute inflammation phase of wounds. Although PGE$_2$ was detected in rat wound fluid at 5 days and exogenous PGE$_2$ increased local blood flow (Lundberg and Gerdin, 1984), inhibition of prostaglandin synthesis by indomethacin did not affect local blood flow or plasma protein leakage in this later phase of wound repair. This suggests that vessels at this time are dilated by other chemical vasodilators or that the intrinsic tone of the vessels is low.

As discussed in section 4.6., corticosteroids are able to inhibit phospholipases and these drugs, like non-steroid antiinflammatory compounds, can therefore suppress inflammatory edema by inhibiting the generation of vasodilator, edema-potentiating prostaglandins. Corticosteroids also appear to have other inhibitory effects on blood vessels and their responses to mediators. This action is probably independent of phospholipase inhibition, but is dependent (like phospholipase inhibition) on the synthesis of an endogenous anti-inflammatory protein (Tsurufuji et al., 1979). Steroids may suppress vascular changes during wound healing by this mechanism as these drugs, unlike non-steroidal compounds, have been observed to reduce both blood flow and plasma protein leakage in rat skin 5 days after injury (Lundberg and Gerdin, 1984).

Sympathomimetics can have marked effects on inflammatory edema. As α-adrenoreceptors are important in the control of arteriolar tone, exogenous nor-epinephrine can reverse the potentiating effect of prostaglandins and inhibit edema formation (Williams and Peck, 1977; Williams et al., 1984). Sym-pathomimetics can also act directly on microvascular endothelial cells and attenuate responses to inflammatory mediators. Thus, it has been shown that β_2-agonists, such as isoproterenol and terbutaline, can inhibit plasma protein leakage induced by histamine and bradykinin (Svenjso et al., 1977; O'Donnell and Persson, 1978; Dobbins et al., 1982). In the tissues of some species, inhibition of leakage by β_2-agonists is marked, although in others (e.g., rabbit skin), the vasodilator effect of these agents predominates, thus causing enhanced edema formation (Kenawy et al., 1978).

6.3. Increased Permeability Induced by Leukocyte Chemoattractants

Depletion of circulating neutrophils reduces inflammatory edema in a number of models (Stetson, 1951; Humphrey, 1955; Cochrane et al., 1965; Phelps and McCarty, 1966), giving rise to the concept that phagocytosing neutrophils in the tissue release proteolytic enzymes that damage microvascular endothelial cells, thereby increasing vascular permeability. The importance of this mechanism was disputed because it was observed that the major phase of increased permeability preceded that of neutrophil accumulation (Hurley, 1963). However, instillation of C5 fragments into the airways in rabbits did induce histologic evidence of edema, concomitant with neutrophil emigration (Shaw et al., 1980).

In contrast to edema in the lung, which was not detected before 1 hr, studies in rabbit skin showed that complement-activated plasma or C5a, in the presence of a vasodilator prostaglandin, induced local edema within 5–6 min when injected intradermally (Williams, 1978; Jose et al., 1978; Wedmore and Williams 1981a). Although the edema response to intradermally injected C5a or C5a des Arg was apparent within minutes, leakage was completely dependent on neutrophils. Edema formation was entirely suppressed by depletion of circulating neutrophils, although edema responses to histamine, bradykinin, and PAF were unaffected (Wedmore and Williams, 1981a,b; Issekutz, 1981). Thus, local extravascular C5a appears to increase microvascular permeability by inducing a rapid interaction between neutrophils and microvascular endo-

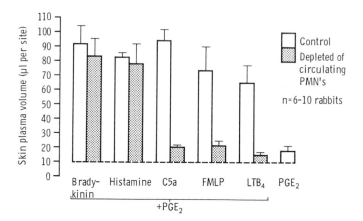

Figure 3. Effect of depletion of circulating polymorphonuclear leukocytes on local edema induced by intradermally injected bradykinin, histamine, C5a des Arg, f-Met-Leu-Phe (FMLP) and leukotriene B$_4$, each agent mixed with PGE$_2$. Doses used per site were bradykinin 8×10^{-12} moles, histamine 10^{-11} moles, rabbit C5a des Arg 2×10^{-11} moles, FMLP 3×10^{-12}, LTB$_4$ 2×10^{-10} moles, and PGE$_2$ 3×10^{-10} moles. Responses were measured using intravenous [^{125}I]albumin, as described for Fig. 2. Open columns represent responses in control rabbits; shaded columns represent responses in rabbits 4 days after an intravenous dose of nitrogen mustard 1.75 mg/kg to deplete circulating polymorphonuclear (PMN) leukocytes. Note the dependence of responses to C5a des Arg, FMLP, and LTB$_4$ on PMN leukocytes, and the independence of responses to bradykinin and histamine. Responses are expressed as mean $\pm$SEM for N = 4–16 rabbits.

thelial cells. These findings show that histamine release by C3a and C5a is not the only link between the complement system and the microvasculature. Human C5a has been shown to induce wheal and flare reactions in human skin (Yancey et al., 1985), and a requirement for neutrophils has been determined (Williamson et al., 1986). Other chemoattractants were also shown to behave in a similar manner to C5a in rabbit skin. Thus, FMLP and LTB$_4$ induce little edema alone but are potent when mixed with PGE$_2$. Again, depletion of circulating neutrophils abolishes these responses (Wedmore and Williams, 1981b) (see Fig. 3). A topographic study of the hamster cheek pouch, using intravital microscopy, showed that LTB$_4$ induced leakage from larger vessels in addition to those postcapillary venules affected by histamine (Björk et al., 1982).

Experiments using agents that activate neutrophils intravascularly have implicated oxygen-derived radicals in injury to the lung microvasculature. Thus, catalase, which inactivates hydrogen peroxide, suppresses such injury in vivo (Till et al., 1982; Johnson and Ward, 1981) and suppresses injury to cultured endothelial cells in contact with activated neutrophils (Sacks et al., 1978; Martin, 1984). By contrast, chemoattractants are normally generated extravascularly in tissues as an essential part of local host defence. Recently, however, it has been discovered that local reactions to extravascular chemoattractants are also suppressed by catalase given intravenously (Rampart and

Williams, 1985). Thus, edema response to intradermally injected C5a, LTB$_4$, or FMLP in the rabbit are suppressed by catalase, whereas the responses to histamine, bradykinin, and PAF are not affected (all agents in combination with PGE$_2$). These results suggest that either catalase blocks neutrophil/endothelial cell reactions by an unknown mechanism, or that within the microvessel lumen, local extravascular chemoattractants trigger a low-level respiratory burst in neutrophils that results in hydrogen peroxide generation.

There is compelling evidence to implicate neutrophil–endothelial cell interactions in edema formation for different sorts of inflammatory reactions including the early phase of wound repair. The contribution of neutrophil-dependent edema to later phases of wound healing remains to be determined.

7. Conclusion

In this chapter, an overview of some of the chemicals generated in a tissue responding to infection and injury has been presented. With limited space, it is impossible to give a fully comprehensive list of known mediators; many mediators (perhaps the most important) must await discovery. I have attempted to discuss the mediators that have been the subject of most intensive study, describing how these mediators act and interact to induce changes in tone and permeability of microvessels and facilitate leukocyte accumulation. Clearly, most of the research quoted investigated acute models of inflammation. Of particular interest are the observations of receptors on vascular tissue induced by noxious stimuli (see Section 5.4), dilatation induced by endothelial cell/smooth muscle cell interactions (see Section 4.2), and increased microvascular permeability induced by neutrophil/endothelial cell interaction (see Section 6.3).

The relationship between wound healing and inflammation was discussed in Section 1. Studies on mediator generation and actions during wound healing specifically have been infrequent. However, it is possible to piece together the changes that may occur in tissue undergoing an acute inflammatory reaction important to wound healing. A representation of some of the mediators involved in a local reaction is shown in Fig. 4. It follows that effective suppression of the inflammatory response may be deleterious to host defense and wound healing. Such a suppression may limit acute tissue injury, but it may also retard tissue remodeling and/or inhibit the elimination of necrotic tissue masses. Errors in mechanisms controlling the transition from inflammation to healing may be involved in proliferative diseases, such as psoriasis, in which persistent inflammation is associated with aberrant tissue cell replication. Similarly, connective tissue diseases, such as scleroderma, may result from a failure of healing control systems. Knowledge of inflammatory mediators and their mechanisms of action is a first step in the understanding of the inductive phase of wound healing.

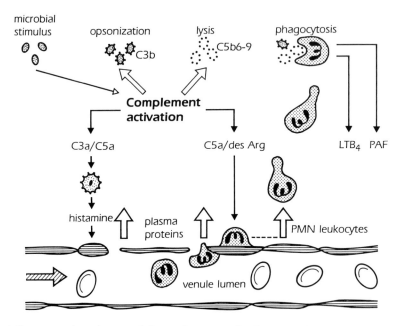

Figure 4. Representation of some of the mediators involved in controlling the supply of plasma proteins and polymorphonuclear (PMN) leukocytes from the blood to an infected tissue. The microbial cell walls or cell walls complexed with antibody trigger complement activation in extracellular tissue fluid resulting in opsonization by C3b and (for some microbes) lysis by C5b6–9. The anaphylatoxins C3a and C5a are generated as by-products of complement activation. These polypeptides can release mast cell histamine, which may contribute to an early phase of vasodilatation and plasma protein leakage. C5a and its more physiologically stable product C5a des Arg induce emigration of PMN leukocytes. This emigration (mainly of neutrophils in the early stages) results in some way in increased vascular permeability, which may be responsible for plasma protein leakage starting at 5–6 min and lasting several hours. The leukocytes phagocytose the opsonized microbes and may secrete LTB$_4$ and PAF, both of which may contribute to continuing leukocyte accumulation and plasma protein leakage. All these mechanisms have the effect of controlling the supply of blood proteins (containing complement, antibodies, and fibrinogen) and phagocytic cells to an infected tissue in order to facilitate local host-defense processes.

References

Abelous, J. E., and Bardier, E., 1909, De l'action hypotensive et myotique de l'urine humaine normales, *C. R. Soc. Biol. (Paris)* **66:**876.

Amara, S. G., Jonas, V., Rosenfeld, M. G., Ong, E. S., and Evans, R. M., 1982, Alternative RNA processing in calcitonin gene expression generates mRNAs encoding different polypeptide products, *Nature (Lond.)* **298:**240–244.

Amelang, E., Prasad, C. M., Raymond, R. M., and Grega, G. J., 1981, Interactions among inflammatory mediators on edema formation in the canine forelimb, *Circ. Res.* **49:**298–306.

Anand, P., Bloom, S. R., and McGregor, G. P., 1983, Topical capsaicin pretreatment inhibits axon reflex vasodilatation caused by somatostatin and vasoactive intestinal polypeptide in human skin, *Br. J. Pharmacol.* **77:**505–509.

Armstrong, J. M., Lattimer, N., Moncada, S., and Vane, J. R., 1978, Comparison of the vasodepressor effects of prostacyclin and 6-oxo-prostaglandin $F_{1\alpha}$ with those of prostaglandin E_2 in rats and rabbits, Br. J. Pharmacol. **62:**125–130.

Arnout, M. A., Tod III, R. F., Dana, N., Melamed, J., Schlossman, S. F., and Colten, H. R., 1983, Inhibition of phagocytosis of complement C3 or immunoglobulin G-coated particles and of C3bi binding by monoclonal antibodies to a monocyte–granulocyte membrane glycoprotein (Mo-1), J. Clin. Invest. **72:**171–179.

Arthurson, G., 1979, Microvascular permeability to macromolecules in thermal injury, Physiol. Scand. (Suppl.) **463:**111–122.

Ash, A. S. F., and Schild, H. O., 1966, Receptors mediating some actions of histamine, Br. J. Pharmacol. **27:**427–439.

Atherton, A., and Born, G. V. R., 1973, Relationship between the velocity of rolling granulocytes and that of blood flow in venules, J. Physiol. (Lond.) **233:**157–165.

Bayliss, W. M., 1901, On the origin from the spinal cord of the vasodilator fibres of the hind limb, and on the nature of these fibres, J. Physiol. (Lond.) **26:**173–209.

Benveniste, J., Tence, M., Varenne, P., Bidault, J., Boullet, C., and Polonsky, J., 1979, Semi-synthèse et structure proposée du facteur activant les plaquettes (P.A.F.): PAF-acether, un alkyl ether analogue de la lysophosphatidylcholine, C. R. Acad. Sci. Paris **289:**1037–1042.

Bergstrom, S., Duner, H., von Euler, U. S., Pernow, B., and Sjovall, J., 1959, Observations on the effects of infusion of prostaglandin E in man, Acta Physiol. Scand. **45:**145–151.

Bisgaard, H., Kristensen, J., and Sondergaard, J., 1982, The effect of leukotriene C_4 and D_4 on cutaneous blood flow in humans, Prostaglandins **23:**797–801.

Björk, J., and Smedegard, G., 1983, Acute microvascular effects of PAF-Acether, as studied by intravital microscopy, Eur. J. Pharmacol. **96:**87–94.

Björk, J., Hedqvist, P., and Arfors, K-E., 1982, Increase in vascular permeability induced by leukotriene B_4 and the role of polymorphonuclear leukocytes, Inflammation **6:**189–200.

Björk, J., Hugli, T. E., and Smedegard, G., 1983, Microvascular effects of anaphylatoxins C3a and C5a, J. Immunol. **134:**1115–1119.

Black, J. W., Duncan, W. A. M., Durant, C. J., Ganellin, C. R., and Parsons, E. M., 1972, Definition and antagonism of histamine H_2-receptors, Nature (Lond.) **236:**385–390.

Black, J. W., Owen, D. A. A., and Parsons, M. E., 1975, An analysis of the depressor responses to histamine in the cat and dog: Involvement of both H_1- and H_2-receptors, Br. J. Pharmacol. **54:**319–324.

Blank, M. L., Snyder, F., Byers, L. W., Brooks, B., and Muirhead, E. E., 1979, Antihypertensive activity of an alkyl ether analog of phosphatidylcholine, Biochem. Biophys. Res. Commun. **90:**1194–1200.

Bloom, S. R., and Polack, J. M., 1983, Regulatory peptides and the skin, Clin. Exp. Dermatol. **8:**3–18.

Boxer, L. A., Allen, J. M., Schmidt, M., Yoder, M., and Baehner, R. L., 1980, Inhibition of polymorphonuclear leukocyte adherence by prostacyclin, J. Lab. Clin. Med. **95:**672–678.

Boyce, M. J. and Wareham, K., 1980, Histamine H_1- and H_2-receptors in the cardiovascular system of man, in: H_2-antagonists (A. Torsoli, P. E. Lucchelli, and R. W. Brimblecombe, eds.), pp. 280–294, Excerpta Medica, Amsterdam.

Brain, S. D., and Williams, T. J., 1985, Inflammatory oedema induced by synergism between calcitonin gene-related peptide (CGRP) and mediators of increased vascular permeability, Br. J. Pharmacol. **86:**855–860.

Brain, S. D., Williams, T. J., Tippins, J. R., Morris, H. R., and MacIntyre, I., 1985, Calcitonin gene-related peptide is a potent vasodilator, Nature (Lond.) **313:**54–56.

Brocklehurst, W. E., 1960, The release of histamine and formation of a slow-reacting substance (SRS-A) during anaphylactic shock, J. Physiol. (Lond.) **151:**416–435.

Brown, K. A., and Collins, A. J., 1977, Action of nonsteroidal, anti-inflammatory drugs on human and rat peripheral leukocyte migration in vitro, Ann. Rheum. Dis. **36:**239–243.

Chahl, L. A., 1977, Interactions of substance P with putative mediators of inflammation and ATP, Eur. J. Pharmacol. **44:**45–49.

Cherry, P. D., Furchgott, R. F., Zawadzki, J. V., and Jothianandan, D., 1982, Role of endothelial cells in relaxation of isolated arteries by bradykinin, *Proc. Natl. Acad. Sci. USA* **72:**2106–2110.

Chipman, P., and Glover, W. E., 1976, Histamine H_2-receptors in the human peripheral circulation, *Br. J. Pharmacol.* **56:**494–496.

Clark, E. R., and Clark, E. L., 1935, Observations on changes in blood vascular endothelium in the living animal, *Am. J. Anat.* **57:**385–438.

Cochrane, C. G., Unanue, E. R., and Dixon, F. J., 1965, A role of polymorphonuclear leukocytes and complement in nephrotoxic nephritis, *J. Exp. Med.* **122:**99–114.

Colditz, I. G., and Movat, H. Z., 1984a, Desensitization of acute inflammatory lesions to chemotaxins and endotoxin, *J. Immunol.* **133:**2163–2168.

Colditz, I. G., and Movat, H. Z., 1984b, Kinetics of neutrophil accumulation in acute inflammatory lesions induced by chemotaxins and chemotaxinigens, *J. Immunol.* **133:**2169–2173.

Coste, H., Gaspach, C., and Abita, J.-P., 1981, Effect of indomethacin on the binding of the chemotactic peptide formyl-Met-Leu-Phe on human polymorphonuclear leukocytes, *FEBS Lett.* **132:**85–88.

Dahindin, C., and Fehr, J., 1980, Receptor-directed inhibition of chemotactic factor-induced neutrophil hyperactivity by Pyrazolon Derivatives, *J. Clin. Invest.* **66:**884–891.

Dahlen, S.-E., Bjork, J., Hedqvist, P., Arfors, K. E., Hammarstrom, S., Lindgren, J.-A., and Samuelsson, B., 1981, Leukotrienes promote plasma leakage and leukocyte adhesion in postcapillary venules: In vivo effects with relevance to the acute inflammatory response, *Proc. Natl. Acad. Sci. USA* **78:**3887–3891.

Dale, H. H., 1913, The anaphylactic reaction of plain muscle in the guinea pig, *J. Pharmacol. Exp. Ther.* **4:**167.

Dale, H. H., and Laidlaw, P. P., 1910, The physiological action of β-iminazolylethylamine, *J. Physiol. (Lond.)* **41:**318–344.

Damerau, B., and Vogt, W., 1976, Effect of hog anaphylatoxin (C5a) on vascular permeability and leukocyte emigration in vivo, *Naunyn Schmiedeberg's Arch. Pharmacol.* **255:**237–241.

Davies, J. M., and Williams, K. I., 1984, Endothelial-dependent relaxant effects of vasoactive intestinal polypeptide and arachidonic acid in rat aortic strips, *Prostaglandins* **27:**195–202.

Demopoulos, C. A., Pinckard, R. N., and Hanahan, D. J., 1979, Evidence for 1-0-alkyl-2-acetyl-sn-glyceryl-3-phosphorylcholine as the active component (a new class of lipid chemical mediators), *J. Biol. Chem.* **254:**9355–9358.

Desai, U., Kreutzer, D. L., Showell, H., Arroyave, C. V., and Ward, P. A., 1979, Acute inflammatory pulmonary reactions induced by chemotactic factors, *Am. J. Pathol.* **96:**71–84.

Dobbins, D. E., Solika, C. Y., Premen, A. J., Grega, G. J., and Dabney, J. M., 1982, Blockade of histamine and bradykinin-induced increases in lymph flow, protein concentration, and protein transport by terbutaline in vivo, *Microcirculation* **2/2:**127–150.

Drazen, J. M., Austen, K. F., Lewis, R. A., Clark, D. A., Goto, G., Marfat, A., and Cory, E. J., 1980, Comparative airway and vascular activites of leukotrienes C-I and D in vivo and in vitro, *Proc. Natl. Acad. Sci. USA* **77:**4354–4358.

Ebbecke, U., 1923, Über Gewebsreizung und Gefässreaktion, *Pfluger's Arch.* **199:**197–216.

Feldberg, W., and Kellaway, C. H., 1938, Liberation of histamine and formation of a lysocithin-like substance by cobra venom, *J. Physiol. (Lond.)* **94:**187–226.

Fernandez, H. N., and Hugli, T. E., 1978, Primary structural analysis of the polypeptide portion of human C5a anaphylatoxin, *J. Biol. Chem.* **253:**6955–6964.

Feuerstein, G., 1984, Leukotrienes and the cardiovascular system, *Prostaglandins* **27:**781–802.

Fisher, L.A., Kikkawa, D. O., Rivier, J. E., Amara, S. G., Evans, R. M., Rosenfeld, M. G., Vale, W. W., and Brown, M. R., 1983, Stimulation of noradrenergic sympathetic outflow by calcitonin gene-related peptide, *Nature (Lond.)* **305:**534–536.

Flynn, P. J., Becker, W. K., Vercellotti, G. M., Weisdord, D. J., Craddock, P. R., Hammerschmidi, D. E., Lillehei, R. C., and Jacob, H. S., 1984, Ibuprofen inhibits granulocyte responses to inflammatory mediators: A proposed mechanism for reduction of experimental myocardial infact size, *Inflammation* **8:**33–44.

Folkow, B., Haeger, K., and Kahlson, G., 1948, Observations on reactive hyperaemia as related to histamine on drugs antagonising vasodilatation induced by histamine and on vasodilator properties of adenosine triphosphate, *Acta Physiol. Scand.* **15**:264–278.

Ford-Hutchinson, A. W., Bray, M. A., Doig, M. V., Shipley, M. E., and Smith, M. J. H., 1980, Leukotriene B, a potent chemokinetic and aggregating substance released from polymorphonuclear leukocytes, *Nature (Lond.)* **286**:264–265.

Foreman, J. C., Jordan, C. C., Oehme, P., and Renner, H., 1983, Structure–activity relationships for some substance P-related peptides that cause wheal and flare reactions in human skin, *J. Physiol. (Lond.)* **335**:449–465.

Forrest, M. J., Jose, P. J., and Williams, T. J., 1986, Kinetics of the generation and action of chemical mediators in zymosan-induced inflammation of the rabbit peritoneal cavity, *Br. J. Pharmacol.* **89**:719–730.

Frey, E. K., and Kraut, H., 1928, Ein neues Kreislaufhormon und seine Wirking, *Arch. Exp. Pathol. Pharmakol.* **133**:1–56.

Friedberger, E., 1910, Weitere Untersuchungen über Eiweissanaphylaxie, *Z. Immunitaetsforsch.* **4**:636.

Furchgott, R. F., 1981, The requirement for endothelial cells in the relaxation of arteries by acetylcholine and some other vasodilators, *Trends Pharmacol. Sci.* **2**:173–176.

Furchgott, R. F., and Zawadzki, J. V., 1980, The obligatory role of endothelial cells in the relaxation of arterial smooth muscle by acetylcholine, *Nature (Lond.)* **288**:373–376.

Gallin, J. I., 1980, Degranulating stimuli decrease the negative surface charge and increase the adhesiveness of human neutrophils, *J. Clin. Invest.* **65**:298–306.

Gallin, J. I., and Quie, P. G., 1978, *Leukocyte Chemotaxis: Methods, Physiology and Clinical Implications*, Raven, New York.

Gerard, C., and Hugli, T. E., 1981, Identification of classical anaphylatoxin as the des-Arg form of the C5a molecule: Evidence of a modulator role for the oligosaccharide unit in human des-Arg[74]-C5a, *Proc. Natl. Acad. Sci. USA* **78**:1833–1837.

Goetzl, E. J., Brash, A. R., Tauber, A. I., Oates, J. A., and Hubbard, W. C., 1980, Modulation of human neutrophil function by mon-hydroxy-eicosatetraenoic acids, *Immunology* **39**:491–501.

Goldblatt, M. W., 1935, Properties of human seminal fluid, *J. Physiol. (Lond.)* **84**:208–218.

Greutter, C. A., Barry, B. K., McNamara, D. B., Greutter, D. Y., Kadowitz, P. J., and Ignarro, L. J., 1979, Relaxation of bovine coronary artery and activation of coronary arterial guanylate cyclase by nitric oxide, nitroprusside and a carcinogenic nitrosoamine, *J. Cyclic Nucleotide Res.* **5**:211–224.

Griffith, T. M., Edwards, D. H., Lewis, M. J., Newby, A. C., and Henderson, A. H., 1984, The nature of the endothelium-derived vascular relaxant factor, *Nature (Lond.)* **308**:645–647.

Hagermark, O., Hokfelt, T., and Pernow, B., 1978, Flare and itch induced by substance P in human skin, *J. Invest. Dermatol.* **71**:233–235.

Hahn, F., and Oberdorf, A., 1950, Antihistaminica and anaphylaktoide, *Z. Immunitaetsforsch.* **107**:528–538.

Halonen, M., Palmer, J. D., Lohman, I. C., McManus, L. M., and Pinckard, R. N., 1980, Respiratory and circulatory alterations induced by acetyl glyceryl ether phosphorylcholine (AGEPC), a mediator of IgE anaphylaxis in the rabbit, *Am. Rev. Respir. Dis.* **122**:915–924.

Halpern, B. N., 1942, Les antihistaminiques de synthèse: Essais de chimiotherapie des états allergiques, *Arch. Int. Pharmacodyn. Ther.* **68**:339–408.

Hamberg, M., Svensson, J., and Samuelsson, B., 1975, Thromboxanes: A new group of biologically active compounds derived from prostaglandin endoperodixes, *Proc. Natl. Acad. Sci. USA* **72**:2994–2998.

Heltianu, C., Simionescu, M., and Simionescu, N., 1982, Histamine receptors of the microvascular endothelium revealed *in situ* with a histamine–ferritin conjugate: characteristic high-affinity binding sites in venules, *J. Cell Biol.* **93**:357–364.

Henson, P. M., Larsen, G. L., Webster, R. O., Mitchell, R. C., Goins, A. J., and Henson, J. E., 1982, Pulmonary microvascular alterations and injury induced by complement fragments: Synergistic effect of complement activation, neutrophils sequestration, and prostaglandins, *Ann. NY Acad. Sci.* **384**:287–300.

Higgs, G. A., 1984, The effects of lipoxygenase inhibitors in anaphylactic and inflammatory responses in vivo, *Prostaglandins Leukotrienes Medicine* **13**:89–92.

Higgs, G. A., Flower, R. J., and Vane, J. R., 1979, A new approach to anti-inflammatory drugs, *Biochem. Pharmacol.* **28**:1959–1981.

Higgs, G. A., Eakins, K. E., Mugridge, K. G., Moncada, S., and Vane, J. R., 1980, The effects on nonsteroid anti-inflammatory drugs on leukocyte migration in carragheenin-induced inflammation, *Eur. J. Pharmacol.* **66**:81–86.

Holmdahl, G., Hakanson, R., Leander, S., Roseel, S., Folders, F., and Sundler, F., 1981, A substance P antagonist, (D-Pro 2, D-Trp 7,9), inhibits inflammatory responses in the rabbit eye, *Science* **214**:1029–1031.

Holzmann, S., 1982, Endothelium-induced relaxation by acetylcholine associated with larger rises in cyclic GMP in coronary arterial strips, *J. Cyclic Nucleotide Res.* **8**:409–419.

Hoover, R. L., Folger, R., Haering, W. A., Ware, B. R., and Karrovs, M. J., 1980, Adhesion of leukocytes to endothelium: Roles of divalent cations, surface charge, chemotactic agents and substrate, *J. Cell. Sci.* **45**:73–86.

Hoover, R. L., Karnovsky, M. J., Auster, K. F., Corey, E. J., and Lewis, R. A., 1984, Leukotriene B_4 action on endothelium mediates augmented neutrophil/endothelial adhesion, *Proc. Natl. Acad. Sci. USA* **81**:2191–2193.

Huey, R. Kawahara, M. S., and Hugli, T. E., 1983, Potentiation of the anaphylatoxins in vivo using an inhibitor of serum carboxypeptidase N(SCPN), *Am. J. Pathol.* **112**:48–60.

Humphrey, J. H., 1955, The mechanism of Arthus reactions. 1. The role of polymorphonuclear leukocytes and other factors in reversed passive Arthus reactions in rabbits, *Br. J. Exp. Pathol.* **36**:268–282.

Humphrey, D. M., Hanahan, D. J., and Pinckard, R. N., 1982, Induction of leukocytic infiltrates in rabbit skin by acetyl glyceryl ether phosphorylcholine, *Lab. Invest.* **47**:227–234.

Hunter, 1794, A treatise on the blood, in: *Inflammation and Gun-shot Wounds*, G. Nicol, London.

Hurley, J. V., 1963, An electron microscopic study of leukocyte emigration and vascular permeability in rat skin, *Aust. J. Exp. Biol. Med. Sci.* **41**:171–186.

Hurley, J. V., Edwards, B., and Ham, K. N., 1970, The response of newly formed blood vessels in healing wounds to histamine and other permeability factors, *Pathology* **2**:133–145.

Ignarro, L. J., Burke, T. M., Wood, K. S., Wolin, M. S., and Kadowitz, P. J., 1984, Association between cyclic GMP accumulation and acetylcholine-elicited relaxation of bovine intrapulmonary artery, *J. Pharmacol. Exp. Ther.* **228**:682–690.

Issekutz, A. C., 1981, Vascular responses during acute neutropholic inflammation. Their relationship to in vivo neutrophil emigration, *Lab. Invest.* **45**:435–441.

Issekutz, A. C., and Bhimji, S., 1982, The effect of nonsteroidal anti-inflammatory agents on E. coli induced inflammation, *Immunopharmacology* **42**:11–22.

Issekutz, A. C., and Movat, H. Z., 1979, The effect of vasodilator prostaglandins on polymorphonuclear leukocyte infiltration and vascular injury, *Pathology* **107**:300–309.

Johnson, K. J., and Ward, P. E., 1981, Role of oxygen metabolites in immune complex injury of lung, *J. Immunol.* **126**:2365–2369.

Johnston, M. G., Hay, J. B., and Movat, H. Z., 1976, The modulation of enhanced vascular permeability by prostaglandins through alterations in blood flow, *Agents Actions* **6**:705–711.

Jones, G., and Hurley, J. V., 1984, The effect of prostacyclin on the adhesion of leukocytes to injured vascular endothelium, *J. Pathol.* **142**:51–59.

Joris, I., Majno, G., and Ryan, G. B., 1972, Endothelial contraction in vivo: A study of the rat mesentery, *Virchows Arch. [B]* **12**:73–83.

Jose, P. J., Peck, M. J., Robinson, C., and Williams, T. J., 1978, Characterization of a histamine-independent vascular permeability-increasing factor generated on exposure of rabbit plasma to zymosan, *J. Physiol. (Lond.)* **281**:13–14.

Jose, P. J., Forrest, M. J., and Williams, T. J., 1983, Detection of the complement fragment C5a in inflammatory exudates from the rabbit peritoneal cavity using radioimmunoassay, *J. Exp. Med.* **158**:2177–2182.

Juhlin, S., and Michaelsson, G., 1969, Cutaneous vascular reactions to prostaglandins in healthy subjects and in patients with urticaria and atopic dermatitis, *Acta Derm. Venereol. (Stockh.)* **49:**251–261.

Kahlson, G., and Rosengren, E., 1971, New approaches to the physiology of histamine, *Physiol. Rev.* **48:**155–196.

Kangawa, K., Minamino, N., Fukada, N., and Matsuo, H., 1983, Neuromedin K: A novel mammalian tachykinin identified in porcine spinal cord, *Biochem. Biophys. Res. Commun.* **114:**533–540.

Kaplan, B. K., Edelson, H. S., Korchak, H. M., Given, W. P., Abrahamson, S., and Weissmann, G., 1984, Effects of non-steroidal anti-inflammatory agents on human neutrophil functions *in vitro* and *in vivo, Biochem. Pharmacol.* **33:**371–378.

Katsuki, S., Arnold, W., Mittal, C. K., and Murad, F., 1977, Stimulation of guanylate cyclase by sodium nitroprusside, nitroglycerin and nitric oxide in various tissue preparations and comparison to the effects of sodium azide and hydroxylamine, *J. Cyclic Nucleotide Res.* **3:**23–25.

Kenaway, S. A., Lewis, G. P., and Williams, T. J., 1978, The effects of α- and β-adrenoceptor agonists on inflammatory exudation in rabbit and guinea pig skin, *Br. J. Pharmacol.* **64:**447–448.

Kimura, H., Mittal, C. K., and Murad, F., 1975, Activation of guanylate cyclase from rat liver and other tissues by sodium azide, *J. Biol. Chem.* **250:**8016–8022.

Kraut, H., Frey, E. K., and Werle, E., 1930, Der Nachweis eines Kreislaufhormons in der Pankeasdruse. IV. Mitt. uber dieses kreislaufhormon, *Z. Physiol. Chem.* **189:**97–106.

Kurzrok, R., and Lieb, C. C., 1930, Biochemical studies of human semen. II. The action of semen on the human uterus, *Proc. Soc. Exp. Biol. Med.* **28:**268–272.

Lembeck, F., and Holzer, P., 1979, Substance P as neurogenic mediator of antidromic vasodilation and neurogenic plasma extravasation, *Naunyn Schmiedeberg Arch. Pharmacol.* **310:**175–183.

Lembeck, F., Donnerer, J., and Bartho, L., 1982, Inhibition of neurogenic vasodilation and plasma extravasation by substance P antagonists, somatostatin and (D-met 2,pro5) enkephalinamide, *Eur. J. Pharmacol.* **85:**171–176.

Levi, R., Owen, D. A. A., and Trzeciakowski, J., 1982, Actions of histamine on the heart and vasculature, in: *Pharmacology of Histamine Receptors* (C. R. Ganellin and M. E. Parsons, eds.), pp. 236–297, PSG-Wright, London.

Lewis, T., 1927, *The Blood Vessels of the Human Skin and Their Responses,* Shaw & Sons, London.

Lewis, T., and Grant, R. I., 1924, Vascular reactions of the skin to injury. Part II. The liberation of a histamine-like substance in injured skin; the underlying cause of factitious urticaria and of wheals produced by burning, and observations upon the nervous control of certain skin reactions, *Heart* **11:**209–265.

Lin, A. H., Morton, D. R., and Gorman, R. R., 1982, Acetyl glyceryl ether phosphorylcholine stimulates leukotriene B_4, synthesis in human polymorphonuclear leukocytes, *J. Clin. Invest.* **70:**1058–1065.

Lo, T. N., Almeida, A.P., and Beaven, M. A., 1984, Effect of indomethacin on generation of chemotactic activity in inflammatory exudates induced by carrageenan, *Eur. J. Pharmacol.* **99:**31–43.

Lundberg, C., and Gerdin, B., 1984, The inflammatory reaction in an experimental model of open wounds in the rat. The effect of arachidonic acid metabolites, *Eur. J. Pharmacol.* **97:**229–238.

Lundberg, J. M., and Saria, A., 1983, Capsaicin-induced desensitization of airway mucosa to cigarette smoke, mechanical and chemical irritants, *Nature (Lond.)* **302:**251–253.

Lundberg, J. M., Saria, A., Brodin, E., Rosell, S., and Folkers, K., 1983, A substance P antagonist inhibits vagally induced increase in vascular permeability and bronchial smooth muscle contraction in the guinea pig, *Proc. Natl. Acad. Sci. USA* **80:**1120–1124.

MacGregor, R. R., Spognuolo, P. J., and Lentnek, A. L., 1974, Inhibition of granulocyte adherence by ethanol, prednisone, and aspirin, measured with an assay system, *N. Engl. J. Med.* **29:**642–646.

Maderazo, E. G., Breaux, S. P., and Woronick, C. L., 1984, Inhibition of human polymorphonuclear leukocyte cell responses by ibuprofen, *J. Pharm. Sci.* **19:**1403–1406.

Majno, G., and Palade, G. E., 1961, Studies on inflammation. I. The effect of histamine and serotonin on vascular permeability: An electron microscopic study, *J. Biol. Phys. Biochem. Cytol.* **11:**571–605.

Majno, G., Schoefl, G. I., and Palade, G., 1961, Studies on inflammation. II. The site of action of histamine and serotonin on the vascular tree; a topographic study, *J. Biophys. Biochem. Cytol.* **11**:607–626.

Majno, G., Shea, S. M., and Leventhal, M., 1969, Endothelial contraction induced by histamine-type mediators. An electron microscopic study, *J. Cell Biol.* **42**:647–672.

Marasco, W. A., Phan, S. H., Krutzsch, H., Showell, H. J., Feltner, D. E., Nairn, R., Becker, E. L., and Ward, P. A., 1984, Purification and identification of formyl-methionyl-leucyl-phenylalanine as the major peptide neutrophil chemotactic factor produced by Escherichia coli, *J. Biol. Chem.* **259**:5430–5439.

Martin, W. J., 1984, Neutrophils kill pulmonary endothelial cells by a hydrogen-peroxide dependent pathway. An *in vitro* model of neutrophil-mediated lung injury, *Am. Rev. Respir. Dis.* **130**:209–213.

Martin, W., Villani, G. M., Jothianandan, D., and Furchgott, R. F., 1985, Selective blockade of endothelim-dependent and glyceral trinitrate-induced relaxation by hemoglobin and methylene blue in rabbit aorta, *J. Pharmacol. Exp. Ther.* **232**:708–716.

Matzner, Y., Drexler, R., and Levy, M., 1984, Effect of dipyrone, acetylsalicylic acid and acetaminophen on human neutrophil chemotaxis, *Eur. J. Clin. Invest.* **14**:440–443.

McManus, L. M., Pinckard, R. N., Fitzpatrick, F. F., O'Rourke, R. A., Johanson, W. G., and Hanahan, D. J., 1981, Acetyl glyceryl ether phosphorylcholine (AGEPC): Intravascular alterations following intravenous infusion in the baboon, *Lab. Invest.* **45**:303–307.

Menkin, V., 1938a, Studies in inflammation. XIV. Isolation of the factor concerned with increased capillary permeability in injury, *J. Exp. Med.* **67**:129–144.

Menkin, V., 1938b, Studies on inflammation. XVI. On the formation of a chemotactic substance by enzymic actions, *J. Exp. Med.* **67**:153–158.

Miki, N., Kawabe, Y., and Kuriyama, K., 1977, Activation of cerebral guanylate cyclase by nitric oxide, *Biochem. Biophys. Res. Commun.* **75**:851–856.

Moncada, S. (ed.), 1983, Prostacyclin, thromboxane and leukotrienes, *Br. Med. Bull.* **39**(3):209–300.

Moncada, S., Ferreira, S. H., and Vane, J. R., 1973, Prostaglandins, aspirin-like drugs and the oedema of inflammation, *Nature (Lond.)* **246**:217–219.

Morris, H. R., Taylor, G. W., Piper, P. J., and Tippins, J. R., 1980, The structure elucidation of slow-reacting substance of anaphylaxis (SRS-A) from guinea pig lung, *Nature (Lond.)* **285**:104–106.

Morris, H. R., Panico, M., Etienne, T., Tippins, J. R., Girgis, S. I., and MacIntyre, I., 1984, Isolation and characterization of human calcitonin gene-related peptide, *Nature (Lond.)* **308**:746–748.

Murphy, R. C., Hammerstrom, S., and Samuelsson, B., 1979, Leukotriene C: A slow-reacting substance from murine mastocytoma cells, *Proc. Natl. Acad. Sci. USA* **76**:4275–4279.

Myers, B., and Rightor, M., 1978, Augmentation of wound tensile strength in rats by induction of inflammation with autogenous blood, *Surgery* **83**:78–82.

Nawa, H., Kotani, H., and Nakanishi, S., 1984, Tissue-specific generation of two prepro-tachykinin mRNAs from one gene by alternative RNA splicing, *Nature (Lond.)* **312**:729–734.

O'Donnell, S. R., and Persson, C. G. A., 1978, -adrenoceptor mediate inhibition by terbutaline of histamine effects on vascular permeability, *Br. J. Pharmacol.* **62**:321–324.

Pavek, K. P., and Smedegard, G., 1979, Anaphylatoxin-induced shock and two patterns of anaphylactic shock hemodynamics and mediators, *Acta Physiol. Scand.* **105**:393–403.

Peck, M. J., and Williams, T. J., 1978, Prostacyclin (PGI$_2$) potentiates bradykinin-induced plasma exudation in rabbit skin, *Br. J. Pharmacol.* **62**:464–465.

Peck, M. J., Piper, P. J., and Williams, T. J., 1981, The effect of leukotrienes C$_4$ and D$_4$ on the microvasculature of guinea pig skin, *Prostaglandins* **21**:315–321.

Perez, H. D., Goldstein, I. M., Chernoff, D., Webster, R. O., and Henson, P. M., 1980, Chemotactic activity of C5a des Arg: Evidence for a requirement for an anionic peptide "helper factor" and inhibition by a cationic protein in serum from patients with systemic lupus erythematosus, *Mol. Immunol.* **17**:163–169.

Pham Huy, D., Roch-Arveiller, M., Muntaner, O., and Girand, J. P., 1985, Effect of some anti-inflammatory drugs on FMLP-induced chemotaxis and random migration of rat polymorphonuclear leukocytes, *Eur. J. Pharmacol.* **111**:251–256.

Phelps, P., and McCarty, D. J., 1966, Crystal-induced inflammation of canine joints. II. Importance of polymorphonuclear leukocytes, *J. Exp. Med.* **124**:115–125.

Rampart, M., and Williams, T. J., 1986, Suppression of inflammatory oedema by ibuprofen involving a mechanism independent of cyclo-oxygenase inhibition, *Biochem. Pharmacol.* **35**:581–586.

Pinckard, R. N., McManus, L. M., and Hanahan, D. J., 1982, Chemistry and biology of acetyl glyceryl ether phosphorylcholine (platelet-activating factor), in: *Advances in Inflammation Research*, Vol. 4 (G. Weissmann, ed.), pp. 147–180, Raven, New York.

Rampart, M., and Williams, T. J., 1985, Inhibition of PMN-dependent oedema formation in rabbit skin by systemic treatment with catalase and 15-methyl PGE$_2$, *Br. J. Pharmacol.* **85**:274.

Ramsdell, S. G., 1928, The use of tryphan blue to demonstrate the immediate skin reaction in rabbits and guinea pigs, *J. Immunol.* **15**:305–311.

Rapoport, R. M., Draznin, M. B., and Murad, F., 1983, Endothelium-dependent relaxation in rat aorta may be mediated through cyclic GMP-dependent protein phosphorylation, *Nature (Lond.)* **306**:174–176.

Rapport, M. M., Green, A. A., and Page, I. H., 1948, Serum vasoconstrictor (serotonin). IV. Isolation and characterization, *J. Biol. Chem.* **176**:1243–1251.

Regoli, D., and Barabe, J., 1980, Pharmacology of bradykinin and related kinins, *Pharmacol. Rev.* **32**:1–46.

Regoli, D., Barabe, J., and Park, W. K., 1977, Receptors for bradykinin in rabbit aorta, *Can. J. Physiol. Pharmacol.* **55**:855–867.

Regoli, D., Marcaeu, F., and Barabe, J., 1978, De novo formation of vascular receptors for bradykinin, *Can. J. Physiol. Pharmacol.* **56**:674–677.

Rocha e Silva, M., Beraldo, W. T., and Rosenfeld, G., 1949, Bradykinin a hypotensive and smooth muscle stimulating factor released from plasma globulin by snake venom and by trypsin, *Am. J. Physiol.* **156**:261–273.

Rosenfeld, M. G., Mermod, J. J., Amara, S. G., Swanson, L. W., Sawchenko, P. E., Rivier, J., Vale, W. W., and Evans, R. M., 1983, Production of a novel neuropeptide encoded by the calcitonin gene via tissue-specific RNA processing, *Nature (Lond.)* **304**:129–135.

Sacks, T., Moldow, C. F., Craddock, P. R., Bowers, T. K., and Jacob, H. S., 1978, Oxygen radicals mediate endothelial cell damage by complement-stimulated granulocytes. An *in vitro* model of immune vascular damage, *J. Clin. Invest.* **61**:1161–1167.

Said, S. I., and Mutt, V., 1970, Polypeptide with broad biological activity: Isolation from small intestine, *Science* **169**:1217–1218.

Saldeen, T., 1983, Vasoactive peptides derived from degradation of fibrinogen and fibrin, *Ann. NY Acad Sci.* **408**:424–437.

Saria, A., and Lundberg, J. M., 1985, Neurogenic inflammation, in: *Inflammatory Mediators* (G. A. Higgs, and T. J. Williams, eds.), pp. 73–85, Macmillan, New York.

Schayer, R. W., 1965, Histamine and circulatory homeostasis, *Fed. Proc. Fed. Am. Soc. Exp. Biol.* **24**:1295–1297.

Schiffmann, E., Corcoran, B. A., and Wahl, S. A., 1975, N-formylmethionyl peptide as chemoattractants for leukocytes, *Proc. Natl. Acad. Sci. USA* **72**:1059–1062.

Schoefl, G. I., 1963, Studies on inflammation. III. Growing capillaries: Their structure and permeability, *Virchows Arch. [A]* **337**:97–141.

Schultz, H. E., 1910, Physiological studies in anaphylaxis. I. The reaction of smooth muscle of the guinea pig sensitised with horse serum, *J. Pharmacol. Exp. Ther.* **1**:549.

Shaw, J. O., Henson, P. M., Henson, J., and Webster, R. O., 1980, Lung inflammation induced by complement-derived chemotactic fragments in the alveolus, *Lab. Invest.* **42**:547–558.

Showell, H. J., Freer, R. J., Zigmond, S. H., Schiffmann, E., Aswanikumar, S., Corcoran, B., and Becker, E. L., 1976, The structure–activity relations of synthetic peptides as chemotactic factors and inducers of lysosomal enzyme secretion for neutrophils, *J. Exp. Med.* **143**:1154–1169.

Snyderman, R., Phillips, J., and Mergenhagen, S. E., 1970, Polymorphonuclear leukocyte chemotactic activity in rabbit serum and guinea pig serum treated with immune complexes: Evidence for C5a as the major chemotactic factor, *Infect. Immun.* **1**:521–525.

Sondergaard, J., and Greaves, M. W., 1971, Prostaglandin E₁: Effect on human cutaneous vasculature and skin histamine, Br. J. Dermatol. **84**:424–428.

Spilberg, I., and Mehta, J., 1979, Demonstration of a specific neutrophil receptor for a cell-derived chemotactic factor, J. Clin. Invest. **63**:85–88.

Springer, T. A., Teplow, D. B., and Dreyer, W. J., 1985, Sequence homology of the LFA-1 and the Mac-1 leukocyte adhesion glycoproteins and unexpected relation to leukocyte interferon, Nature (Lond.) **314**:540–542.

Stetson, C. A., 1951, Similarities in the mechanisms determining the Arthus and Schwartzman Phenomena, J. Exp. Med. **94**:347–358.

Stimler, N. P., Bach, M. K., Bloor, C. M., and Hugli, T. E., 1982, Release of leukotrienes from guinea pig lung stimulated by C5a des Arg anaphylatoxin, J. Immunol. **128**:2247–2252.

Sugio, K., and Daly, J. W., 1984, Adenosine analogs: Potentiation of bradykinin-induced plasma exudation in rat skin and prevention by caffeine and theophylline, Life Sci. **35**:1575–1583.

Svensjo, E., Persson, C. G. A., and Rutili, G., 1977, Inhibition of bradykinin induced macromolecular leakage from postcapillary venules by a β₂-adrenoceptor stimulant, terbutaline, Acta Physiol. Scand. **101**:504–506.

Terragno, N. A., Lonigro, A. J., Malik, K. U., and McGiff, J. C., 1972, The relationship of the renal vasodilator action of bradykinin to the release of a prostaglandin E-like substance, Experientia **28**:437–439.

Till, G. O., Johnson, K. J., Kunkel, R., and Ward, P. A., 1982, Intravascular activation of complement and acute lung injury. Dependency on neutrophils and toxic oxygen metabolites, J. Clin. Invest. **69**:1126–1135.

Tonnesen, M. G., Smedley, L., Goins, A., and Henson, P. M., 1982, Interaction between neutrophils and vascular endothelial cells in: Agents and Actions, Cologne Atherosclerosis Conference, Vol. XI, pp. 25–38, (M. J. Parnham, and J. Winkelmann, eds.), Birkhauser Verlag, Basel.

Tonnesen, M. G., Smedley, L. A., and Henson, P. M., 1984, Neutrophil–endothelial cell interactions. Modulation of neutrophil adhesiveness induced by complement fragments C5a and C5a des Arg and Formyl-methionyl-leucyl-phenylalaline in vitro, J. Clin. Invest. **74**:1581–1592.

Tregear, G. W., Niall, H. D., Potts, J. T. Jr., Leeman, S. E., and Chang, M. M., 1971, Synthesis of substance P, Nature (New Biol.) **232**:870–889.

Tsurufuji, S., Sugio, K., and Takemasa, F., 1979, The role of glucocorticoid receptor and gene expression in the anti-inflammatory action of dexamethasone, Nature **280**:408–410.

Turner, S. R., Trainer, J. A., and Lynn, W. S., 1975, Biogenesis of chemotactic molecules by the arachidonate lipoxygenase system of platelets, Nature (Lond.) **257**:680–681.

Van de Coorde, J., and Leusen, I., 1983, Role of endothelium in the vasodilator response of rat thoracic aorta to histamine, Eur. J. Pharmacol. **87**:113–120.

Vargaftig, B. B., and Ferreira, S. H., 1981, Blockade of the inflammatory effects of platelet-activating factor by cyclo-oxygenase inhibitors, Br. J. Med. Res. **14**:187–189.

Voelkel, N. F., Worthen, S., Reeves, J. T., Henson, P. M., and Murphy, R. C., 1982, Nonimmunological production of leukotrienes induced by platelet-activating factor, Science **218**:286–288.

von Euler, U. S., 1936, On the specific vasodilating and plain muscle stimulating substance from accessory genital glands in man and certain animals (prostaglandin and vesiglandin), J. Physiol. (Lond.) **88**:213–234.

von Euler, U. S., and Pernow, B. (eds.), 1977, Substance P, Raven, New York.

Wedmore, C. V., and Williams, T. J., 1981a, Platelet-activating factor (PAF), a secretory product of polymorphonuclear leukocytes, increases vascular permeability in rabbit skin, Br. J. Pharmacol. **74**:916–917.

Wedmore, C. V., and Williams, T. J., 1981b, Control of vascular permeability by polymorphonuclear leukocytes in inflammation, Nature (Lond.) **289**:646–650.

Werle, E., 1937, Uber die Wirkung des Kallikreins auf den isolierten Darm and uber eine neue dermakontrahierende Substanz, Biochem. Z. **289**:217–233.

Wilkinson, P. C., 1982, Chemotaxis and Inflammation, **2nd ed.**, Churchill Livingstone, London.

Williams, T. J., 1976, The pro-inflammatory activity of E-, A-, D- and F-type prostaglandins and analogues 16, 16-dimethyl-PGE₂ and (15S)-15-methyl-PGE₂ in rabbit skin; the relationship between potentiating of plasma exudation and local blood flow changes, *Br. J. Pharmacol.* **56**:341–352.

Williams, T. J., 1978, A proposed mediator of increased vascular permeability in acute inflammation in the rabbit, *J. Physiol. (Lond.)* **281**:44–45.

Williams, T. J., 1979, Prostaglandin E_2, prostaglandin I_2 and the vascular changes in inflammation, *Br. J. Pharmacol.* **65**:517–524.

Williams, T. J., 1982, Vasoactive intestinal polypeptide is more potent than prostaglandin E_2 as a vasodilator and oedema potentiator in rabbit skin, *Br. J. Pharmacol.* **77**:505–509.

Williams, T. J., and Jose, P. J., 1981, Mediation of increased vascular permeability after complement activation: Histamine-independent action of rabbit C5a, *J. Exp. Med.* **153**:136–153.

Williams, T. J., and Morley, J., 1973, Prostaglandins as potentiators of increased vascular permeability in inflammation, *Nature (Lond.)* **246**:215–217.

Williams, T. J., and Peck, M. J., 1977, Role of prostaglandin-mediated vasodilatation in inflammation, *Nature (Lond.)* **270**:530–532.

Williams, T. J., and Piper, P. J., 1980, The action of chemically pure SRS-A on the microcirculation *in vivo*, *Prostaglandins* **19**:779–789.

Williams, T. J., Jose, P. J., Forrest, L. H., Smaje, L. H., and Clough, G. F., 1984, Inflammatory oedema induced by synergism between prostaglandins and C5a: The importance of the interaction between neutrophils and venular endothelial cells, in: *Progress in Microcirculation Research.* Vol. II (F. C. Courtice, D. G. Garlick, and M. A. Perry, eds.), pp. 439–448, Committee in Postgraduate Medical Education, University of New South Wales, Sydney.

Williamson, L. M., Sheppard, K., Davies, J. M., and Fletcher, J., 1986, Neutrophils are involved in the increased vascular permeability produced by activated complement in man, *Br. J. Haemotol.* **64**:375–384.

Yancey, K. B., Hammer, C. H., Harvath, L., Renfer, L., Frank, M. M., and Lawley, T. J., 1985, Studies of human C5a as a mediator of inflammation in normal human skin, *J. Clin. Invest.* **75**:486–495.

Chapter 6

Neutrophil Emigration, Activation, and Tissue Damage

MARCIA G. TONNESEN, G. SCOTT WORTHEN, and
RICHARD B. JOHNSTON, JR.

1. Introduction

The early inflammatory phase of wound healing is characterized by a rapid accumulation of neutrophils. Despite this observation, the neutrophil does not appear to play a central or essential role in the wound healing process per se. The classic study by Simpson and Ross (1972), in which wound repair was monitored in guinea pigs depleted of neutrophils by the administration of antineutrophil serum, failed to demonstrate that either wound debridement or formation of granulation tissue is dependent on the presence of neutrophils.

Neutrophils are attracted to sites of tissue injury by a variety of chemotactic factors (Wilkinson, 1982) generated as a result of blood vessel disruption with concomitant blood extravasation and coagulation, platelet aggregation, and complement activation. Such chemotactic factors include kallikrein from the activated Hageman Factor (HF) pathway, fibrinopeptides produced during fibrin clot formation (see Chapters 3 and 4), C5a from complement activation, leukotriene B_4 released by activated neutrophils, bacterial formyl-methionyl peptides, and platelet-release products (see Chapters 2 and 5). The process of neutrophil egress from the bloodstream and migration to the wounded tissue involves a sequence of biologic events depicted in Fig. 1, that constitute the central theme of this chapter. The emigrating neutrophil must first adhere to the microvascular endothelium adjacent to the wound, migrate between endothelial cells, penetrate the endothelial basement membrane and blood vessel wall, and then migrate through the interstitial connective tissue in a directed fashion in response to a gradient of chemotactic factor. Once at the site of tissue injury, the neutrophil fulfills its major function as the first line of defense

MARCIA G. TONNESEN • Department of Pediatrics, National Jewish Center for Immunology and Respiratory Medicine, and Dermatology Service, Veterans' Administration Medical Center, Denver, Colorado 80206.   G. SCOTT WORTHEN • Department of Medicine, National Jewish Center for Immunology and Respiratory Medicine, Denver, Colorado 80206.   RICHARD B. JOHNSTON, JR. • Department of Pediatrics, The University of Pennsylvania School of Medicine and The Children's Hospital of Philadelphia, Philadelphia, Pennsylvania 19104.

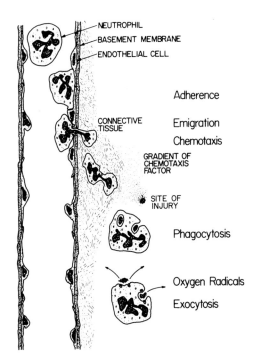

Figure 1. Scheme depicting the various stages of neutrophil accumulation and participation in the early inflammatory phase of wound healing.

against infection by the phagocytosis and intracellular killing of microorganisms. Extracellular release of toxic oxygen metabolites, granule proteolytic enzymes, and cationic proteins, accompanying the phagocytic event, may potentiate the tissue injury and prolong the acute inflammatory phase. The neutrophil then meets its fate at the wound site. This end-stage nonrecirculating cell is believed to be cleared from the tissue by inflammatory macrophages (see Chapter 7).

This chapter reviews in some depth the current knowledge regarding the mechanisms by which neutrophils adhere to vascular endothelium, penetrate blood vessel walls, migrate through interstitial connective tissues, kill microorganisms, and potentially contribute to tissue injury.

2. Adherence of Neutrophils to Vascular Endothelium

Neutrophil adherence to the endothelium of the microvasculature (Fig. 2) is the initial step in diapedesis, the process by which leukocytes migrate through blood vessels to accumulate at a site of injury in the surrounding tissue. The first description of white blood cell emigration has been attributed to Dutrochet (1824), who reported in 1824 on his microscopic observations of the movement of blood in the transparent tadpole tail (Grant, 1973). Despite intense interest and investigation into the nature of the leukocyte–endothelial

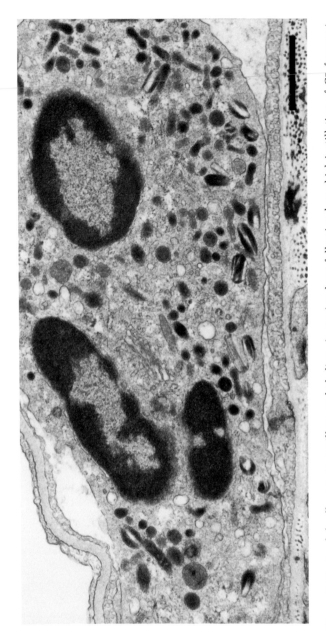

Figure 2. Neutrophil adherent to capillary endothelium in canine lung following bronchial instillation of C5 fragment preparation. Bar = 1 μm.

interaction during the ensuing century and a half, the mechanisms involved still have not been completely elucidated.

2.1. *In Vivo* Observations

Using a system similar to that of Dutrochet to visualize directly the microvasculature of the tadpole tail, Clark and Clark (1935) documented that adhesion of leukocytes to the endothelium regularly precedes emigration (Figs. 1 and 2). Since localized leukocyte adherence to the endothelium clearly could occur in the absence of subsequent migration through the vessel wall, they attributed leukocyte sticking to a transient alteration in the consistency of the endothelial cells. By contrast, Metchnikoff (1893) had proposed in 1893 that diapedesis was the result of the response of leukocytes to chemotactic attraction from outside the vessel wall. The concept that the leukocyte–vascular interaction is influenced by products of tissue damage that diffuse to the vessel wall from a nearby site of injury (Fig. 3) gained credence from the classic observation by Allison *et al.* (1955) that adherence of leukocytes to the microvascular endothelium, induced by thermal injury in the rabbit ear chamber, first occurred on the side of the vessel closest to the site of injury. Thus, the stage was set for further elucidation of the contribution of inflammatory mediators to neutrophil–endothelial adhesion. However, the controversy persisted as to whether enhanced adhesiveness of the leukocyte or the endothelial cell is

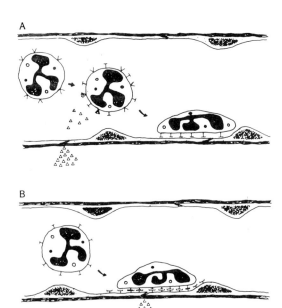

Figure 3. Scheme depicting enhanced neutrophil adherence to endothelium mediated by soluble factor(s) (triangles) which diffused to the vessel wall from a nearby site of tissue injury. The factor(s) might act on the neutrophil (A) or on the endothelial cell (B) to enhance adhesiveness.

primarily responsible for the initial interaction (Fig. 3). Even the elegant electron microscopic studies by Florey and Grant (1961) and Marchesi and Florey (1960) of inflammation induced in the rabbit ear and rat mesentery failed to resolve the issue, since no specific morphologic alterations were detected in either cell type and no intercellular "cement" substance appeared to be present (Fig. 2).

2.2. Inflammatory Mediators and Biochemical Mechanisms

Relatively recent advances in tissue culture technology facilitating the isolation and culture of vascular endothelial cells from a variety of species, including humans (Ryan et al., 1980; Gimbrone, 1976; Kern et al., 1983), have permitted delineation of some of the factors governing the adhesive interaction between neutrophils and endothelial cells. In vitro, neutrophils adhere preferentially to cultured endothelial cells, compared with other cell types, including fibroblasts and smooth muscle cells (Lackie and DeBono, 1977; MacGregor et al., 1978; Hoover et al., 1978; Beesley et al., 1978; Tonnesen et al., 1984). Human neutrophils demonstrate a baseline level of spontaneous adhesion to endothelial cells, which is dependent on divalent cations (Hoover et al., 1978), and ranges from 20 to 55%, depending on the donor and the assay system employed (MacGregor et al., 1978; Hoover et al., 1978; Tonnesen et al., 1984). Such spontaneous adhesion in vitro may be a manifestation of in vivo neutrophil margination—a pool of intravascular neutrophils reversibly associated with the vascular endothelial surface (Athens et al., 1961).

It has now been clearly shown that human neutrophil adherence to cultured endothelial monolayers in vitro can be enhanced by a variety of inflammatory mediators and that both the neutrophil and the endothelial cell may actively contribute to the adhesive interaction, depending on the stimuli employed (Fig. 3). Chemotactic peptides, such as formyl-methionyl-leucyl-phenylalanine (FMLP) and the chemotactically active fragment of the fifth component of complement (C5a), and lipid mediators, such as platelet-activating factor (PAF) and leukotriene B_4 (LTB$_4$), appear to act primarily on the neutrophil to increase its adhesion to endothelium. The initial evidence supporting an effect on neutrophil adhesiveness following stimulation by chemotactic factors resulted from (1) comparative adherence studies in which stimulated neutrophils adhered to protein-coated surfaces and to a variety of cultured cell types to the same degree as they adhered to endothelial cells (Tonnesen et al., 1984), and (2) pretreatment studies in which pretreatment of the neutrophil, but not the endothelial cell, with chemotactic peptides produced increased adhesion (Tonnesen et al., 1984). More conclusive evidence derives from the recent definition of the critical role of leukocyte surface-adhesive glycoproteins in a variety of neutrophil adherence-dependent functions (Anderson et al., 1984), including adherence to cultured human umbilical vein and microvascular endothelial cells (Harlan et al., 1985; Tonnesen et al., 1986a,b).

The best-studied leukocyte surface adhesive glycoprotein complex, termed

154

CDw18 by the Second International Workshop on Leukocyte Differentiation Antigens (Bernstein et al., 1985) or Mac-1 Glycoprotein Family by Springer and co-workers (Sanchez-Madrid et al., 1983; Springer et al., 1984) is composed of a family of three structurally and functionally related glycoproteins: Mac-1 (the C3bi complement receptor), LFA-1 (lymphocyte function associated antigen), and p150,95. Each of the three glycoproteins is composed of an α- and a β-subunit, which are noncovalently associated (Sanchez-Madrid et al., 1983). The β-subunits are immunologically identical, while the three α-subunits are immu-nologically distinct (Sanchez-Madrid et al., 1983). Only hematopoietic precur-sor cells and white blood cells have thus far been shown to express this glycopro-tein family (Anderson and Springer, 1987). In unstimulated blood neutrophils, Mac-1 and p150,95 are present in an intracellular vesicular compartment as well as on the cell surface (Springer et al., 1984; Todd et al., 1984; Anderson et al., 1985). Chemotactic factors including FMLP, C5a, LTB_4, and PAF, as well as phorbol myristate acetate (PMA) and the calcium ionophore A23187, stimulate a rapid 2–10-fold increase in cell-surface expression (Springer et al., 1984; Todd et al., 1984; Arnaout et al., 1984; Harlan et al., 1985; Anderson et al., 1985; Tonnesen et al, 1986a,b). This upregulation of expression of a portion of the glycoprotein family on the surface of stimulated neutrophils appears to be critical to the development of increased adhesiveness for endothelium, since neutrophils from patients with a genetic deficiency of the Mac-1 glycoprotein family, termed leukocyte adhesion deficiency (LAD) (Anderson and Springer, 1987), exhibit strikingly diminished adherence in vitro to cultured human endothelial cells compared with normal control neutrophils when stimulated with chemotactic peptides (Tonnesen et al., 1986a), lipid mediators (Tonnesen et al., 1986b), or PMA (Harlan et al., 1985). In addition, monoclonal antibodies to the common β-subunit of the glycoprotein family markedly inhibit the increased adhesion of normal neutrophils to cultured endothelial cells stimulated by chemotactic peptides (Tonnesen et al., 1986a), lipid mediators (Tonnesen et al., 1986b), or PMA (Harlan et al., 1985). Figure 4 illustrates the diminished ad-herence response of neutrophils from a patient with LAD, stimulated by FMLP or LTB_4, to adhere to two types of cultured human endothelial cells as well as to serum-coated plastic, and the ability of a monoclonal antibody to the β-subunit to inhibit stimulated adherence of normal neutrophils under the same condi-tions. Although enhanced expression of the adhesive glycoproteins, Mac-1 and p150,95, on the surface of the neutrophil appears essential to the induction of stimulated neutrophil adherence to endothelium, the degree to which these molecules are directly involved in the actual adhesion process remains to be clarified.

The process by which chemotactic peptides and lipid mediators stimulate increased neutrophil adhesiveness should be rapid and readily modulated in order to ensure proper localization of neutrophil interaction with the micro-vascular endothelium adjacent to a site of tissue injury in vivo. Indeed, in vitro studies have shown that the onset of enhanced adherence in response to stim-ulus occurs quickly (onset within 30 sec, maximal in less than 2 min) and can be rapidly modulated, since the capacity for enhanced adhesiveness dimin-

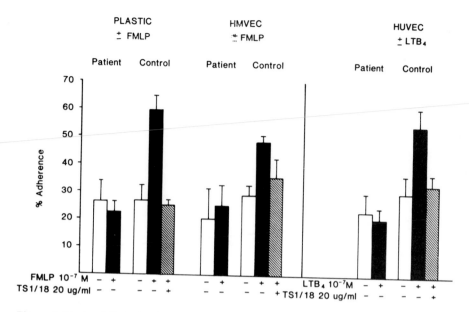

Figure 4. Neutrophils isolated from a patient with leukocyte adhesion deficiency and stimulated with FMLP or LTB$_4$ show diminished adherence to serum-coated plastic and to cultured human microvascular (HMVEC) and umbilical vein (HUVEC) endothelial cells compared with normal control neutrophils. The response of normal neutrophils to FMLP and LTB4 is inhibited by a monoclonal antibody (TS1/18) to the beta subunit of the Mac-1 glycoprotein family.

ishes markedly upon removal of the stimulus (Tonnesen *et al.*, 1984). Thus *in vivo*, presumably those neutrophils already near the surface of the endothelium would adhere in response to local stimuli generated at a nearby site of tissue injury, mediated by a rapid increase in neutrophil surface expression of the Mac-1 glycoprotein family. The critical importance to the neutrophil–endo-thelial interaction of enhanced adhesiveness on the part of the neutrophil is exemplified *in vivo* by patients with LAD whose neutrophils lack the Mac-1 glycoprotein family. Such patients are characterized by their inability to mobilize neutrophils (and monocytes) to injured and infected tissues, resulting in recurrent or progressive soft tissue infections (see Section 6), diminished pus formation, impaired wound healing, and early demise (Anderson *et al.*, 1984, 1985; Anderson and Springer, 1987; Arnaout *et al.*, 1982; Bowen *et al.*, 1982; Crowley *et al.*, 1980; Ross *et al.*, 1985). The ability of bone marrow transplantation to correct the defect and cure patients with this genetic abnormality (Fischer *et al.*, 1983) strongly suggests that enhanced adhesivity induced in the neutrophil by inflammatory mediators plays a primary role in neutrophil emigration and accumulation at sites of tissue injury.

Endothelial cells may also be activated to contribute to the neutrophil–endothelial interaction, although with a delayed time course. The human cytokines, interleukin-1 (IL-1) and tumor necrosis factor (TNF), as well as bacterial lipopolysaccharide (LPS), induce cultured human umbilical vein endo-thelial cells to increase their adhesivity for human neutrophils through a process that is time dependent, requiring 4–6 hr for maximal response, reversible, and appears to require *de novo* RNA and protein synthesis, since it is inhibited by actinomycin D or cycloheximide (Bevilacqua *et al.*, 1985; Gamble *et al.*, 1985). Neutrophil adherence to IL-1-, TNF-, or LPS-activated endothelial cells may occur by a mechanism dependent in part upon the CDw18/Mac-1 glycoprotein complex, since monoclonal antibodies to the common β-subunit also inhibit such adherence, although to a lesser degree than antibody inhibition of chemotactic factor-stimulated neutrophil adherence to nonactivated endothelial cells (Pohlman *et al.*, 1986; Tonnesen *et al.*, unpublished observations). In addition, treatment of umbilical vein endothelial cells with thrombin (Zimmerman *et al.*, 1985) or leukotrienes C_4 and D_4 (McIntyre *et al.*, 1986) will also increase adhesivity for neutrophils by a mechanism possibly related to increased synthesis of PAF by the endothelial cells.

Thus, it is now known that neutrophil adherence to endothelial cells *in vitro* occurs spontaneously (possibly related to the marginating pool), increases rapidly upon neutrophil stimulation by chemotactic peptides and lipid mediators (mediated by increased surface expression of the Mac-1 glycoprotein family), and may be more slowly enhanced through participation of the endothelium after activation by cytokines or LPS.

2.3. Hemodynamic and Physical Effects

Although the biochemical mechanisms that mediate neutrophil adherence to endothelial cells are beginning to be recognized, the physical principles that govern neutrophil behavior within the microvasculature are still unclear. Current evidence provides the following simplified scheme. In vessels without geometric constraints, theoretical (Schmid-Schonbein *et al.*, 1975) and *in vivo* (Atherton and Born, 1973) data suggest that a balance exists between shear stress (or velocity gradient) and neutrophil adhesiveness in determining adherence to endothelium. Neutrophil viscoelasticity also plays a role in determining the torque or force exerted on the neutrophil by the flowing blood (Gaehtgens *et al.*, 1984).

The effects of hydrodynamic parameters on neutrophil adherence have begun to be studied *in vitro*. Doroszewski and colleagues (Doroszewski *et al.*, 1977), studying the effect of shear rate on adherence of leukemic leukocytes to glass, noted that adherence decreased as shear rate increased. Forrester and Lackie (1984) calculated that the adhesive interaction between neutrophils and an albumin-coated surface in a flow chamber is sufficient to resist a distractive force of 4×10^{-11} N. Using a device similar to a cone-in-plate viscometer (van Grondelle *et al.*, 1984), we have subjected neutrophils and pulmonary artery endothelial cells to shear stress during the process of adherence. Low values of shear stress were sufficient to markedly reduce adherence with or without stimulus, unless the neutrophils were allowed to preadhere. Preadherence of neutrophils to the endothelial monolayer for 6 min permitted some of the stimulated cells to resist subsequently applied shear stress. This requirement for a period of static adherence in order for neutrophil stimuli to increase the "strength" of adherence is of considerable interest, particularly in light of the likelihood of vasodilation and subsequent possible static contact in the microvasculature near a site of tissue injury (see Chapter 5).

Thus, neutrophil adherence to endothelium is a complex and as yet incompletely understood process, apparently involving active participation by both the neutrophil and the endothelial cell, and modulated by local hemodynamic and physical effects. Much remains to be delineated. Is the Mac-1 glycoprotein family directly involved in adhesion, or are other steps required? What is the nature of the adhesive site on the endothelial surface? How are the adhesive sites modulated to permit subsequent neutrophil migration between endothelial cells? How important a role does shear stress play in vivo in determining the localization of neutrophil adherence and diapedesis near a site of tissue injury?

3. Migration of Neutrophils through Vascular Endothelium

Once adherent to the vessel wall, neutrophils must migrate through the vascular endothelium to gain access to the wounded tissue. Despite early microscopic observations permitting direct visualization of the process of leukocyte diapedesis, remarkably little has yet been elucidated concerning the mechanisms involved. The postcapillary venule is the usual site of leukocyte diapedesis in most organs, except the lung, where the capillary has been shown to be a common site of emigration (Shaw, 1980; Damiano et al., 1980; Lipscomb et al., 1983). However, it is important to emphasize that neutrophils can pass through the endothelium of even large arteries in vivo, given appropriate stimuli and physical conditions. For example, C5 fragments applied to the exposed adventitial surface of the carotid artery in an anesthetized rabbit induces significant adherence of neutrophils to the endothelium and migration through the arterial wall (Tonnesen et al., 1982).

It is generally believed that neutrophils leave the circulation and migrate to a site of tissue injury in response to chemoattractant molecules which are generated in the damaged tissue and diffuse to form a chemotactic gradient (Wilkinson, 1982). These molecules (discussed in depth in Chapter 5) include the biologically active fragment of the fifth component of complement (C5a), bacterially related formyl peptides such as FMLP, LTB_4, and PAF. Neutrophil diapedesis can be induced in vivo by the installation of one of these chemotactic factors as demonstrated, for example, in rabbit skin with FMLP and PAF (Colditz and Movat, 1984), in the hamster cheek pouch with PAF (Björk et al., 1983) and LTB_4 (Lindbom et al., 1982), and in the lung by C5 fragments (Shaw et al., 1980; Shaw, 1980), C5a and C5a des arg (Larsen et al., 1980). Neutrophil chemotaxis in vitro induced by chemotactic factors is addressed in Chapter 10.

158

3.1. *In Vivo* Observations

Clark and Clark (1935) described and depicted schematically the emigration of individual leukocytes through the microvascular endothelium of the tadpole tail and the rabbit ear, a process that took 2–9 min. These workers commented that no preformed hole in the vessel wall was ever seen, but rather that the effect was that of one gel pushing through a slightly softer gel, usually with no evidence of injury to the endothelium. Subsequent ultrastructural studies in the rat mesentery (Marchesi, 1961) and in the rabbit lung (Shaw, 1980) determined that neutrophils migrate between endothelial cells, first extending pseudopods and then passing through the intercellular junctions in close apposition to the endothelial cell plasma membrane. Endothelial intercellular junctions immediately re-form behind the migrating cells (Marchesi and Florey, 1960; Shaw, 1980). The absence of holes, special channels, or visible alterations in the endothelium suggested to Marchesi (1961) that neutrophil emigration is an active process on the part of the migrating blood cell. However, Shaw (1980) and Williamson and Grisham (1961) observed endothelial cytoplasmic extensions partially enveloping migrating leukocytes, perhaps indicating an active role for the endothelium in the process of diapedesis.

3.2. Effect of Inflammatory Mediators and Participation by the Endothelium

Further evidence for active participation by the endothelium in neutrophil emigration comes from an *in vitro* study in which Niedermeyer *et al.* (1984) measured granulocyte adherence to, and migration into, bovine pulmonary artery intimal explants placed in chemotaxis chambers with the endothelium facing toward the upper chamber. Granulocyte migration through the endothelium and into the explant was enhanced by chemotactic stimulation and did not injure the endothelium, as assessed by lactate dehydrogenase release. Physical removal of the endothelium did not change the degree of migration. However, glutaraldehyde fixation of the explant, producing an intact but nonviable endothelium, resulted in more tightly adherent granulocytes and significantly less migration, suggesting that granulocyte diapedesis across a vascular wall is an interactive process between granulocytes and the endothelium and that intact, viable endothelium facilitates granulocyte migration. Using the same system, Meyrick *et al.* (1984) demonstrated that granulocyte migration in response to zymosan-activated plasma does not detectably alter permeability of the explants to radiolabeled sucrose, water, or albumin, indicating the presence of a tight apposition between the plasma membranes of the migrating neutrophil and the endothelial cells, in agreement with the *in vivo* ultrastructural observations described above. Thus, neutrophil migration and vascular permeability appear to be independent phenomena; this concept is considered in depth in Chapter 5.

Neutrophils rapidly migrate (within 15–30 sec) beneath cultured endothelial monolayers grown *in vitro* (Beesley *et al.*, 1979; Tonnesen *et al.*, 1984) in the presence or absence of added stimuli. The process of neutrophil migration through endothelium *in vitro* morphologically resembles that *in vivo*, since there is close apposition of cell membranes as the neutrophil moves between two endothelial cells (Fig. 5).

Several investigators have grown monolayers of endothelial cells on chemotaxis filters to begin to study mechanisms of neutrophil migration (Taylor *et al.*, 1981; Smedly *et al.*, 1983; Hopkins *et al.*, 1984; Cramer *et al.*, 1984). In the absence of a chemotactic stimulus, neutrophils preferentially migrate through bovine endothelial cell monolayers compared to migration through fibroblasts, smooth muscle cells, or filters alone (Smedly *et al.*, 1983), once again suggesting that the endothelium may facilitate neutrophil diapedesis. The addition of a chemotactic stimulus such as FMLP (Smedly *et al.*, 1983; Taylor *et al.*, 1981), C5 fragments (Smedly *et al.*, 1983), LTB$_4$ (Hopkins *et al.*, 1984), or PAF (Hopkins *et al.*, 1984) to the abluminal surface of such endothelial monolayers markedly enhances neutrophil migration; however, the preferential effect of the endothelium is eliminated (Smedly *et al.*, 1983). Although endothelial monolayers, either bovine aortic (Taylor *et al.*, 1981) or human umbilical vein (Hopkins, *et al.*, 1984), grown on chemotaxis filters have been shown to provide a functional barrier to the passage of radiolabeled albumin, potentially more relevant *in vivo* modeling has been attempted by using connective tissue derived from human amnion as a substrate for the cultured endothelial cells. Confluent monolayers of human umbilical vein endothelial cells grown on amnion develop a measurable transendothelial electrical resistance—an assessment of endothelial permeability—as high as 50 Ω/cm^2 (Cramer *et al.*, 1984). Using this model system, Cramer *et al.* (1984) demonstrated that lipid mediators (LTB$_4$) and chemotactic peptides (FMLP) can directly, in the absence of serum and connective tissue factors, mediate neutrophil adherence to and migration through the endothelial monolayer, penetration of the basal lamina, and migration into the connective tissue of the amnion.

Despite the elegant *in vivo* observations and *in vitro* models outlined, many fascinating questions remain concerning the actual mechanism of neutrophil migration through the vascular endothelium. Does the endothelium actively contribute to the process of emigration, perhaps by opening intercellular junctions? Does the neutrophil provide a signal to initiate this process? How does the endothelial junctional complex interact with the neutrophil surface to enable the neutrophil to slip or crawl between endothelial cells and to prevent increased endothelial permeability? What triggers the reformation of the junction once the neutrophil has passed through?

4. Migration of Neutrophils through Connective Tissue

Once the neutrophil has passed between vascular endothelial cells, it must then traverse basement membrane and interstitial connective tissue on its journey to a site of tissue injury. The mechanisms by which the neutrophil moves

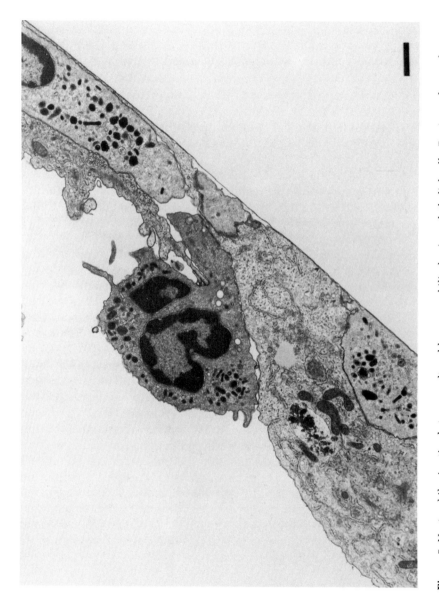

Figure 5. Neutrophil migrating between cultured human umbilical vein endothelial cells. Portions of two other neutrophils that already migrated beneath the monolayer are visible in this section. Bar = 1 μm.

through connective tissue are currently under intense investigation but are as yet poorly understood. However, the three-step theory of invasion proposed by Liotta (1984) to describe the sequence of biochemical events during tumor cell invasion of the extracellular matrix may well apply to the migration of neutrophils to sites of tissue injury. Step 1 would be neutrophil attachment to basement membrane, possibly mediated through specific glycoproteins such as laminin, via neutrophil plasma membrane receptors. Step 2 would involve secretion of hydrolytic enzymes by the attached neutrophil that could locally degrade basement membrane and extracellular matrix constituents, including the attachment glycoproteins. Step 3 would be neutrophil locomotion through the extracellular matrix. The enusing discussion considers experimental evidence pertaining to each of these steps.

4.1. *In Vivo* Observations

In vivo morphologic evidence suggests that the vascular basement membrane presents a significant barrier to neutrophil migration. Marchesi and Florey (1960), studying neutrophil migration to a site of mild mechanical trauma in the rat mesentery, noted that emigrating neutrophils were detained in the subendothelial space prior to streaming out into the surrounding connective tissue. After traversing the venular endothelium in the rabbit ear chamber in response to ultraviolet (UV) light injury, neutrophils, as though meeting a resistance, turned and moved parallel to the endothelium and formed a layer in the subendothelium before escaping into the interstitium (Florey and Grant, 1961). Shaw (1980), investigating leukocyte diapedesis in rabbit lung induced by chemotactic factors, documented a holdup of neutrophils at the subendothelial basement membrane, followed by migration into the interstitium through a small opening in the vascular basement membrane. This phenomenon was also noted in a model of neutrophil emigration into mouse lung in response to an inoculation of *Staphylococcus aureus* into the bronchus (Lipscomb et al., 1983).

4.2. Attachment to Vascular Basement Membrane

The initial step in neutrophil penetration of vascular basement membrane may be attachment to membrane components. Recent studies have suggested that neutrophil interaction with laminin, an ubiquitous basement membrane glycoprotein (see Chapters 19 and 20), may be important (Terranova et al., 1986; Yoon et al., 1987). Laminin increases the attachment of dispase-treated rabbit peritoneal exudate neutrophils to type IV collagen-coated plastic, which is inhibitable by antilaminin and associated with specific granule secretion (Terranova et al., 1986). Laminin surface-receptor expression increases when human neutrophils are stimulated with PMA or FMLP (Yoon et al., 1987). Laminin also stimulates chemotaxis of rabbit neutrophils in a Boyden chamber assay, and antibody to laminin blocks this effect as well as inhibiting neutrophil migration through human amnion in response to FMLP (Terranova *et al.*, 1986).

4.3. Degradation of Vascular Basement Membrane

It has been widely postulated but insufficiently documented that neutrophil penetration of basement membrane and connective tissue barriers is accomplished by proteolytic digestion (Senior and Campbell, 1983). This hypothesis derives from several lines of experimental evidence. Experimental models of tumor cell metastasis using human amnion strongly suggest that proteolysis of basement membrane and extracellular matrix is an important pathogenetic mechanism (Liotta *et al.*, 1980; Thorgeirsson *et al.*, 1982; Liotta, 1984). Some (Williamson and Grisham, 1961), but not all (Shaw, 1980), morphologic studies describe disintegration of the vascular basement membrane in the course of neutrophil emigration to the extravascular space. Neutrophil granule extracts damage vascular basement membrane when injected into animal tissues *in vivo* (Janoff and Zeligs, 1968), and neutrophils or neutrophil granule extracts are able to degrade basement membranes *in vitro* (Cochrane and Aikin, 1966; Janoff and Zeligs, 1968). These effects are blocked by inhibitors of proteolysis (Janoff and Zeligs, 1968). The neutral proteinases contained within human neutrophils (see Section 6.3 and Table I) can cleave many of the constituents of basement membrane and extracellular matrix, including collagen types I through V as well as denatured collagen, elastin, laminin, fibronectin, and proteoglycans (reviewed by Senior and Campbell, 1983).

An *in vitro* model of neutrophil migration through human amnion (simulating vascular basement membrane and interstitial connective tissue) in a modified chemotaxis chamber has been used by Russo *et al.* (1981) to demonstrate that human neutrophils can penetrate the full thickness of the amnion in response to a chemoattractant (FMLP). Focal dissolution of the basement mem-

Table I. Neutrophil Products Capable
of Producing Tissue Injury

Oxygen metabolites
   Superoxide anion (O_2^-)
   Hydrogen peroxide (H_2O_2)
   Hydroxyl radical ($\cdot OH$)
   Hypochlorous acid (HOCl)
   N-chloramines
Neutral proteases
   Collagenase (active on types I, II, and III collagen)
   Elastase (also active on type IV collagen)
   Gelatinase (active on type V collagen)
   Cathepsin G
Nonenzymatic cationic proteins

brane was observed at the front of neutrophil contact. Sibille *et al.* (1986) extended the amnion model to investigate neutrophil-induced injury to extracellular matrix. PMA-stimulated neutrophils caused injury to the basement membrane surface of the amnion as assessed by fibronectin release and by transmission electron microscopy. This injurious effect was inhibited by a chloromethylketone elastase inhibitor but not by superoxide dismutase (SOD) and catalase, suggesting that elastase rather than oxygen radicals solubilizes fibronectin from the matrix. Similarly, neutrophils can rapidly degrade subendothelial matrices *in vitro* (produced by cultured human umbilical vein endothelial cells) by a process which is enhanced by stimulation with PMA and dependent on elastase but not oxygen metabolites (Weiss and Regiani, 1984).

A probable role for elastase in neutrophil migration through elastin-rich barriers was suggested by Sandhaus and Henson (Personal communication, 1987) who showed that neutrophils migrating through chemotaxis filters coated with insoluble elastin in response to FMLP degrade the elastin, as assessed by solubilization of tritiated elastin fragments. Both elastin degradation and neutrophil migration through the elastin barrier are blocked by a specific chloromethylketone inhibitor of neutrophil elastase. Figure 6 illustrates a neutrophil making its way through the internal elastic lamina of the carotid artery of an anesthetized rabbit in response to C5 fragments applied to the adventitial surface of the artery (Tonnesen *et al.*, 1982), perhaps by a similar elastase-dependent mechanism.

4.4. Locomotion through Extracellular Matrix

Cell motility is addressed in depth in Chapter 10 and is discussed here only in relationship to neutrophil movement through the extracellular matrix. Directed neutrophil migration through tissues toward a site of injury in response to chemoattractants requires that neutrophils be invasive cells in that they must not be inhibited from migrating on foreign cellular or matrix substrata. Indeed, Armstrong and Lackie (1975) elegantly demonstrated that neutrophils do not exhibit contact paralysis of locomotion (defined as the cessation of forward extension of pseudopods of a cell as a result of its collision with another cell) upon collision with fibroblasts. In addition, neutrophil locomotion through tissue involves interaction with three-dimensional lattices containing aligned or complex patterns of fibrous tissue rather than solely with two-dimensional planar surfaces. Wilkinson and co-workers (Wilkinson *et al.*, 1982; Wilkinson and Lackie, 1983) studied the influence of contact guidance (responses in which the direction of orientation or locomotion of cells is determined by the shape, alignment, or curvature of the substratum) on locomotion and chemotaxis of human neutrophils, using serum-coated glass chambers with grooves and aligned hydrated collagen or fibrin gels. Neutrophils show contact guidance, which appears to be a response to the three-dimensional nonplanar shape of the substratum. In addition, chemotaxis of neutrophils is more efficient if the cells are moving along the axis of fiber alignment than if they have to cross the aligned fibers, suggesting that tissue architecture may be

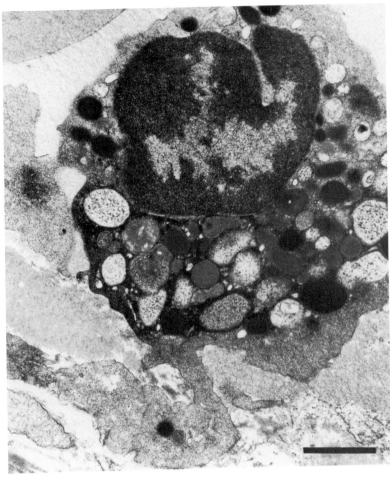

Figure 6. Neutrophil penetrating the internal elastic lamina of a rabbit carotid artery in response to the application of C5 fragments on the adventitial surface of the artery in vivo. Bar = 1 μm.

a significant determinant of the efficiency of cellular mobilization to injured or infected sites. Another important factor is that tissue architecture (and thus its effects) may vary considerably from tissue to tissue, from organ to organ.

Several investigators have studied the characteristics and mechanisms of neutrophil movement through three-dimensional hydrated collagen gels. Grinnell (1982) determined that the basic pattern of migration of neutrophils in collagen is similar to that observed on planar surfaces, i.e., a cycle of cell extension and cytoplasmic flow into the leading extension. However, neutrophils in collagen are less spread and lack thin lamellipodia and tail-end retraction fibers. As seen by scanning electron microscopy (SEM), no destruction or distortion of collagen fibrils is observed as neutrophils migrate through the lattice. Brown (1982) contrasted the poor adherence and failure to locomote of neutrophils on collagen-coated glass with the ready ability of neutrophils to invade three-dimensional matrices of collagen fibers and deduced that invasion is largely independent of adhesion. SEM was also unable to display any apparent changes in the structure of the collagen gels after invasion by neutrophils. This observation, coupled with the inability of the protease inhibitors α_1-antitrypsin or α_2-macroglobulin to inhibit neutrophil movement, led Brown to conclude that invasion of collagen gels by neutrophils is not dependent on proteolytic digestion of the collagen matrix.

The concept that two-dimensional locomotion is adherence dependent while three-dimensional locomotion is largely adherence independent has been confirmed and extended by Schmalstieg et al. (1986) studying patients with LAD who are unable to mobilize neutrophils from the microvasculature to peripheral sites of inflammation. Patient neutrophils exhibit profound impairment of movement stimulated by FMLP over a two-dimensional planar surface under agarose. Less impairment of movement is apparent in three-dimensional chemotaxis through cellulose filters, and no deficiency occurs in collagen gels. In addition, antibodies to the common beta subunit of the glycoprotein family block the two-dimensional but not the three-dimensional migration. Thus, emigration of neutrophils from the vascular space appears to be adherence dependent, while migration through extravascular tissues may be adherence independent.

Clearly, much remains to be learned about the mechanism by which neutrophils move through basement membrane and interstitial connective tissue. How closely do the in vitro model systems discussed mimic the in vivo setting? What interactions are occurring at the level of the cell membrane between migrating neutrophils and matrix molecules? Are enzymes secreted by or expressed on the surface of neutrophils in sufficient amounts and are they necessary for cell migration? If so, what signals and regulatory mechanisms are involved?

5. Phagocytic Killing of Microorganisms by Neutrophils

Once the neutrophil has reached the site of tissue injury, it forms a primary line of defense against infection by the phagocytosis and intracellular killing of microorganisms.

The Phagocytosis-Associated Respiratory Burst

That phagocytic cells can produce toxic metabolites of oxygen was first reported in 1961 by Iyer et al. (1961), who detected hydrogen peroxide (H_2O_2) in the medium after exposure of neutrophils to particles. It had previously been reported that neutrophils exposed to opsonized microorganisms consumed oxygen from the surrounding buffer in a nonmitochondrial (cyanide-insensitive) event (Baldridge and Gerard, 1933; Sbarra and Karnovsky, 1959). Thus, it was proposed that the oxygen consumed in this phagocytosis-dependent respiratory burst was converted to an agent capable of killing ingested microorganisms (Karnovsky, 1968). That this impressive event was in fact pertinent to phagocytic killing of microorganisms was demonstrated convincingly by the experiment of nature chronic granulomatous disease, in which absence of the respiratory burst was associated with markedly deficient killing of most bacteria (Baehner and Nathan, 1967; Quie et al., 1967) and with life-threatening infections by those bacteria (Johnston and Baehner, 1971).

The list of oxygen metabolites generated in the phagocytosis-dependent respiratory burst subsequently expanded to include additional toxic agents. These include hypohalides, superoxide anion, and hydroxyl radical.

Hypohalides, especially hypochlorite anion (OCl^-) (Klebanoff and Hamon, 1972), are generated through activity of myeloperoxidase:

$$Cl^- + H_2O_2 \xrightarrow{\text{myeloperoxidase}} OCl^- + H_2O$$

Superoxide anion (O_2^-) (Babior et al., 1973), now recognized to be the initial conversion product of the consumed oxygen, generated through activity of a plasma membrane-associated enzyme or enzyme complex termed NADPH oxidase, reduces oxygen univalently using NADPH as electron donor (Babior, 1984):

$$O_2 + NADPH \xrightarrow[\text{oxidase}]{\text{NADPH}} O_2^- + NADP^+ + H^+$$

Most of this O_2^- is thought to react with itself in a dismutation reaction to form H_2O_2 and oxygen.

Hydroxyl radical ($\cdot OH$) (Johnston et al., 1973, 1975; Weiss et al., 1977), a highly potent oxidant formed by the interaction between O_2^- and H_2O_2 in the presence of iron or copper (Haber–Weiss reactions), is summarized as:

$$O_2^- + H_2O_2 \xrightarrow{\text{Fe or Cu}} \cdot OH + OH^- + O_2$$

or by the interaction between H_2O_2 and iron—the Fenton reaction (Babior, 1984).

More recently identified toxic agents are chloramines, formed by the reaction of hypochlorite with ammonia or amines (Thomas, 1979). Other microbicidal products of the reduction of oxygen may be formed, but these have not yet been well substantiated.

The evolving knowledge of phagocytosis-associated oxidative metabolism was considered in the perspective of microbicidal activity, the unexamined assumption being that the products of the respiratory burst were released primarily into the phagocytic vacuole with the captured microorganisms.

During the mid-1970s, it became clear that a substantial fraction of the phagocytosis-stimulated oxygen metabolites was released to the outside of neutrophils (Goldstein et al., 1975). An in vitro model of tissue-bound immune complexes had played a central role in forming the concept that tissue damage at sites of inflammation might be attributable to release by neutrophils of toxic granule constituents to the outside of the cell (Henson, 1971). Using this same model, it could be demonstrated that both neutrophils (Johnston and Lehmeyer, 1976) and monocytes (Johnston et al., 1976) can release large amounts of toxic oxygen species to the outside without undergoing cell lysis. Thus, the experimental basis for hypothesizing that granule enzymes and cationic proteins are involved in tissue injury was extended to invoke the possibility that toxic oxygen metabolites might be involved as well (Johnston and Lehmeyer, 1976). More direct demonstration of the participation of oxygen by-products in tissue damage has ensued, as will be seen (see also Fantone and Ward, 1982; Henson and Johnston, 1987).

The strong evidence supporting the importance of the respiratory burst in phagocytic killing does not preclude a role for nonoxidative mechanisms in this process (reviewed by Gabay et al., 1986). However, these nonoxidative microbicidal processes have not been clearly defined, and their role in vivo remains to be proved. The possible involvement of proteases and cationic proteins in tissue injury is discussed in Sections 6.3 and 6.4, respectively.

6. Neutrophil Secretion and the Potential for Tissue Injury

The accumulation of neutrophils at a wound or other inflammatory site has been discussed in light of the mechanisms by which neutrophils adhere and migrate across vascular and connective tissue boundaries. Presumably, they do so in response to the complex array of mediators generated by the coagulation and complement pathways (see Chapters 3 and 5), modulated perhaps by the hemodynamic conditions accompanying an acute inflammatory response (see Section 2.3; see also Chapter 5). The precise role played by neutrophil accumulation in the natural history of the wound remains unclear. Neutrophils, absent infection, appear to contribute little to the process by which wound repair occurs. Studies by Simpson and Ross (1972) demonstrated that the rate of wound closure is similar in neutrophil-depleted guinea pigs compared with normal wounded controls, although there is a higher incidence of infection, and wounds in neutrophil-depleted animals demonstrate less interstitial edema. Similarly, studies by Anderson et al. (1978) on healing of oral wounds in guinea pigs showed no difference in rate of reepithelialization between neutrophil-depleted animals and controls, but there is a higher incidence of deep wound infections. Indeed, neutrophils and their contents may prevent reepithelialization of corneal wounds (Wagoner et al., 1984).

Other workers, however, notably Carrel (1924), in some classic early studies, as well as Alexander et al. (1971), noted an increase in wound connective tissue if neutrophil stimuli or new irritants are added; Carrel (1922) also suggested that fibroblast growth in vitro is enhanced by neutrophils or their lysates. Nonetheless, the weight of evidence clearly suggests that neutrophils play little role in the wound healing process itself. This should not be interpreted to mean, however, that neutrophils cannot modulate the healing process. That the role of neutrophils might be more complex than hitherto suspected may be inferred from the work of Barcikowski and colleagues, who have suggested that ion-exchange chromatography of neutrophil lysates separates fractions that inhibit wound healing from those that may be stimulatory (Barcikowski et al., 1978).

If neutrophils play no role in abetting wound healing, then (teleologically) they must accumulate to prevent infectious complications of breaking skin barriers. Leukocyte adhesion deficiency (see Section 2.2) represents an experiment of nature with regard to the vital importance of neutrophil influx to the resolution of an infected wound. Neutrophils of patients with this genetic disorder are unable to adhere to vascular endothelium (Tonnesen et al., 1986a,b; Harlan et al., 1985) and thus to mobilize in response to tissue injury, and also to produce a respiratory burst to particulate stimuli and possibly to microorganisms (Arnaout et al., 1982; Ross et al., 1985). Such patients suffer from recurrent or progressive soft tissue infections, diminished pus formation, and impaired wound healing. The infections include skin abscesses, cellulitis, otitis media, ulcerative stomatitis/pharyngitis, gingivitis/periodontitis, pneumonitis, peritonitis, and septicemia; typically the pathogens are species of such microorganisms as Staphylococcus, Pseudomonas, Escherichia coli, Klebsiella, and Proteus (Anderson et al., 1985; Anderson and Springer, 1987; Bowen et al., 1982; Crowley et al., 1980). The severity of clinical infectious complications among moderate and severely deficient patients was shown to be directly related to the degree of neutrophil glycoprotein deficiency (Anderson et al., 1985). The susceptibility of these patients to infectious complications in wounds may be due both to the inability of neutrophils to accumulate at the injury site as well as to a putative defect in uptake of particulate stimuli, possibly also dependent on localized neutrophil adhesiveness (Ross et al., 1985).

In these patients, then, the delay in normal healing represents the end result of a complex interaction between minimal neutrophil accumulation, perhaps diminished microbicidal activity (leading to chronic ongoing infections), and diminished monocyte influx. The oxidant mechanisms which form the principal response employed by neutrophils against microorganisms have been discussed above. (See Chapters 7 and 8, which explore the role of monocytes in the wound.)

Accepting as given a wound characterized by neutrophil accumulation, edema, and the panoply of mediators suggested in other chapters, this section explores the consequences of that wound becoming infected. A number of studies have emphasized the increased tissue injury and subsequent scarring that characterizes the infected wound, especially during the preantibiotic era (Edwards and Dunphy, 1958). Although a complete mechanistic understanding of these events eludes us, there are enough suggestions from the literature to construct a reasonable scheme. This scheme requires the introduction of a new actor: the microorganism. The microorganisms that either colonize or invade wounds may be of many types, including both gram-negative and -positive species, each of which may produce a variety of agents that modulate neutrophil function. So as to simplify an extraordinarily extensive list, bacterial endotoxins are used as a model system.

The lipopolysaccharides (LPS), a unique class of compounds extractable from the walls of gram-negative bacteria, constitute along with protein and lipid components bacterial endotoxin (Morrison and Ulevitch, 1978). It has been known for 100 years that endotoxins have potent effects on man and animals (Westphal et al., 1977); many of these properties can be attributed to the lipid A-containing lipopolysaccharide portion of the molecule (Galanos et al., 1977). This chapter largely discusses work employing purified LPS preparations, recognizing that one must be careful about generalizing from the actions of such purified LPS preparations to the behavior of endotoxins.

Mammals live in symbiosis with gram-negative bacteria and have evolved a wide array of defenses against, and reaction to, these organisms. Many of these responses are initiated by recognition of the LPS portion of the bacterial cell wall. It has been suggested by a number of workers that the host response to LPS may be a deleterious one, but only recently have the mechanisms of LPS interactions with cells and humoral mediation systems begun to become known.

We suggest that the defenses evoked by LPS are of several types, characterized by an enhanced response by the neutrophil to other inflammatory mediators, with the resulting pathogenetic sequence: LPS enhances neutrophil adherence to endothelium and also primes the neutrophil to respond more vigorously to the effects of other inflammatory mediators. Exposure of the primed neutrophil to chemotactic factors and secretagogues may then result in enhanced release of oxygen radicals, neutral proteases, and lipid mediators. The action of these released products may be to contribute to further tissue injury.

6.1. Effects of LPS on Neutrophils

One of the most widely studied effects of LPS is the acute neutropenia that quickly follows an intravenous injection. Stetson (1951) described the time course and site of localization (lung as well as other capillary beds) of neutrophil disappearance in rabbits given endotoxin. The mechanism by which this disappearance occurs is not clear even now, although it has been documented in all species including human beings, in whom studies have confirmed the localization of neutrophils to the marginating pool (Athens et al., 1961). Since C5a has been shown to promote neutropenia in vivo (McCall et al., 1974) and increased neutrophil adherence in vitro (Webster et al., 1980), many workers have argued that neutropenia is due to complement activation. However, several lines of evidence suggest that LPS-induced neutropenia may occur by complement-independent mechanisms. A number of groups have shown that neutropenia in rabbits (Fong and Good, 1971), guinea pigs (Kane et al., 1973), or rhesus monkeys (Ulevitch et al., 1978) is unchanged by complement depletion with cobra venom factor (CVF), suggesting that an intact complement system is not required. LPS-induced neutropenia studied in C4-deficient guinea pigs (Kane et al., 1973) and C6-deficient rabbits (Muller-Berghaus and Lohmann, 1974) appears identical to that seen in congenic complement-sufficient counterparts. Finally, recent observations indicate that neutrophils can be stimulated by endotoxin in the presence of heat-inactivated plasma to increase adherence to plastic surfaces (Dahinden et al., 1983) and in the absence of plasma to increase adherence to cultured endothelial monolayers (Tonnesen et al., 1987).

Adherence is not the only neutrophil activity that may be stimulated by endotoxin. LPS enhances bacterial killing and phagocytosis (Cohn and Morse, 1960), and neutrophils treated with LPS release lysosomal enzymes (Bannatyne et al., 1977). LPS increases hexose monophosphate shunt activity and NBT reduction (Goihman-Yahr et al., 1975) by neutrophils. Dahinden and colleagues (1983) demonstrated the ability of LPS to induce neutrophil lysosomal enzyme release and superoxide production in vitro. Of considerable importance is the recent observation by Guthrie et al. (1984) in which LPS was shown to prime neutrophils such that they respond with greatly enhanced secretion of superoxide anion upon subsequent stimulation by FMLP. Haslett et al. (1985) demonstrated that trace concentrations of LPS present during isolation may dramatically alter neutrophil shape change, lysosomal enzyme release, and chemotaxis.

The nature of the interaction between LPS and neutrophils remains obscure. It appears that LPS is bound to neutrophils by glycerophosphatides (Adye and Springer, 1977) and is probably a passive event (Gimber and Rafter, 1969), although specific binding to monocytes has been described (Haeffner-Cavaillon et al., 1985). The neutrophil, perhaps by virtue of lipases (Graham et al., 1967), is capable of inactivating LPS. However, other studies suggest that the amount of LPS actually bound to neutrophils in vivo is exceedingly small (Herring et al., 1963).

These results, taken together, suggest that LPS can increase adherence of neutrophils and prime them for enhanced release of oxygen radicals and lysosomal enzymes.

6.2. Oxygen Radicals and Tissue Injury

Neutrophils, monocytes, and macrophages respond to both soluble and phagocytic stimuli by the production of a family of reactive oxygen species (see Section 5.1). These metabolites have a variety of injurious effects (Fantone and Ward, 1982). The precise relative roles of these different reactive species in leukocyte-mediated tissue injury are unclear, but considerable data exist to implicate oxygen radical species.

Oxygen radicals released from leukocytes have been shown in studies in vitro to be toxic to endothelial cells (Sacks et al., 1978), fibroblasts (Simon et al., 1981), and epithelial cells (Martin et al., 1981). Clear-cut evidence for the involvement of these oxygen metabolites in tissue injury in an infected wound is elusive, but the involvement of oxygen species in vascular injury in other systems is suggestive that similar mechanisms may occur in wounds. Studies by McCormick *et al.* (1981) show that in animal models of acute vasculitis in the skin and lung secondary to the deposition of immune complexes, injury may be attenuated by the local installation of SOD, which converts superoxide to hydrogen peroxide. SOD appears to exert its effect in this system largely by diminishing the magnitude of neutrophil accumulation. Although not well understood, the mechanism may involve the ability of superoxide to react with plasma arachidonic acid so as to generate a potent neutrophil chemotactic activity (Petrone *et al.*, 1980). Thus, the generation of superoxide may be another example of a positive feedback loop in the inflammatory process whereby neutrophil production of superoxide results in the generation of new chemotactic factors thereby attracting more neutrophils. Such a mechanism might explain how one inflammatory mediator (in this case, immune complexes) may result in the final product measured as tissue injury. As an important contrast, injury to the lung secondary to the local installation of immune complexes can also be abrogated by the presence of catalase, which converts H_2O_2 into water and oxygen (Johnson and Ward, 1981). Importantly, the use of this agent does not diminish the intensity of the neutrophil influx but does diminish the intensity of the subsequent lung injury. These data suggest a role of H_2O_2 in mediating tissue injury, although whether the effect of H_2O_2 is due to its own properties or to its conversion to other toxic species (including hydroxyl radical) remains unclear.

Toxic metabolites may also be formed from the oxidation of fatty acids. Formation of hydroperoxy fatty acids may lead on the one hand to the formation of biologically active leukotrienes, which exert potent pro-inflammatory actions, and on the other hand to both monohydroperoxy and dihydroperoxy fatty acids, which facilitate production of hydroxyl radicals (Mead, 1976). This pathway may be important in light of the recent evidence that lipid peroxidation within cell membranes may directly promote cell and tissue injury by altering membrane fluidity and increasing the permeability to ions, thereby changing ionic potentials, ultimately leading to cellular swelling (Maridonneau *et al.*, 1983). Calcium influx has been observed in cells injured by free radicals; this accumulation may then lead to activation of phospholipases and protein kinase C (Farber, 1982). It is to be expected that many other toxic species generated by the action of oxygen radicals on cellular constituents will be identified in years to come.

Oxygen radicals may promote tissue injury by mechanisms that do not involve direct toxic injury to cells. Certain oxygen species may oxidize and inactivate circulating antiproteinases, permitting proteolytic enzymes to act in an unrestrained fashion (Carp and Janoff, 1979). The ability of superoxide anion to generate chemotactic factors is another such example. Hydrogen peroxide has been shown to alter basement membrane and connective tissue such that it renders the connective tissue more easily degraded by proteolytic enzymes.

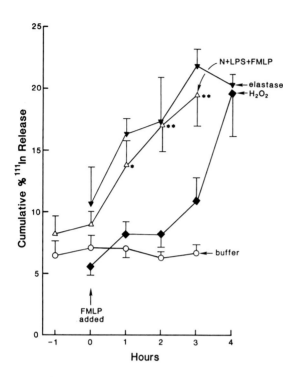

Figure 7. Endothelial injury induced by stimulated neutrophils and isolated components of neutrophils. Human microvascular endothelial cells were labeled with [^{111}In]tropolonate. Spontaneous release of label (○) (buffer) is negligible after the first hour. In the presence of neutrophils incubated with LPS, the addition of the chemotaxin formyl-methionyl-leucyl-phenylalanine (FMLP) results in a rapid release of label (△). This type of injury is mimicked by 5 U/ml human neutrophil elastase (▼) but very different from injury induced by 10^{-4} M H_2O_2 (◆) wherein the release of label is only apparent after a several-hour lag period.

The aforementioned examples illustrate the potential role that oxidants may play in producing tissue injury. In a wound in which bacteria are present, the effect of even small amounts of LPS may be to prime the neutrophil such that when exposed to neutrophil stimuli such as C5a, or even other bacteria-derived peptides such as FMLP, the cell responds with an enhanced release of O_2^- and H_2O_2 (Guthrie et al., 1984). The studies by Guthrie and co-workers indicate that only nanogram amounts of LPS are required for this effect; thus, it may be expected to occur in a wound contaminated by even small numbers of gram-negative bacteria.

In summary, inflammatory cell derived oxygen metabolites have a wide spectrum of activities, including direct injury to cells, potentiation of the action of neutrophil-derived proteases, and generation of new chemotactic activity. It is to be expected that in wounds contaminated by bacteria, the release of such metabolites will be markedly enhanced. The precise role of oxidant injury in inducing damage in the sterile or infected wound remains unclear, and should be an area of fruitful future study.

6.3. Neutral Proteases and Tissue Injury

Neutrophil granules were first isolated by Cohn and Hirsch (1960) and were described as consisting of two types: the azurophil or primary granule and the specific or secondary granule. Recently, the existence of a tertiary granule has been proposed (Dewald et al., 1982). Some of the potentially injurious constituents of neutrophils are shown in Table I. Different species may exhibit markedly different amounts of the components listed. This discussion, however, emphasizes the actions of elastase, cathepsin G, and collagenases as well as enzymatically inactive cationic proteins which have also been isolated from neutrophil granules.

The isolation of elastolytic activity from human neutrophils was first reported by Janoff and Zeligs (1968). Neutrophil elastase is a serine proteinase found in azurophil granules; it has a molecular weight of approximately 35,000 and is capable of degrading a wide range of substrates, including elastin and type IV collagen (Mainardi et al., 1980), as well as fibronectin, fibrinogen, proteoglycans, and immunoglobulins. Of considerable importance is the ability of elastase to degrade the C3 and C5 components of the complement system, generating active phlogistic fragments. Human neutrophils have a high concentration of this substance, particularly when compared with rabbit, the only other species that has been well studied (Janoff, 1985).

To date, elastase has been suggested as an important contributor to several pathologic states. The morphologic and structural alterations in the lung which typify emphysema can be duplicated in animals by the installation of neutrophil-derived elastase, and the lack of endogenous inhibitor (α_1-antiproteinase deficiency) is strongly linked to early development of severe disease (Snider, 1981). Elastolytic activity has been recovered from the bronchoalveolar lavage of patients suffering from adult respiratory distress syndrome (ARDS) in whom acute inflammatory injury to the lung is apparent (Lee et al, 1981). Furthermore, immunoreactive elastase has been found in rheumatoid synovial fluid and synovium (Ekerot and Ohlsson, 1982).

Cathepsin G, like elastase, is extremely cationic with an isoelectric point of pH 11, and a molecular weight of 27,000. It has nearly as broad a spectrum of activities as does neutrophil elastase in that it can degrade fibrinogen, proteoglycans, hemoglobin, complement, immunoglobulin, and other proteins such as casein (Rindler-Ludwig and Braunsteiner, 1975). It has also been suggested that cathepsin G may serve some intracellular functions including the activation of latent enzymes such as collagenase or gelatinase. There is also evidence, however, that the combined action of neutrophil elastase and cathepsin G exerts a more powerful effect on matrix degradation than does either agent alone (Boudier et al,. 1981).

Neutrophils possess an impressive array of collagenases. In addition to elastase, which possesses activity against type IV collagen, neutrophils also contain a collagenase (located in specific granules) and a gelatinase (which may be located within specific or so-called tertiary granules). Each of these collagenases has unique specificity. Collagenase, a metalloenzyme, is capable of degrading collagen types I, II, and III (Hasty et al., 1986), while gelatinase (also a metalloenzyme) is specific for type IV and denatured collagen (Hibbs et al., 1985). Their specificities are thus much more restricted than are those of neutrophil elastase or cathepsin G. These different collagenolytic activities may be released differentially from neutrophils. It has been reported that stimuli capable of causing specific and tertiary granule release may not necessarily produce azurophil granule release, particularly during chemotactic migration (Gallin, 1984). Thus, it is possible that collagenases may serve important functions during neutrophil migration *in vivo* (see Section 4.4).

The role of neutrophil-derived proteinases in inflammation remains unclear. In addition to the data previously presented regarding elastase in lung injury, proteolytic activity has been found in inflamed tissues from patients with ulcerative colitis, serum sickness and rheumatoid arthritis (Bonney and Smith, 1986). In rabbits with nephrotoxic nephritis, the kidney shows evidence of neutrophil degranulation, of alkaline phosphatase activity at inflammatory sites, and of basement membrane fragments and cathepsins in the urine (Henson, 1972; Hawkins and Cochrane, 1968). In addition, extracts of neutrophil granules are capable of producing an inflammatory response (particularly in the joint); treatment of these extracts with proteinase inhibitors abolishes the inflammatory activity. Thomas (1979) injected neutrophil granules into endotoxin-treated rabbits and reproduced a lesion resembling the generalized Shwartzman reaction.

Recent work from several laboratories, including our own, suggests that neutrophil proteinases may play a direct role in cellular injury *in vitro*. For example, Harlan and colleagues (1981) implicated neutrophil proteinases in endothelial cell detachment by stimulated neutrophils. Potential interactions between LPS and stimulated neutrophils are exemplified by a recent study by Smedly *et al.* (1986), in which we demonstrated that neutrophils incubated with endotoxin are more able to injure endothelial cells in culture, and appear to do so by release of neutrophil elastase (figure 7). Despite these findings, it is difficult as yet to unequivocally relate any acute inflammatory state to the action of a particular leukocyte proteinase.

6.4. Nonenzymatic Cationic Proteins and Tissue Injury

Another class of neutrophil-derived product that may contribute to tissue injury are the cationic proteins derived from neutrophil lysosomal granules. Janoff and Zweifach (1964) reported that a cationic protein preparation extracted from the lysosomes of rabbit neutrophils increased vascular permeability. The active agent was purified and found to cause release of mast cell granules. The definitive studies of Ranadive and Cochrane (1970) demonstrated that rabbit neutrophil granules contained at least four distinct cationic proteins that were able to increase vascular permeability, three of which acted by a mechanism independent of mast cells. One of them may be similar to the factor isolated by Janoff and Zweifach. The others are all arginine-enriched highly cationic molecules.

The mechanism by which these proteins increase permeability and thus enhance tissue injury is not clear. A recent study has described localized discrete regions of negative charge on the surface of endothelial cells (Simionescu and Simionescu, 1983). Interaction with highly cationic molecules might alter the charge distribution on the structure of the endothelial cells. If this charge distribution poses a significant barrier to the migration of macromolecules, the result might be marked enhancement in macromolecule leakage without any change in pore size. Indeed, a recent study suggested that polycations such as protamine or polylysine infused into the cerebral circulation markedly alter both charge of the luminal vascular surface and vascular permeability (Nagy *et al.*, 1983). In addition, the cationic proteins described above may be directly toxic to certain cells, particularly the endothelium (Peterson *et al.*, 1985). The neutrophil-derived cationic proteins may thus contribute to tissue injury by several different mechanisms.

Thus, neutrophils contain the machinery to generate a variety of injurious substances that may be released into the wound. Neutrophil release of oxidants, proteases, and cationic proteins may be modulated by a variety of factors, including the panoply of stimuli present at a wound site as well as material from infecting bacteria. However, despite major advances in our understanding of the nature of the toxic substances released from neutrophils, many fundamental questions remain. Does the neutrophil response to a complex mediator environment differ from its response to single (or at most two) agents as tested in the laboratory? What factors govern the secretion of agents from different compartments within the neutrophil? What is the relative contribution of the different oxidant species, the several types of proteases, and other nonenzymatic proteins to neutrophil-induced injury? How do these different agents, each one capable of producing some type of tissue injury, interact with each other so as to produce the final injury?

7. Conclusion

Considerable progress has been made in our understanding of the mechanisms by which neutrophils migrate from the blood stream to sites of tissue injury and, once there, how they engulf and kill microorganisms and potentially contribute to tissue injury. Neutrophil adherence to vascular endothelium enhanced by chemotactic peptides and lipid mediators depends upon the expression of adhesive glycoproteins on the neutrophil surface. Cytokines as well as bacterial lipopolysaccharides may activate the endothelial cell, rendering it more adhesive for neutrophils. Hemodynamic and physical effects such as shear stress, static contact, and viscoelasticity serve to modulate the neutrophil–endothelial adhesive interaction. Neutrophils migrate between endothelial cells by a process that is independent of vascular permeability but that may involve active participation by the endothelium. Neutrophil degradation of vascular basement membrane and directed migration through interstitial connective tissue in response to a chemotactic gradient may be facilitated by proteolytic digestion, enhanced by contact guidance, and independent of adherence. Phagocytic killing of microorganisms by neutrophils is mediated in part by oxygen metabolites generated in the phagocytosis-associated respiratory burst. Toxic products including oxygen radicals, neutral proteases, and nonenzymatic cationic proteins released during the phagocytic event may contribute to tissue injury. This injurious potential may be enhanced through the neutrophil priming effect of bacterial lipopolysaccharides.

The neutrophil is considered the primary line of defense against microorganisms during the acute inflammatory phase of wound healing. In the absence of active wound infection, the role of the neutrophil in the process of wound repair is believed to be minimal but awaits further investigation. In addition, the possibility that neutrophil participation and interaction in the setting of an infected wound may alter the subsequent pattern of healing and influence the final outcome needs to be explored.

References

Adye, J. C., and Springer, G. F., 1977, Binding of endotoxin (LPS) by glycerophosphatides from human platelets and leukocytes, *Naturwissenschaften* **64**:150–151.

Alexander, J. W., Bossert, J. E., McClellan, M. A., and Altemier, W. A., 1971, Stimulants of cellular proliferation in wounds, *Arch. Surg.* **103**:167–174.

Allison, F., Jr., Smith, M. R., and Wood, W. B., 1955, Studies on the pathogenesis of acute inflammation. I. The inflammatory reaction to thermal injury as observed in the rabbit ear chamber, *J. Exp. Med.* **102**:655–668.

Andersen, L., Attstrom, R., and Fejerskov, O., 1978, Effect of experimental neutropenia on oral wound healing in guinea pigs, *Scand. J. Dent. Res.* **86**:237–247.

Anderson, D. C., and Springer, T. A., 1987, Leukocyte adhesion deficiency: An inherited defect in the Mac-1, LFA-1, and p150,95 glycoproteins, *Annu. Rev. Med.* **38**:175–194.

Anderson, D. C., Schmalstieg, F. C., Arnaout, M. A., Kohl, S., Tosi, M. F., Dana, N., Buffone, G. J., Hughes, B. J., Brinkley, B. R., Dickey, W. D., Abramson, J. S., Springer, T. A., Boxer, L. A., Hollers, J. M., and Smith, C. W., 1984, Abnormalities of polymorphonuclear leukocyte function associated with a heritable deficiency of high molecular weight surface glycoproteins (GP138): Common relationship to diminished cell adherence, *J. Clin. Invest.* **74**:536–551.

Anderson, D. C., Schmalstieg, F. C., Finegold, M. J., Hughes, B. J., Rothlein, R., Miller, L. J., Kohl, S., Tosi, M. F., Jacobs, R. L., Waldrop, T. C., Goldman, A. S., Shearer, W. T., and Springer, T. A., 1985, The severe and moderate phenotypes of heritable Mac-1, LFA-1 deficiency: Their quantitative definition and relation to leukocyte dysfunction and clinical features, *J. Infect. Dis.* **152**:668–689.

Armstrong, P. B., and Lackie, J. M., 1975, Studies on intercellular invasion in vitro using rabbit peritoneal neutrophil granulocytes (PMNs). 1. Role of contact inhibition on locomotion, *J. Cell Biol.* **65**:439–462.

Arnaout, M. A., Pitt, J., Cohen, H. J., Melamed, J., Rosen, F. S., and Colten, H. R., 1982, Deficiency of a granulocyte membrane glycoprotein (gp 150) in a boy with recurrent bacterial infections, *N. Engl. J. Med.* **306**:693–699.

Arnaout, M. A., Spits, H., Terhorst, C., Pitt, J., and Todd, R. F., 1984, Deficiency of a leukocyte surface glycoprotein (LFA-1) in two patients with Mo1 deficiency: Effects of cell activation on Mo1/LFA-1 surface experssion in normal and deficient leukocytes, *J. Clin. Invest.* **74**:1291–1300.

Athens, J. W., Haab, O. P., Raab, S. O., Mauer, A. M., Ashenbrucker, H., Cartwright, G. E., and Wintrobe, M. M., 1961, Leukokinetic studies IV. The total blood, circulating and marginal granulocyte pools and the granulocyte turnover rate in normal subjects, *J. Clin. Invest.* **40**:989–995.

✳ Atherton, A., and Born, G. V. R., 1973, Relationship between the velocity of rolling granulocytes and that of the blood flow in venules, *J. Physiol. (Lond.)* **233:**157–165.

Babior, B. M., 1984, The respiratory burst of phagocytes, *J. Clin. Invest.* **73:**599–601.

Babior, B. M., Kipnes, R. S., and Curnutte, J. T., 1973, Biological defense mechanisms: The production by leukocytes of superoxide, a potential bactericidal agent, *J. Clin. Invest.* **52:**741–744.

Baehner, R. L., and Nathan, D. G., 1967, Leukocyte oxidase: Defective activity in chronic granulomatous disease, *Science* **155:**835–836.

Baldrige, C. W., and Gerard, R. W., 1933, The extra respiration of phagocytosis, *Am. J. Physiol.* **103:**235–236.

Bannatyne, R. M., Harnett, N. M., Lee, K. Y., and Biggar, W. D., 1977, Inhibition of the biologic effects of endotoxin on neutrophils by polymyxin B sulfate, *J. Infect. Dis.* **136:**469–474.

Barcikowski, S., Tchorzewski, H., Warno, O., and Dancewicz, R., 1978, Untersuchungen uber die rolle der leukozyten im heilprozess chirurgischer verletzungen, *Z. Exp. Chir.* **11:**371–376.

Beesley, J. E., Pearson, J. D., Carleton, J. S., Hutchings, A., and Gordon, J. L., 1978, Interaction of leukocytes with vascular cells in culture, *J. Cell Sci.* **33:**85–101.

Beesley, J. E., Pearson, J. D., Hutchings, A., Carleton, J. S., and Gordon, J. L., 1979, Granulocyte migration through endothelium in culture, *J. Cell Sci.* **38:**237–248.

Bernstein, I. D., and Self, S., 1986, The joint report of the myeloid section of the Second International Workshop on Human Leukocyte Differentiation Antigens, in: *Leukocyte Typing II: Report of the Second International Workshop on Human Leukocyte Differentiation Antigens,* Vol. 3, *Human Myeloid and Hematopoietic Cells* (E. L. Reinherz, B. S. Haynes, L. M. Nadler, and I. D. Bernstein, eds.), pp. 1–25, Springer-Verlag, New York.

Bevilacqua, M. P., Pober, J. S., Wheeler, M. E., Cotran, R. S., and Gimbrone, M. A., Jr., 1985, Interleukin-1 acts on cultured human vascular endothelium to increase the adhesion of polymorphonuclear leukocytes, monocytes and related leukocyte cell lines, *J. Clin. Invest.* **76:**2003–2011.

Bjork, J., Lindbom, L., Gerdin, B., Smedegard, G., Arfors, K. E., and Benveniste, J., 1983, Paf-acether (platelet-activating factor) increases microvascular permeability and affects endothelium-granulocyte interaction in microvascular beds, *Acta Physiol. Scand.* **119:**305–308.

✳ Bonney, R. J., and Smith, R. J., 1986, Evidence for the role of neutral proteases in chronic inflammatory diseases in humans, *Adv. Inflamm. Res.* **11:**127–133.

Boudier, C., Holle, C., and Bieth, J. G., 1981, Stimulation of the elastolytic activity of leukocyte elastase by leukocyte cathepsin G, *J. Biol. Chem.* **256:**10256–10258.

Bowen, T. J., Ochs, H. D., Altman, L. C., Price, T. H., VanEpps, D. E., Brautigan, D. L., Rosin, R. E., Perkins, W. D., Babior, B. M., Klebanoff, S. J., and Wedgwood, R. J., 1982, Severe recurrent bacterial infections associated with defective adherence and chemotaxis in two patients with neutrophils deficient in a cell-associated glycoprotein, *J. Pediatr.* **101:**932–940.

Brown, A. F., 1982, Neutrophil granulocytes: Adhesion and locomotion on collagen substrata and in collagen matrices, *J. Cell Sci.* **58:**445–467.

Carp, H., and Janoff, A., 1979, In vitro suppression of serum elastase-inhibitory capacity by reactive oxygen species generated by phagocytosing polymorphonuclear leukocytes, *J. Clin. Invest.* **63:**793–797.

Carrel, A., 1922, Growth-promoting function of leukocytes, *J. Exp. Med.* **36:**385–391.

Carrel, A., 1924, Leukocytic trephones, *JAMA* **82:**255–258.

Clark, E. R., and Clark, E. L., 1935, Observations on changes in blood vascular endothelium in the living animal, *Am. J. Anat.* **57:**385–438.

Cochrane, C. G., and Aikin, B. S., 1966, Polymorphonuclear leukocytes in immunologic reactions. The destruction of vascular basement membrane in vivo and in vitro, *J. Exp. Med.* **124:**733–752.

Cohn, Z. A., and Hirsch, J. G., 1960, The isolation and properties of the specific cytoplasmic granules of rabbit polymorphonuclear leucocytes, *J. Exp. Med.* **112:**983–1004.

Cohn, Z. A., and Morse, S. I., 1960, Functional and metabolic properties of polymorphonuclear leukocytes. II. The influence of a lipopolysaccharide endotoxin, *J. Exp. Med.* **111:**689–704.

Colditz, I. G., and Movat, H. Z., 1984, Kinetics of neutrophil accumulation in acute inflammatory lesions induced by chemotaxins and chemotaxinigens, *J. Immunol.* **133:**2169–2173.

Cramer, E. B., Migliorisi, G., Pologe, L., Abrahams, E., Pawlowski, N. A., Cohn, Z., and Scott, W. A., 1984, Effect of leukotrienes on endothelium and the transendothelial migration of neutrophils, *J. Allergy Clin. Immunol.* **74:**386–390.

Crowley, C. A., Curnutt, J. T., Rosin, R. E., Andre-Schwartz, J., Gallin, J. I., Klempner, M., Snyderman, R., Southwick, F. S., Stossel, T. P., and Babior, B. M., 1980, An inherited abnormality of neutrophil adhesion: Its genetic transmission and its association with a missing protein, *N. Engl. J. Med.* **302:**1163–1168.

Dahinden, C., Galanos, C., and Fehr, J., 1983, Granulocyte activation by endotoxin. I. Correlation between adherence and other granulocyte functions, and role of endotoxin structure on biologic activity, *J. Immunol.* **130:**857–862.

Damiano, V. V., Cohen, A., Tsang, A. L., Batra, G., and Petersen, R., 1980, A morphologic study of the influx of neutrophils into dog lung alveoli after lavage with sterile saline, *Am. J. Pathol.* **100:**349–364.

Dewald, B., Bretz, U., and Baggiolini, M., 1982, Release of gelatinase from a novel secretory compartment of human neutrophils, *J. Clin. Invest.* **70:**518–525.

Doroszewski, J., Skierski, J., and Przadka, L., 1977, Interaction of neoplastic cells with glass surface under flow conditions, *Exp. Cell Res.* **104:**335–343.

Dutrochet, M. H., 1824, *Recherches anatomiques et physiologiques sur la structure intime des animaux et des végétaux, et sur leur motilité*, Bailliere et Fils, Paris.

Edwards, L. C., and Dunphy, J. E., 1958, Wound healing. I. Injury and normal repair, *N. Engl. J. Med.* **259:**224–233.

Ekerot, L., and Ohlsson, K., 1982, Immunoreactive granulocyte elastase in rheumatoid synovial fluid and membrane, *Scand J. Plast. Reconstr. Surg.* **16:**117–122.

Fantone, J. C., and Ward, P. A., 1982, Role of oxygen-derived free radicals and metabolites in leukocyte-dependent inflammatory reactions, *Am. J. Pathol.* **107:**397–418.

Farber, J. L., 1982, Biology of disease: membrane injury and calcium homeostasis in the pathogenesis of coagulative necrosis, *Lab. Invest.* **47:**114–123.

Fischer, A., Descamps-Latscha, B., Gerota, I., Scheinmetzler, C., Virelizier, J. L., Trung, P. H., Lisowska-Grospierre, B., Perez, N., Durandy, A., and Griscelli, C., 1983, Bone-marrow transplantation for inborn error of phagocytic cells associated with defective adherence, chemotaxis and oxidative response during opsonised particle phagocytosis, *Lancet* **2:**473–476.

Florey, H. W., and Grant, L. H., 1961, Leukocyte migration from small blood vessels stimulated with ultraviolet light: An electron-microscope study, *J. Pathol.* **82:**13–17.

Fong, J. S. C., and Good, R. A., 1971, Prevention of the localized and generalized Shwartzman reactions by an anticomplementary agent, cobra venom factor, *J. Exp. Med.* **135:**642–655.

Forrester, J. V., and Lackie, J. M., 1984, Adhesion of neutrophil leucocytes under conditions of flow, *J. Cell Sci.* **70:**93–110.

Gabay, J. E., Heiple, J. M., Cohn, Z. A., and Nathan, C. F., 1986, Subcellular location and properties of bactericidal factors from human neutrophils, *J. Exp. Med.* **164:**1407–1421.

Gaehtgens, P., Pries, A. R., and Nobis, U., 1984, Flow behavior of white cells in capillaries, in: *White Cell Mechanics: Basic Science and Clinical Aspects*, (J. Meiselman, M. A. Lichtman, P. L. LaCelle, eds.), pp. 147–158, Alan R. Liss, New York.

Galanos, C., Luderitz, O., Rietschel, E., and Westphal, O., 1977, New aspects of the chemistry and biology of bacterial lipopolysaccharides with special reference to their Lipid A component, in: *Biochemistry of Lipids. II*, Vol. 14 (*International Review of Biochemistry*), (T. W. Goodwin, ed.), pp. 239–335, University Park Press, Baltimore.

Gallin, J. I., 1984, Neutrophil specific granules: A fuse that ignites the inflammatory response, *Clin. Res.* **32:**320–328.

Gamble, J. R., Harlan, J. M., Klebanoff, S. J., and Vadas, M. A., 1985, Stimulation of the adherence of neutrophils to umbilical vein endothelium by human recombinant tumor necrosis factor, *Proc. Natl. Acad. Sci. USA* **82:**8667–8671.

Gimber, P. E., and Rafter, G. W., 1969, The interaction of *Escherichia coli* endotoxin with leukocytes, *Arch. Biochem.* **135:**14–20.

Gimbrone, M. A., Jr., 1976, Culture of vascular endothelium, *Prog. Hemost. Thromb.* **3:**1–28.

Goihman-Yahr, M., Rodriguez-Ochoa, G., Aranzazu, N., and Convit, J., 1975, Polymorphonuclear activation in leprosy. I. Spontaneous and endotoxin-stimulated reduction of nitroblue tetrazolium: Effects of serum and plasma on endotoxin-induced activation, *Clin. Exp. Immunol.* **20**:257–264.

Goldstein, I. M., Roos, D., Kaplan, H. B., and Weissmann, G., 1975, Complement and immunoglobulins stimulate superoxide production by human leukocytes independently of phagocytosis, *J. Clin. Invest.* **56**:1155–1163.

Graham, R. C., Jr., Karnovosky, M. J., Shafer, A. W., Glass, E. A., and Karnovsky, M. L., 1967, Metabolic and morphological observations on the effect of surface-active agents on leukocytes, *J. Cell. Biol.* **32**:629–647.

Grant, L., 1973, The sticking and emigration of white blood cells in inflammation, in: *The Inflammatory Process*, Vol. II (B. W. Zweifach, L. Grant, and R. T. McCluskey, eds.), pp. 205–249, Academic Press; New York.

Grinnell, F., 1982, Migration of human neutrophils in hydrated collagen lattices. *J. Cell Sci.* **58**:95–108.

Guthrie, L. A., McPhail, L. C., Henson, P. M., and Johnston, R. B., Jr., 1984, Priming of neutrophils for enhanced release of oxygen metabolites by bacterial lipopolysaccharide: Evidence for increased activity of the superoxide-producing enzyme, *J. Exp. Med.* **160**:1656–1671.

Haeffner-Cavaillon, N., Cavaillon, J.-M., Etievant, M., Lebbar, S., and Szabo, L., 1985, Specific binding of endotoxin to human monocytes and mouse macrophages: Serum requirement, *Cell Immunol.* **91**:119–131.

Harlan, J. M., Killen, P. D., Harker, L. A., Striker, G. E., and Wright, D. C., 1981, Neutrophil-mediated endothelial injury *in vitro*. Mechanisms of cell detachment, *J. Clin. Invest.* **68**:1394–1403.

Harlan, J. M., Killen, P. D., Senecal, F. M., Schwartz, B. R., Yee, E. K., Taylor, R. F., Beatty, P. G., Price, T. H., and Ochs, H. D., 1985, The role of neutrophil membrane glycoprotein GP-150 in neutrophil adherence to endothelium *in vitro*, *Blood* **66**:167–178.

Haslett, C., Guthrie, L. A., Kopaniak, M. M., Johnston, R. B., Jr., and Henson, P. M., 1985, Modulation of multiple neutrophil functions by preparative methods or trace concentrations of bacterial lipopolysaccharides, *Am. J. Pathol.* **119**:101–110.

Hasty, K. A., Hibbs, M. S., Kang, A. H., and Mainardi, C. L., 1986, Secreted forms of human neutrophil collagenase, *J. Biol. Chem.* **261**:5645–5650.

Hawkins, D., and Cochrane, C. G., 1968, Glomerular basement membrane damage in immunological glomerulonephritis, *Immunology* **14**:665–681.

Henson, P. M., 1971, The immunologic release of constituents from neutrophil leukocytes. II. Mechanisms of release during phagocytosis, and adherence to nonphagocytosable surfaces, *J. Immunol.* **107**:1547–1557.

Henson, P. M., 1972, Pathologic mechanisms in neutrophil-mediated injury, *Am. J. Pathol.* **68**:593–612.

Henson, P. M., and Johnston, R. B., Jr., 1987, Tissue injury in inflammation: Oxidants, proteinases and cationic proteins, *J. Clin. Invest.* **79**:669–674.

Herring, W. B., Herion, J. C., Walter, R. I., and Palmer, J. G., 1963, Distribution and clearance of circulating endotoxin, *J. Clin. Invest.* **42**:79–87.

Hibbs, M. S., Hasty, K. A., Seyer, J. M., Kang, A. H., and Mainardi, C. L., 1985, Biochemical and immunological characterization of the secreted forms of human neutrophil gelatinase, *J. Biol. Chem.* **260**:2493–2500.

Hoover, R. L., Briggs, R. T., and Karnovsky, M. J., 1978, The adhesive interaction between polymorphonuclear leukocytes and endothelial cells *in vitro*, *Cell* **14**:423–428.

Hopkins, N. K., Schaub, R. G., and Gorman, R. R., 1984, Acetyl glyceryl ether phosphorylcholine (PAF-Acether) and leukotriene B_4-mediated neutrophil chemotaxis through an intact endothelial cell monolayer, *Biochim. Biophys. Acta* **805**:30–36.

Iyer, G. Y. N., Islam, D. M. F., and Quastel, J. H., 1961, Biochemical aspects of phagocytosis, *Nature (Lond.)* **192**:535–541.

Janoff, A., 1985, Elastase in tissue injury, *Annu. Rev. Med.* **36**:207–216.

Janoff, A., and Zeligs, J. D., 1968, Vascular injury and lysis of basement membrane in vitro by neutral protease of human leukocytes, *Science* **161**:702–704.

Janoff, A., and Zweifach, B. W., 1964, Production of inflammatory changes in the microcirculation by cationic proteins extracted from lysosomes, *J. Exp. Med.* **120**:747–764.

Johnson, K. J., and Ward, P. A., 1981, Role of oxygen metabolites in immune complex injury of lung, *J. Immunol.* **126**:2365–2369.

Johnston, R. B., Jr., and Baehner, R. L., 1971, Chronic granulomatous disease: Correlation between pathogenesis and clinical findings, *Pediatrics* **48**:730–739.

Johnston, R. B., Jr., and Lehmeyer, J. E., 1976, Elaboration of toxic oxygen by-products by neutrophils in a model of immune complex disease, *J. Clin. Invest.* **57**:836–841.

Johnston, R. B., Jr., Keele, B., Webb, L., Kessler, D., and Rajagopalan, K. V., 1973, Inhibition of phagocytic bactericidal activity by superoxide dismutase: A possible role for superoxide anion in the killing of phagocytized bacteria, *J. Clin. Invest.* **52**:44a.

Johnston, R. B., Jr., Keele, B. B., Jr., Misra, H. P., Lehmeyer, J. E., Webb, L. S., Baehner, R. L., and Rajagopalan, K. V., 1975, The role of superoxide anion generation in phagocytic bactericidal activity: Studies with normal and chronic granulomatous disease leukocytes, *J. Clin. Invest.* **55**:1357–1372.

Johnston, R. B., Jr., Lehmeyer, J. E., and Guthrie, L. A., 1976, Generation of superoxide anion and chemiluminescence by human monocytes during phagocytosis and on contact with surface-bound immunoglobulin G, *J. Exp. Med.* **143**:1551–1556.

Kane, M. A., May, J. E., and Frank, M. M., 1973, Interactions of the classical and alternate complement pathways with endotoxin lipopolysaccharide. Effect on platelets and blood coagulation, *J. Clin. Invest.* **52**:370–376.

Karnovsky, M. L., 1968, The metabolism of leukocytes, *Semin. Hematol.* **5**:156–165.

Kern, P. A., Knedler, A., and Eckel, R. H., 1983, Isolation and culture of microvascular endothelium from human adipose tissue, *J. Clin. Invest.* **71**:1822–1829.

Klebanoff, S. J., and Hamon, C. B., 1972, Role of myeloperoxidase-mediated antimicrobial systems in intact leukocytes, *J. Reticuloendothel. Soc.* **12**:170–196.

Lackie, J. M., and DeBono, D., 1977, Interactions of neutrophil granulocytes and endothelium in vitro, *Microvasc. Res.* **13**:107–112.

Larsen, G. L., McCarthy, K., Webster, R. O., Henson, J., and Henson, P. M., 1980, A differential effect of C5a and C5a des arg in the induction of pulmonary inflammation, *Am. J. Pathol.* **100**:179–188.

Lee, C. T., Fein, A. M., Lippmann, M., Holtzman, H., Kimbel, P., and Weinbaum, G., 1981, Elastolytic activity in pulmonary lavage fluid from patients with adult respiratory-distress syndrome, *N. Engl. J. Med.* **304**:192–196.

Lindbom, L., Hedqvist, P., Dahlen, S. E., Lindgren, J. A., and Arfors, K. E., 1982, Leukotriene B$_4$ induces extravasation and migration of polymorphonuclear leukocytes in vivo, *Acta Physiol. Scand.* **116**:105–108.

Liotta, L. A., 1984, Tumor invasion and metastases: Role of the basement membrane, *Am. J. Pathol.* **117**:339–348.

Liotta, L. A., Tryggvason, K., Garbisa, S., Hart, I., Foltz, C. M., and Shafie, S., 1980, Metastatic potential correlates with enzymatic degradation of basement membrane collagen, *Nature (Lond.)* **284**:67–68.

Lipscomb, M. F., Onotrio, J. M., Nash, E. J., Pierce, A. K., and Toews, G. B., 1983, A morphological study of the role of phagocytes in the clearance of *Staphylococcus aureus* from the lung, *J. Reticuloendothel. Soc.* **33**:429–442.

MacGregor, R. R., Macarak, E. J., and Kefalides, N. A., 1978, Comparative adherence of granulocytes to endothelial monolayers and nylon fiber, *J. Clin. Invest.* **61**:697–702.

Mainardi, C. L., Dixit, S. N., and Kang, A. H., 1980, Degradation of type IV (basement membrane) collagen by a protease isolated from human polymorphonuclear leukocyte granules, *J. Biol. Chem.* **255**:5435–5441.

Marchesi, V. T., 1961, The site of leukocyte emigration during inflammation, *Q. J. Exp. Physiol.* **46**:115–118.

Marchesi, V. T., and Florey, H. W., 1960, Electron micrographic observations on the emigration of leukocytes, *Q. J. Exp. Physiol.* **45**:343–348.

Maridonneau, I., Braquet, P., and Garay, R. P., 1983, Na$^+$ and K$^+$ transport damage induced by oxygen free radicals in human red-cell membranes, *J. Biol. Chem.* **258**:3107–3113.

Martin, W. J., Gadek, J. E., Hunninghake, G. W., and Crystal, R. G., 1981, Oxidant injury of lung parenchymal cells, *J. Clin. Invest.* **68**:1277–1288.

McCall, C. E., DeChatelet, L. R., Brown, D., and Lachman, P., 1974, New biological activity following intravascular activation of the complement cascade, *Nature (Lond.)* **249**:841–842.

McCormick, J. R., Harkin, M. M., Johnson, K. J., and Ward, P. A., 1981, Suppression by superoxide dismutase of immune-complex-induced pulmonary alveolitis and dermal inflammation, *Am. J. Pathol.* **102**:55–61.

McIntyre, T. M., Zimmerman, G. A., and Prescott, S. M., 1986, Leukotrienes C_4 and D_4 stimulate human endothelial cells to synthesize platelet-activating factor and bind neutrophils, *Proc. Natl. Acad. Sci. USA* **83**:2204–2208.

Mead, J. F., 1976, Free radical mechanisms of lipid damage and consequences for cellular membranes, in: *Free Radicals in Biology*, Vol. I (W. A. Pryor, ed.), pp. 51–70, Academic Press, New York.

Metchnikoff, E., 1893, *Lectures on the Comparative Pathology of Inflammation*, Kegan, Paul, Trench, Trubner, London.

Meyrick, B., Hoffman, L. H., and Brigham, K. L., 1984, Chemotaxis of granulocytes across bovine pulmonary artery intimal explants without endothelial injury, *Tissue Cell* **16**:1–16.

Morrison, D. C., and Ulevitch, R. J., 1978, The effects of bacterial endotoxin on host mediation systems, *Am. J. Pathol.* **93**:527–617.

Muller-Berghaus, G., and Lohmann, E., 1974, The role of complement in endotoxin-induced disseminated intravascular coagulation: Studies in congenitally C6-deficient rabbits, *Br. J. Haematol.* **28**:403–418.

Nagy, Z., Peters, H., and Huttner, I., 1983, Charge-related alterations of the cerebral endothelium, *Lab. Invest.* **49**:662–671.

Niedermeyer, M. E., Meyrick, B., Parl, F. F., and Brigham, K. L., 1984, Facilitation of granulocyte migration into bovine pulmonary artery intimal explants by intact viable endothelium, *Am. J. Pathol.* **117**:252–261.

Peterson, M. W., Clark, R., Stone, P., and Shasby, D. M., 1985, Neutrophil cationic protein increases endothelial albumin transport, *Am. Rev. Respir. Dis.* **131**(Suppl.):A421.

Petrone, W. F., English, D. K., Wong, K., and McCord, J. M., 1980, Free radicals and inflammation: The superoxide dependent activation of a neutrophil chemotactic factor in plasma, *Proc. Natl. Acad. Sci. USA* **77**:1159–1163.

Pohlman, T. H., Stanness, K. A., Beatty, P. G., Ochs, H. D., and Harlan, J. M., 1986, An endothelial cell surface factor(s) induced in vitro by lipopolysaccharide, interleukin-1, and tumor necrosis factor increases neutrophil adherence by a CDw18-dependent mechanism, *J. Immunol.* **136**:4548–4553.

Quie, P. G., White, J. G., Holmes, B., and Good, R. A., 1967, In vitro bactericidal capacity of human polymorphonuclear leukocytes: Diminished activity in chronic granulomatous disease of childhood, *J. Clin. Invest.* **46**:668–679.

Ranadive, N. S., and Cochrane, C. G., 1970, Basic proteins in rat neutrophils that increase vascular permeability, *Clin. Exp. Immunol.* **6**:905–911.

Rindler-Ludwig, R., and Braunsteiner, H., 1975, Cationic proteins from human neutrophil granulocytes. Evidence for their chymotrypsin-like properties, *Biochim. Biophys. Acta* **379**:606–617.

Ross, G. D., Thompson, R. A., Walport, M. J., Springer, T. A., Watson, J. V., Ward, R. H. R., Lida, J., Newman, S. L., Harrison, R. A., and Lachmann, P. J., 1985, Characterization of patients with an increased susceptibility to bacterial infections and a genetic deficiency of leukocyte membrane complement receptor type 3 and the related membrane antigen LFA-1, *Blood* **66**:882–890.

Russo, R. G., Liotta, L. A., Thorgeirsson, U., Brundage, R., and Schiffmann, E., 1981, Polymorphonuclear leukocyte migration through human amnion membrane, *J. Cell Biol.* **91**:459–467.

Ryan, U. S., Mortara, M., and Whitaker, C., 1980, Methods for microcarrier culture of bovine pulmonary artery endothelial cells avoiding the use of enzymes, *Tissue Cell* **12**:619–635.

Sacks, T., Moldow, C. F., Craddock, P. R., Bowers, T. K., and Jacob, H. S., 1978, Oxygen radicals mediate endothelial cell damage by complement-stimulated granulocytes: An *in vitro* model of immune vascular damage, *J. Clin. Invest.* **61**:1161–1167.

Sanchez-Madrid, F., Nagy, J. A., Robbins, E., Simon, P., and Springer, T. A., 1983, A human leukocyte differentiation antigen family with distinct alpha subunits and a common beta subunit: The lymphocyte function-associated antigen (LFA-1), the C3bi complement receptor (OKM1/Mac-1) and the p150,95 molecule, *J. Exp. Med.* **158**:1785–1803.

Sbarra, A. J., and Karnovsky, M. L., 1959, The biochemical basis of phagocytosis. I. Metabolic changes during the ingestion of particles by polymorphonuclear leukocytes, *J. Biol. Chem.* **234**:1355–1362.

Schmalstieg, F. C., Rudloff, H. E., Hillman, G. R., and Anderson, D. C., 1986, Two-dimensional and three-dimensional movement of human polymorphonuclear leukocytes: Two fundamentally different mechanisms of locomotion, *J. Leukocyte Biol.* **40**:677–691.

Schmid-Schonbein, G. W., Fung, Y. C., and Zweifach, B. W., 1975, Vascular endothelium–leukocyte interaction; sticking shear force in venules, *Circ. Res.* **36**:173–184.

Senior, R. M., and Campbell, E. J., 1983, Neutral proteinases from human inflammatory cells: A critical review of their role in extracellular matrix degradation, *Clin. Lab. Med.* **3**:645–666.

Shaw, J. O., 1980, Leukocytes in chemotactic-fragment-induced lung inflammation, *Am. J. Pathol.* **101**:283–291.

Shaw, J. O., Henson, P. M., Henson, J., and Webster, R. O., 1980, Lung inflammation induced by complement-derived chemotactic fragments in the alveolus, *Lab. Invest.* **42**:547–558.

Sibille, Y., Lwebuga-Mukasa, J. S., Polomski, L., Merrill., W. W., Ingbar, D. H., and Gee, J. B. L., 1986, An in vitro model for polymorphonuclear-leukocyte-induced injury to an extracellular matrix, *Am. Rev. Respir. Dis.* **134**:134–140.

Simon, R. H., Scoggin, C. H., and Patterson, D., 1981, Hydrogen peroxide causes fatal injury to human fibroblasts exposed to oxygen radicals, *J. Biol. Chem.* **256**:7181–7186.

Simionescu, D., and Simionescu, M., 1983, Differentiated distribution of the cell surface charge on the alveolar-capillary unit. Characteristic paucity of anionic sites on the air–blood barrier, *Microvasc. Res.* **25**:85–100.

Simpson, D. M., and Ross, R., 1972, The neutrophilic leukocyte in wound repair. A study with antineutrophil serum, *J. Clin. Invest.* **51**:2009–2023.

Smedly, L. A., Tonnesen, M. G., Worthen, G. S., Mason, R. J., and Henson, P. M., 1983, Neutrophil recognition of endothelial cells: Preferential adherence and transmigration, *Fed. Proc.* **42**:386.

Smedly, L. A., Tonnesen, M. G., Sandhaus, R. A., Haslett, C., Guthrie, L. A., Johnston, R. B., Jr., Henson, P. M., and Worthen, G. S., 1986, Neutrophil-mediated injury to endothelial cells: Enhancement by endotoxin and essential role of neutrophil elastase, *J. Clin. Invest.* **77**:1233–1243.

Snider, G. L., 1981, Pathogenesis of emphysema and chronic bronchitis, *Med. Clin. North Am.* **65**:647–665.

Springer, T. A., Thompson, W. S., Miller, L. J., Schmalstieg, F. C., and Anderson, D. C., 1984, Inherited deficiency of the Mac-1, LFA-1, p150,95 glycoprotein family and its molecular basis, *J. Exp. Med.* **160**:1901–1918.

Stetson, C. A., Jr., 1951, Studies on mechanism of Shwartzman phenomenon. Certain factors involved in the production of the local hemorrhagic necrosis, *J. Exp. Med.* **93**:489–504.

Taylor, R. F., Price, T. H., Schwartz, S. M., and Dale, D. C., 1981, Neutrophil–endothelial cell interactions on endothelial monolayers grown on micropore filters, *J. Clin. Invest.* **67**:584–587.

Terranova, V. P., DiFlorio, R., Hujanen, E. S., Lyall, R. M., Liotta, L. A., Thorgeirsson, U., Siegal, G. P., and Schiffmann, E., 1986, Laminin promotes rabbit neutrophil motility and attachment, *J. Clin. Invest.* **77**:1180–1186.

Thomas, E. L., 1979, Myeloperoxidase, hydrogen peroxide, chloride antimicrobial system: Nitrogen-chlorine derivatives of bacterial components in bactericidal action against *Escherichia coli, Infect. Immun.* **23**:522–531.

Thorgeirsson, U. P., Liotta, L. A., Kalebic, T., Margulies, I. M., Thomas, K., Rios-Candelore, M., and Russo, R. G., 1982, Effect of natural protease inhibitors and a chemoattractant on tumor cell invasion in vitro, *J. Natl. Cancer Inst.* **69**:1049–1054.

Todd, R. F., Arnaout, M. A., Rosin, R. E., Crowley, C. A., Peters, W. A., and Babior, B. M., 1984, Subcellular localization of the large subunit of Mo1 (Mo1α; formerly gp 110), a surface glycoprotein associated with neutrophil adhesion, *J. Clin. Invest.* **74**:1280–1290.

Tonnesen, M. G., Smedly, L., Goins, A., and Henson, P. M., 1982, Inteaction between neutrophils and vascular endothelial cells, in: *Agents and Actions*, Vol. 11, *Cologne Atherosclerosis Conference* (M. J. Parnham and J. Winkelmann, eds.), pp. 25–38, Birkhauser Verlag, Basel.

Tonnesen, M. G., Smedly, L. A., and Henson, P. M., 1984, Neutrophil–endothelial cell interactions: Modulation of neutrophil adhesiveness induced by complement fragments C5a and C5a des arg and formyl-methionyl-leucyl-phenylalanine in vitro, *J. Clin. Invest.* **74**:1581–1592.

Tonnesen, M. G., Anderson, D. C., Springer, T. A., Knedler, A., Avdi, N. J., and Henson, P. M., 1986a, MAC-1 glycoprotein family mediates adherence of neutrophils to endothelial cells stimulated by chemotactic peptides, *Clin. Res.* **34**:419 (abst.).

Tonnesen, M. G., Anderson, D. C., Springer, T. A., Knedler, A., Avdi, N. J., and Henson, P. M., 1986b, MAC-1 glycoprotein family mediates adherence of neutrophils to endothelial cells stimulated by leukotriene B$_4$ and platelet activating factor, *Fed. Proc.* **45**:379.

Tonnesen, M. G., Anderson, D. C., Springer, T. A., Knedler, A., Avdi, N., and Henson, P. M., 1987, Endotoxin directly enhances neutrophil adherence to endothelial cells by a Mac-1 glycoprotein-dependent mechanism, *Clin. Res.* **35**:722 (abst.).

Ulevitch, R. J., Cochrane, C. G., Bangs, K., Herman, C. M., Fletcher, J. R., and Rice, C. L., 1978, The effect of complement depletion on bacterial lipopolysaccharide (LPS)-induced hemodynamic and hemostatic changes in the Rhesus monkey, *Am. J. Pathol.* **92**:227–240.

van Grondelle, A., Worthen, G. S., Ellis, D., Mathias, M. M., Murphy, R. C., Strife, R. J., Reeves, J. T., and Voelkel, N. F., 1984, Altering hydrodynamic variables influences PGI$_2$ production by isolated lungs and endothelial cells, *J. Appl. Physiol.* **57**:388–395.

Wagoner, M. D., Kenyon, K. R., Gipson, I. K., Hanninen, L. A., and Seng, W. L., 1984, Polymorphonuclear neutrophils delay corneal epithelial wound healing in vitro, *Invest. Ophthalmol. Vis. Sci.* **25**:1217–1220.

Webster, R. O., Hong, S. R., Johnston, R. B., Jr., and Henson, P. M., 1980, Biological effects of the human complement fragments C5a and C5a desarg on neutrophil function, *Immunopharmacology* **2**:201–219.

Weiss, S. J., and Regiani, S., 1984, Neutrophils degrade subendothelial matrices in the presence of alpha-1-proteinase inhibitor, *J. Clin. Invest.* **73**:1297–1303.

Weiss, S. J., King, G. W., and LoBuglio, A. F., 1977, Evidence for hydroxyl radical generation by human monocytes, *J. Clin. Invest.* **60**:370–373.

Westphal, O., Westphal, U., and Sommer, T., 1977, History of pyrogen research, in: *Microbiology 1977* (D. Schlessinger, ed.), pp. 221–228, The American Society for Microbiology, Washington, D.C.

Wilkinson, P. C., 1982, *Chemotaxis and Inflammation*, 2nd ed., Churchill Livingstone, New York.

Wilkinson, P. C., and Lackie, J. M., 1983, The influence of contact guidance on chemotaxis of human neutrophil leukocytes, *Exp. Cell Res.* **145**:255–264.

Wilkinson, P. C., Shields, J. M., and Haston, W. S., 1982, Contact guidance of human neutrophil leukocytes, *Exp. Cell Res.* **140**:55–62.

Williamson, J. R., and Grisham, J. W., 1961, Electron microscopy of leukocyte margination and emigration in acute inflammation in dog pancreas, *Am. J. Pathol.* **39**:239–256.

Yoon, P. S., Boxer, L. A., Mayo, L. A., Yang, A. X., and Wicha, M. S., 1987, Human neutrophil laminin receptors: Activation-dependent receptor expression, *J. Immunol.* **138**:259–265.

Zimmerman, G. A., McIntyre, T. M., and Prescott, S. M., 1985, Thrombin stimulates the adherence of neutrophils to human endothelial cells in vitro, *J. Clin. Invest.* **76**:2235–2246.

Chapter 7

Resolution of Inflammation

CHRISTOPHER HASLETT and PETER M. HENSON

1. Introduction

For centuries, the inflammatory response has been regarded as an important consequence of injury and one that normally leads to repair and restoration of function. From the battlefield observations of John Hunter in 1794 to the elegant vascular studies of Cohnheim (1889) and the descriptions of cell migration by Metchnikoff (1891) a century later, the reiterated theme was that inflammation is a salutary response to injury. The clear-cut implication of these observations is the close connection between the inflammatory process and repair. More recently, however, it has become apparent that inflammation, paradoxically, may contribute to the pathogenesis of a large number of diseases, irrespective of the tissue in which the process is initiated. For example, in Arthus and Schwartzmann phenomena, the inflammatory process, especially neutrophil infiltration, contributes to tissue injury and necrosis. Many human disorders are recognized in which the inflammatory process may play a key pathogenetic role. These include the adult respiratory distress syndrome (ARDS) and fibrosing alveolitis in the lung, as well as various forms of glomerulonephritis that may lead to scarring in the kidney. A relationship between inflammation and scarring has been recognized in such disorders for some time. Scar tissue formation represents an alternate result of inflammation. Extensive scarring or fibrosis of any organ can cause catastrophic loss of function of that organ.

Simplistically then, inflammatory disease processes involve either abnormalities of resolution mechanisms and/or such a severe insult from the initiating factors that the tissue cannot repair itself satisfactorily. Understanding the mechanisms involved in resolution of inflammation is therefore an important goal for determining the interrelationship between tissue injury and repair. In fact, it is our contention that we will be unable to determine the reasons for persistence of inflammation in many important diseases without first under-

CHRISTOPHER HASLETT • Department of Medicine, Royal Postgraduate Medical School, Hammersmith Hospital, London W12 OHS, England.   PETER M. HENSON • Department of Pediatrics, National Jewish Center for Immunology and Respiratory Medicine, Denver, Colorado 80206.

standing how the normal inflammatory reaction resolves. Resolution of inflammation is the focus of this chapter.

Despite the importance of resolution of inflammation, it has received remarkably little attention in research. Much more emphasis has been placed on the initiation of the process than on its resolution. Accordingly, the material presented herein is sketchy at best, conceptual to a considerable degree, but it is hoped that will serve as a motivation for further investigation. To a large extent, we use the lung as an arena in which to discuss these events, since this is the organ we know best. However, it is important to emphasize at the outset that we predict that resolution of inflammation follows comparable pathways in all tissues. This is not to underemphasize effects of local architecture or unique patterns of vascularization, but rather to suggest that these provide an overlay on the basic mechanisms.

2. The Inflammatory Response

In order to discuss resolution of inflammation we must first, briefly, consider the inflammatory process. A simple sequence of inflammatory events is depicted histologically (in the lung) in Fig. 1. It is important to recognize that these events are dynamic and variable and that histology provides only static snapshots of the process. Furthermore, these static views give no indication of changes in physiologic parameters such as hemodynamics, neural responses, or functional changes. These various aspects of the inflammatory reaction are discussed in greater detail in Chapters 2–6 and 8. Here we wish to emphasize the following sequence in acute inflammation, which is considered throughout the rest of the chapter, within the context of resolution: (1) production of mediators; (2) adhesion of granulocytes to the vascular endothelium and migration through the endothelium, basement membranes (and epithelia) into the tissues or organ spaces (or in lung, gut, and skin to the external environment); (3) altered vascular permeability, with increased passage of fluid and plasma components into the tissues; (4) granulocyte release of biologically active materials and granulocyte phagocytosis of invading organisms or cell debris; (5) emigration of monocytes (and perhaps local multiplication of mononuclear phagocyte precursors); and (6) maturation of monocytes to inflammatory macrophages, removal of the components of inflammation, and return to normal.

It is now commonplace to see the inflammatory process defined as a complex interplay of cellular changes controlled by a network of interacting mediators. Here, mediators are seen as molecules derived from one cell (or from biologic fluid constituents) which act on another cell by way of specific receptors. They usually have a tissue life-span intermediate between neurotransmitters and hormones, in general limiting their sphere of influence to a local site. This can be emphasized by the observation that placement of chemoattractant C5 fragments (C5f) into the air spaces of the lung of a dog produces a complete inflammatory response at that site but leaves portions of that same lung lobe no more than 2 cm away, completely unaffected both hemodynamically and cellularly (Lien *et al.*, 1987*b*). However, the distinction between short-acting neu-rotransmitters and mediators is becoming blurred as individual molecules are suspected of playing roles both in the central nervous system (CNS) and in inflammatory responses.

It is also important to emphasize that, in the sequence outlined above, each stage significantly overlaps the others and usually depends on the initiation of other stages. Thus, vascular permeability in acute inflammation is often associ-ated with granulocyte involvement, and macrophage emigration and function is clearly important for subsequent reparative processes (see Chapter 8). It is also evident that we have ignored some other important players in many in-flammatory responses, namely, the contribution of tissue "signaling" cells, e.g., mast cells, and resident tissue macrophages, and the important and complex series of lymphocytic effects on cells. However, even by focusing on a sup-posedly simple, acute, self-limited, lymphocyte-independent, inflammatory re-sponse, resolution of the reaction is a complex enough area for discussion and should suffice to outline some concepts and possibilities for further investigation.

3. Resolution of Inflammation

A simplistic sequence of criteria should therefore be met during resolution of inflammation: (1) mediator dissipation; (2) cessation of granulocyte in-flux;(3) return of normal vascular permeability; (4) control of phagocyte secre-tion of biologically toxic materials and enzymes; (5) monocyte migration, matu-ration into macrophages, and cessation of further monocyte influx; and (6) removal of fluid, proteins, bacterial and cellular debris, neutrophils, and finally macrophages. With the resolution of these processes, the stage should be set for recovery of normal tissue architecture and function or, at the least, for the initiation of fibroplasia and scarring.

3.1. Mediator Dissipation

It is not our purpose to discuss the myriad of mediators thought to play a role in inflammation. Rather, we need to consider how they are removed, inactivated, or rendered impotent, since it seems reasonable to suggest that continued action would lead to continued inflammation. The following general mechanisms would seem to be important: (1) spontaneous decay, (2) inactiva-tion or inhibition of the mediator, (3) reduction of local mediator concentration by dilution or diffusion, (4) alteration of the responsiveness of the target cells to the action of such a mediator, and (5) antagonism of the effect of the mediator. A further requirement in the case of most of these removal mechanisms is that production of the mediator must cease as well.

Examples are known, at least *in vitro*, that exemplify each of these pro-cesses. Thromboxane A_2 and endothelial cell-derived relaxing factor are spon-

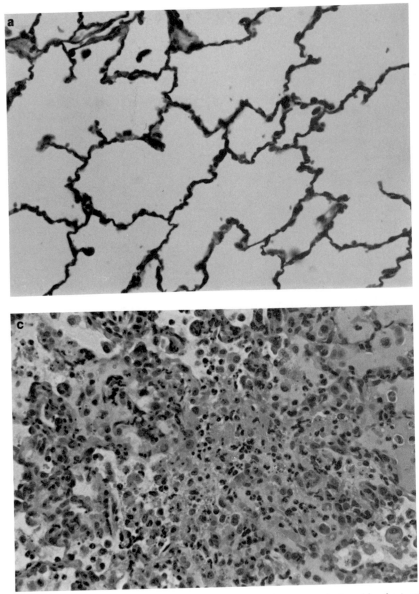

Figure 1. An acute pulmonary inflammatory response. The lesion was induced by the instillation of C5f into the lungs of rabbits (Larsen *et al.*, 1980). (a) A control lung given saline, (b) an early reaction, i.e., at the point of neutrophil emigration and increased vascular permeability (here manifested by intraalveolar edema fluid), (c) a reaction at 48 hr showing granulocyte removal and mononuclear phagocyte accumulation, and (d) the 'lesion' at 5 days, i.e., after resolution is complete.

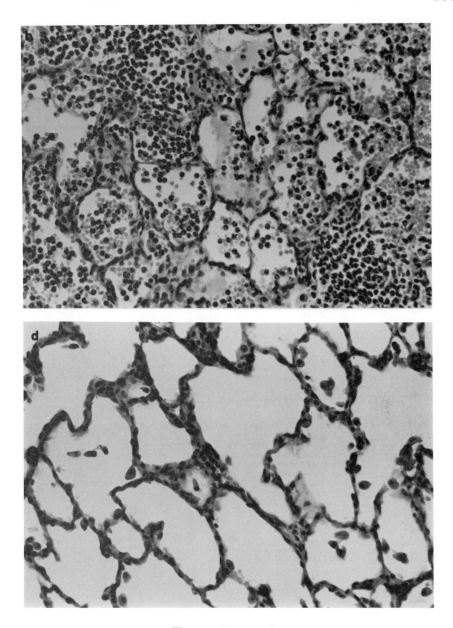

Figure 1. (Continued)

taneously unstable. Specific inactivating enzymes are known for platelet-activating factor (PAF) and histamine and less specific but equally effective peptidases inactivate C5a and bradykinin. If proteases are considered mediators, examples of inhibitors abound. Reduction of mediator concentration would be expected to occur as a result of local edema, and diffusion of low-molecular-weight molecules into blood and lymph is also expected. Downregulation of receptors is a well-known cellular response to receptor–ligand interactions. An appropriate example is the desensitization observed in neutrophil responses to most stimuli (Henson *et al.*, 1981).

Whether such downregulation actually serves to limit responses *in vivo* is unclear and requires further study. An interesting new twist on such unresponsiveness is suggested by the recent experiments of Vicker and colleagues (1986) in which neutrophils are claimed to respond chemotactically only to gradients of chemoattractant that are actually in the process of forming while standing gradients are not recognized. If applicable *in vivo*, a new way of providing a limitation on cellular migration is implied. In any event, the many gaps between our understanding of possible processes *in vitro* and effective mechanisms *in vivo* are readily apparent.

Finally, we suggest that it is most appropriate to think of mediators involved in inflammation as functioning within a network (Murphy and Henson, 1985). In fact, a spider web serves as an effective analogy. In most circumstances, multiple molecules produced at the local site can act as a positive signal to the participating cell (whether a mobile inflammatory cell or a sessile, responsive, tissue cell). These may act in concert (if they act through different receptors) or can act synergistically (e.g., Guthrie *et al.*, 1984; Haslett *et al.*, 1985). In addition, mediators providing negative signals are usually present in inflammatory sites and would be expected to balance the effects of the positive stimuli. Specific examples might be prostaglandins, cortisol, or less well-defined molecules, such as neutrophil-immobilizing factor (NIF) (Goetzl *et al.*, 1973) or macrophage migration inhibition factor (MIF). We would argue for a balanced impact of negative and positive stimuli on each cell in the inflammatory site, with the outcome (cell by cell, and ultimately for the whole tissue) dependent on the dynamic alterations in this balance.

However easy the mediator network idea is to conceptualize, it is difficult to prove. *In vitro*, one may add combinations of mediators to a population of cells and show enhancement and inhibition of responses (Chapter 5). In particular, currently most cellular activities have been studied both with and without the addition of a cyclo-oxygenase antagonist such as indomethacin, to determine the dampening (or enhancing) effect of simultaneous production of prostanoids. *In vivo*, however, the situation is much more complex. It is currently popular to sample local inflammatory fluid, bronchoalveolar lavage fluid (BALF) in the lung, and to measure the content of mediators. BALF certainly shows us what might be present, but failure to observe a mediator does not prove its absence. First, few laboratories are able to assay the wide spectrum of potential mediators. Second, the problems of quantification are enormous, especially of ephemeral molecules in complex fluids. Third, of necessity, the samples include only those molecules not bound to cells or consumed in the reactions. Fourth, sampling procedures do not generally gain access to the precise sites of inflammation. Finally, fluid samples represent average concentrations and in no way address local gradients, geographic restraints, and direct effects on the cells producing or responding to the associated stimuli. These are serious problems that will no doubt exercise the minds of numerous scientists during the next few years. However, the complexity of the inflammatory system should not discourage necessary first forays into important areas for study. Furthermore, it is apparent that studies of mediator networks must include combinations of highly specific antagonists as well as measurement of concentrations.

In any event, we suggest within the context of this chapter that inflammation wanes when the balance of mediators tips toward the inhibitory rather than the stimulatory, due (presumably) to a combination of the different mechanisms suggested above (Fig. 2). More specifically, in terms of resolution of the inflammatory response, it seems likely that the acute hemodynamic alterations in the area of tissue subjected to the insult are largely controlled by the mediator network. Thus, an altered balance of stimuli would reasonably be expected, by itself, to restore the blood flow and the proportion of involved vessels back to normal. The ability to reverse local hemodynamic changes in inflammation with drugs (Allison *et al.*, 1955; Williams, 1979; Issekutz, 1981) (see Chapter 5) suggests the transient and reversible nature of these

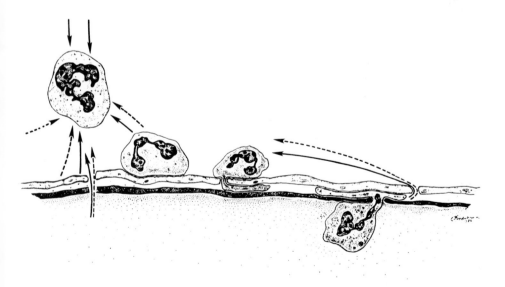

Figure 2. Depiction of the proposed mediator network in the context of inflammatory cell emigration from the vasculature. (———) Likely positive stimuli; (---) corresponding inhibitory influences. Note that the addition to the scheme of hemodynamic effects (and their control by additional sets of mediators) would add even more complexity to this interactive process.

responses. In more chronic inflammatory reactions in which significant alterations in vascular architecture occur, including neovascularization and invoca-
tion of collateral vessels, restoration of normality, if it can occur at all, is much
more complex, little understood, and outside the realm of this discussion.

The cessation of cellular influx presumably also reflects the balance of
appropriate stimuli. By contrast, removal of inflammatory cells may involve
intrinsic changes within the cells themselves. In general, however, the alteration in soluble signal factors (mediators) directs and controls the outcome of
the inflammatory process as emphasized throughout this chapter.

3.2. Cessation of Granulocyte Influx

Mechanisms responsible for the cessation of granulocyte migration into
tissues during resolution of inflammation are not understood. It is impossible
to obtain an accurate appraisal of granulocyte influx kinetics from static counts
of cells in histologic sections of tissue. For example, the presence of just a few
cells in an inflamed tissue might suggest a low level of granulocyte influx, but if
a rapid disposal process was operating, it would also be consistent with a much
greater influx of cells. Similarly, if granulocyte removal in tissues was delayed,
static counts of cells would not reflect a recent cessation of migration. Until the
tissue fate of such cells and factors controlling the mechanisms responsible are
elucidated, our knowledge of granulocyte kinetics and their time of residence
in tissues will remain incomplete.

Recent studies using radiolabeled cells have given a clearer picture of
neutrophil influx kinetics. These indicate that cessation of influx may be an
early event in the evolution of the inflammatory process. After a single injection of a variety of inflammatory agents into rabbit skin (Colditz and Movat,
1984a,b) the migration of intravenously infused labeled neutrophils had effectively ceased within 6 hr. In the rabbit knee joint, injection of C5 fragments
caused a brisk inflammatory reaction with large numbers of neutrophils present (as detected by lavage) from 2 to 24 hr. Monocytes accumulated from 6 hr
onward, and there was virtual resolution of the lesion by 48 hr (Haslett et al.,
1987). However, if radiolabeled neutrophils were injected intravenously at 6 hr
after induction of the arthritis, there was minimal migration of these labeled
cells. Thus, despite the continued presence of neutrophils at the site, influx
had effectively ceased by 6 hr after initiation. In addition to emphasizing the
point that static cell counts may not give a true representation of cell influx,
these studies provide an opportunity to investigate mechanisms that lead to the
cessation of migration. Several theoretical mechanisms may contribute to the
cessation of neutrophil migration (Fig. 3):

1. The cellular barriers to neutrophil migration could alter so as to impede
the passage of new cells. From classic ultrastructural studies (Marchesi and
Florey, 1960) neutrophils appear to pass between endothelial or epithelial cells
during migration. This does not appear to cause cell injury in vivo (Milks and

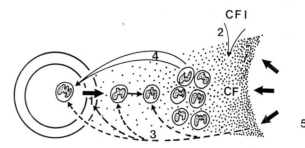

Figure 3. Possible mechanisms in cessation of neutrophil migration. 1, altered cell barriers to migration; 2, chemotactic inhibitory factors; 3, deactivation; 4, negative feedback; and 5, cessation of chemotactic factors' (CF) production and/or removal of chemoattractants.

Cramer, 1984) and neutrophils can migrate through epithelial monolayers *in vitro* without altering their barrier properties (Parsons *et al.*, 1985). How intercellular junctions of barrier cells are unlocked during neutrophil migration and locked again afterwards is unknown. An intriguing speculation is that the endothelial or epithelial cell plays an active rather than a passive role during migration (see Chapter 6).

2. Chemotactic factor inhibitory systems could develop and inactivate chemotactic factors locally. Chemotactic factor inactivators (CFIs) have been isolated from plasma and shown to inactivate C5-related chemotactic activity *in vitro* (Berenberg and Ward, 1973). When injected (in microgram quantities) into inflammatory sites, CFIs inhibit neutrophil migration (Johnston *et al.*, 1977). An appealing concept is that CFIs are generated from plasma proteins that leak into the extravasculature space during the phase of increased vascular permeability. However, CFIs have not been isolated, characterized, and quantified from inflammatory lesions, and a plasma protein-derived CFI is unlikely to be responsible for cessation of neutrophil migration when extravascular protein leakage is minimal or absent.

3. Deactivation or desensitization of migrating neutrophils could occur locally at the inflammatory site or distantly in the bloodstream. By this mechanism, neutrophils become unresponsive to further chemotactic factor stimulation (Ward and Becker, 1967). This phenomenon might be expected to occur in sites of inflammation where the concentration of chemotactic factors is high and has been suggested as a possible mechanism in the control of neutrophil chemotaxis *in vitro*, but its role *in vivo* is uncertain.

4. A negative feedback loop might operate by which further neutrophil influx is prevented by the neutrophils that have already accumulated at the inflammatory site. Although there are numerous precedents for the importance of feedback loops in biology, there is no good evidence of such a mechanism in the control of inflammatory cell influx.

5. Turnoff of neutrophil influx may simply be secondary to cessation of chemotactic factor generation and its subsequent dissipation at the inflammatory site.

The relative importance of these different mechanisms has been investigated by quantifying the migration of a pulse of labelled neutrophils delivered intravenously after a second consecutive injection of inflammatory agent injected into an inflammatory site (timed to coincide with cessation of neutrophil migration induced by an earlier injection of phlogistin). If a chemotactic factor inhibitory system was operating, migration of labeled neutrophils in response to a second injection of a dissimilar agent would be greatly reduced, as compared with migration to a single challenge of inflammatory agent. If a specific desensitization mechanism was operating, however, labeled neutrophil migration to the second challenge would only occur if the identical agent were used for both injections. This design has been used in experimental skin inflammation (Colditz and Movat, 1984b) and a rabbit model of acute arthritis (Haslett et al., 1986).

Repeated injection of a variety of inflammatory agents into rabbit skin caused progressively reduced migration of neutrophils in a stimulus-specific fashion for most phlogistins used (Colditz and Movat, 1984b). This suggested a specific desensitization process. However, not all agents provoked a reduced response to the second injection (a second injection of casein caused an enhanced migration), and reduced influx was not always stimulus specific (endotoxin-treated sites were also desensitized to an injection of FMLP). Unfortunately, specific desensitization does not provide a unifying mechanism to explain cessation of neutrophil flux into skin in response to all acute inflammatory stimuli. In a C5f-induced model of arthritis, neutrophil influx in response to a single injection had effectively ceased by 2–6 hr after challenge (Haslett et al., 1987). In repsonse to a second injection of C5f into the same joint, either 6 or 24 hr later, there was no evidence of reduced migration but a slight, but consistent, enhancement. This observation was not consistent with mechanisms 1, 2, or 3 (Fig. 3). Cessation of neutrophil influx did, however, coincide with a marked reduction in chemoattractant activity within the joint, most pronounced at 2–6 hr after C5a injection. This suggested that cessation of migration might simply have been the result of disappearance or exhaustion of chemoattractants. The fact that the profile of disappearance of chemoattractant activity after C5f injection was almost identical in neutrophil-depleted animals (with no nuetrophil migration in response to C5f injection) suggested that neutrophil accumulation itself was not involved in the disappearance of chemoattractant activity.

In conclusion, it seems likely that mechanisms responsible for cessation of neutrophil influx vary with the stimulus, and possibly with the site of injury also. Clearly, considerably more work is required in this area, particularly because control of neutrophil influx is an early event in resolution of inflammation, and an important kinetic parameter determining neturophil load to tissues.

3.3. Restoration of Normal Microvascular Permeability

Cohnheim deduced that increased permeability to fluid occurred in inflamed blood vessels almost a century before abnormalities could be shown by electron microscopy. Even today, most of the factors contributing to increased microvascular permeability and how the microvasculature recovers during the resolution phase are uncertain. However, the following mechanisms appear to contribute.

3.3.1. Endothelial Intercellular Gaps

During the early 1960s, gaps between endothelial cells were observed by electron microscopy in inflammatory reactions (Majno and Palade, 1961). They appeared to lie within intercellular junctions and to occur transiently and were not associated with overt endothelial cell damage. Gaps occurred in venules rather than capillaries and were not uniform throughout the vasculature; for example, they were seen in the bronchial but not the pulmonary microvessels of the lung (Majno et al., 1969). The more recent demonstration that neutrophils interact preferentially with the capillary endothelium in the pulmonary circulation but with the venular endothelium in the systemic circulation (Lien et al., 1987a,b) adds weight to the concept that these two microvascular beds differ in their contribution to inflammatory reactions. However, whether this represents intrinsic cellular differences, hemodynamic effects or both remains uncertain (see Chapter 6). Experimentally, endothelial intercellular gaps can be induced by short-term mediators such as histamine or bradykinin. Gap opening (and presumably closing) involves cytoskeletal changes (Majno et al., 1969), is rapidly responsive and reversible, and may provide a control point for leakage of fluid and protein into the inflamed site.

3.3.2. Endothelial and Epithelial Cell Injury

Even in relatively mild injury such as experimentally controlled minimal thermal injury, there is morphologic evidence of endothelial cell damage ranging from cytoplasmic vacuolization and nuclear smudging to total destruction (R. A. F. Clark and B. R. Reed, unpublished observations). In areas of chemotactic factor-induced experimental pneumonia (Larson et al., 1980) or human lobar pneumococcal pneumonia, both of which eventually resolve completely, there is also evidence of gross epithelial injury and fluid leakage into the alveolar spaces (Fig. 1). In many instances of increased vascular permeability and associated cell injury, neutrophils appear to be involved in the injurious process (Heflin and Brigham, 1981). Stimulated neutrophils certainly may injure endothelial cells in vitro by generation of oxygen radicals (Sacks et al., 1978; Yamada et al., 1981) and release of enzymes (Harlan et al., 1981; Smedly et al., 1986). While neutrophil migration through cell barriers itself does not necessarily cause cell injury (Milks and Cramer, 1984; Parsons et al., 1985), the state and degree of activation of neutrophils (Smedly et al., 1986) and degree and extent of their contact with endothelial or epithelial cells (Parsons et al., 1985) are important parameters determining the likelihood of injury. To simplify, we might predict a whole range of severity of injury to endothelial cells from minor individual cell perturbation to areas of cell destruction and denudation and yet the cell sheet retains the capacity to repair completely (see Chapters 14 and 16).

Although cellular mechanisms are discussed elsewhere, two possible repair mechanisms should be mentioned: (1) sublethal cell injury followed by complete recovery of individual cells, and (2) destruction of cells requiring their replacement by local proliferation.

Little is known about recovery of endothelial cells after sublethal injury. However, epithelial cells *in vitro* appear to recover after sublethal injury by oxidants. For example, Parsons *et al.* (1984) showed that H_2O_2 (a product of activated neutrophils and macrophages) caused marked reduction in trans-epithelial electrical resistance of monolayers *in vitro*, but this effect reversed within 30 min by a mechanism that appeared to require protein synthesis.

A number of investigators have demonstrated the marked ability of endothelial cells to reform monolayers that have been deliberately wounded *in vitro* (Haudenschild *et al.*, 1979). Similarly, in massive lung injury, sheets of epithelium can be regenerated by division of type II pneumonocytes. However, it has been hypothesized that if epithelial denudation is too extensive and especially if basement membrane is disrupted, healing occurs by fibrosis (Hakkinen *et al.*, 1982), and the geometry of re-epithelialization may be deranged (Fukuda *et al.*, 1985).

3.4. Control of Inflammatory Cell Secretion

It may reasonably be argued that the mere accumulation of inflammatory cells into the tissues has little significance; rather, it is what they secrete or release into the site that results in inflammatory injury. Mechanisms by which these secretory events are downregulated or terminated therefore are important considerations in the context of resolution. However, at the outset it is critical to indicate that little is known of these control mechanisms *in vivo*. The simplest concept—that the cells discharge their contents until mediators are exhausted—clearly is incorrect, since cells examined in, or from, inflammatory sites still contain granules, lysosomes, proteases, and so forth. In fact, such cells in some instances can be induced to secrete mediators when stimulated *in vitro*, clearly indicating that their *capacity* for response still exists (Zimmerli *et al.*, 1986). What is not known in such circumstances is whether they had ceased their secretory activities in the lesion whence they came. The obvious technical problems are enhanced by the fact that we look at cell populations, whereas the changes are occurring in individual cells.

A great deal is known about stimulation and modulation of inflammatory cell secretory reactions *in vitro* (Henson *et al.*, 1987). In general, these events follow the stimulus–secretion coupling pathways that have been delineated in a wide variety of secretory cells.

As discussed for adhesive and chemotactic responses, the predominant controlling influences of mediator secretion are likely to be the combination of stimulatory and inhibitory mediators to which the cells are exposed. In particular, but by no means exclusively, the prostaglandins PGI_1 and PGE_2 are of interest as inhibitors of inflammatory cell responses through their stimulation of adenylate cyclase. Some of the many potential important additional influences include (1) exhaustion of intracellular supplies of the secreted product (unlikely); (2) exhaustion of intracellular secretory processes (e.g., energy supplies) (3) receptor downregulation; (4) death of the cell; (5) removal, inactivation, or inhibition of stimuli; (6) developing dominance of inhibitory factors; and (7) removal of the cells themselves. This area seems ripe for fruitful research. Most investigators who have studied secretory processes in cells taken from inflammatory lesions have placed the cells in buffers or media entirely different from the environment surrounding the cells *in vivo*. Although highly complex, it would seem possible with appropriately labeled cells and currently available analytic and separation techniques to begin to determine (1) whether inflammatory cells cease their secretory processes before they are removed from the lesion, and (2) the mechanisms by which the control is engineered.

3.5. Monocyte Migration and Maturation

Macrophages, which can produce chemotactic factors (Merrill *et al.*, 1980) and thereby initiate the inflammatory response, can also play a critical role in its resolution. The inflammatory macrophage is a professional scavenger but also has the potential to release mediators that can amplify or downregulate the inflammatory response, and generate growth factors that influence fibroblast and possibly epithelial cell proliferation and matrix deposition (see Chapter 9). The cell is therefore pivotally placed and equipped to orchestrate either resolution or progression of inflammation.

3.5.1. Initiation of Monocyte Influx

It has been recognized for some time that tissue macrophages are largely derived from circulating monocytes of bone marrow origin. Metchnikoff observed the sequential localization of neutrophils and macrophages at sites of tissue injury. Originally suspected on morphologic grounds, macrophage origin from monocytes was later confirmed by tagging peripheral blood monocytes with carbon (Markham and Florey, 1951) or [³H]thymidine (Volkman and Gowans, 1965). We suggest that the sequential migration of monocytes and their subsequent maturation into macrophages is a critical sequence in the normal resolution of inflammation. However, factors controlling monocyte migration and its inevitable cessation during the resolution phase are even less well understood than those for the neutrophil. The apparent sequential migration of monocytes after infiltration of tissue with neutrophils and the explanation thereof are still a matter of contention. Several possible mechanisms could account for this apparent sequence: (1) Neutrophils and monocytes respond and migrate to the same stimuli, but monocytes are slower overall; (2) neutrophils and monocytes accumulate in local blood vessels simultaneously, but monocytes take longer to migrate through tissue barriers; (3) monocytes commence migration with neutrophils but their accumulation initially is obscured by sheer weight of neutrophil numbers (monocyte migration would then become more apparent later, when short-lived neutrophils disappeared while monocyte migration persisted) and (4) monocyte migration occurs later and is due to different stimuli, possibly initiated, facilitated, or amplified as a result of earlier neutrophil migration.

In experimental skin inflammation, it was generally thought that monocytes migrated later than neutrophils. In vitro, it certainly seems that monocytes are slower to respond to chemotaxins (E. Cramer, 1987, personal communication). However, Paz and Spector (1962) reported that neutrophils and monocytes appear in perivascular tissue at the same time but suggested that monocytes tend to be obscured by the greater number of neutrophils migrating at that time. This observation was supported by Issekutz et al. (1981) using radiolabeled monocytes. They also contrasted prolonged monocyte migration with short-lived neutrophil influx. Thus, in skin, the apparent sequential accumulation of neutrophils may be explained by massive early neutrophil migration which is short-lived and overtaken by the more persistent monocyte migration.

However, in an interesting and elegant series of experiments, Page and Good (1958) examined the relationship between the migration of neutrophils and mononuclear cells in the skin and suggested that mononuclear cell migration may depend on neutrophil migration. Although their results were expressed semiquantitatively, and accumulating mononuclear cells were interpreted as lymphocytes (but were almost certain to have been monocytes), an interesting relationship between neutrophils and monocytes was nevertheless suggested. In a patient with cyclic neutropenia, these workers showed that mononuclear cell accumulation in response to an inflammatory stimulus occurred only when neutrophils were present. They proceeded to model the problem in the rabbit and confirmed that mononuclear cell migration to skin inflammatory sites did not occur in rabbits treated with nitrogen mustard (to deplete neutrophils) but went on to show that the mononuclear cell response could be reconstituted by replenishment of mustard-treated animals with neutrophils from donor rabbits.

However, other skin window experiments in neutropenic patients have not permitted confirmation of their observations (Dale and Wolf, 1971), and monocyte migration into healing wounds did not appear to be inhibited in guinea pigs rendered neutropenic by antineutrophil serum. However, antineutrophil serum may destroy the neutrophils, and it seems possible that neutrophil products thus liberated may act hormonally themselves to attract monocytes. In inflammation of body cavities, such as pleural space (Hurley et al., 1966), synovial cavity (Haslett et al., 1987), and lung air spaces, the delay between early neutrophil influx and later mononuclear cell accumulation is clearer. In inflammation of the lung, we have also observed that monocytes fail to migrate in rabbits depleted in circulating neutrophils by nitrogen mustard, an effect that was reversed by neutrophil replenishment (J. Ordal, unpublished observations; Doherty et al., 1987). In summary, the dependence of monocyte migration on neutrophils clearly requires further investigation, particularly with regard to mechanism.

If monocyte migration is indeed dependent on neutrophils, it is possible that neutrophil migration could facilitate monocyte passage through tissue barriers or lead to the generation of chemotaxins for monocytes. Any such putative chemoattractant would need to be highly specific for monocytes, as neutrophil migration is ceasing at the time monocyte migration is at its peak. Most chemotaxins appear to attract both cell types *in vitro*. However, fragments of fibronectin (Norris *et al.*, 1982) and of other connective tissue proteins (Senior *et al.*, 1980; Postlethwaite and Kang, 1976) do appear to be relatively specific chemotactic factors for monocytes. Such fragments could be generated *in vivo* by neutrophil proteolytic enzymes.

Mechanisms responsible for the cessation of monocyte influx, which inevitably must occur during resolution of inflammation, remain entirely obscure, although the same principles applied above to the neutrophil, pertain. An appealing hypothesis is that monocyte migration terminates as the local enzymatic and secretory activity declines and cleavage of local connective tissue proteins ceases.

3.5.2. Monocyte Maturation and Modulation

Macrophages from inflammatory sites display features of activation. They tend to be larger than resident macrophages and have more secondary lysosomes, vacuoles, and mitochondria (Mackaness, 1970). Inflammatory macrophages are functionally more active than resident cells. They have a greatly increased pinocytic rate (Edelson *et al.*, 1975), enhanced phagocytic capability (Bianco *et al.*, 1975), and, upon direct stimulation, secrete enhanced amounts of enzymes and active oxygen species (Johnston *et al.*, 1978). The inflammatory macrophage may therefore be considered not only to be in optimal condition for uptake and destruction of microorganisms, but also to play its role in resolution of inflammation by phagocytosis of debris and removal of enzymes and other proteins by endocytosis (see Section 3.6).

It is generally believed that the inflammatory macrophage population is mostly composed of recently migrated monocytes (Bursuker and Goldman, 1979), the rest deriving from local cell division (Bouwens *et al.*, 1985; Blusse van Oud Alblas *et al.*, 1981). The fully activated state of the inflammatory macrophage is probably arrived at by a combination of maturation of monocytes into macrophages and modulation of recently matured macrophages by local factors (e.g., interferon) such that their functions are amplified. Edelson (1980) considers maturation as a genetically determined irreversible sequence leading to monocyte transformation into a macrophage, whereas reversibility of the amplification effect by removal of the modulatory influence is implicit in a modulation mechanism.

Monocyte maturation into macrophages can be followed *in vitro*, when classic features of the inflammatory macrophage develop (discussed in more detail in Chapter 4i and 4ii). These include loss of membrane 5-nucleotidease, increased pinocytosis, the development of functional complement receptors (Newman *et al.*, 1980), increased enzyme content and greatly enhanced release of superoxide anion and lysosomal enzymes upon stimulation (see Musson and

Henson, 1984). Of great relevance to the resolution of inflammation, the maturing monocyte gains the ability to recognize and ingest senescent granulocytes (Newman *et al.*, 1982).

Modulators, which amplify a variety of macrophage functions, include γ-interferon (IF$_\gamma$) and bacterial products such as lipopolysaccharide and muramyldipeptide (Pabst *et al.*, 1982). These agents are active in miniscule amounts, concentrations that may be expected to occur at some inflammatory sites, particularly where lipopolysaccharide enters skin wounds or may be delivered by plasma low-density lipoproteins during the phase of increased vascular permeability. Since the early observations that interferons enhance endocytosis (Huang *et al.*, 1971) and phagocytosis (Hamberg *et al.*, 1978) IF$_\gamma$ has been shown to modulate a wide variety of macrophage metabolic and surface-receptor functions (Ezekowitz and Gordon, 1986). Modulating agents such as IF$_\gamma$ also amplify the responses of resident–resident peritoneal macrophages when tested *in vitro*. However, in a comparison between the responsiveness of resident murine Kupffer cells, and the recently migrated liver macrophages in murine listeriosis, the newly recruited cells appeared to be greatly responsive to modulated respiratory burst activity, whereas the initial resident cells appeared to be relatively refractory to interferon stimulation (Lepay *et al.*, 1985a,b). Thus most evidence indicates that it is the newly migrated monocytes, which by a process of maturation and modulation by local amplification factors form the bulk of activated macrophages at the inflammatory site. The distinction between modulation and maturation may be somewhat artificial, however. For example, bacterial products such as lipopolysaccharide (1 pg/ml) and muramyldipeptide (1 ng/ml) may be necessary not only for a maximal superoxide generating capacity but for maintenance of viability and maturation of monocytes in tissue culture as well (Pabst *et al.*, 1982).

It should be stressed that activated oxygen species and enzymes such as elastase and collagenase (Werb and Gordon 1975a,b), which are released in enhanced amounts by activated macrophages, are potentially injurious to local tissues. Therefore, the control of secretion, deactivation of macrophages, or further maturation into a less active cell, together with the removal of modulating agents, are of great importance in limitation of local injury and subsequent resolution of inflammation. It is also possible that other modulatory systems may develop which have downregulatory effects on macrophages. *In vitro*, corticosteroids have marked inhibitory effects. Macrophages have a dexamethasone receptor (Werb and Gordon, 1975a) and dexamethasone inhibits general metabolic activity and release of macrophage enzymes. Therefore, during the resolution phase of inflammation, agents with steroidlike effects could downmodulate activated macrophages.

3.6. Clearance Removal of Fluid, Proteins, Debris, and Cells

In order for complete resolution to occur, fluid, proteins, fibrin, debris, and inflammatory cells must be disposed of effectively. Important mechanisms are lymphatic drainage and phagocytosis by scavenging macrophages.

3.6.1. Fluid, Proteins, and Debris

Most fluid is removed by lymph drainage, although restoration of normal hemodynamics may initially play a role by reconstituting the balance of hydrostatic and osmotic forces in small blood vessels, resulting in an increase in fluid absorption at the venous end of the capillary. Lymphatic vessels become widely distended as lymphatic removal of fluid and proteins increases. Fibrinolysis, mediated by proteolytic enzymes from plasma and inflammatory cells breaks down fibrin clots (see Chapter 18). Products of this digestion are drained in the lymph. However, the inflammatory macrophage may also phagocytose fibrinaceous material (see Chapter 3) and remove other proteins and fluid selectively by endocytosis.

The macrophage is considered to be of critical importance in the clearance phase of inflammation. Maturing macrophages increase in size, protein content, and synthetic and secretory ability. It has long been recognized that they also have greatly increased endocytic potential. This is reflected by increased uptake of particles coated with immunoglobulin or complement proteins (Bianco et al., 1975) associated with increased surface Fc and C3 receptors. Thus, the uptake of opsonized (and also nonopsonized) large particles at inflammatory sites is enhanced. Pinocytosis is also greatly enhanced. Pinocytic rate is increased fivefold in activated macrophages (Edelson et al., 1975), which is equivalent to a volume uptake of 25% of the cell per hour and internalization of 3% of the surface of the cell per minute (Steinman et al., 1976). An enormously efficient membrane turnover process exists in activated macrophage, which is of great importance in the recycling of surface receptors. The contents of pinocytic vesicles (if digestible) are degraded completely with first-order kinetics (Steinman and Cohn, 1972), and there is early fusion with lysosomes (Steinman et al., 1974). Therefore, the process provides an important mechanism for the removal of pro-inflammatory agents at inflammatory sites such as enzymes and other large proteins (e.g., α_2-macroglobulin–protease complexes (Kaplan and Nielsen, 1979), antibodies, and immune complexes (Steinman and Cohn, 1972). Endocytosis may also disarm the activated macrophage by reducing the number of surface receptors. For example, macrophage Fc receptors can be downregulated by endocytosis of antibody-coated erythrocyte ghosts (Mellman et al., 1983).

3.6.2. Neutrophils

Despite the potential of neutrophils for inducing tissue injury by the action of enzymes, oxygen metabolites, and toxic proteins (Janoff, 1970; Henson and Johnston, 1987), the fate of neutrophils at inflammatory sites has received little formal study. Neutrophil disposal is a prerequisite for the resolution of inflammation, and the rate of disposal is an important kinetic parameter determining residence time of neutrophils in tissues (see Fig. 6). The fate of most neutrophils probably occurs at the inflammatory lesion itself; there is no evidence that neutrophils return to the bloodstream and minimal indication that lymphatic drainage is an important disposal route. Most pathology textbooks either

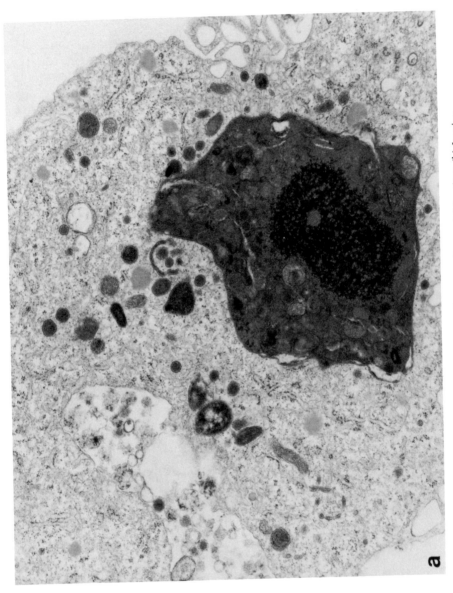

Figure 4. Neutrophil phagocytosis by macrophages. (a) *In vitro.* (b) *In vivo.*

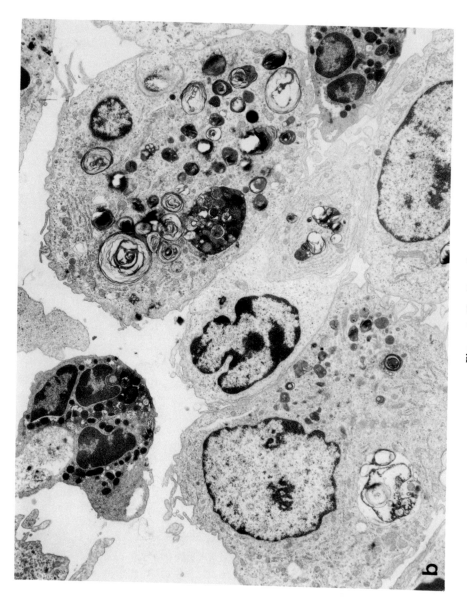

Figure 4. (Continued)

do not refer to this aspect of inflammation or suggest that neutrophils disrupt and their fragments are removed by macrophages. In this regard, Hurley (1983) stated:

> Some polymorphs may leave the damaged area via lymphatics or tissue spaces and finally die at some distance from the site of inflammation. However, most die locally, disintegrate and liberate their granules and cytoplasmic enzymes into adjacent tissue spaces. The remnants of the dead cells are then engulfed by macrophages.

If this is the rule, healthy tissues would be exposed to the injurious effects of neutrophil contents. Alternatively, a disposal process for intact effete neutrophils would tend to limit local injury. We suggest that there is significant evidence that inflammatory macrophages can recognize intact senescent neutrophils in a process that leads to phygocytosis and digestion. We hypothesize that it is this process that is the rule at self-limited inflammatory sites (particularly those that do not involve cytolytic bacterial products) rather than neutrophil disruption with its potentially damaging consequences.

Neutrophil ingestion by phagocytes was first observed by Metchnikoff (1891a) in studies of inflammation in tadpole tails, when he noted them to become englobed by other phagocytes. He also observed this process in inflammation caused by streptococci (Metchnikoff, 1891b): "the streptococci are englobed by polynuclear leukocytes, and are never taken up by the macrophages, which, however, carry out the entire work of absorption and even englobe the microphages [neutrophils]." Since those seminal observations, the apparent ingestion of neutrophils by macrophages has been noted in various disease states (Chandra et al., 1975; Kadri et al., 1975) as well as by macrophages in healthy bone marrow (Dresch et al., 1980). Phagocytosis of neutrophils by mouse (Heifets et al., 1980) and guinea pig macrophages (Brewer, 1964) has been shown. We have carried out studies of this interaction, using human peripheral blood neutrophils and macrophages derived from blood monocytes in vitro. Mature macrophages, but not monocytes, had the capacity to recognize and engulf neutrophils (Fig. 4) aged in tissue culture. By contrast, they did not phagocytose freshly isolated neutrophils (Newman et al., 1982). Resident alveolar macrophages did not appear to recognize aged neutrophils, but macrophages lavaged from inflamed lungs avidly engulfed such cells. Thus it appears that macrophages from sites of inflammation or monocyte-derived macrophages (which show many similarities to inflammatory macrophages) are able to recognize a change that occurs in senescent but otherwise intact and viable neutrophils. The actual recognition mechanism is under investigation. However, it does not seem to be the same mechanism by which macrophages recognize senescent erythrocytes (Kay, 1975), because neutrophil aging and uptake occurred in the absence of immunoglobulin. Preliminary inhibition studies with sugars suggest a specific recognition process (J. S. Savill, P. M. Henson, and C. Haslett, unpublished data).

3.6.3. Macrophages

Having played the leading cellular role in the resolution of inflammation, macrophages are themselves reduced in number and the tissue complement of

macrophages usually returns toward normal. Whether macrophages are removed by other phagocytes at the inflammatory site and/or in lymph nodes or
whether they disappear by some other mechanism is entirely unknown.

4. Summary

Despite incomplete knowledge of the actual mechanisms involved, the
normal resolution of inflammation sets the stage for repair and restoration of
function. We suggest the following speculative scheme by which a variety of
initiating events provokes a stereotyped sequence of responses (Fig. 5) that
results in resolution of inflammation. Injury to cellular barriers is minimal (in
self-limited acute inflammation) but is associated with a leak of fluid and
proteins. Reconstitution of normal microvascular permeability occurs by re-
forming of junctions and regeneration of endothelial cells, where necessary.
Neutrophil influx ceases early in acute inflammation and is closely linked to
cessation of local chemoattractant generation and removal. Monocyte migration is often dependent on neutrophil influx and ceases by unknown mechanisms. Monocytes mature into inflammatory macrophages, which are professional scavengers, removing cellular and bacterial debris. Neutrophils are

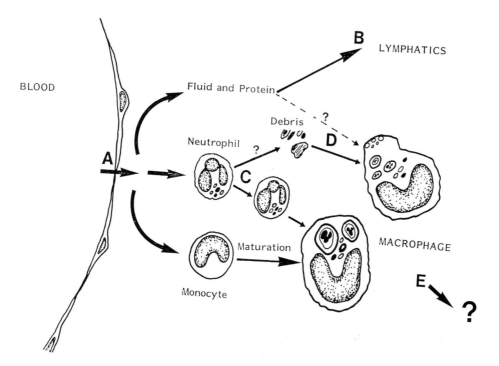

Figure 5. Scheme for resolution of inflammation. A, Restoration of normal hemodynamics; B,
drainage of fluid and proteins by lymphatics; C, recognition and disposal of senescent cells by
macrophages; D, macrophage scavenging of debris and pinocytosis of fluid; and E, macrophage
disposal.

primarily removed by a process in which inflammatory macrophages recognize specific surface markers that develop on the aging but otherwise intact neutrophil. Fluid is removed by lymphatics and to some degree by pinocytosing macrophages. The final event in setting the stage for return to normality is deactivation and removal of excess macrophages by unknown mechanisms. It must be stressed that these events are part of a continuum rather than discrete temporal steps. For example, fluid removal by lymphatics is occurring while monocytes are migrating, and healing of cellular barriers is progressing, while macrophages are removing debris.

5. Speculation

5.1. Importance of Resolution Mechanisms in Host Defense against Injury

Tissue injury in inflammatory processes is generally perceived as a balance between the injurious influences and tissue protective mechanisms. During neutrophil migration and phagocytosis, for example, there appears to be an obligatory release of proteases and oxygen metabolites which have the potential to injure tissues. Tissue defenses, however, include antiproteases and scavengers of oxygen metabolites and it is considered that the balance is normally heavily weighted toward protection, rather than toward injury. For example, the discovery of the genetic accident, α_1-antiprotease deficiency (Laurell and Eriksson, 1963) and its association with lung emphysema led to the protease-antiprotease theory of emphysema pathogenesis. Much is now known about tissue defenses. However, the factors that control the load of neutrophils and thus of their potentially injurious contents are also an important part of the balance (Fig. 6). These factors are much less well understood and have been discussed briefly. For example, we conceptualize neutrophil load as being determined both by the total number of neutrophils and their time of residence in tissues. The time of residence would be determined by the rate of neutrophil influx and the subsequent rate of neutrophil disposal. Factors controlling neutrophil influx and disposal may therefore be crucial in tissue defense against injury.

5.2. Termination of Inflammation by Processes Other Than Resolution

In his discussions of termination of inflammation, Hurley (1983) described suppuration, fibrosis, and chronic inflammation as alternative modes of termination. Factors that determine which terminating pathway is followed have not been identified. However, consideration of our speculative scheme (Fig. 5) for the normal resolution of acute inflammation reveals several steps at which the resolution process could go astray. Experimental modeling of these steps to

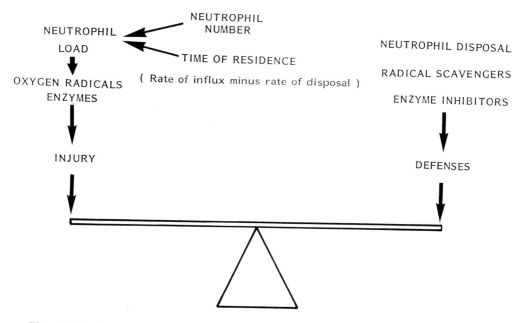

Figure 6. The importance of neutrophil load and its determinants in the balance between injurious influence and tissue protection.

understand the mechanisms involved should give important insight into the mechanisms by which chronic inflammation and fibrosis may develop out of the acute inflammatory process and result in permanent injury and loss of function.

ACKNOWLEDGMENTS. This work was carried out in the F. L. Bryant, Jr., Research Laboratory at the National Jewish Center for Immunology and Respiratory Medicine, and supported by grants HL27353, GM 24834, and HL 33058 from the National Institutes of Health. Dr. C. Haslett was supported in part by a MRC Travelling Fellowship.

References

Allison, F., Jr., Smith, M. R., and Wood, W. B., Jr., 1955, Studies on the pathogenesis of acute inflammation. I. The inflammatory reaction to thermal injury as observed in the rabbit ear chamber, *J. Exp. Med.* **102:**655–674.

Berenberg, J. L., and Ward, P. A., 1973, Chemotactic factor inactivator in normal human serum, *J. Clin. Invest.* **52:**1200–1207.

Blusse van Oud Alblas, A., van der Linden-Schrever, B., and van Furth, R., 1981, Origin and kinetics of pulmonary macrophages during an inflammatory reaction induced by intravenous administration of heat-killed Bacillus Calmette-Guérin, *J. Exp. Med.* **154:**235–252.

Bouwens, L., and Wisse, E., 1985, Proliferation kinetics and fate of monocytes in rat liver zymosan-induced inflammation, *J. Leukocyte Biol.* **37:**531–544.

Bursuker, I., and Goldman, R., 1979, Derivation of resident and inflammatory peritoneal macrophages from percursor cells differing in 5'-nucleotidase activity, *J. Reticuloendothel. Soc.* **26**:205–208.

Bianco, C., Griffin, F. M., and Silverstein, S. C., 1975, Studies of the macrophage complement receptor. Alteration of receptor function upon macrophage activation, *J. Exp. Med.* **141**:1278–1290.

Brewer, D. B., 1964, Electron-microscope phagocytosis of neutrophil polymorphonuclear leukocytes by macrophages, *J. Pathol.* **88**:307–309.

Chandra, P., Chaudhery, S. A., Rosner, F., and Kagem, M., 1975, Transient histocytosis with striking phagocytosis of platelets, leukocytes and erythrocytes, *Arch. Intern. Med.* **135**:989–991.

Colditz, I. G., and Movat, H. Z., 1984a, Chemotactic factor-specific desensitization of skin to infiltration by polymorphonuclear leukocytes, *Immunol. Lett.* **8**:83–87.

Coditz, I. G., and Movat, H. Z., 1984b, Desensitization of acute inflammatory lesions to chemotaxins and endotoxin, *J. Immunol.* **133**:2163–2168.

Conheim, J., 1889, *Lectures on General Pathology*, 2nd ed. [German transl.], Vol. 1, The New Sydenham Society, London, 1882.

Dale, D. C., and Wolff, S. M., Skin window studies of the acute inflammatory responses of neutropenic patients, *Blood* **38**:138–142.

Doherty, D. E., Downey, G., Worthen, G. S., Haslett, C., and Henson, P. M., 1987, Monocyte retention and accumulation in pulmonary inflammation: Requirements for neutrophils, submitted for publication.

Dresch, C. E., Flandrin, E., and Breton-Gorius, J., 1980, Phagocytosis of neutrophil polymorphonuclears by macrophages in human bone marrow: Importance in granulopoiesis, *J. Clin. Pathol.* **33**:1110–1113.

Edelson, P. J., 1980, Monocytes and macrophages: Aspects of their cell biology, in: *Handbook of Inflammation*, Vol. 2 (G. Weissman, ed.), pp. 469–495, Elsevier/North-Holland Biomedical Press, New York.

Edelson, P. J., Zwiebel, R., and Cohn, Z. A., 1975, The pinocytic rate of activated macrophages, *J. Exp. Med.* **142**:1150–1164.

Ezekowitz, R. A. B., and Gordon, S., 1986, Interaction and regulation of macrophage receptors, *Ciba Foundation Symposium* **118**:127–136.

Fukuda, Y., Ferrans, V. J., Schoenberger, C. I., Rennard, S. I., and Crystal, R. G., 1985, Patterns of pulmonary structural remodeling after experimental paraquat toxicity. The morphogenesis of intraalveolar fibrosis, *Am. J. Pathol.* **118**:452–475.

Goetzl, E. J., Gigli, I., Wasserman, S., and Austen, K. F., 1973, A neutrophil mobilizing factor derived from human leukocytes. II. Specificity of action on polymorphonuclear leukocyte mobility, *J. Immunol.* **111**:938–945.

Guthrie, L. A., McPhail, L. C., Henson, P. M., and Johnston, Jr., R. B., 1984, The priming of neutrophils for enhanced release of superoxide anion and hydrogen peroxide by bacterial lipopolysaccharide: Evidence for increased activity of the superoxide-producing enzyme, *J. Exp. Med.* **160**:1656–1671.

Hakkinen, J. P., Whiteley, J. W., and Witschi, H. P., 1982, Hyperoxia but not thoracic irradiation potentiates bleomycin- and cyclophosphamide-induced damage in mice, *Am. Rev. Respir. Dis.* **126**:281–285.

Ham, K. M., and Hurley, J. V., 1968, An electron-microscopic study of the vascular response to mild thermal injury in the rat, *J. Pathol.* **95**:175–183.

Hamburg, S. I., Manejias, R. E., and Rabinovitch, 1978, Macrophage activation: Increased ingestion of IgG-coated erythrocytes after adminisration of interferon inducers to mice, *J. Exp. Med.* **147**:593–598.

Harlan, J. M., Killen, P. D., Harker, L. A., and Striker, G. E., 1981, Neutrophil-mediated endothelial injury *in vitro*, *J. Clin. Invest.* **68**:1394–1403.

Haslett, C., Guthrie, L. A., Kopaniak, M. M., Johnston, R. B., and Henson, P. M., 1985, Modulation multiple neutrophil functions by preparative methods and trace amounts of bacterial lipopolysaccharide, *Am. J. Pathol.* **119**:101–110.

Haslett, C., Giclas, P. C., and Henson, P. M., 1987, Mechanisms leading to cessation of neutrophil migration in acute experimental arteritis, submitted for publication.

Haudenschild, C. L., and Schwartz, S. M., 1979, Endothelial regeneration. II. Restitution of endothelial continuity, *Lab. Invest.* **41**:407–418.

Heflin, A. C., and Brigham, K., 1981, Prevention by granulocyte depletion of increased vascular permeability in sheep lung following endotoxemia, *J. Clin. Invest.* **68**:1253–1260.

Heifets, L., Imai, K., and Goren, M. B., 1980, Expression of peroxidase-dependent iodination by macrophages ingesting neutrophil debris, *J. Reticuloendothel. Soc.* **28**:391–404.

Henson, P. M., and Johnston, R. B., Jr., 1987, Tissue injury in inflammation: Oxidants, proteinases and cations, *J. Clin. Invest.* **79**(3):669–674.

Henson, P. M., Schwartzmann, N. A., and Zanolari, B., 1981, Intracellular control of human neutrophil secretion. II. Stimulus specificity of desensitization induced by six different soluble and particulate stimuli, *J. Immunol.* **127**:754–759.

Huang, K., Donahoe, R. M., Gordon, F. B., and Dressler, H. R., 1971, Enhancement of phagocytosis by interferon-containing preparations, *Infection Immun.* **4**:581–588.

Hunter, J., 1974, *The Works of John Hunter FRS with Notes*, Vol. III (J. F. Palmer, ed.), Longman, Rees, Orme, Green and Longman, London.

Hurley, J. V., 1983, Termination of acute inflammation. I. Resolution, in: *Acute Inflammation*, 2nd Ed., (J. V. Hurley, ed.), pp. 109–117, Churchill Livingstone, London.

Hurley, J. V., Ryan, G. B., and Friedman, A., 1966, The mononuclear response to intrapleural injection in the rat, *J. Pathol.* **91**:575–587.

Issekutz, A. C., 1981, Vascular responses during acute neutrophilic inflammation. Their relationship to in vivo neutrophil emigration, *Lab. Invest.* **45**:435–441.

Issekutz, T. B., Issekutz, A. C., and Movat, H. Z., 1981, The *in vivo* quantitation and kinetics of monocyte migration into acute inflammatory tissue, *Am. J. Pathol.* **103**:47–55.

Janoff, A., 1970, Mediators of tissue damage in human polymorphonuclear neutrophils, *Sci. Haematol.* **3**:96–130.

Johnston, K. J., Anderson, T. P., and Ward, R. A., 1977, Suppression of immune complex-induced inflammation by the chemotactic factor inactivator, *J. Clin. Invest.* **59**:951–958.

Johnston, R. B., Godzik, C. A., and Cohn, Z. A., 1978, Increased superoxide anion production by immunologically activated and chemically-elicited macrophages, *J. Exp. Med.* **148**:115–127.

Kadri, A., Noinuddim, M., and De Leeuw, N. K., 1975, Phagocytosis of blood cells by splenic macrophages in thrombotic thrombocytopenic purpura, *Ann. Intern. Med.* **82**:799–802.

Kaplan, J., and Nielsen, M. L., 1979, Analysis of macrophage surface receptors. I. Binding of α_2-macroglobulin–protease complexes to rabbit alveolar macrophages, *J. Biol. Chem.* **254**:7323–7328.

Kay, M. M. B., 1975, Mechanism of removal of senescent cells by human macrophages *in situ*, *Proc. Natl. Acad. Sci. USA* **72**:3521–3525.

Larson, G. L., McCarthy, K., Webster, R. O., Henson, J. E., and Henson, P. M., 1980, A differential effect of C5a and C5a des arg in the induction of pulmonary inflammation, *Am. J. Pathol.* **100**:179–192.

Laurell, C. B., and Eriksson, S., 1963, The electrophoretic α-1-globulin pattern of serum in α-1 antitrypsin deficiency, *Scand. J. Clin. Lab. Invest.* **15**:132–140.

Lepay, D. A., Steinman, R. M., Mattan, C. F., Murray, H. W., and Cohn, Z. A., 1985a, Liver macrophages in murine listerosis. Cell mediated immunity is correlated with an influx of macrophages capable of generating active oxygen intermediates, *J. Exp. Med.* **161**:1503–1512.

Lepay, D. A., Nathan, C. F., Steinman, R. M., Murray, H. W., and Cohn, Z. A., 1985b, Murine Kupffer cells. Mononuclear phagocytes deficient in generation of reactive oxygen intermediates, *J. Exp. Med.* **161**:1079–1096.

Lien, D. C., Bethel, R. A., Henson, P. M., and Worthen, G. S., 1987c, Platelet activating factor causes rapid neutrophil sequestration in the canine trachea, in preparation.

Lien, D. C., Wagner, W. W., Capen, R. L., Haslett, C., Hanson, W. L., Hofmeister, S. E., Henson, P. M., and Worthen, G. S., 1987a, Physiologic neutrophil sequestration in the lung: visual evidence for localization in capillaries, *J. Appl. Physiol.* **62**:1236–1243.

Lien, D. C., Worthen, G. S., Capen, R. L., Gillespie, M. M., Hanson, W. L., Hofmeister, S. E., Wagner,

W. W., Jr., and Henson, P. M., 1987b, The acute inflammatory process in the lung: direct observation of neutrophil behavior in response to C5 fragments, submitted for publication.

Mackaness, G. B., 1970, The monocyte in cellular immunity, *Semin. Haematol.* **7:**172–184.

Majno, E., and Palade, G. E., 1961, Studies on Inflammation I. The effect of histamine and serotinin on vascular permeability: An electron microscopic study, *J. Biol. Phys. Biochem. Cytol.* **11:**571–605.

Majno, E.. Shea, S. M., and Leventhall, M., 1969, Endothelial contraction induced by histamine-type mediators. An electron microscopic study, *J. Cell. Biol.* **42:**647–672.

Marchesi, V. T., and Florey, H. W., 1960, Electron micrographic observations on the emigration of leukocytes, *Q. J. Exp. Physiol.* **45:**343–348.

Markham, M. P., and Florey, H. W., 1951, The effect of experimental tuberculosis on the intravenous injection of insoluble substances: Experiments with carbon, *Br. J. Exp. Pathol.* **46:**50–61.

Mellman, I. S., Plutner, H., Steinman, R. M., Unkeless, J. C., and Cohn, Z. A., 1983, Internalisation and degradation of macrophage Fc receptors during receptor-mediated phagocytosis, *J. Cell. Biol.* **96:**887–895.

Merrill, W. W., Naegel, G. P., Matthay, R. A., and Reynolds, H. Y., 1980, Alveolar macrophage-derived chemotactic factor. Kinetics of in vitro production and partial characterization, *J. Clin. Invest.* **65:**268–276.

Metchnikoff, E., 1891a, Lectures on the Comparative Pathology of Inflammation. Lecture VII, Delivered at the Pasteur Institute in 1891 (F. A. Starling and E. H. Starling, transl.), Dover, New York, 1968.

Metchnikoff, E., 1891b, Lectures on the Comparative Pathology of Inflammation. Lecture XII. Delivered at the Pasteur Institute in 1891 (F. A. Starling and E. H. Starling, transl.), Dover, New York. 1968.

Milks, L., and Cramer, E., 1984, Transepithelial electrical resistance studies during in vitro neutrophil (PMN) migration, *Proc. Fed. Am. Soc. Exp. Biol.* **43:**777.

Murphy, R. C., and Henson, P. M., 1985, Mediator network, in: *Leukotrienes and Immediate Hypersensitivity.* 9e Forum D'Immunologie, Volume 136D, ed? Ann. Inst. Pasteur/Immunol. Elsevier, Paris, pp. 175–228.

Musson, R. A., and Henson, P. M., 1984, Phagocytic cell, in: *Immunology of the Lung* (J. Bienenstock, ed.), pp. 119–138, McGraw-Hill, New York.

Newman, S. L., Musson, R. A., and Henson, P. M., 1980, Development of functional macrophage receptors during in vitro maturation of human monocytes into macrophages, *J. Immunol.* **125:**2236–2244.

Newman, S. L., Henson, J. E., and Henson, P. M., 1982, Phagocytosis of senescent neutrophils by human monocyte-derived macrophages and rabbit inflammatory macrophages, *J. Exp. Med.* **156:**430–442.

Norris, D. A., Clark, R. A. F., Swigart, L. M., Huff, J. C., Weston, W. L., and Howell, S. E., 1982, Fibronectin fragments are chemotactic for human peripheral blood monocytes, *J. Immunol.* **129:**1612–1618.

Pabst, M. J., Hedegaard, H. B., and Johnston, R. B., Jr., 1982, Cultured human monocytes require exposure to bacterial products to maintain an optimal oxygen radical response, *J. Immunol.* **128:**123–128.

Page, A. R., and Good, R. A., 1958, A clinical and experimental study of the function of neutrophils in the inflammatory response, *Am. J. Pathol.* **34:**645–657.

Parsons, P. E., Cott, G. R., Mason, R. J., and Henson, P. M., 1984, Reversible oxidant "injury" of an epithelial monolayer, *Proc. Fed. Am. Soc. Exp. Biol.* **43:**777.

Parsons, P. E., Sugahara, K., Mason, R. J., and Henson, P. M., 1985, The effect of neutrophil migration and prolonged neutrophil contact on epithelial permeability, *Proc. Fed. Am. Soc. Exp. Biol.* **44:**1919.

Paz, R. A., and Spector, W. E., 1962, The mononuclear cell response to injury, *J. Pathol.* **84:**85–103.

Postlethwaite, A. E., and Kang, A. H., 1976, Collagen and collagen peptide-induced chemotaxis of human blood monocytes, *J. Exp. Med.* **143:**1299–1307.

Sacks, T., Moldow, C. F., Craddock, P. R., Bower, T. K., and Jacob, H. S., 1978, Oxygen radicals mediate endothelial cell damage by complement-stimulated granulocytes, *J. Clin. Invest.* **61**:1161–1167.

Senior, R. M., Griffin, G. T., and Mecham, R. P., 1980, Chemotactic activity of elastin-derived peptides, *J. Clin. Invest.* **66**:859–862.

Smedly, L. A., Tonnesen, M. G., Sandhaus, R. A., Haslett, C., Guthrie, L. A., Johnston, R. B., Henson, P. M., and Worthen, G. S., 1986, Neutrophil-mediated injury to endothelial cells: Enhancement by endotoxin and essential role of neutrophil elastase, *J. Clin. Invest.* **77**:1233–1243.

Steinman, R. M., and Cohn, Z. A., 1972, The uptake, distribution and fate of horseradish peroxidase–antiperoxidase complexes in mouse peritoneal macrophages *in vitro. J. Cell. Biol.* **55**:186–204.

Steinman, R. M., Silver, J. M., and Cohn, Z. A., 1974, Pinocytosis in fibroblasts: quantitative studies *in vitro, J. Cell. Biol.* **63**:949–969.

Steinman, R. M., Brodie, S. E., and Cohn, Z. A., 1976, Membrane flew during pinocytosis—A sterologic analysis, *J. Cell Biol.* **68**:665–687.

Vicker, M. G., Lackie, J. M., and Schill, W., 1986, Neutrophil leucocyte chemotaxis is not induced by a spatial gradient of chemoattractant, *J. Cell Sci.* **84**:263–280.

Volkman, A., and Gowans, J. L., 1965, The production of macrophages in the rat, *Br. J. Exp. Pathol.* **46**:50–61.

Ward, P. A., and Becker, E. L., 1967, The deactivation of rabbit neutrophils by chemotactic factor and the nature of the activatable esterase, *J. Exp. Med.* **127**:693–709.

Werb, Z., and Gordon, S., 1975a, Elastase secretion by stimulated macrophages. Characterisation and regulation, *J. Exp. Med.* **142**:361–377.

Werb, Z., and Gordon, S., 1975b, Secretion of a specific collagenase by stimulated macrophages, *J. Exp. Med.* **142**:346–360.

Williams, T. J., 1979, Prostaglandin E_2, prostaglandin I_2 and the vascular changes of inflammation, *Br. J. Pharmacol.* **65**:517–524.

Yamada, O., Moldow, C. F., Sacks, T., Craddock, P. R., Boogaerts, M. A., and Jacob, H. S., 1981, Deleterious effects of endotoxin on cultured endothelial cells: An *in vitro* model of vascular injury, *Inflammation* **5**:115–126.

Zimmerli, W., Seligmann, B., and Galin, I. J., 1986, Exudation primes human and guinea pig neutrophils for subsequent responsiveness to the chemotactic peptide N-formylmethionyl leucylphenylamine and increases complement component C3bi receptor expression, *J. Clin. Invest.* **77**:925–933.

Chapter 8

The Multiple Roles of Macrophages in Wound Healing

DAVID W. H. RICHES

1. Introduction

The process of wound healing is associated with dynamic changes in the type and density of various infiltrating cell populations (Ross and Benditt, 1961). Tissue injury, in response to a variety of agents (e.g., surgical trauma or burns), rapidly induces a nonspecific inflammation probably as a result of blood coagulation, with accompanying platelet aggregation and activation of the complement and kinin systems (see Chapters 2 and 3). The first blood leukocytes to be attracted and demobilized at the site of tissue injury are neutrophils, the number of which increases steadily before peaking at 24–48 hr (see Chapter 6). The main function of neutrophils is apparently to destroy bacteria introduced into the tissue during injury. However, in the absence of gross infection, depletion of circulating neutrophils in guinea pigs by treatment with antineutrophil serum has no effect on the subsequent healing of experimentally induced wounds (Simpson and Ross, 1972).

As the number of wound neutrophils begins to decline, the macrophage population increases, replacing the neutrophil as the predominant professional wound phagocyte. For many years, the primary function of macrophages was thought to be the removal and degradation of injured tissue debris in anticipation of the reparative process. However, studies reported by Leibovich and Ross (1975) showed that the combined depletion of circulating blood monocytes and local tissue macrophages in guinea pigs resulted not only in a severe retardation of tissue debridement but also in a marked delay in fibroblast proliferation and subsequent wound fibrosis. Thus, the data indicate that wound macrophages play a key role in the orchestration and execution of both the degradative and reparative phases of wound healing. As a result of further investigations during the 1970s, it is now recognized that wound macrophages secrete growth factors that stimulate the proliferation of fibroblasts, smooth muscle cells, and endothelial cells. The reduced oxygen tension in the avascular

DAVID W. H. RICHES • Department of Pediatrics, National Jewish Center for Immunology and Respiratory Medicine, Denver, Colorado 80206.

wound is thought to stimulate wound macrophages to secrete an angiogenesis factor (or factors) that, in conjunction with mesenchymal cell growth factors, stimulates neovascularization (i.e., the directed outgrowth of new capillaries) of the wound space. Furthermore, evidence is beginning to emerge that factors secreted by wound macrophages may control the synthesis of connective tissue proteins, specifically collagen, by other cell types within the healing wound.

The objective of this chapter is to provide an overview of the multiple roles of the macrophage in both the degradative and reparative phases of wound healing. As a basis for understanding the multiple responses of this adaptable cell, the origin of wound macrophages (Section 2), the signals involved in their emigration from the vasculature (Section 3), and the mechanisms underlying the differentiation of monocytes into macrophages (Section 4) are discussed. Also, the role of these cells in tissue debridement is discussed with particular reference to the secreted and intracellular proteolytic enzymes that are thought to be preeminently involved in this process (Section 5). In consideration of the reparative phase, the focus is mainly on the characteristics and conditions under which mitogenic and angiogenic factors are secreted by macrophages (Section 6). Regrettably, but out of necessity, this chapter largely excludes the important and frequently overlapping roles of other cells (e.g., the platelet) in the process of wound healing (see Chapter 2).

2. Origin and Kinetics of Macrophages

The ontogeny of mononuclear phagocytes has been studied in great depth during the past 20 years. Early studies in the mouse by van Furth and colleages (beginning with van Furth and Cohn, 1968) have revealed the nature and turnover kinetics of two cells located in bone marrow that are precursors of the circulating blood monocyte, namely the monoblast (Goud et al., 1975, Goud and van Furth, 1975) and the promonocyte (van Furth et al., 1973). These investigations were complemented by other studies on the characterization of specific mononuclear phagocyte lineage growth factors, such as colony-stimulating factor-1 (CSF-1), reviewed by Nicola and Metcalf (1986). Together, these studies revealed much about the characteristics and conditions of growth of mononuclear phagocytes and their precursors, under both steady-state conditions and in response to inflammation.

While there appears to be little doubt concerning the origin of the circulating blood monocyte, there continues to be considerable debate as to the origin of tissue macrophages, such as the resident peritoneal macrophage and the alveolar and interstitial macrophages of the lung. Evidence presented indicates that tissue macrophages are simply derived by the demobilization of circulating blood monocytes, whereas contradicting evidence argues that tissue macrophages proliferate locally. The objective of this section is to discuss the role of locally produced and monocyte-derived macrophages under steady-state and inflammatory conditions.

2.1. Steady-State Conditions

The origin of tissue macrophages (local production versus monocyte influx) appears to vary according to tissue/organ type and whether the measurements were made under steady-state or inflammatory conditions. For example, current evidence for the lung suggests that a major proportion of the pulmonary alveolar macrophage population (70%) may be sustained, under steady-state conditions, by local macrophage proliferation. This conclusion is based on several lines of evidence, including (1) the maintenance of the size of the alveolar macrophage population during periods of monocytopenia induced either by sytemic hydrocortisone administration (Lin *et al.*, 1982), or by external or internal bone marrow irradiation (Tarling and Coggle, 1982; Sawyer *et al.*, 1982); (2) the large reduction of the pulmonary alveolar macrophage population following irradiation of the thorax (Tarling and Coggle, 1982); (3) a more accurate appreciation of the turnover time of pulmonary alveolar macrophages (Coggle and Tarling, 1984); and (4) an analysis of the alveolar macrophage populations in parabiotic mice (Sawyer, 1986). Indeed, the contribution of locally proliferated pulmonary macrophages has now been recognized by van Furth *et al.* (1985a) in revised calculations of the origin and kinetics of these cells.

The Kupffer cells of the liver, however, appear to be more dependent on the circulating blood monocyte for the repletion of senescent cells under steady-state conditions with perhaps only about 8% derived by local division (van Furth *et al.*, 1985a). Evidence from the scanning electron microscope (Satodate *et al.*, 1985) indicates the importance of the sinusoidal fenestration for the settlement of blood monocytes on the sinusoidal surfaces of the liver, again pointing to the monocytic origin of the Kupffer cell.

In all likelihood, the resident tissue macrophages originate from two sources, despite the polarized views presented. The picture emerging is that macrophage replenishment in the steady state results from both local division and monocyte influx, with the proportions of cells derived from each pathway varying according to the tissue or organ studied. Thus, it is conceivable that the division of tissue macrophages provides cells with a tissue-specific function, while the monocyte-derived cells perform some of the more generic functions of macrophages, after adapting to the local conditions that prevail in the tissue to which they have migrated (for review, see Ginsel *et al.*, 1985.)

2.2. Inflammatory Conditions

Unlike the question of the origin of resident tissue macrophages, there is now little doubt that under inflammatory conditions circulating blood monocytes are actively recruited into organs and tissues, where they further differentiate into macrophages. This recruitment has been demonstrated for the inflammatory response in the peritoneal cavity following intraperitoneal injection of mild sterile inflammatory agents, such as latex spherules and newborn calf serum (van Furth et al., 1973); in the lung following the intrabronchial instillation of bacillus Calmette-Guérin (BCG) (Blusse van Oud Alblas et al., 1983); and in the liver following the intravenous administration of inflammatory stimuli such as zymosan particles (Bouwens and Wisse, 1985) or glucan (Deimann and Fahima, 1980). However, after the initial influx of circulating blood monocytes, local macrophages frequently develop mitotic activity. Daems (1980) suggested that under steady-state conditions, blood monocytes rapidly migrate through the vasculature of tissues and organs for the purposes of surveillance, while under inflammatory or other insultory conditions the monocytes accumulate in the tissues, where they differentiate into macrophages and assist in the activities of the resident tissue macrophages. An obvious implication of Daems's idea is that the responsive adaptable circulating blood monocyte can differentiate into a macrophage whose functional properties are determined by the prevailing conditions it encounters at the site of demobilization (e.g., in response to stimuli such as bacteria, activated complement components, connective tissue breakdown products, oxygen tension). On the basis of work conducted in vivo and in vitro, the ability of the monocyte to undergo stimulus-dependent differentiation into macrophages with markedly differing functional properties is likely to be of great significance to understanding both the beneficial and deleterious aspects of macrophage involvement in health and disease. (Monocyte maturation and differentiation are discussed in Section 4.)

As a tissue, the skin generally contains very few macrophages, although during an inflammatory response the number of cells increases quite strikingly. Evidence first presented by Leibovich and Ross (1975) showed that the increase in the number of macrophages during an inflammatory response (wound healing) is derived from circulating blood monocytes. These investigators found that the systemic administration of hydrocortisone (an inducer of monocytopenia) resulted in a 66% reduction in the number of macrophages associated with experimentally induced skin wounds in the guinea pig. Locally administered antimacrophage serum had no effect on the number of circulating monocytes, nor did it affect the number of wound macrophages.

Similar conclusions have been drawn concerning the bone marrow origin of macrophages in healing wounds of humans by Stewart et al. (1981). By observing the karyotype (sex chromosome markers) of macrophages and fibroblasts emigrating from explants of a 5-day skin wound, derived from a 9-year-old girl who had recently received a bone marrow graft from her 11-year-old brother, it was found that the fibroblasts had the karyote of the recipient, while the macrophages bore the karotype of the donor. Thus, the data suggest that the macrophages of the healing wound were derived from bone marrow while the fibroblasts were presumed to originate in local tissue.

In an attempt to gain information about the origin and kinetics of macrophages in the skin under inflammatory conditions in the mouse, van Furth et al. (1985b) measured the rate of appearance of mononuclear phagocytes onto a subcutaneously inserted glass coverslip (the inflammatory stimulus). Removal and examination of the coverslips 3–6 hr postinsertion revealed a large influx of granulocytes. However, when the coverslips were removed after 6–8 hr, the granulocytes had been replaced by mononuclear cells, which visually and functionally resembled blood monocytes. The number of mononuclear phagocytes that attached to the glass coverslips correlated directly with the time the coverslips were left in place. On the basis of (1) similarities in the [³H]thymidine-labeling indices of circulating blood monocytes and the mononuclear phagocytes that became attached to the glass coverslips; and (2) the fact that the induction of a monocytopenia, by systemic administration of hydrocortisone prior to the insertion of the glass coverslips, resulted in a large reduction in the accumulation of mononuclear phagocytes onto the surface of the coverslip; the investigators also concluded that the increase in the number of macrophages during this type of inflammatory response in the skin was almost exclusively (99%) due to an influx of circulating blood monocytes, with little or no proliferation of local tissue macrophages.

Thus, to summarize, the evidence seems to indicate that under steady state conditions, the macrophage content of organs and tissues is replenished predominantly by local macrophage proliferation, although there is also a contribution by the blood-borne monocyte. Under inflammatory conditions, the rapid increase in macrophage numbers is due principally to the emigration of monocytes from the vasculature. The obvious next question is, what triggers the migration of monocytes from the vasculature to the extravascular space during an inflammatory response?

3. Monocyte Migration and the Role of Connective Tissue Components

3.1. Multiplicity of *in Vivo* Monocyte Chemotactic Factors

From the discussion in Section 2.2, it is clear that macrophage involvement in wound healing is dependent on an influx and accumulation of circulating blood monocytes in the affected tissue (see Chapter 3). The emigration of these cells from the vasculature to the extravascular compartment appears to be effected by many different endogenous and exogenous chemotactic agents which are probably generated within the extravascular compartment. In this context, one can envisage a sequence of events leading to the generation of neutrophil and monocyte chemotactic factors. Disruption of capillaries will lead to the extravasation of blood plasma and formed elements, platelet aggregation and activation, blood coagulation, and the generation of activated complement components and kinins. Many of these elements behave as strong chemotactic factors for inflammatory cells (see Chapter 5). In addition, other monocyte chemotactic agents may be generated by degradation of the connective tissue matrix. A list of some monocyte chemotactic factors that may be active *in vivo* can be found in Table I. However, this discussion is limited to some selected factors of relevance to monocyte migration to the skin under inflammatory (as opposed to immune) circumstances.

Table I. Monocyte Chemotactic Factors

Factors	Investigators
Plasma-derived factors	
Complement-derived peptides C5a and C5a des Arg	Marder *et al.* (1985)
Fibrinopeptides	Kay *et al.* (1973)
IgG-proteolytic fragments	Ishida *et al.* (1978)
Macrophage chemotactic factor from skin (MCFS-1)	Kambara *et al.* (1977)
Thrombin	Bar-Shavit *et al.* (1983)
Extracellular matrix-derived factors	
Collagen/collagen fragments	Postlethwaite and Kang (1976)
Elastin/elastin fragments	Senior *et al.* (1980)
Fibronectin fragments	Norris *et al.* (1982)
Cell-derived factors	
Leukotriene B_4	Ford-Hutchinson *et al.* (1980)
Platelet factor 4	Deuel *et al.* (1981)
Arterial smooth muscle cell factor	Jauchem *et al.* (1982)
Bacterial-derived factors	
Formyl methionyl peptides	Snyderman and Fudman (1980)
N-Acetylmuramyl-L-alanyl-D-isoglytamine	Ogawa *et al.* (1983)

3.2. Complement Component Fragments C5a and C5a des Arg

Activation of either the classic or alternative pathway of the complement system results in cleavage of the N-terminal region of the α-chain of C5, thereby generating C5a, a basic, 11 kD glycopeptide possessing potent inflammatory properties. C5a behaves as a vasodilatory agent, as an anaphylatoxin (releasing histamine and other granule constituents from mast cells), as well as a chemotactic factor for neutrophils and monocytes (Chapter 5). When injected into skin, nanogram quantities of human C5a induce a wheal-and-flare reaction within seconds, peaking in intensity 10–30 min after injection but essentially disappears 60 min after injection (Yancey *et al.*, 1985). The changes in vascular permeability induced by C5a injection are probably due to an effect (that appears to be neutrophils dependent) on the vascular endothelium, as well as a vasodilatory effect caused by C5a-dependent prostaglandin production (Wedmore and Williams, 1981).

C5a is rapidly converted to C5a des Arg by serum carboxypeptidase N, which largely inactivates its anaphylatoxic properties and inhibits its neutrophil chemotactic activity by a factor of 10–15-fold. Interestingly, and of considerable significance to the migration of circulating blood monocytes to sites of inflammation, the conversion of C5a to C5a des Arg apparently has no effect on the activity of this molecule as a monocyte chemotactic factor, with maximal chemotactic responses to both peptides seen at a concentration of 3.6 $\times 10^{-9}$ M (Marder et al., 1985). Curiously, however, in investigating the binding of [^{125}I]-C5a and [^{125}I]-C5a des Arg to purified monocytes it was found that C5a des Arg, while apparently binding to the same receptor as C5a, binds with an affinity approximately 100-fold weaker than that observed with C5a (Marder et al., 1985). A second significant trait of C5a and C5a des Arg is their ability to stimulate in vitro adherence of purified human peripheral blood monocytes to monolayers of human microvascular endothelial cells (Doherty et al., 1987). The latter process is essential for monocyte diapedesis through blood vessel walls en route to the site of attraction in the extravascular compartment.

3.3. Connective Tissue Matrix Proteins

Purified components of the connective tissue matrix also express chemotactic activity in vitro for monocytes and fibroblasts. These connective tissue components include major structural proteins such as collagen and elastin as well as less abundant proteins such as fibronectin. Interestingly, small proteolytic cleavage fragments of collagen, elastin, and fibronectin are also chemotactic for fibroblasts and monocytes.

Type I collagen, the major structural protein of skin, is chemotactic for monocytes and fibroblasts, though not for neutrophils (Postlethwaite and Kang, 1976; Postlethwaite et al., 1978). This chemotactic property is expressed by native collagen as well as by cyanogen bromide and proteolytically derived collagen fragments varying in molecular size from small oligopeptides (3–10-amino acids) to larger fragments the size of ovalbumin (43,000 M_r). Senior and colleagues (1980) also found that oligopeptides (14,000–20,000 M_r), derived by digestion of human aortic elastin and bovine ligament elastin with human neutrophil elastase, are also preferentially chemotactic for monocytes. More recent studies localized the chemotactic activity of elastin to the repeating peptide sequence Val-Gly-Val-Ala-Pro-Gly (Senior et al., 1984).

Fibronectin is also deposited at inflammatory sites and areas of wound healing. This 440,000-M_r glycoprotein, produced by a variety of cell types, such as fibroblasts, endothelial cells, and mononuclear phagocytes, associates with fibrin and collagen fibrils and appears to be derived both from local synthesis as well as from blood plasma. Once deposited, fibronectin exhibits several functions: it behaves as an anchor protein for fibroblasts (see Chapter 10) and mononuclear phagocytes (Bevilacqua et al., 1981; Clark et al., 1984; Horsburgh et al., 1987) and directs the migration of epidermal cells during wound re-epithelization (see Chapters 13 and 14). The intact fibronectin molecule was found to be chemotactically inactive (Clark et al., 1985). However, studies have shown that proteolytic fragments derived from plasma fibronectin may serve as potent chemotactic factors for circulating blood monocytes, although not for neutrophils or lymphocytes (Norris et al., 1982). The chemotactic activity of fibronectin fragments (produced spontaneously during the purification of plasma fibronectin) is bimodal, with genuine chemotaxis observed at low protein concentrations (1–100 μg/ml), while at higher concentrations (300–600 μg/ml) a chemokinetic response appears to contribute to the enhanced migration of the monocytes through the nucleopore filters. In more recent studies, the chemotactic active site has been localized to a 120,000-M_r fibronectin fragment that contains the RGDS fibroblastic cell binding site (Clark et al., 1984). It is also significant that fibronectin fragments are chemotactic for fibroblasts (Postlethwaite et al., 1981).

If connective tissue fragments are chemotactically active in vivo, this raises the question of how are they generated, since it implies that some degradation of the connective tissue matrix must take place before monocytes can be attracted to the area. One possibility is that neutrophils, whose accumulation at an inflammatory site generally precedes that of monocytes, promote some limited degradation of the connective tissue matrix, thereby generating monocyte chemotactic factors. Consistent with this notion is the finding that neutrophil granules contain both elastase (Murphy et al., 1977) and collagenase (Robertson et al., 1972), activities capable of degrading insoluble collagen and elastin to soluble (and therefore potentially chemotactic) fragments. Human granulocyte elastase and cathepsin G have also been reported to degrade fibronectin (McDonald and Kelley, 1980; Vartio, 1982). In seeming contradiction to this hypothesis, Simpson and Ross (1972) found that neutrophil depletion of guinea pigs with antineutrophil serum had no effect on the migration of monocytes to a site of inflammation in the skin. However, in tissue injury, proteases are generated from sources other than neutrophils. For example, plasmin is generated from plasma-derived plasminogen by plasminogen activator (see Chapter 21) and degrades fibronectin (Jilek and Hormann, 1977).

3.4. Interactions with Multiple Chemotactic Factors

The nature and characteristics of just a few of the many chemotactic factors that might be generated during an inflammatory response in vivo have been discussed, raising the important issue of whether different chemotactic factors attract different subpopulations of monocytes or whether monocytes express multiple receptors for different chemotactic factors. In conventional chemotaxis assays using a Boyden chamber, it was consistently found that only a proportion (40–60%) of peripheral blood monocytes migrate through nucleopore filters in response to chemotactic agents such as C5a, N-formyl-methionyl-leucyl-phenylalanine (FMLP), or T-cell-derived lymphokines. This observation led to the question of whether there are different subpopulations of migrating monocytes with different chemotaxin receptors or combinations of receptors on the surface of each monocyte? By showing that the cells that migrate into a nucleopore filter in response to one chemotactic factor could then migrate out of the filter in the reverse direction when the chemotactic factor was removed from the lower chamber, and a second chemotactic factor was placed in the upper chamber, it became apparent that a migrating population of monocytes could respond to more than one chemotactic factor. Furthermore, stimulus-specific desensitization to one stimulus (FMLP) did not inhibit the migration of cells to another stimulus (activated serum) when chemotactic factors were employed at low concentration (although high doses of single chemotactic agents will induce cross-desensitization to other stimuli) (Cianciolo and Snyderman, 1981). Thus, the evidence documented by two independent laboratories (Falk and Leonard, 1980; Cianciolo and Snyderman, 1981) indicates that monocytes express multiple receptors for different chemotactic factors.

The implications are (1) that the multiple chemotactic factors generated during an inflammatory response potentially all play a role in the attraction of monocytes to that site; and (2) that the responding monocyte population is relatively homogeneous.

4. Monocyte Maturation and Differentiation

4.1. Monocyte–Macrophage Maturation

After migrating from the vasculature into the tissues in response to an inflammatory stimulus, monocytes rapidly differentiate into cells with characteristics that lie somewhere between those of the monocyte and the resident tissue macrophage. These cells, which are often referred to as inflammatory macrophages, have been studied extensively *in vitro*. They can be obtained in relatively large quantities by irritation of the peritoneal cavity of laboratory animals with sterile stimuli, such as thioglycollate medium, proteose peptone, mineral oil, heterologous serum, and endotoxin. Macrophages isolated from experimentally-induced inflammatory granulomas also express the phenotype of the inflammatory macrophage (Bonney *et al.*, 1978).

Some of the properties and characteristics of inflammatory macrophages are illustrated in Table II. Many of these capacities are suggestive of the pre-

Table II. Properties of Inflammatory Macrophages

Receptors
    Increased expression of IgG–Fc receptor
    Increased expression of transferrin receptors
    Ingestion of iC3b-sensitized targets via the CR3 receptor

Secreted products
    Induction of elastase secretion
    Induction of collagenase secretion
    Induction of plasminogen activator secretion

Intracellular products
    Increased activities of lysosomal acid hydrolases
    Increased levels of tissue transglutaminase
    Increased activity of creatine kinase
    Increased activity of cAMP-dependent protein kinase 1

sumed function of macrophages in the inflammatory response, that is, as a predominant mediator of tissue debridement. Notable traits include increased levels of lysosomal enzymes, enhanced capacities for endocytosis, the ability to ingest particulate material via C3b and iC3b receptors, and the secretion of the neutral proteases plasminogen activator and elastase. The roles of some of the macrophage's altered capacities in the process of tissue debridement are discussed in Section 5.

The differentiation of human monocytes into macrophages can be stimulated (and thus studied) simply by culturing purified peripheral blood monocytes in the presence of autologous (Musson, 1983) or heterologous serum (Zuckermann et al., 1979) for 5–7 days. In the absence of a serum source, monocytes remain in their undifferentiated state. The process of differentiation is associated with many phenotypic changes similar to those seen in in vivo-derived inflammatory macrophages, including (1) the increased expression of cell-surface receptors for complement component iC3b (Newman et al., 1980), IgG–Fc (Jungo and Hafner, 1986) and transferrin (Hirata et al., 1986); (2) the enhanced expression of intracellular enzymes such as α-hexosaminidase (Musson et al., 1980, creatine kinase (Loike et al., 1984), tissue tranglutaminase (Murtaugh et al., 1984), and cAMP-dependent protein kinase 1 (Wenger and O'Dorisio, 1985); and (3) the downregulation of the capacity to secrete hydrogen peroxide and superoxide anion (Nakagawara et al., 1981). In addition, the differentiation of monocytes into macrophages is apparently negatively regulated by γ-interferon (Lee and Epstein, 1980; Becker, 1984) and by corticosteroids (Rinehart et al., 1982).

The mechanisms responsible for driving the differentiation of monocytes into inflammatory macrophages are unclear. In vitro studies have indicated that several serum constituents may be implicated, including 1,25-dihydroxyvitamin D_3 (Proveddini et al., 1986; Tanaka et al., 1983). In the context of wound healing, an attractive theory for the extravascular differentiation of monocytes has stemmed from experiments in which the effect of fibronectin binding to monocytes was investigated. Circulating blood monocytes express a high-avidity magnesium-dependent plasma membrane receptor for surface-bound fibronectin (Bevilacqua et al., 1981; Hosein and Bianco, 1985). The receptor facilitates the attachment of monocytes to extracellular matrix, probably by recognizing the sequence Arg-Gly-Asp-Ser of fibronectin (Wright and Meyer, 1985). Engagement of fibronectin receptors by surface-bound ligands induces several functional changes within the monocyte, the most significant of which, in terms of monocyte differentiation, is the activation of the C3b and iC3b receptors for phagocytosis (Wright et al., 1983), and the ability to secrete plasminogen activator and elastase following stimulation by nonspecific phagocytosis (Bianco, 1983). Thus, monocytes binding insolubilized fibronectin assume some of the characteristics of inflammatory macrophages. In other words, the mere process of binding monocytes to connective tissue fibronectin may, by itself, be sufficient to drive the differentiation of monocytes into inflammatory macrophages (Hosein et al., 1985). The finding that the binding of soluble fibronectin to monocytes is minimal suggests a control mechanism to limit monocyte differentiation to areas of fibronectin deposition (Clark *et al.*, 1984). This mechanism does not exclude other possible mechanisms for the induction of monocyte differentiation.

4.2. Macrophage Phenotypic Differentiation and Activation

The inflammatory macrophage has also been referred to as a responsive macrophage. At this stage of differentiation, the macrophage possesses all the machinery to permit it to participate actively in the degradation of the connective tissue matrix and the subsequent process of tissue remodeling. In all probability, at least in a sterile wound, the responsive macrophage does not differentiate any further.

However, the term responsive indicates another important property of these cells, namely, their ability to respond to signals which can further change the functional and phenotypic properties of the inflammatory macrophage. Macrophages respond to these signals in a two-step process, termed macrophage activation (Fig. 1). In the first step, responsive macrophages interact with a primary stimulus, usually α-, β-, or γ-interferon. This first step converts responsive macrophages to primed macrophages. The primed macrophages show an enhanced ability to interact with neoplastic target cells, but are unable to destroy them. In the second step, a triggering stimulus, usually a bacterial or viral product, such as lipopolysaccharide or double-stranded RNA, drives the primed macrophage to the fully activated phenotype. Macrophages now express full competence to lyse tumor cells, as well as enhanced microbicidal activity. Macrophages cannot be triggered to express the activated phenotype in the absence of a priming signal. The fully activated macrophage phenotype might be advantageous for effective containment of virulent microorganisms in

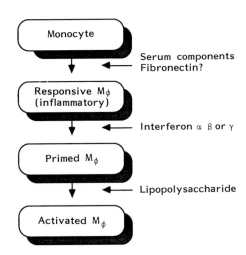

Figure 1. The pathway of differentiation of monocytes to macrophages and subsequent activation by exogenous and endogenous environmental stimuli.

an infected wound (Adams and Hamilton, 1983). (The issue of macrophage phenotypes is raised again in Section 6.2.)

5. Role of Mononuclear Phagocytes in Tissue Debridement

It is apparent that one must consider the role of both the monocyte and the inflammatory macrophage in the process of tissue debridement, since mononuclear phagocytes initially enter an inflammatory site with the phenotype of a monocyte, and differentiate into macrophages only later. Monocytes begin to arrive at the inflammatory site several hours after the initial neutrophil influx. [Not only do neutrophils ingest and kill bacteria, they also can destroy tissue by the generation of oxygen radicals, which could damage adjacent tissue cells, and the secretion of granule constituents, such as lysosomal enzymes, which might degrade connective tissue matrix (see Chapter 6).] Upon arrival at the inflammatory site, monocytes probably undertake operations similar to those of neutrophils, i.e., bacterial killing, and secretion of lysosomal enzymes and oxygen radicals, although the time it takes monocytes to liberate these enzymes and oxygen radicals is somewhat longer than the time it takes for neutrophils. A significant question regarding the role of lysosomal enzymes in the degradation of the connective tissue matrix is whether the pH of the local pericellular microenvironment can be reduced sufficiently to allow the predominantly acid pH-optimal lysosomal enzymes to become active. Evidence presented indicates that under certain conditions cells can acidify their immediate local environment. This appears to be true for the chrondrocyte during cartilage breakdown (Dingle et al., 1975) and the osteoclast during bone resorption (Schenk, 1974). Indeed, Etherington (1980) indicated that the pH level at the attachment site of a macrophage to its substratum can fall below 5. In general, lysosomal enzymes have pH optima in the 3.5–5.5 range. Thus, one might expect that under conditions of low pH, lysosomal enzymes will be active at least for a limited period in the microenvironment. However, extracellular degradation by lysosomal enzymes is probably a minor contribution of the mononuclear phagocyte to the process of tissue debridement. As discussed below, after their differentiation into macrophages, mononuclear phagocytes are considerably more active as effector cells in the process of connective tissue breakdown.

5.1. Degradation of the Connective Tissue Matrix

Put simply, the connective tissue matrix consists of a crosslinked supporting framework of collagen fibrils that endow the tissue with the properties of tensile strength. Added to this is a crosslinked network of elastin fibers that provide the tissue with elastic properties. Finally, the mesh of collagen and elastin fibrils is saturated with a filler substance composed of proteoglycans (consisting of a protein backbone with long-chain glycosaminoglycans attached) and other glycoproteins such as laminin and fibronectin (see Chapters

18–20). Successful breakdown of the connective tissue matrix requires enzymes capable of degrading these major constituents.

There is abundant evidence to implicate the macrophage as one of the major effector cells involved in the removal and degradation of damaged connective tissue at inflammatory sites, prior to the initiation of tissue reconstruction. Responsive macrophages synthesize and secrete several neutral pH-optimum proteolytic enzymes that play an instrumental role in this catabolic process. These proteolytic enzymes are capable of degrading collagen and elastin, as well as the ground substance proteoglycans and their constituent glycosaminoglycans. Increasing evidence also indicates that the fibroblast may be a major source of collagenase (see Chapter 21). It seems likely that some cleavage of the connective tissue matrix is initiated extracellularly, thereby generating smaller fragments of tissue debris which can subsequently be ingested by macrophages and degraded intracellularly by the lysosomal system.

5.2. Extracellular Degradation of the Connective Tissue Matrix

The macrophage has been found to synthesize several enzymes that are involved in the extracellular degradation of the connective tissue matrix (Table II). The degradation can, to some extent, be considered a softening-up process, to produce smaller pieces of connective tissue matrix for subsequent ingestion and intracellular degradation by the lysosomal system.

Investigations initiated during the mid-1970s identified three inducible secreted neutral proteases of macrophages as elastase, collagenase, and plasminogen activator. Plasminogen activator itself has little proteolytic activity but in the presence of plasminogen, the potent proteolytic enzyme, plasmin, is generated (see Chapter 21). Resident mouse peritoneal macrophages constitutively secrete almost undetectable amounts of these enzymes, while responsive macrophages constitutively secrete relatively abundant quantities of all three enzymes (Unkeless et al., 1974; Werb and Gordon, 1975a,b).

The role of these macrophage-derived enzymes in the degradation of connective tissue matrices has been studied in vitro, using the extracellular connective tissue matrix that is deposited on the surfaces of Petri dishes by vascular smooth muscle cells, endothelial cells, or fibroblasts as a physiologic substrate (Jones and Scott-Burden, 1979; Werb et al., 1980a). This system is unique since the cells involved in the deposition of the connective tissue matrix can be cultured in the presence of radioactivity-labeled amino acid and sugar precursors, thereby internally labeling the connective tissue matrix. This system provides a significant amount of information about the characteristics of the macrophage populations involved in the breakdown of the connective tissue matrix, as well as the relative importance of the various enzymes that are secreted or retained within these cells.

Highly purified mouse macrophage elastase degraded both the elastin and glycoprotein components of the connective tissue matrix, while plasmin, a product of macrophage plasminogen activation, degraded 50–70% of the glycoprotein component, but had no effect on collagen or elastin (Werb et al., 1980a). Highly purified fibroblast collagenase (mouse macrophage collagenase has not been purified for functional analysis) was found to be specific for the collagenous component of the matrices. Degradation of all three components of the connective tissue matrix was accomplished when responsive macrophages were cultured on the connective tissue matrices, a property shared with conditioned medium from these cells. However, by comparison with fibroblast collagenase, the collagenolytic potential of the conditioned medium appeared to be low (Jones and Werb, 1980).

The elastinolytic activity of the mononuclear phagocyte changes as the monocyte differentiates into the responsive macrophage. Isolated human blood monocytes express a serine-esterase type elastase activity that is biochemically and antigenically indistinguishable from human neutrophil elastase (Sandhaus et al., 1983). However, as monocytes differentiate into macrophages in vitro, the elastinolytic activity changes from a serine esterase to that of a metalloproteinase. The time course of change to this latter elastase activity coincides with that of monocyte differentiation into the responsive macrophage. Thus, the conversion of the elastase activity from the initial serine esterase to a metalloproteinase appears to be a maturationally linked event. The metalloproteinase elastase of mouse responsive macrophages was thoroughly investigated by Banda and Werb (1981). The 22,000-M_r enzyme, optimally active at pH 8.0, is inhibited by α_2-macroglobulin, but not by α_1-antitrypsin. Other studies have indicated that macrophage elastase is also proteolytically active against a variety of nonelastin substrates, including fibrinogen, fibrin, fibronectin, laminin, immunoglobulins, and proteoglycans (Banda et al., 1983, 1985).

Ultrastructural and biochemical observations of the macrophage–connective tissue matrix interactions revealed that the connective tissue components are initially degraded extracellularly in the immediate vicinity of the cells. Degradation of the matrix can sometimes extend several millimeters from the macrophages (Werb et al., 1980b). This process may be mediated by secreted proteases and by membrane-associated proteases, including elastase (Lavie et al., 1980). In general, extracellular degradation of the connective tissue matrix in this in vitro system, generated fragments with molecular weights greater than 5000. It seems likely that some degradation of the proteoglycan and glycoprotein components precedes the initiation of elastin or collagen degradation, in order to allow elastase and collagenase access to their respective substrates (Anderson, 1976; Jones and Werb, 1980).

5.3. Intracellular Degradation of the Connective Tissue Matrix

While in vitro investigations show that connective tissue matrices can be almost completely degraded extracellularly (Werb et al., 1980b, Jones and Werb, 1980), other studies of connective tissue matrix breakdown in vivo (using the postpartum mouse uterus as a model) show macrophages to be actively engaged in the phagocytosis of stromal collagen fibers (Parakkal, 1972) that are considerably larger than the fragments generated in in vitro studies (discussed in Section 5.2). Furthermore, by localizing the lysosomal enzyme acid phosphatase to the collagen-containing organelles, collagen fibers were concluded to be localized in secondary lysosomes (Parakkal, 1972). Since the collagen fibers were only discernible for 24–48 hr, it was evident that the ingested collagen was rapidly digested. The reasons for the differences in the reported sizes of the connective tissue fragments produced in these two studies are unclear; however, the studies differ fundamentally in several ways. There are two notable discrepancies: (1) the composition of the connective tissue matrices produced in vitro may be significantly different from those laid down in vivo; and (2) differences almost certainly exist in the diffusional capacity, and the enzyme:substrate ratios of secreted enzymes in the two models. The discrepancies may result in significant differences in the rate of extracellular and intracellular degradation.

The characteristics of two lysosomal enzymes implicated in the intracellular degradation of collagen fragments have been studied by Etherington and colleagues. Named cathepsin B and cathepsin N, both enzymes are thiol-dependent proteinases that are optimally active at pH 3.5, with negligible activity seen above pH 4.5. Both appear to cleave the collagen molecule in the nonhelical N-telopeptide region (Etherington, 1976). The fragments produced by the action of cathepsins B and N are then presumed to be further degraded by other lysosomal endo- and exopeptidases. However, the identity of these enzymes is unclear. There is little evidence in the literature regarding acid optimal collagenases, with the exception of a recently reported acid collagenase in osteoclasts (Blair et al., 1986).

Irrespective of the differences in these experimental systems, the clear indication from these studies is that macrophage-dependent degradation of the connective tissue matrix probably represents a two step process in which some degradation is initiated extracellularly, thereby producing fragments which are subsequently ingested and digested intracellularly.

The mechanism of uptake of connective tissue fragments by macrophages remains largely speculative. Over recent years, a number of receptors, previously described as nonspecific receptors, were identified. It is conceivable that these and other macrophage cell surface receptor systems may be involved in the uptake of fragments of the connective tissue matrix. For example, the scavenger receptor, believed to mediate the uptake of acetylated low-density lipoproteins, also binds sulfated polysaccharides such as dextran sulfate and maleylated albumin (Brown et al., 1980). It is conceivable that this receptor may also mediate the uptake of connective tissue fragments via their constituent glycosaminoglycans (which are also sulfated polysaccharides). Locally deposited fibronectin, which binds to denatured collagen more readily than native collagen, may also facilitate this process by promoting macrophage phagocytosis (Gudewicz et al., 1980).

5.4. Regulation of Fibroblast Collagenase Secretion by Macrophages

Although responsive macrophages have been shown to synthesize and secrete an extracellularly acting collagenase activity (Werb and Gordon,

1975a), the amounts of enzyme produced are relatively low and appear to contribute little to the in vitro degradation of experimental connective tissue matrices (Werb et al., 1980a). Rapidly accumulating evidence points to the fibroblast as perhaps the major connective tissue cell involved in collagen breakdown under physiologic and pathologic conditions. The secretion of collagenase is not a constitutive property of fibroblasts, but rather is an inducible response dependent on de novo protein synthesis and which appears tightly controlled by factors secreted by macrophages (see Chapter 21).

Early evidence of macrophage regulation of fibroblast collagenase secretion was obtained by Huybrechts-Godin et al. (1979). They observed that coincubation of macrophages and fibroblasts on a ^{14}C-labeled collagen film led to a more rapid and extensive degradation of the collagen matrix, when compared with either fibroblasts or macrophages alone. Similarly, conditioned medium from macrophages stimulated the degradation of the collagen films by fibroblasts. These early investigations suggest that the secretion of the factor (or factors) responsible for inducing collagenase secretion by fibroblasts was constitutively secreted by macrophages in culture. In more recent studies from the same laboratory, rabbit bone marrow macrophages were cultured for various periods of time; conditioned medium was then tested for the induction of collagenase secretion in cultures of human, rabbit. and mouse dermal fibroblasts. Maximum collagenase secretion was noted on the third day of culture and thus appears synchronized with the appearance of the responsive macrophage phenotype and with the production of plasminogen activator and elastase by inflammatory macrophages (see Chapter 18). Thus, the most recent studies indicate that the secretion of the macrophage regulatory factor is developmentally regulated.

Other recent investigations have focused on the identity of the monokine responsible for the induction of fibroblast collagenase synthesis. On the basis of similarities in the physical characteristics of the purified monokine, several independent laboratories concluded that the active material is interleukin-1 (IL-1) (Postlethwaite et al., 1983; Huybrechts-Godin et al., 1985). IL-1 is not only secreted by bone marrow macrophages, but is also the mononuclear cell factor (MCF) involved in the control of collagenase synthesis by rheumatoid synovial fibroblasts and rabbit articular chondrocytes (Dayer et al., 1979, 1986; Mizel et al., 1981). Thus, macrophages play a pivotal role in the process of tissue debridement by secreting both tissue degrading proteolytic enzymes as well as factors that regulate the secretion of the enzyme collagenase by fibroblasts.

6. Macrophage Involvement in Tissue Remodeling

Experiments conducted by Leibovich and Ross (1975) showed mononuclear phagocyte depletion of guinea pigs to be associated with an impairment of wound healing, providing the first concrete evidence that macrophages are essential to the final phase of wound healing, i.e., the process of tissue repair and remodeling. Subsequent studies in several different experimental systems have provided further evidence of the association of macrophages with cell proliferation during the granulation tissue phase of wound healing (e.g., Hunt et al., 1984; Miller et al., 1986).

Macrophages are now known to participate in at least three aspects of tissue remodeling: (1) as a source of growth factors for fibroblasts and other mesenchymal cells; (2) as a source of angiogenic factors involved in the neo-vascularization of the healing wound; and (3) as a source of factors that can modulate the production of connective tissue matrix proteins by other cells (e.g., fibroblasts) within the local microenvironment.

6.1. Macrophage-Derived Growth Factor

Several lines of evidence initially suggested that macrophages may play a role in the proliferation of fibroblasts, smooth muscle cells, and other mesenchymal cells. After the demonstration that in vivo depletion of circulating monocytes and local tissue macrophages in guinea pigs, by treatment with hydrocortisone and antimacrophage serum, respectively, resulted in an inhibition of both fibroblast proliferation and connective tissue formation (Leibovich and Ross, 1975), subsequent studies showed that macrophages actively secrete a factor (or factors) that induce the proliferation of quiescent fibroblasts (Leibovich and Ross, 1976). These growth factors are collectively known as macrophage-derived growth factor (MDGF) but, unlike platelet-derived growth factor (PDGF), MDGF is not retained intracellularly but is synthesized by macrophages and directly secreted to the extracellular environment.

In vitro investigations indicate that the secretion of MDGF is a constitutive property of monocytes and macrophages. However, the level of MDGF secretion can be significantly increased following stimulation of macrophages with a variety of agents including bacterial endotoxin, concanavalin A (Glenn and Ross, 1981), fibronectin (Martin et al., 1983), and phorbol diesters (Leslie et al., 1984). The exact nature of MDGF remains to be determined and it almost certainly represents multiple growth factors. Similarities have been reported to exist among MDGF and PDGF (Shimokado et al., 1984), IL-1 (Schmidt et al., 1985), and pituitary fibroblast growth factor (Baird et al., 1985).

Macrophage-derived growth factor also stimulates the in vitro proliferation of other mesenchymal cells, specifically smooth muscle cell and vascular endothelial cells (Martin et al., 1981; Polverini et al., 1977). It also appears likely that these are the responses to multiple growth factors in macrophage conditioned medium. In support of this concept is the finding that interleukin 1, which originally was identified as a macrophage-derived T-cell growth factor, is mitogenic for fibroblasts and T cells but not for arterial smooth muscle cells or vascular endothelial cells (Libby et al., 1985).

6.2. Macrophage Involvement in Tissue Neovascularization

Studies initiated in the mid-1970s showed that another significant role of the macrophage in the process of wound healing is the contribution of an-

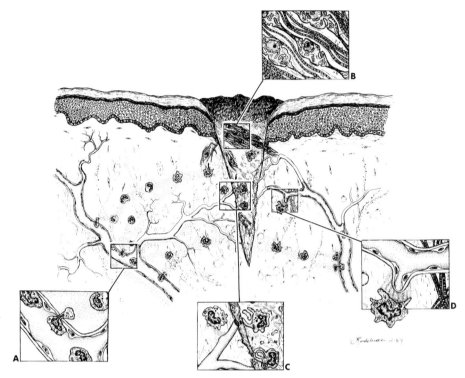

Figure 2. Schematic representation of the phases of macrophage involvement in wound repair. (a) Emigration of a blood-borne monocyte from the vasculature to the extravascular tissue. Under the influence of chemotactic factors generated at the site of injury, the monocyte is initially thought to adhere to the vascular endothelium before migrating through the wall of the blood vessel. (b) Having arrived at the inflammatory site, the monocyte differentiates into a macrophage. One of the early functions of the macrophage is to control the process of tissue debridement. This is achieved by the secretion of proteolytic enzymes, and by the secretion of a factor (probably interleukin-1), which stimulates wound fibroblasts to secrete collagenase. After debridement is complete, fibroblases secrete collagen (a process that is under macrophage control) as part of the reparative process. (c) Macrophages also participate in the reparative phase by secreting angiogenesis factor(s) that stimulate the directed outgrowth of endothelial cells from adjacent capillaries. (d) Angiogenesis probably proceeds in the form of budding from nearby capillaries. Ultimately, a new network of capillaries will be established to restore the circulation in the healing wound area.

giogenesis factors which stimulate the directed outgrowth of new capillaries (neovascularization) towards a specific stimulus of the avascular, collagen–fibroblast meshwork of the wound space. The new capillary growth is thought to result from the ability of angiogenesis factors to induce the directed migration of endothelial cells, as well as perhaps stimulating the proliferation of endothelial, smooth muscle, and other mesenchymal cells involved in the formation of new blood capillaries. Early evidence suggested the involvement of macrophages in wound tissue neovascularization, since macrophages isolated from wound fluids were potently angiogenic when injected into rat corneas (Greenburg and Hunt, 1978; Thakral et al., 1979). Similarly, the culture supernatants of wound macrophages were found to be angiogenic, indicating that these factors were secreted products of macrophages.

Several investigations established that responsive mouse peritoneal macrophages secrete angiogenesis factors (Polverini et al., 1977), suggesting that this response is a general capacity of inflammatory macrophages. Consistent with this idea are the following findings. First, recently migrated peripheral blood monocytes probably acquire the same phenotype as thioglycollate-induced inflammatory macrophages as they differentiate and mature. Second, macrophages isolated from solid tumors also secrete angiogenesis factors (Polverini et al., 1984), but here as part of an inflammatory response to the tumor. Third, macrophages isolated from human rheumatoid synovia, another inflammatory condition, are potent inducers of neovascularization (Koch et al., 1986). Unstimulated monocytes or macrophages, as well as neutrophils and lymphocytes, fail to secrete angiogenesis factors. It is conceivable that in all these situations recently migrated blood monocytes encountered the same exogenous or endogenously derived stimuli which induced the secretion of angiogenesis factors.

The nature of these putative stimuli are largely unknown. However, Knighton et al. (1983), on the basis of their findings that rabbit bone marrow-derived macrophages secrete angiogenesis factors during periods of hypoxia, suggested that the reduced oxygen tension found in the center of a healing wound triggers newly recruited macrophages to secrete angiogenesis factors. Elimination of the oxygen gradient from the hypoxic core of a wound to the oxygenated edge inhibits neovascularization of the wound (Knighton et al., 1981). Since the secretion of angiogenesis factors is stopped when macrophages are returned to 20% oxygen, it might be expected that the secretion of angiogenesis factors is self limiting, i.e., the response is downregulated once the neovascularization of the wound is complete.

Other conditions that induce angiogenesis factor secretion by macrophages were elucidated by in vitro studies. For example, Polverini et al. (1977) found that the phagocytosis of Latex spheres by resident macrophages was sufficient to induce angiogenesis factor secretion, while Koch et al. (1986) demonstrated that incubation of purified populations of human peripheral blood monocytes secrete angiogenesis factors when exposed to high concentrations of bacterial endotoxin (5 μg/ml) or concanavalin A (25 μg/ml). These latter conditions probably drive macrophages to the fully activated state (see Section 4). However, in all probability, these macrophages began secreting angiogenesis factors at the responsive stage through which they pass on the pathway to the fully activated phenotype.

Some physical properties of macrophage angiogenesis factor(s) have emerged. Banda *et al.* (1982) purified an angiogenic component of rabbit wound fluid some 9600-fold. The factor, believed to be proteinaceous in nature, was found to stimulate neovascularization in a rabbit corneal implant assay when employed at concentrations as low as 200 ng/ml. The purified factor was also found to induce the directed migration of brain capillary endothelial cells *in vitro*, but it failed to induce DNA-synthesis or endothelial cell proliferation, indicating that other factors (e.g., MDGF or PDGF) are probably involved in stimulating proliferation of the cells involved in tissue neovascularization.

6.3. Macrophages and the Regulation of Connective Tissue Matrix Synthesis

Evidence is beginning to emerge that the macrophage may also regulate the remodeling phase of wound healing by controlling the synthesis of connective tissue matrix proteins by other cell types. Leibovich and Ross (1975) observed that treatment of guinea pigs with hydrocortisone and antimacrophage globulin resulted in a marked delay in fibrosis in experimental wounds. At the time, these results were hypothetically attributed to an impaired production of MDGF, which would result in a reduced number of fibroblasts, hence a reduced level of collagen production. More recent studies, however, have shown that wound macrophages also secrete factors that can increase collagen synthesis in an *in vivo* corneal assay system (Hunt *et al.*, 1984). Moreover, the effect of wound macrophages on collagen synthesis was doubled when these cells were incubated in a high concentration of endotoxin (1 μg/ml) for 30 min prior to injection into rat corneas.

7. Concluding Comments

The data discussed establish that the blood-derived mononuclear phagocyte is essential to the execution of both the degradative and reparative phases of wound healing. At the risk of oversimplifying their contribution, Fig. 2 summarizes some of the more significant aspects of macrophage involvement in wound healing.

How the various aspects of macrophage involvement in wound healing are regulated is not discussed here, simply because virtually nothing is known about it. Speculatively, since the process of debridement and tissue reconstruction are mutually antagonistic, one must presume that these processes can be differentiated on a time scale on which debridement is completed before reconstruction commences. One could obviously make a strong technical argument that continued connective tissue degradation during tissue reconstruction would be counterproductive and clearly not in the best interests of biosynthetic economy, although this can happen in pathologic states such as the chronic rheumatoid joint. In practice, wound healing is probably a continuous process in which debridement of a small area of the wound is completed and repair commences, while at the same time, debridement is taking place in another part of the injured tissue. In this type of model, one might hypothesize that macrophages respond to a signal(s) that instruct them to stop secreting neutral proteases and other factors (e.g., IL-1) involved in the extracellular degradation of the connective tissue matrix. Perhaps the same signal, or another signal then instructs the macrophage to become involved in tissue reconstruction.

Alternatively, tissue debridement may be limited by substrate availability. Here one could envisage that the macrophage, upon encountering and recognizing damaged tissue, automatically expresses enzymes and factors necessary to degrade that damaged connective tissue, in a fashion analogous to the ability of microorganisms to express enzymes capable of using alternative energy sources when grown in their presence. Once all the damaged tissue is removed (i.e., the effective substrate is exhausted), the macrophage may respond by repressing the synthesis of the enzymes and factors that are required for tissue debridement. Based on the evidence given in Section 6.2, which indicates that the reduced oxygen tension in the avascular wound can stimulate the secretion of angiogenesis factor by macrophages, the prevailing conditions in the wound after debridement is complete, may be all that is necessary for the macrophage to begin its role as a modulator of tissue repair.

ACKNOWLEDGMENT. This work was conducted in the F. L. Bryant, Jr., Research Laboratory for the study of the mechanisms of Lung Disease and was supported by grant GM 24834 from the Public Health Service. The author wishes to thank Dr. Claus Fittschen for helpful discussions regarding the involvement of proteases in tissue debridement, and Leigh Landskroner and Barry Silverstein for the excellent artwork and photography, respectively.

References

Adams, D. O., and Hamilton, T. A., 1984, The cell biology of macrophage activation, *Annu. Rev. Immunol.* **2:**283–318.

Anderson, J. C., 1976, Glycoproteins of the connective tissue matrix, *Int. Rev. Connect. Tissue Res.* **7:**251–322.

Baird, A., Mormede, P., and Bohlen, P., 1985, Immunoreactive fibroblast growth factor in cells of peritoneal exudate suggests its identity with macrophage-derived growth factor, *Biochem. Biophys. Res. Commun.* **126:**358–364.

Banda, M. J., and Werb, Z., 1981, Mouse macrophage elastase. Purification and characterization as a metalloproteinase, *Biochem. J.* **193:**589–605.

Banda, M. J., Knighton, D. R., Hunt, and Werb, Z., 1982, Isolation of a nonmitogenic angiogenesis factor from wound fluid, *Proc. Natl. Acad. Sci. USA* **79:**7773–7777.

Banda, M. J., Clark, E. J., and Werb, Z., 1983, Selective proteolysis of immunoglobulins by mouse macrophage elastase, *J. Exp. Med.* **157:**1184–1196.

Banda, M. J., Clark, E. J., and Werb, Z., 1985, Macrophage elastase: Regulatory consequences of the proteolysis of non-elastin substrates, in: *Mononuclear Phagocytes: Characteristics, Physiology and Function* (R. van Furth, ed.), pp. 295–300, Martinus Nijhoff, Dordrecht, Holland.

Bar-Shavit, R., Kahn, A., Fenton, J. W., and Wilner, G. D., 1983, Chemotactic response of monocytes to thrombin, *J. Cell Biol.* **96:**282–285.

Becker, S., 1984, Interferons as modulators of a human monocyte–macrophage differentiation. I. Interferon-γ increases HLA-DR expression and inhibits phagocytosis of zymosan, *J. Immunol.* **132:**1249–1354.

Bevilacqua, M. P., Amrani, D., Mosesson, M. W., and Bianco, C., 1981, Receptors for cold insoluble globulin (plasma fibronectin) on human monocytes, *J. Exp. Med.* **153:**42–60.

Bianco, C., 1983, Fibrin, fibronectin and macrophages, *Ann. NY Acad. Sci.* **408:**602–609.

Blair, H. C., Kahn, A. J., Crouch, E. C., Jeffrey, J. J., and Teitelbaum, S. L., 1982, Isolated osteoclasts resorb the organic and inorganic components of bone, *J. Cell Biol.* **102:**1164–1172.

Blusse van Oud Alblas, A., van der Linden-Schrever, B., and van Furth, R., 1981, Origin and kinetics of pulmonary macrophages during an inflammatory reaction induced by intravenous administration of heat-killed bacillus Calmette-Guérin, *J. Exp. Med.* **154:**235–252.

Blusse van Oud Alblas, A., van der Linden-Schrever, B., and van Furth, R., 1983, Oirgin and kinetics of pulmonary macrophage during an inflammatory reaction induced by intra-alveolar administration of aerosolized heat-killed BCG, *Am. Rev. Respir. Dis.* **128:**276–281.

Bonney, R. J., Gery, I., Lin, T. Y., Meyenhofer, M. F., Acevedo, W., and Davies, P., 1978, Mononuclear phagocytes from carrageenan-induced granulomas. Isolation, cultivation, and characterization, *J. Exp. Med.* **148:**261–275.

Bouwens, L., and Wisse, E., 1985, Proliferation, kinetics, and fate of monocytes in rat liver during zymosan-induced inflammation, *J. Leukocyte Biol.* **37:**531–544.

Brown, M. S., Basu, S. K., Falck, J. R., Ho, Y. K., and Goldstein, J. L., 1980, The scavenger cell pathway for lipoprotein degradation: Specificity of the binding site that mediates the uptake of negatively-charged LDL by macrophages, *J. Supramol. Struct.* **13:**67–81.

Cianciolo, G. J., and Snyderman, R., 1981, Monocyte responsiveness to chemotactic stimuli is a property of a subpopulation of cells that can respond to multiple chemoattractants, *J. Clin. Invest.* **67:**60–68.

Clark, R. A. F., Horsburgh, R. C., Hoffman, A. A., Dvorak, H. F., Mosesson, M. W., and Colvin, R. B., 1984, Fibronectin deposition in delayed-type hypersensitivity, *J. Clin. Invest.* **74:**1011–1016.

Clark, R. A. F., Wilkner, N. E., Norris, D. A., and Howell, S. E., 1985, Cryptic chemotactic activity for human monocytes resides in the cell-binding domain of fibronectin, *J. Cell. Biol.* **101:**217a.

Coggle, J. E., and Tarling, J. D., 1984, The proliferation kinetics of pulmonary alveolar macrophages, *J. Leukocyte Biol.* **35:**317–327.

Crofton, R. W., Diesselhoff-den Dulk, M. M. C., and van Furth, R., 1978, The origin, kinetics, and characteristics of the Kupffer cells in the normal steady state, *J. Exp. Med.* **148:**1–17.

Daems, W. T., 1980, Peritoneal macrophages, in: *The Reticuloendohelial System, A Comprehensive Treatise: Morphology*, Vol. 1 (I. Carr and W. T. Daems, eds.), pp. 57–127, Plenum, New York.

Dayer, J. M., Breard, J., Chess, L., and Krane, S. M., 1979, Participation of monocyte–macrophages and lymphocytes in the production of a factor that stimulates collagenase and prostaglandin release by rheumatoid synovial cells, *J. Clin. Invest.* **64:**1386–1392.

Dayer, J. M., deRochemonteix, B., Burrus, B., Demczuk, S., and Dinarello, C. A., 1986, Human recombinant interleukin 1 stimulates collagenase and prostaglandin E_2 production by human synovial cells, *J. Clin. Invest.* **77:**645–648.

Deimann, W., and Fahimi, D., 1980, Hepatic granulomas induced by glucan. An ultrastructural and peroxidase-cytochemical study, *Lab. Invest.* **43:**172–181.

Deuel, T. F., Senior, R. M., Chang, D., Griffin, G. L., Heinrikson, R. L., and Kaiser, E. T., 1981,

Platelet factor 4 is chemotactic for neutrophils and monocytes, *Proc. Natl. Acad. Sci. USA* **78:**4584–4587.

Dingle, J. T., 1975, The secretion of enzymes into the pericellular environment, *Philos. Trans. R. Soc. Lond. B Biol. Sci.* **271:**315–324.

Doherty, D. E., Haslett, C., Tonneson, M. G., and Henson, P. M., 1987, The adhesion of human peripheral monocytes *in vitro* is enhanced by chemotactic peptides, *J. Immunol.* **138:**1762–1771.

Etherington, D. J., 1976, Bovine spleen cathepsin B1 and collagenolytic cathepsin: a comparative study of the properties of the two enzymes in the degradation of native collagen, *Biochem. J.* **153:**199–209.

Falk, W., and Leonard, E. J., 1980, Human monocyte chemotaxis: Migrating cells are a subpopulation with multiple chemotaxin specificities on each cell, *Infect. Immun.* **29:**953–959.

Ford-Hutchinson, A. W., Bray, M. A., Doig, M. V., Shipley, M. E., and Smith, M. J., 1980, Leukotriene B, a potent chemokinetic and aggregating substance released from polymorphonuclear leukocytes, *Nature (Lond.)* **286:**264–265.

Ginsel, L. A., Rijfkogel, L. P., and Daems, W. T., 1985, A dual origin of macrophages? Review and hypothesis, in: *Macrophage Biology* (S. Reichard and M. Kojima, eds.), pp. 621–649, Alan R. Liss, New York.

Glenn, K. C., and Ross, R., 1981, Human monocyte-derived growth factor(s) for mesenchymal cells: Activation of secretion by endotoxin and concanavalin A, *Cell* **25:**603–615.

Goud, T. J. L. M., and van Furth, R., 1975, Proliferative characteristics of monoblasts grown in vitro, *J. Exp. Med.* **142:**1200–1217.

Goud, T. J. L. M., Schotte, C., and van Furth, R., 1975, Identification and characterization of the monoblast in mononuclear phagocyte colonies grown *in vitro*, *J. Exp. Med.* **142:**1180–1198.

Greenberg, G. B., and Hunt, T. K., 1978, The proliferation response *in vitro* of vascular endothelial and smooth muscle cells exposed to wound fluid and macrophages, *J. Cell. Physiol.* **97:**353–360.

Gudewicz, P. W., Molnar, J., Lai, M. Z., Beezhold, D. W., Siefring, G. E., Jr., Credo, R. B., and Lorand, L., 1980, Fibronectin-mediated uptake of gelatin-coated latex particles by peritoneal macrophages, *J. Cell Biol.* **87:**427–433.

Hirata, T., Bitterman, P. B., Mornex, J-F., and Crystal, R. G., 1986, Expression of the transferrin receptor gene during the process of mononuclear phagocyte maturation, *J. Immunol.* **136:**1339–1345.

Horsburgh, C. R., Clark, R. A. F., and Kirkpatrick, C. H., 1987, Lymphokines and platelets promote human monocyte adherence to fibrinogen and fibronectin in vitro, *J. Leukocyte Biol.* **41:**14–24.

Hosein, B., and Bianco, C., 1985, Monocyte receptors for fibronectin characterized by a monoclonal antibody that interferes with receptor activity, *J. Exp. Med.* **112:**157–170.

Hosein, B., Mosessen, M. W., and Bianco, C., 1985, Monocyte receptors for fibronectin, in: *Mononuclear Phagocytes: Characteristics, Physiology, and Function* (R. van Furth, ed.), pp. 723–730, Martinus Nijhoff, Dordrecht, Holland.

Hunt, T. K., Knighton, D. R., Thakral, K. K., Goodson, W. H., and Andrews, W. S., 1984, Studies on inflammation and wound healing: Angiogenesis and collagen synthesis stimulated *in vivo* by resident and activated wound macrophages, *Surgery* **96:**48–54.

Huybrechts-Godin, G., Hauser, P., and Vaes, G., 1979, Macrophage–fibroblast interaction in collagenase production and cartilage degradation, *Biochem. J.* **184:**643–650.

Huybrechts-Godin, G., Peeters-Joris, C., and Vaes, G., 1985, Partial characterization of the macrophage factor that stimulates fibroblasts to produce collagenase and to degrade collagen, *Biochim. Biophys. Acta* **846:**51–54.

Ishida, M., Honda, M., and Heyashi, H., 1978, In vitro macrophage chemotactic generation from serum immunoglobulin G by neutrophil neutral seryl protease, *Immunology* **35:**167–176.

Jauchem, J. R., Lopez, M., Sprague, E. A., and Schwartz, C. J., 1982, Mononuclear cell chemoattractant activity from cultured arterial smooth muscle cells, *Exp. Mol. Pathol.* **37:**166–174.

Jilek, F., and Hormann, H., 1977, Cold insoluble globulin. II. Plasminolysis of cold insoluble globulin, *Hoppe Seylers Z. Physiol. Chem.* **358:**133–136.

Jones, P. A., and Scott-Burden, T., 1979, Activated macrophages digest the extracellular matrix proteins produced by cultured cells, *Biochem. Biophys. Res. Commun.* **86:**71–77.

Jones, P. A., and Werb, Z., 1980, Degradation of connective tissue matrices by macrophages. II. Influence of matrix composition on proteolysis of glycoproteins, elastin and collagen by macrophages in culture, *J. Exp. Med.* **152:**1527–1536.

Jungo, T. W., and Hafner, S., 1986, Quantitative assessment of Fc receptor expression and function during in vitro differentiation of human monocytes to macrophages, *Immunology* **58:**131–137.

Kambara, T., Ueda, K., and Maeda, S., 1977, The chemical mediation of delayed hypersensitivity skin reactions. I. Purification of a macrophage-chemotactic factor from bovine gamma-globulin induced skin reactions in guinea pigs, *Am. J. Pathol.* **87:**359–374.

Kay, A. B., Pepper, D. S., and Ewart, M. R., 1973, Generation of chemotactic activity for leukocytes by the action of thrombin of human fibrinogen, *Nature (Lond.)* **243:**56–57.

Knighton, D. R., Silver, I. A., and Hunt, T. K., 1981, Regulation of wound-healing angiogenesis— Effect of oxygen gradients and inspired oxygen concentration, *Surgery* **90:**262–270.

Knighton, D. R., Hunt, T. K., Scheuenstuhl, H., Halliday, B. J., Werb, Z., and Banda, M. J., 1983, Oxygen tension regulates the expression of angiogenesis factor by macrophages, *Science* **221:**1283–1285.

Koch, A. E., Polverini, P. J., and Leibovitch, S. J., 1986, Induction of neuvascularization by activated human monocytes, *J. Leukocyte Biol.* **39:**233–238.

Lavie, G., Zucker-Franklin, D., and Franklin, E. C., 1980, Elastase-type proteases on the surface of human blood monocytes: Possible role in amyloid formation, *J. Immunol.* **125:**175–180.

Lee, S. H. S., and Epstein, L., 1980, Reversible inhibition of the maturation of human peripheral blood monocytes to macrophages, *Cell Immunol.* **50:**177–190.

Leibovich, S. J., and Ross, R., 1975, The role of the macrophage in wound repair. A study with hydrocortisone and antimacrophage serum, *Am. J. Pathol.* **78:**71–100.

Leibovich, S. J., and Ross, R., 1976, A macrophage-dependent factor that stimulates the proliferation of fibroblasts in vitro, *Am. J. Pathol.* **84:**501–513.

Leslie, C. C., Musson, R. R., and Henson, P. M., 1984, Production of growth factor activity for fibroblasts by human monocyte-derived macrophages, *J. Leukocyte Biol.* **36:**143–160.

Libby, P., Wyler, D. J., Janicka, M. W., and Dinarello, C. A., 1985, Differential effects of human interleukin 1 on growth of human fibroblasts and vascular smooth muscle cells, *Atherosclerosis* **5:**186–191.

Lin, H. S., Kuhn, C., and Chen, D. M., 1982, Effects of hydrocortisone acetate on pulmonary alveolar macrophage colony-forming cells, *Ann. Rev. Respir. Dis.* **125:**712–715.

Loike, J. D., Kozler, V. F., and Silverstein, S. C., 1984, Creatine kinase expression and creatine phosphate accumulation are developmentally regulated during differentiation of mouse and human monocytes, *J. Exp. Med.* **159:**746–757.

Marder, S. R., Chenoweth, D. E., Goldstein, I. M., and Perez, H. D., 1985, Chemotactic responses of human peripheral blood monocytes to the complement-derived peptides C5a and C5a des Arg, *J. Immunol.* **134:**3325–3331.

Martin, B. M., Gimbrone, M. A., Unanue, E. R., and Cotran, R. S., 1981, Stimulation of nonlymphoid mesenchymal cell proliferation by a macrophage-derived growth factor, *J. Immunol.* **126:**1510–1515.

Martin, B. M., Gimbrone, M. A., Majeau, G. R., Unanue, E. R., and Cotran, R. S., 1983, Stimulation of human monocyte/macrophage-derived growth factor (MDGF) production by plasma fibronectin, *Am. J. Pathol.* **111:**367–373.

McDonald, J. A., and Kelley, D. G., 1980, Degradation of fibronectin by human leukocyte elastase, *J. Biol. Chem.* **255:**8848–8858.

Miller, B., Miller, H., Patterson, R., and Ryan, S. J., 1986, Retinal wound healing. Cellular activity at the vitreoretinal interface, *Arch. Ophthalmol.* **104:**281–285.

Mizel, S. B., Dayer, J. M., Krane, S. M., and Mergenhagen, S. E., 1981, Stimulation of rheumatoid synovial cell collagenase and prostaglandin production by partially purified lymphocyte-activating factor (interleukin 1), *Proc. Natl. Acad. Sci. USA* **78:**2474–2477.

Murphy, G., Reynolds, J. J., Bretz, U., and Baggiolini, M., 1977, Collagenase is a component of the specific granules of human neutrophil leukocytes, *Biochem. J.* **162:**195–197.

Murtaugh, M. P., Arend, W. P., and Davies, P. J. A., 1984, Induction of tissue transglutaminase in human peripheral blood monocytes, *J. Exp. Med.* **159:**114–125.

Musson, R. A., 1983, Human serum induces maturation of human monocytes *in vitro*, *Am. J. Pathol.* **111:**331–340.

Musson, P. A., Shafran, H., and Henson, P. M., 1980, Intracellular and stimulated release of lysosomal enzymes from human peripheral blood monocytes and monocyte-derived macrophages, *J. Reticuloendothel. Soc.* **28:**249–264.

Nakagawara, A., Nathan, C. F., and Cohn, Z. A., 1981, Hydrogen peroxide metabolism in human monocytes during differentiation *in vitro*, *J. Clin. Invest.* **68:**1243–1252.

Newman, S. L., Musson, R. A., and Henson, P. M., 1980, Development of functional complement receptors during *in vivo* maturation of human monocytes into macrophages, *J. Immunol.* **125:**2236–2244.

Nicola, N. A., and Metcalf, D., 1986, Specificity of action of colony-stimulating factors in the differentiation of granulocytes and macrophages, *Ciba Found. Symp.* **118:**7–22.

Norris, D. A., Clark, R. A. F., Swigart, L. M., Huff, J. C., Weston, W. L., and Howell, S. E., 1982, Fibronectin fragment(s) are chemotactic for human peripheral blood monocytes, *J. Immunol.* **129:**1612–1618.

Ogawa, T., Kotani, S., Kusumoto, S., and Shiba, T., 1983, Possible chemotaxis of human monocytes by N-acetylmuramyl-L-ananyl-D-isoglutamine, *Infect. Immun.* **39:**449–451.

Parakkal, P. F., 1972, Macrophages: The time course and sequence of their distribution in the postpartum uterus, *J. Ultrastruct. Res.* **40:**284–291.

Polverini, P. J., Cotran, R. S., Gimbrone, M. A., and Unanue, E. R., 1977, Activated macrophages induce vascular proliferation, *Nature (Lond.)* **269:**804–806.

Polverini, P. J., and Leibovich, S. J., 1984, Induction of neuvascularization *in vivo* and endothelial cell proliferation *in vitro* by tumor-associated macrophages, *Lab. Invest.* **51:**635–642.

Postlethwaite, A. E., and Kang, A. H., 1976, Collagen- and collagen peptide-induced chemotaxis of human blood monocytes, *J. Exp. Med.* **143:**1299–1307.

Postlethwaite, A. E., Seyer, J. M., and Kang, A. H., 1978, Chemotactic attraction of human fibroblasts to type I, II, and III collagens and collagen-derived peptides, *Proc. Natl. Acad. Sci. USA* **75:**871–875.

Postlethwaite, A. E., Keski-Oja, J., Bahan, G., and Kang, A. H., 1981, Induction of fibroblast chemotaxis by fibronectin, *J. Exp. Med.* **153:**494–499.

Postlethwaite, A. E., Lachman, L. B., Mainardi, C. L., and Kang, A. H., 1983, Interleukin 1 stimulation of collagenase production by cultured fibroblasts, *J. Exp. Med.* **157:**801–806.

Proveddini, D. M., Deftos, L. J., and Manolagas, S. C., 1986, 1,25-dihydroxyvitamin D_3 promotes *in vitro* morphologic and enzymatic changes in normal human monocytes consistent with their differentiation into macrophages, *Bone* **7:**23–28.

Rinehart, J. J., Wuest, D., and Ackerman, G. A., 1982, Corticosteroid lateration of human monocyte to macrophage differentiation, *J. Immunol.* **129:**1436–1440.

Robertson, P. B., Ryel, R. B., Taylor, R. E., Shyu, K. W., and Fullmer, H. M., 1972, Collagenase: Localization in polymorphonuclear leukocyte granules in the rabbit, *Science* **177:**64–65.

Ross, R., and Benditt, E. P., 1961, Wound healing and collagen formation. I. Sequential changes in components of guinea pig skin wounds observed in the electron microscope, *J. Biophys. Biochem. Cytol.* **11:**677–700.

Sandhaus, R. A., McCarthy, K. M., Musson, R. A., and Henson, P. M., 1983, Elastinolytic proteinases of the human macrophage, *Chest* **83S:**60S–62S.

Satodate, R., Madarame, T., Monma, N., Masuda, T., Oikawa, K., and Sato, S., 1985, Importance of the sinusoidal fenestration for blood monocytes to settle on the sinusoidal surface of the liver, in: *Macrophage Biology: Progress in Leukocyte Biology*, Vol. 4 (S. Reichard and M. Kojima, eds.), pp. 651–658, Alan R. Liss, New York.

Sawyer, R. T., Strausbach, P. H., and Volkman, A., 1982, Resident macrophage proliferation in mice depleted of blood monocytes by strontium-89, *Lab. Invest.* **46:**165–170.

Sawyer, R. T., 1986, The ontogeny of pulmonary alveolar macrophages in parabiotic mice, *J. Leukocyte Biol.* **40:**347–354.

Schenk, R. K., 1974, The ultrastructure of bone (report), *Verh. Dtsch. Ges. Pathol.* **58:**72–83.

Schmidt, J. A., Oliver, C. N., Lepe-Zuniga, J. L., Green, I., and Gery, I., 1984, Silica-stimulated monocytes release fibroblast proliferation factors identical to interleukin 1. A potential role for interleukin 1 in the pathogenesis of silicosis, *J. Clin. Invest.* **73**:1462–1472.

Senior, R. M., Griffin, G. L., and Mecham, R. P., 1980, Chemotactic activity of elastin-derived peptides, *J. Clin. Invest.* **66**:859–862.

Senior, R. M., Griffin, G. L., Mecham, R. P., Wrenn, D. S., Prasad, K. U., and Urry, D. W., 1984, Val-Gly-Val-Ala-Pro-Gly, a repeating peptide in elastin, is chemotactic for fibroblasts and monocytes, *J. Cell Biol.* **99**:870–874.

Shimokado, K., Raines, E. W., Madtes, D. K., Barrett, T. B., Benditt, E. P., and Ross, R., 1985, A significant part of macrophage-derived growth factor consists of at least two forms of PDGF, *Cell* **43**:277–288.

Simpson, D. M., and Ross, R., 1972, The neutrophilic leukocyte in wound repair, *J. Clin. Invest.* **51**:2009–2023.

Snyderman, R., and Fudman, E. J., 1980, Demonstration of a chemotactic factor receptor on macrophages, *J. Immunol.* **124**:2754–2757.

Stewart, R. J., Duley, J. A., Dewdney, J., Allardyce, R. A., Beard, M. E. J., and Fitzgerald, P. H., 1981, The wound fibroblast and macrophage. II. Their origin studied in a human after bone marrow transplantation, *Br. J. Surg.* **68**:129–131.

Tanaka, H., Abe, E., Miyaura, C., Shiina, Y., and Suda, T., 1983, 1,25-dihydroxyvitamin D_3 induces differentiation of human promyelocytic leukemia cells (HL-60) into monocyte–macrophages, but not into granulocytes, *Biochem. Biophys. Res. Commun.* **117**:86–92.

Tarling, J. D., and Coggle, J. E., 1982, Evidence for the pulmonary origin of alveolar macrophages, *Cell Tissue Kinet.* **15**:577–584.

Thakral, K. K., Goodson, W. H., and Hunt, T. K., 1979, Stimulation of wound blood vessel growth by wound macrophages, *J. Surg. Res.* **26**:430–436.

Unkeless, J. C., Gordon, S., and Reich, E., 1974, Secretion of plasminogen activator by stimulated macrophages, *J. Exp. Med.* **139**:834–850.

van Furth, R., and Cohn, Z. A., 1968, The origin and kinetics of mononuclear phagocytes, *J. Exp. Med.* **128**:415–435.

van Furth, R., Diesselhoff-den Dulk, M. M. C., and Mattie, H., 1973, Quantitative study on the production and kinetics of mononuclear phagocytes during an acute inflammatory reaction, *J. Exp. Med.* **138**:1314–1330.

van Furth, R., Diesselhoff-den Dulk, M. M. C., Sluiter, W., and van Dissel, J. T., 1985a, New perspectives on the kinetics of mononuclear phagocytes, in: *Mononuclear Phagocytes: Characteristics, Physiology and Function* (R. van Furth, ed.), pp. 201–208, Martinus Nijhoff, Dordrecht, Holland.

van Furth, R., Nibberin, P. H., van Dissel, J. T., and Disselhoff-den Dulk, M. M. C., 1985b, The characterization, origin, and kinetics of skin macrophages during inflammation, *J. Invest. Dermatol.* **85**:398–402.

Vartio, T., 1981, Characterization of the binding domains in the fragments cleaved by cathepsin G from human plasma fibronectin, *Eur. J. Biochem.* **123**:223–233.

Wedmore, C. V., and Williams, T. J., 1981, Control of vascular permeability by polymorphonuclear leukocytes in inflammation, *Nature (Lond.)* **289**:646–650.

Wenger, G. D., and O'Dorisio, M. S., 1985, Induction of cAMP-dependent protein kinase I during human monocyte differentiation, *J. Immunol.* **134**:1836–1843.

Werb, Z., and Gordon, S., 1975a, Secretion of a specific collagenase by stimulated macrophages, *J. Exp. Med.* **142**:346–360.

Werb, Z., and Gordon, S., 1975b, Elastase secretion by stimulated macrophages. Characterization and regulation, *J. Exp. Med.* **142**:361–377.

Werb, Z., Banda, M. J., and Jones, P. A., 1980a, Degradation of connective tissue matrices by macrophages. I. Proteolysis of elastin, glycoproteins and collagen by proteinases isolated from macrophages, *J. Exp. Med.* **152**:1340–1357.

Werb, Z., Bainton, D. F., and Jones, P. A., 1980b, Degradation of connective tissue matrices by macrophages. III. Morphological and biochemical studies on extracellular, pericellular and intracellular events in macrox proteolysis by macrophages in culture, *J. Exp. Med.* **152**:1537–1553.

Wright, S. D., Craigmyle, L. S., and Silverstein, S. C., 1983, Fibronectin and serum amyloid P component stimulate C3b- and C3bi-mediated phagocytosis in cultured human monocytes, *J. Exp. Med.* **158**:1339–1343.

Wright, S. D., and Meyer, B. C., 1985, Fibronectin receptor of human macrophages recognizes the sequence Arg-Gly-Asp-Ser, *J. Exp. Med.* **162**:762–767.

Yancey, K. B., Hammer, C. H., Harvath, L., Renfer, L., Frank, M. M., and Lawley, T. J., 1985, Studies of human C5a as a mediator of inflammation in normal human skin, *J. Clin. Invest.* **75**:486–495.

Zuckerman, S. H., Ackerman, S. K., and Douglas, S. D., 1979, Long term human peripheral blood monocyte cultures: Establishment, metabolism, and morphology of primary human monocyte–macrophage cultures, *Immunology* **38**:401–411.

Part II

Granulation Tissue Formation

Chapter 9

The Role of Growth Factors in Tissue Repair I

Platelet-Derived Growth Factor

JUNG SAN HUANG, THOMAS J. OLSEN, and
SHUAN SHIANG HUANG

1. Introduction

Wound healing is a complex biologic phenomenon that as been the subject of much investigation (Ross, 1968; Ross and Glomset, 1976). This process can be divided into three overlapping phases, namely inflammatory, proliferative, and remodeling (see Chapter 1). Upon injury, hemorrhage occurs. Along with the formation of fibrin clots, platelets aggregate and become activated with release of granule contents. Following degranulation of platelets, the appearance and subsequent activation of neutrophils and monocytes at the injury sites constitute the major events in the inflammatory phase. In the proliferative phase, fibroblasts (in most organs) or smooth muscle cells (in large blood vessels) are recruited to the injury sites and proliferate. The formation of new extracellular matrix leads to completion of the remodeling phase.

It is evident that cellular migration, activation, and proliferation are important events in the process of wound healing. The mechanisms controlling this organized and coordinated pattern of migration and proliferation are not well understood. The chemical and biologic characterization of chemoattractants and mitogens first released from human platelets and later synthesized and secreted by macrophages at injury sites should increase our understanding of those control mechanisms. Chapter 9 discusses the properties of human platelet-derived growth factor (PDGF), which possesses both chemotactic and mitogenic activities and is believed to play an important role in wound healing. Subsequent chapters review other growth factors that may have significant roles in wound repair, such as epidermal growth factor (Chapter 10), fibroblast growth factor (Chapter 11), and transforming growth factor β (Chapter 12).

JUNG SAN HUANG, THOMAS J. OLSEN, and SHUAN SHIANG HUANG • E. A. Doisy Department of Biochemistry, St. Louis University School of Medicine, St. Louis, Missouri 63014.

2. Identification and Properties of Platelet-Derived Growth Factor

The observation of a requirement for serum by cultured fibroblasts (Balk, 1971) led to the recognition that the growth-promoting activity in serum is derived from platelets (Kohler and Lipton, 1974; Ross et al., 1974). This activity was later localized to α-granules (Witte et al., 1978; Kaplan et al., 1979a,b) and called PDGF (Ross and Vogel, 1978). The serum concentration of human PDGF is estimated to be 15–50 ng/ml (Singh et al., 1982; Huang et al., 1983; Bowen-Pope et al., 1984a). During the hemostatic response to injury, platelets release PDGF when degranulation occurs, either after exposure to thrombin or following exposure to fibrillar collagen. PDGF has been purified from human platelets or platelet plasma and resolved into two active proteins, PDGF I and PDGF II, which are present in human serum in a molar ratio of 1:2.5. They have similar amino acid composition and identical mitogenic activity and immunoreactivity (Antoniades, 1981; Deuel et al., 1981; Heldin et al., 1981a; Rains and Ross, 1982). Each has 16 half-cysteine residues, all in disulfide linkages. PDGF II is probably a degradation product of PDGF I. Treatment of PDGF with reducing agents yields two polypeptide chains, the A-chain (124 amino acid residues) and the B-chain (160 amino acid residues), with concomitant loss of biologic activity (Betsholtz et al., 1986). The A- and B-chain genes have been localized to chromosomes 7 and 22, respectively (Beltsholtz et al., 1986; Dalla-Favera et al., 1982). The gene coding for a polypeptide precursor of the B chain is identical with c-sis, the cellular homologue of v-sis, the transforming gene of simian sarcoma virus (SSV) (Doolittle et al., 1983; Waterfield et al., 1983; Chiu et al, 1984; Joseph et al., 1984; Johnsson et al., 1984).

PDGF-like molecules are produced by SSV-transformed fibroblasts and by a number of tumor and normal cells. SSV, a retrovirus, causes fibrosarcoma in the woolly monkey (Thielen et al., 1971). It possesses an oncogene, v-sis, coding for the putative transforming protein, p28[v-sis], which forms a homodimer in SSV-transformed fibroblasts (Robbins et al., 1983). The amino acid sequence of p28[v-sis] is 93% homologous to the B-chain of human PDGF. Both p28[v-sis] and PDGF bind to the same receptor in fibroblasts (Deuel et al., 1983; Bowen-Pope et al., 1984b; Huang et al., 1984b; Owen et al., 1984; Garrett et al., 1984; Johnsson et al., 1985a) and show essentially identical mitogenic and chemotactic activities to fibroblasts and inflammatory cells (R. M. Senior, personal communication). An autocrine stimulation of SSV-transformed cells by p28[v-sis] may be the mechanism for transformation of these cells (Deuel et al., 1983; Bowen-Pope et al., 1984b; Huang et al., 1984b; Owen et al., 1984; Garrett et al., 1984; Johnsson et al., 1985b).

Human osteosarcoma cells (U-2 OS) secrete a PDGF-like molecule that has been identified as a homodimer of the A chain of PDGF (Heldin et al., 1986). A homodimer of the B chain of PDGF is expressed in some osteosarcoma cells and glioblastoma cells (Huang and Huang, 1985). Cultured endothelial cells also secrete a PDGF-like molecule, the release of which can be enhanced by treatment with thrombin (Dicorleto and Bowen-Pope, 1983; Harlan et al., 1986).

This PDGF-like molecule is possibly a homodimer of the B chain of PDGF. Cultured arterial smooth muscle cells from newborn rats, but not 3-month-old rats (Seifert *et al.*, 1984), or from the intima of injured arteries (Walker *et al.*, 1986) secrete a PDGF-like molecule recently identified as a homodimer of the A chain of PDGF (Sejersen *et al.*, 1986).

Human blood monocytes, when activated by a variety of stimuli, release a molecule similar to PDGF in biochemical and immunologic properties (Martinet *et al.*, 1986). Resting monocytes do not release this factor. Alveolar macrohpages secrete growth factor activity of which a significant portion is attributed to a PDGF-like molecule (Shimokado *et al.*, 1985; Mornex *et al.*, 1986). These PDGF-like molecules appear to bind to the same PDGF receptor in fibroblasts and exhibit mitogenic activity similar to PDGF. Interestingly, Stroobant and Waterfield (1984) recently identified porcine PDGF as a homodimer of the B-chain.

3. Mitogenic Activity of Platelet-Derived Growth Factor

PDGF is the most potent mitogen in serum for cells of mesenchymal origin, including fibroblasts, glial cells, and smooth muscle cells (Ross and Vogel, 1978; Deuel and Huang, 1983, 1984a,b; Heldin and Westermark, 1984; Ross *et al.*, 1986). PDGF stimulates cell growth through interaction with specific high-affinity receptors on the cell surface of target cells. The dissociation constant K_d and receptor number of PDGF in responsive cells are 1×10^{-9} M and $1-4 \times 10^5$ receptors/cell, respectively (Heldin *et al.*, 1981b; Bowen-Pope and Ross, 1982; Huang *et al.*, 1982; Williams *et al.*, 1982). The receptor protein is an 18,000-M_r glycoprotein with intrinsic and PDGF-stimulated protein tyrosine kinase activity (Ek and Heldin, 1982; Nishimura *et al.*, 1982; Huang *et al.*, 1984c; Daniel *et al.*, 1985). The receptor kinase activity is believed to generate a mitogenic signal leading to DNA synthesis. The gene for the PDGF receptor has been cloned and localized to chromosome 5 (Yarden *et al.*, 1986). The PDGF receptor/protein tyrosine kinase is not found in unresponsive cells such as epithelial and endothelial cells.

4. Chemotactic Activity of Platelet-Derived Growth Factor

PDGF has been shown to be chemotactic for a variety of cells. PDGF is a potent chemoattractant for inflammatory cells that do not respond mitogenically to the growth factor. Maximum neutrophil chemotaxis occurs at PDGF concentrations of 1–5 ng/ml, whereas maximum monocyte chemotaxis occurs at concentration of 20 ng/ml (Deuel *et al.*, 1982). At higher concentrations (20–40 ng/ml), PDGF activates human neutrophils, resulting in superoxide synthesis, release of granule content, and neutrophil aggregation (Tzeng *et al.*, 1984). At similar concentrations, human peripheral monocytes also activated as well (Tzeng *et al.*, 1985). Smooth muscle cells and fibroblasts are strongly attracted to low concentrations of PDGF (10–20 ng/ml) (Grotendorst et al., 1982; Seppa et al., 1982; Senior et al., 1983). The structural determinants of PDGF that mediate chemotaxis may be different from those that mediate mitogenesis (Williams et al., 1983; Senior et al., 1985).

The chemotactic receptors for PDGF in monocytes and neutrophils appear to be different from the PDGF receptor/protein tyrosine kinase found in fibroblasts and smooth muscle cells with respect to kinetics and thermodynamics of ligand binding. No protein tyrosine kinase activity is found in PDGF chemotactic receptors in inflammatory cells. The dissociation constant K_d and receptor number of PDGF in inflammatory cells are 1–4×10^{-9} M and 2000–6000 receptors/cell, respectively (Kimura et al., 1983).

5. Role of Platelet-Derived Growth Factor in Wound Healing

The expression of both chemotactic and mitogenic activities by PDGF suggests that PDGF may play an important role in the wound-healing process. PDGF and other granule proteins mediate recruitment of inflammatory and connective tissue cells into injury sites initiating the process. The orderly progression of neutrophils, macrophages, and then fibroblasts correlates reasonably well with the concentration of PDGF required for maximum chemotaxis (Deuel and Huang, 1984b). Neutrophils can be activated by PDGF to release lysosomal enzymes and neutral proteases to remove damaged tissues and superoxide anions to kill microorganisms. Monocytes are activated as well. Following the inflammatory response, cellular proliferation is the next major step in repair. PDGF released from platelets and PDGF-like molecules produced locally by activated macrophages, smooth muscle cells, and endothelial cells are important in stimulating the proliferation of fibroblasts in skin injury or of smooth muscle cells in vascular injury. PDGF also stimulates fibroblasts to secrete collagenase which may be involved in the removal of damaged collagen tissues or in the remodeling of tissues. Synthesis and secretion of new extracellular matrix by fibroblasts or smooth muscle cells and remodeling represent the final stage of repair (Fig. 1).

6. Plasma Clearance and Inhibitor of Platelet-Derived Growth Factor

Excess PDGF released from activated platelets during blood clotting and vessel injury forms a complex with α_2-macroglobulin (α_2M) (Huang et al., 1984a). The complex formation between PDGF and α_2M is a very fast reaction with a half-life ($t\frac{1}{2}$) of 4 min. The PDGF–α_2M complex may be recognized by the high-affinity α_2M receptors found in the parenchymal cells of liver and thus cleared from the plasma (Huang et al., 1987). The $t\frac{1}{2}$ of [^{125}I]-PDGF injected into plasma was estimated to be 2 min (Bowen-Pope et al., 1984a).

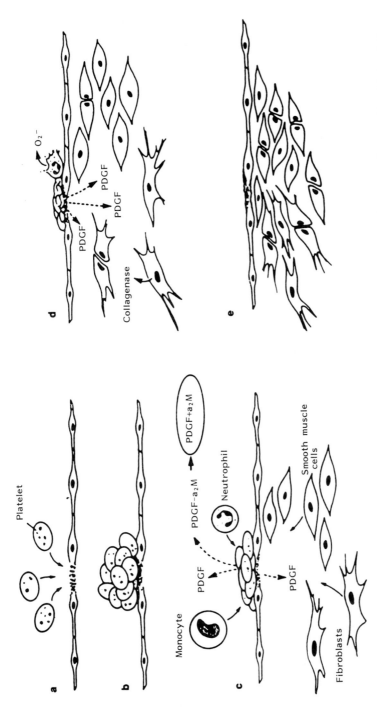

Figure 1. Potential roles of PDGF in wound healing. PDGF is released after injury (a) and platelet adherence and aggregation at injured sites occurs (b). The PDGF released locally stimulates the migration of neutrophils, monocytes, fibroblasts, and smooth muscle cells (in vessel wall injury) into the wounded sites; PDGF released into the systemic circulation is complexed to α_2M (c). At the higher concentrations of PDGF proximal in the wound, PDGF activates neutrophils to generate the release of superoxide and stimulates fibroblasts to synthesize and release superoxide and also collagenase. PDGF also stimulates cellular proliferation of fibroblasts and smooth muscle cells (d). Remodeling and reorganization follow (e). (From Deuel and Huang, 1984b.)

Protamine has been shown to be a potent inhibitor of PDGF mitogenic and chemotactic activities (Deuel et al., 1982; Huang et al., 1982, 1984d). The inhibitor activity of protamine is partially neutralized in the presence of plasma proteins.

7. Conclusions

PDGF is the most potent mitogen in serum for fibroblasts, smooth muscle cells, and glial cells and is also a potent chemoattractant and activator for monocytes and neutrophils. The possession of both of these properties by PDGF, together with the release of PDGF from platelets and its possible local production by other cell types, makes this growth factor a potential wound-healing hormone.

ACKNOWLEDGMENTS. We thank Dr. William S. Sly for his encouragement, Dr. Catherine M. Nolan for review, and Mrs. Kerner for preparing this manuscript.

References

Antoniades, H. N., 1981, Human platelet-derived growth factor (PDGF): Purification of PDGF-I and PDGF-II and separation of their reduced subunits, Proc. Natl. Acad. Sci. USA **78**:7314–7317.

Balk, S. D., 1971, Calcium as a regulator of the proliferation of normal, but not of transformed, chicken fibroblasts in a plasma-containing medium, Proc. Natl. Acad. Sci. USA **68**:271–275.

Betsholtz, C., Johnsson, A., Heldin, C.-H., Westermark, B., Lind, P., Urdea, M. S., Eddy, R., Shows, T. B., Philpott, K., Mellor, A. L., Knott, T. J., and Scott, J., 1986, cDNA sequence and chromosomal localization of human platelet-derived growth factor. A-chain and its expression in tumour cell lines, Nature (Lond.) **320**:695–699.

Bowen-Pope, D. T., and Ross, R., 1982, Platelet-derived growth factor II. Specific binding to culture cells, J. Biol. Chem. **257**:5161–5171.

Bowen-Pope, D. F., Malpass, T. W., Foster, D. M., and Ross, R., 1984a, Platelet-derived growth factor in vivo: Levels, activity, and rate of clearance, Blood **64**:458–469.

Bowen-Pope, D. F., Vogel, A., and Ross, R., 1984b, Production of platelet-derived growth factor-like molecules and reduced expression of platelet-derived growth factor receptors accompany transformation by a wide spectrum of agents, Proc. Natl. Acad. Sci. USA **81**:2396–2400.

Chiu, I.-M., Reddy, E. P., Givol, D., Robbins, K. C., Tronick, S. R., and Aaronson, S. A., 1984, Nucleotide sequence analysis identifies the human c-sis proto-oncogene as a structural gene for platelet-derived growth factor, Cell **37**:123–129.

Dalla-Favera, R., Gallo, R. C., Giallango, A., Crocer, and Croce, C. M., 1982. Chromosomal localization of the human humologs (c-sis) of the simian sarcoma virus one gene, Science **218**:686–688.

Daniel, T. O., Tremble, P. M., Frankelton, A. R. J., and Williams, L. T., 1985, Purification of the platelet-derived growth factor receptor by using an anti-phosphotyrosine antibody, Proc. Natl. Acad. Sci. USA **82**:2684–2687.

Deuel, T. F., and Huang, J. S., 1983, Platelet-derived growth factor: Purification, properties, and biological activities, Prog. Hematol. **13**:201–221.

Deuel, T. F., and Huang, J. S., 1984a, Roles of growth factor activities in oncogenesis, Blood **64**:951–958.

Deuel, T. F., and Huang, J. S., 1984b, Platelet-derived growth factor: Structure, function, and roles in normal and transformed cells, J. Clin. Invest. **74**:669–676.

Deuel, T. F., Huang, J. S., Proffitt, R. T., Baenziger, J. U., Chang, D., and Kennedy, B. B., 1981, Human platelet-derived growth factor: Purification and resolution into two active protein fractions, *J. Biol. Chem.* **256**:8896–8899.

Deuel, T. F., Senior, R. M., Huang, J. S., and Griffin, G. L., 1982, Chemotaxis of monocytes and neutrophils to platelet-derived growth factor, *J. Clin. Invest.* **69**:1046–1049.

Deuel, T. F., Huang, J. S., Huang, S. S., Stroobant, P., and Waterfield, M. D., 1983, Expression of a platelet-derived growth factor-like protein in simian sarcoma virus transformed cells, *Science* **221**:1348–1350.

DiCorleto, P. E., and Bowen-Pope, D. F., 1983, Cultured endothelial cells produce a platelet-derived growth factor-like protein, *Proc. Natl. Acad. Sci. USA* **80**:1919–1923.

Doolittle, R. F., Hunkapillar, M. W., Hood, L. E., Devare, S. G., Robbins, K. C., Aaronson, S. A., and Antoniades, H. N., 1983, Simian sarcoma virus onc gene, v-sis, is derived from the gene (or genes) encoding a platelet-derived growth factor, *Science* **221**:275–277.

Ek, B., and Heldin, C.-H., 1982, Characterization of a tyrosine-specific kinase activity in human fibroblast membranes stimulated by platelet-derived growth factor, *J. Biol. Chem.* **257**:10486–10492.

Garrett, J. S., Coughlin, S. R., Niman, H. L., Tremble, P. J., Giels, G. M., and Williams, L. T., 1984, Blockade of autocrine stimulation in simian sarcoma virus-transformed cells reverses down-regulation of platelet-derived growth factor receptors, *Proc. Natl. Acad. Sci. USA* **81**:7466–7470.

Grotendorst, G. R., Chang, T., Seppa, H. E. J., Kleinman, H. K., and Martin, G. R., 1982, Platelet-derived growth factor is a chemoattractant for vascular smooth muscle cells, *J. Cell. Physiol.* **113**:261–266.

Harlan, J. M., Thompson, P. J., Ross, R., and Bowen-Pope, D. F., 1986, α-thrombin induces release of PDGF-like molecule(s) by cultured human endothelial cells, *J. Cell Biol.* **103**:1129–1133.

Heldin, C.-H., and Westermark, B., 1984, Growth factors: Mechanism of action and relation to oncogenes, *Cell* **37**:9–20.

Heldin, C.-H., Westermark, B., and Wasteson, A., 1981a, Platelet-derived growth factor: Isolation by a large-scale procedure and analysis of subunit composition, *Biochem. J.* **193**:907–913.

Heldin, C.-H., Westermark, B., and Wasteson, A., 1981b, Specific receptors for platelet-derived growth factor on cells derived from connective tissue and glia, *Proc. Natl. Acad. Sci. USA* **78**:3664–3668.

Heldin, C.-H., Johnsson, A., Wennergren, S., Wernstedt, C., Betsholtz, C., and Westermark, B., 1986, A human osteosarcoma cell line secretes a growth factor structurally related to a homodimer of PDGF A-chains, *Nature (Lond.)* **319**:511–514.

Huang, J. S., and Huang, S. S., 1985, Role of growth factors in oncogenesis: Growth factor-proto-oncogene pathways of mitogenesis, *Ciba Found. Symp.* **116**:46–65.

Huang, J. S., Huang, S. S., Kennedy, B. B., and Deuel, T. F., 1982, Platelet-derived growth factor: Specific binding to target cells, *J. Biol. Chem.* **257**:8130–8136.

Huang, J. S., Huang, S. S., and Deuel, T. F., 1983, Human platelet-derived growth factor: Radioim-munoassay and discovery of a specific plasma-binding protein, *J. Cell Biol.* **97**:383–388.

Huang, J. S., Huang, S. S., and Deuel, T. F., 1984a, Specific covalent binding of platelet-derived growth factor to human plasma α_2-macroglobulin, *Proc. Natl. Acad. Sci. USA* **81**:342–346.

Huang, J. S., Huang, S. S., and Deuel, T. F., 1984b, Transforming protein of simian sarcoma virus stimulates autocrine growth of SSV-transformed cells through PDGF cell-surface receptors, *Cell* **39**:79–87.

Huang, S. S., Huang, J. S., and Deuel, T. F., 1984c, The platelet-derived growth factor receptor protein is a tyrosine specific protein kinase, *Cancer Cell* **1**:43–49.

Huang, J. S., Nishimura, J., Huang, S. S., and Deuel, T. F., 1984d, Protamine inhibits platelet-derived growth factor receptor activity, but not epidermal growth factor activity, *J. Cell Biochem.* **26**:205–226.

Huang, S. S., O'Grady, P., Olsen, T., and Huang, J. S., Characterization of covalent complex formation between human platelet-derived growth factor and α_2-macroglobulin, submitted for publication.

Johnsson, A., Heldin, C.-H., Wasteson, A., Westermark, B., Deuel, T. F., Huang, J. S., Seeburg, H.,

Gray, A., Ulrich, A., Scrace, G., Stroobant, P., and Waterfield, M. D., 1984, The c-sis gene encodes a precursor of the B chain of platelet-derived growth factor, *EMBO J.* **3:**921–928.

Johnsson, A., Betsholtz, C., von der Helm, K., Heldin, C.-H., and Westermark, B., 1985a, Platelet-derived growth factor agonist activity of a secreted form of v-sis oncogene product, *Proc. Natl. Acad. Sci. USA* **82:**1721–1725.

Johnsson, A., Betscholtz, C., and Westermark, B., 1985b, Antibodies against platelet-derived growth factor inhibit acute transformation by simian sarcoma virus, *Nature (Lond.)* **317:**438–440.

Josephs, S. F., Guo, C., Ratner, L., and Wong-Staal, F., 1984, Human protooncogene nucleotide sequences corresponding to the transforming regionof simian sarcoma virus, *Science* **223:**487–491.

Kaplan, D. R., Chao, F. C., Stiles, C. D., Antoniades, H. N., and Scher, C. D., 1979a, Platelet-alpha granules contain a growth factor for fibroblasts, *Blood* **53:**1043–1052.

Kaplan, K. L., Broekman, M. J., Chernoff, A., Lesznik, G. R., and Drillings, M., 1979b, Platelet-alpha granule proteins: Studies on release and subcellular localization, *Blood* **53:**604–616.

Kimura, A., Huang, J. S., and Deuel, T. F., 1983, Specific binding of the platelet-derived growth factor to chemotactically active inflammatory cells, *Fed. Proc.* **42:**1830 (abst.).

Kohler, N., and Lipton, A., 1974, Platelets as a source of fibroblast growth-promoting activity, *Exp. Cell Res.* **87:**297–301.

Martinet, Y., Bitterman, P. B., Mornex, J.-F., Grotendorst, G. R., Martin, G. R., and Crystal, R. G., 1986, Activated human monocytes express the c-sis protocogene and release a mediator showing PDGF-like activity, *Nature (Lond.)* **319:**158–160.

Mornex, J. F., Martinet, Y., Yamauchik, K., Bitterman, P. B., Grotendorst, G. R., Chytil-Weir, A., Martin, G. R., and Crystal, R. G., 1986, Spontaneous expression of the c-sis gene and release of a platelet-derived growth factor-like molecule by human alveolar macrophage, *J. Clin. Invest.* **78:**61–66.

Nishimura, J., Huang, J. S., and Deuel, T. F., 1982, Platelet-derived growth factor stimulates tyrosine specific protein kinase activity in Swiss mouse 3T3 cell membranes, *Proc. Natl. Acad. Sci. USA* **79:**4303–4307.

Owen, A. J., Pantazis, P., and Antoniades, H. N., 1984, Simian sarcoma virus-transformed cells secrete a mitogen identical to platelet-derived growth factor, *Science* **225:**54–56.

Raines, E. W., and Ross, R., 1982, Platelet-derived growth factor I. High yield purification and evidence for multiple forms. *J. Biol. Chem.* **257:**5154–5160.

Robbins, K. C., Antoniades, H. N., Devare, S. G., Hunkapiller, M. W., and Aaronson, S. A., 1983, Structural and immunological similarities between simian sarcoma virus gene product(s) and human platelet-derived growth factor, *Nature (Lond.)* **305:**605–606.

Ross, R., 1968, The fibroblast and wound repair, *Biol. Rev.* **43:**51–96.

Ross, R., and Glomset, J. A., 1976, The pathogenesis of atherosclerosis, *N. Engl. J. Med.* **295:**369–377, 420–425.

Ross, R., and Vogel, A., 1978, The platelet-derived growth factor, *Cell* **14:**203–210.

Ross, R., Glomset, J. A., Kartya, B., and Harker, L., 1974, A platelet-dependent serum factor that stimulates the proliferation of arterial smooth muscle cells *in vitro, Proc. Natl. Acad. Sci. USA* **71:**1207–1210.

Ross, R., Raines, E. W., and Bowen-Pope, D. F., 1986, The biology of platelet-derived growth factor, *Cell* **45:**155–169.

Seifert, R. A., Schwartz, S. M., and Bowen-Pope, D. F., 1984, Developmentally regulated production of platelet-derived growth factor-like molecules, *Nature (Lond.)* **311:**669–671.

Sejersen, T., Betsholtz, C., Sjolund, M., Heldin, C.-H., Westermark, B., and Thyberg, J., 1986, Rat skeletal myoblasts and arterial smooth muscle cells express the gene for the A chain, but not the gene for the B chain (c-sis) of platelet-derived growth factor (PDGF) and produce a PDGF-like protein, *Proc. Natl. Acad. Sci. USA* **83:**6844–6848.

Senior, R. M., Griffin, G. L., Huang, J. S., Walz, D. A., and Deuel, T. F., 1983, Chemotactic activity of platelet alpha granule proteins for fibroblasts, *J. Cell Biol.* **96:**382–385.

Senior, R. M., Huang, J. S., Griffin, G. L., and Deuel, T. F., 1985, Dissociation of the chemotactic and mitogenic activities of platelet-derived growth factor by human neutrophil elastase, *J. Cell Biol.* **100:**351–356.

Seppa, H., Grotendorst, G., Seppa, S., Schiffmann, E., and Martin, G. R., 1982, Platelet-derived growth factor is chemotactic for fibroblasts, *J. Cell Biol.* **92:**584–588.

Shimokado, K., Raines, E. W., Madtes, D. K., Barrett, T. B., Benditt, E. P., and Ross, R., 1985, A significant part of macrophage-derived growth factor consists of at least two forms of PDGF, *Cell* **43:**277–286.

Singh, J. P. K., Chaikin, M. A., and Stiles, C. D., 1982, Phylogenetic analysis of platelet-derived growth factor by radio-receptor assay, *J. Cell Biol.* **95:**667–671.

Stiles, C. D., 1983. The molecular biology of platelet-derived growth factor, *Cell* **33:**653–655.

Stroobant, P., and Waterfield, M. D., 1984, Purification and properties of porcine platelet-derived growth factor, *EMBO J.* **3:**2963–2967.

Thielen, G. H., Gould, D., Fowler, M., and Dungworth, D. L., 1971, C-type virus in tumor tissue of woolly monkey (Lagothrix spp.) with fibrosarcoma, *J. Natl. Cancer Inst.* **47:**881–889.

Tzeng, D. Y., Deuel, T. F., Huang, J. S., Senior, R. M., Boxer, L. A., and Baehner, R. L., 1984, Platelet-derived growth factor promotes polymorphonuclear leukocyte activation, *Blood* **64:**1123–1128.

Tzeng, D. Y., Deuel, T. F., Huang, J. S., and Baehner, R. L., 1985. Platelet-derived growth factor promotes human peripheral monocyte activation, *Blood* **66:**179–183.

Walker, L. N., Bowen-Pope, D. F., Ross, R., and Reidy, M. A., 1986, Production of PDGF-like molecules by cultured arterial smooth muscle cells accompanies proliferation after arterial injury, *Proc. Natl. Acad. Sci. USA* **83:**7311–7315.

Waterfield, M. D., Scrace, G. T., Whittle, N., Stroobant, P., Johnsson, A., Wasteson, A., Westermark, B., Heldin, C.-H., Huang, J. S., and Deuel, T. F., 1983, Platelet-derived growth factor is structurally related to the putative transforming protein p28[v-sis] of simian sarcoma virus, *Nature (Lond.)* **304:**35–39.

Williams, L. T., Tremble, P., and Antoniades, H. N., 1982, Platelet-derived growth factor binds specifically to receptors on vascular smooth muscle cells and the binding becomes non-dissociable, *Proc. Natl. Acad. Sci. USA* **79:**5867–5870.

Williams, L. T., Antoniades, H. N., and Goetzl, E. J., 1983, Platelet-derived growth factor stimulates mouse 3T3 cell mitogenesis and leukocyte chemotaxis through different structural determinants, *J. Clin. Invest.* **72:**1759–1763.

Witte, L. D., Kaplan, K. L., Nossel, H. L., Lages, B. A., Weiss, H. J., and Goodman, D. S., 1978, Studies of the release from human platelets of the growth factor for cultured human arterial smooth muscle cells, *Circ. Res.* **42:**402–409.

Yarden, Y., Escobedo, J. A., Kuang, W.-J., Yang-Feng, T. L., Daniel, T. O., Tremble, P. M., Chen, E. Y., Ando, M. E., Harkins, R. N., Francke, U., Freid, V. A., Ullrich, A., and Williams, L. T., 1986, Structure of the receptor for platelet-derived growth factor helps define a family of closely related growth factor receptors, *Nature (Lond.)* **323:**226–232.

Chapter 10

The Role of Growth Factors in Tissue Repair II

Epidermal Growth Factor

ALLEN R. BANKS

1. History

Stanley Cohen described a protein isolated from the submaxillary glands of male mice that caused the premature eyelid opening and tooth eruption in neonatal mice (Cohen, 1962). On the basis of histologically apparent maturation and growth of the epidermis in the treated mouse tissues, Cohen and Elliott (1963) named the active fraction of the gland extract epidermal growth factor (EGF). Gray (1937) described a factor isolated from human urine that inhibited gastric acid secretion and named this factor urogastrone (Gray et al., 1939, 1940). Gregory (1975) reported that the amino acid sequence of urogastrone from human urine was very similar to that of the mouse EGF. Both proteins had cysteines in homologous positions and 27 of the 53 amino acids were identical (Gregory, 1975). Furthermore, the amino acid differences between EGF and urogastrone appeared to be relatively conservative. Because of the apparent functional equivalence of EGF and urogastrone, urogastrone in most instances is called human EGF and is so identified in the following discussion. A number of reviews on EGF have been recently published (King, 1985; Daughaday and Heath, 1984; Gregory, 1985; Stoscheck and King, 1986).

2. Structure

EGF is a single-chain acidic polypeptide with an isoelectric point (pI) of 4.5 (depending on the source) containing 53 amino acid residues. The polypeptide is nonglycosylated and very stable, surviving boiling or treatment with acid (Savage and Cohen, 1972; Planck et al., 1984; Matrisian et al., 1984; Mayo, 1985). It has a wide variety of physiologic effects, including the ability to stimulate the growth of a multitude of cell types and tissues. Six cysteine residues are arranged to form three disulfide bonds that hold the polypeptide chain in the tight rigid tertiary structure required for its biologic activity (Gregory and Preston, 1977).

ALLEN R. BANKS • Amgen, Inc., Thousand Oaks, California 91320.

When isolated from the mouse submaxillary gland, EGF is associated with a serine protease giving rise to a high-molecular-weight form of the growth factor (Taylor *et al.*, 1972, 1974; Hiramatsu *et al.*, 1982). The amino acid sequence of the mouse submaxillary EGF binding protease has high homology to mouse nerve growth-factor-binding protein (Anundi *et al.*, 1982; Lundgren *et al.*, 1984). Analysis of human serum for immunoreactive EGF has shown a 6000-M_r form corresponding to the 53-amino acid polypeptide EGF and a high-molecular-weight complex that can be dissociated to give the low-molecular-weight EGF polypeptide. Thus, EGF may circulate in plasma bound to a carrier protein as is the case for insulin-like growth factor (Zapf *et al.*, 1975; Hintz and Liu, 1977).

Recently, other proteins that bind to the EGF receptor and have effects similar to EGF on living cells have been described. One example is transforming growth factor-α (TGF-α), naturally found in normal tissues that may in fact be a fetal form of EGF (Derynck *et al.*, 1984). A second example is the vaccinia virus growth factor (VVGF) which is made by vaccinia virus infected cells perhaps to increase the growth rate in these infected cells (Reisner, 1985; Twardzik *et al.*, 1985). Both TGF-α and VVGF are similar to EGF in that they have cysteines in homologous positions. Otherwise, the amino acid sequences are quite different from EGF.

3. Sources of Epidermal Growth Factor

Until recently, mouse EGF was isolated from male mouse salivary glands while human EGF or urogastrone was isolated from human urine (Gregory, 1975; Kasselberg *et al.*, 1985; Mattila *et al.*, 1986). Each male mouse submaxillary gland may contain up to 1 mg of EGF (Savage and Cohen, 1972), while an adult human excretes about 50 µg of the factor in the urine per day. The function of such large amounts of EGF in the male mouse submaxillary gland is unknown; however, various roles have been suggested ranging from wound healing to an endocrine function involved in sperm motility (Tsutsumi *et al.*, 1986). EGF is also found in high concentrations in milk (Jansson *et al.*, 1985; Gresik *et al.*, 1984; Thornburg *et al.*, 1984; Petrides *et al.*, 1985) and is secreted by Brunner's glands in the small intestine (Olsen *et al.*, 1985).

4. Molecular Biology

The gene encoding mouse EGF is found on chromosome 3 and is under androgen control, while the gene for human EGF-urogastrone is found on chromosome 4 (Zabel *et al.*, 1985; Brissenden *et al.*, 1984). In humans, the EGF gene is a complex of 24 exons separated by large noncoding regions or introns, yielding an initial transcript of 110 kilobases (kb) of RNA (Bell *et al.*, 1986). After splicing and export from the nucleus, the 5-kb human messenger RNA codes for a 1207-amino acid precursor protein called preproepidermal growth factor. The mouse message codes for 1217 amino acids (Scott *et al.*, 1983, 1985).

There is approximately 75% homology at the nucleotide level between the two messages encoding the preproepidermal growth factor proteins. Approximately two-thirds into the length of the precursor protein the 53-amino acid EGF polypeptide is found. Although the function of the residual amino acid polypeptides is unknown, they have homology to other proteins, including atrial natriuretic peptide, blood coagulation factor X, the low-density-lipoprotein (LDL) receptor, transferrin, interleukin-II, and their respective receptors (Pfeffer and Ullrich, 1985; Bost et al., 1985; Sudhof et al., 1985; Hayashida and Miyata, 1985; Doolittle et al., 1984). From a molecular engineering perspective, it would not be practical to express the entire protein coded by the EGF prepromessage RNA in order to produce a relatively small 53-amino acid fragment. Instead, investigators have chemically constructed synthetic genes coding for the 53-amino acid polypeptide only.

Synthetic genes coding for EGF have been constructed for expression in E. coli, B. subtilis, and yeast (Smith et al., 1982; Flock et al., 1984; Brake et al., 1984; Urdea et al., 1983; Allen et al., 1985; Oka et al., 1985). Small chemically synthesized deoxyoligonucleotides are enzymatically ligated together to form the required coding sequence for expression of the desired polypeptide. Transformation of the suitably controlled synthetic structural gene into the host microorganism permits biosynthesis of the small polypeptide growth factor. This direct expression of EGF in a microbial host eliminates problems associated with expression of a large prepropolypeptide, such as subsequent proteolytic digestion to release the small region of interest.

When gene transcript expression is optimized in *Escherichia coli* by choosing the proper codons, optimizing secondary structure, and selecting a suitable ribosome binding site complementary to the E. coli 16S RNA, the desired protein can exceed one-half the total cellular protein produced by the bacteria. Thus, purification is straightforward as compared with eukaryotic cell expression, where the most highly expressed proteins might represent 1% of the total cellular protein.

Expression of synthetic genes in yeast can be by direct expression or can take advantage of the α-mating factor secretion system. Secretion into the extracellular matrix at high levels can be achieved using the α-factor system. Although proteolysis interferes with protein isolation with the alpha factor system for some proteins, it is the better way to obtain EGF from yeast, since the secreted protein is purified from the extracellular medium rather than from a mixture of intracellular proteins (Bitter et al., 1984). EGF is produced commercially by both E. coli expression and yeast α-factor secretion.

5. Epidermal Growth Factor Receptor

Current evidence suggests that the EGF polypeptide initiates all its effects by receptor binding (Wiley et al., 1985; Hunter, 1984; Carpenter, 1985). EGF receptors are found on virtually all mammalian cell types but are found most abundantly on epithelial cells (Nanney et al., 1984; Green and Couchman, 1984; Toyoda et al., 1986; Chabot et al., 1986). The receptors are also found in large numbers on fibroblasts, endothelial cells, and smooth muscle cells (Lim and Hauschka, 1984). Certain tumors have been shown to have elevated receptor numbers (Stoscheck and King, 1986; Gusterson et al., 1985; Gullick et al., 1986a; Fitzpatrick et al., 1984; Libermann et al., 1984) which may relate to their tumorigenicity. The human EGF receptor is composed of 1210 amino acids (Ullrich et al., 1984). The amino-terminal extracellular ligand-binding domain of 621 amino acids is heavily glycosylated (Moseley and Suva, 1986) and is probably crosslinked with disulfide bonds. There is a small transmembrane domain followed by a cytoplasmic domain composed of the remaining 542 carboxy-terminal amino acids. The human EGF receptor gene resides on chromosome 7. A number of reviews concerning the EGF receptor have been published (Adamson and Rees, 1981; Carpenter, 1984; Carpenter and Zendegui, 1986).

When EGF binds to the large extracellular domain of its transmembrane receptor, the EGF–receptor complex is internalized, and a multitude of sequelae occur (Gullick et al., 1985; Bockus and Stiles, 1984; Mroczkowski et al., 1984; Murthy et al., 1986; Rakowicz-Szulczynska et al., 1986). Experiments designed to demonstrate activity for EGF by internalizing it in some way other than by being bound to its receptor have found that such intracellular EGF lacks biologic activity (Ito et al., 1984). Once the EGF receptor is activated, by binding of EGF to the extracellular binding site, the cytoplasmic domain becomes an active tyrosine kinase, phosphorylating itself (autophosphorylation) (Downward et al., 1984; Bortics and Gill, 1985) as well as other intracellular proteins (Aoyagi et al., 1985; Dunn et al., 1986). The activated receptor enhances turnover of membrane inositol phospholipids and increases cellular pH and free Ca^{2+} (Moolenaar et al., 1984). EGF–receptor complexes are seen to cluster on the cell membrane and are subsequently internalized (Zidovetzki et al., 1986). The internalization of the receptor and the intracellular effects that follow give rise to observable changes in cellular morphology. The cells assume a less differentiated phenotype, grow rapidly, and divide. Generally, cells treated with EGF will temporarily lose their differentiated markers, such as collagen elaboration in the case of fibroblasts, rapidly divide and then return to their differentiated forms on removal or exhaustion of the growth factor supply. The result, in the end, is a larger number of fully active adult cells.

An interesting relationship has been found between the EGF receptor and the viral oncogene v-erb-B carried by the avian erythroblastosis virus. The v-erb-B protein is a truncated version of the EGF receptor lacking the EGF binding domain but retaining the intracellular receptor domain. It leads to a permanent growth-on signal to the cell and may aid in viral propagation (Ullrich et al., 1984; Downward et al., 1984b).

6. *In Vitro* Effects of Epidermal Growth Factor

The major in vitro effect of EGF is cellular growth. Other effects of EGF, beyond the scope of this summary, include gene activation and in some cells, stimulation of hormone secretion (Ikeda *et al.*, 1984; Freemark, 1986; Singh-asa *et al.*, 1985; Richman *et al.*, 1985).

Cell growth is a major effect of EGF. The polypeptide acts as a progression factor in the cell cycle; that is, cells that are competent to proceed through the cell cycle are stimulated to do so by the presence of EGF in the culture medium. EGF works in concert with other factors in various proportions, depending on the cell type. Cells involved in wound healing that are affected by EGF in this manner include epithelial cells, fibroblasts, and endothelial cells (McAuslan *et al.*, 1985; Stanulis-Praeger and Gilchrest, 1986; Nakagawa *et al.*, 1985). This does not mean that other cells are unaffected (Almazan *et al.*, 1985); proliferation of virtually every cell type is stimulated by EGF.

Epidermal growth factor has been shown to have similar effects on tissues in whole-organ culture. Skin grows in cultures supplemented with EGF (Boyce and Ham, 1983). Fetal rat calvaria have been shown to grow and take up nutrients in bone organ culture (Centrella and Canalis, 1985; Canalis and Raisz, 1979). Duodenum in organ culture supplemented with EGF grows and matures (Beaulieu *et al.*, 1985). Fetal lung in culture also has been shown to grow and mature under the influence of EGF (Gross *et al.*, 1986). Other functions of EGF that may relate directly to wound repair include chemotactic stimulation of epithelial cells (Blay and Brown, 1985) and stimulation of fibroblast collagenase production (Chua *et al.*, 1985).

7. *In Vivo* Effects of Epidermal Growth Factor

In vivo effects of EGF related to wound healing are widespread. One of the first effects of EGF demonstrated *in vivo* was the inhibition of gastric acid secretion in animals (Gregory, 1975; Konturek *et al.*, 1984); in fact, intravenous administration of EGF to humans with severe duodenal ulceration (Zollinger-Ellison syndrome) reduced the levels of gastric acid secretion as well as pain (Koffman *et al.*, 1982). Similar reductions in gastric acid levels were seen in normal human subjects (Elder *et al.*, 1975). EGF administered orally at levels found in saliva promote healing of chronic duodenal ulcers in rats, where it appears to be both a cytoprotective and growth-stimulating polypeptide (Olsen *et al.*, 1984, 1986; Thornburg *et al.*, 1984).

Epidermal growth factor has been shown to prevent hyaline membrane disease in fetal lambs (Sundell *et al.*, 1980). Control lambs delivered prematurely developed hyaline membrane disease, while identical twin lambs treated intravenously with EGF did not. EGF also appears to be important in maturation of fetal gut. When administered subcutaneously twice daily, EGF increased intestinal weight, lactase specific activity, and net calcium transport in normal 2-week-old suckling rats (Oka *et al.*, 1983). No effects were observed in weanling rats, which have an essentially mature intestinal tract.

The early observation that EGF accelerates the rate of eyelid opening in neonatal mice may have suggested experiments in eye healing (Cohen, 1962). Increased healing of corneal epithelium has been demonstrated in rats, rabbits, and monkeys (Arturson, 1984; Woost *et al.*, 1985; Brightwell *et al.*, 1985). Stromal healing has been demonstrated in rabbits and monkeys (Woost *et al.*, 1985; Brightwell *et al.*, 1985). EGF administered topically to rabbit eyes increased the tensile strength of full-thickness incisions by 20-fold. Administered to monkeys eyes, EGF increased the rate of epithelial regeneration and the tensile strength of full-thickness stromal incisions. An increase in fibroblast activity and collagen deposition was noted.

Epidermal growth factor may have an important role in bone repair. EGF increases DNA synthesis in bone culture and stimulates the proliferation of periosteal fibroblasts (Canalis and Raisz, 1979). There is a concomitant decrease in collagen synthesis, probably due to loss of the differentiated phenotype during cell replication.

Experiments using wound chambers *in vivo* suggest a role for EGF in deep wound healing, such as surgical wounds. EGF has been shown to stimulate fibroplasia and collagen deposition when administered in a wound chamber model (Laato *et al.*, 1986). Sustained release of EGF from a slow-release pellet implanted subcutaneously in a polyvinyl alcohol sponge "caused a dramatic increase in the extent and organization of the granulation tissue at day 7, a doubling in the DNA content, and 33% increases in protein content and wet weight, as compared with placebo controls" (Buckley *et al.*, 1985).

Skin healing has been demonstrated using a pig model. EGF applied topically to split-thickness skin wounds in pigs was shown to accelerate healing. In one study, 50% of EGF-treated wounds were completely healed on day 2, while placebo-treated wounds required 4 days for 50% of them to heal. Similar effects were seen with partial-thickness burns treated with a cream containing 10 µg/ml EGF (Brown *et al.*, 1986).

8. Summary

The implications for clinical wound repair are clear. Data show that EGF can increase the rate of healing in eye wounds, in skin wounds, and in deep tissue. Organ culture results suggest that EGF may be useful for the healing of bone and skin. EGF has been shown to be effective in the treatment of ulcers, both orally and parenterally. These data coupled with the availability of large quantities of EGF produced by recombinant DNA technology indicate a bright and interesting future in the field of wound healing as augmentation of healing becomes practical through the application of natural growth factors such as EGF.

References

Adamson, E. D., and Rees, A. R., 1981, Epidermal growth factor receptors, *Mol. Cell. Biochem,* **34:**129–152.

Allen, G., Paynter, C. A., and Winther, M. D., 1985, Production of epidermal growth factor in *Escherichia coli* from a synthetic gene, *J. Cell Sci.* **3**(Suppl.):29–38.

Almazan, G., Honegger, P., and Matthieu, J. M., and Guentert-Lauber, B., 1985, Epidermal growth factor and bovine growth hormone stimulate differentiation and myelination of brain cell aggregates in culture, *Brain Res.* **353**:257–264.

Anundi, H., Ronne, H., Peterson, P. A., and Rask, L., 1982, Partial amino-acid sequence of the epidermal growth-factor-binding protein, *Eur. J. Biochem.* **129**:365–371.

Aoyagi, T., Suya, H., Umeda, K., Kato, N., Nemoto, O., Kobayashi, H., and Miura, Y., 1985, Epidermal growth factor stimulates tyrosine phosphorylation of pig epidermal fibrous keratin, *J. Invest. Dermatol.* **84**:118–121.

Arturson, G., 1984, Epidermal growth factor in the healing of corneal wounds, epidermal wounds and partial-thickness scalds, *Scand. J. Plast. Reconstr. Surg.* **18**:33–37.

Beaulieu, J. F., Ménard, D., and Calvert, R., 1985, Influence of epidermal growth factor on the maturation of fetal mouse duodenum in organ culture, *J. Pediatr. Gastroenterol. Nutr.* **4**:476–481.

Bell, G. I., Fong, N. M., Stempien, M. M., Wormsted, M. A., Caput, D., Ku, L., Urdea, M. S., Rall, L. B., and Sanchez-Pescador, R., 1986, Human epidermal growth factor precursor: cDNA sequence, expression *in vitro*, and gene organization, *Nucleic Acids Res.* **14**:8427–8446.

Bertics, P. J., and Gill, G. N., 1985, Self-phosphorylation enhances the protein-tyrosine kinase activity of the epidermal growth factor receptor, *J. Biol. Chem.* **260**:14642–14647.

Bitter, G. A., Chen, K. K., Banks, A. R., and Lai, P. H., 1984, Secretion of foreign proteins from Saccharomyces cerevisiae directed by a-factor gene fusions, *Proc. Natl. Acad. Sci. USA* **84**:5330–5334.

Blay, J., and Brown, K. D., 1985, Epidermal growth factor promotes the chemotactic migration of cultured rat intestinal epithelial cells, *J. Cell Physiol.* **124**:107–112.

Bockus, B. J., and Stiles, C. D., 1984, Regulation of cytoskeletal architecture by platelet-derived growth factor, insulin and epidermal growth factor, *Exp. Cell Res.* **153**:186–197.

Bost, K. L., Smith, E. M., and Blalock, J. E., 1985, Regions of complementarity between the messenger RNA for epidermal growth factor, transferrin, interleukin-2 and their respective receptors, *Biochem. Biophys. Res. Commun.* **128**:1373–1380.

Boyce, S. T., and Ham, R. G., 1983, Calcium-regulated differentiation of normal human epidermal keratinocytes in chemically defined clonal culture and serum-free serial culture, *J. Invest. Dermatol.* **81**(Suppl. 1):33s–40s.

Brake, A. J., Merryweather, J. P., Colt, D. G., Heberlein, U. A., Masiarz, F. R., Mullenbach, G. T., Urdea, M. S., Valenzuela, P., and Barr, P. J., 1984, Alpha-factor-directed synthesis and secretion of mature foreign proteins in *Saccharomyces cerevisiae*, *Proc. Natl. Acad. Sci. USA* **81**:4642–4646.

Brightwell, J. R., Riddle, S. L., Eiferman, R. A., Valenzuela, P., Barr, P. J., Merryweather, J. P., and Schultz, G. S., 1985, Biosynthetic human EGF accelerates healing of neodecadron-treated primate corneas, *Invest. Ophthal. Vis. Sci.* **26**:105–110.

Brissenden, J. E., Ullrick, A., and Francke, U., 1984, Human chromosomal mapping of genes for insulin-like growth factors I and II and epidermal growth factor, *Nature (Lond.)* **310**:781–784.

Brown, G. L., Curtsinger, L. III, Brightwell, J. R., Ackerman, D. M., Tobin, G. R., Polk, H. C., Jr., George-Nascimento, C., Valenzuela, P., and Schultz, G. S., 1986, Enhancement of epidermal regeneration by biosynthetic epidermal growth factor, *J. Exp. Med.* **163**:1319–1324.

Buckley, A., Davidson, J. M., Kamerath, C. D., Wolt, T. B., and Woodward, S. C., 1985, Sustained release of epidermal growth factor accelerates wound repair, *Proc. Natl. Acad. Sci. USA* **82**:7340–7344.

Canalis, E., and Raisz, L. G., 1979, Effect of epidermal growth factor on bone formation in vitro, *Endocrinology* **104**:862–869.

Carpenter, G., 1984, Properties of the receptor for epidermal growth factor, *Cell* **37**:357–358.

Carpenter, G., 1985, Epidermal growth factor: Biology and receptor metabolism, *J. Cell Sci.* **3**(Suppl.):1–9.

Carpenter, G., and Zendegui, J. G., 1986, Epidermal growth factor, its receptor, and related proteins, *Exp. Cell Res.* **164**:1–10.

Centrella, M., and Canalis, E., 1985, Local regulators of skeletal growth: A perspective, *Endocrine Rev.* **6**:544–551.

Chabot, J. G., Walker, P., and Pelletier, G., 1986, Distribution of epidermal growth factor binding sites in the adult rat liver, *Am. J. Physiol.* **250**:G760.

Chua, C. C., Geiman, D. E., Keller, G. H., and Ladda, R. L., 1985, Induction of collagenase secretion in human fibroblast cultures by growth promoting factors, *J. Biol. Chem.* **260**:5213–5216.

Cohen, S., 1962, Isolation of a mouse submaxillary gland protein accelerating incisor eruption and eyelid opening in the new-born animal, *J. Biol. Chem.* **237**:1555–1562.

Cohen, S., and Elliot, G. A., 1963, The stimulation of epidermal keratinization by a protein isolated from the submaxillary gland of the mouse, *J. Invest. Dermatol.* **40**:1–5.

Daughaday, W. H., and Heath, E., 1984, Physiological and possible clinical significance of epidermal and nerve growth factors, *Clin. Endocrinol. Metab.* **13**:207–226.

Derynck, R., Roberts, A. B., Winkler, M. E., Chen, E. Y., and Gueddel, D. V., 1984, Human transforming growth factor-α: Precursor structure and expression in *E. coli, Cell* **38**:287–297.

Doolittle, R. F., Feng, D. F., and Johnson, M. S., 1984, Computer-based characterization of epidermal growth factor precursor, *Nature (Lond.)* **307**:558–560.

Downward, J., Parker, P., and Waterfield, M. D., 1984, Autophosphorylation sites on the epidermal growth factor receptor, *Nature (Lond.)* **311**:483–485.

Downward, J., Yarden, Y., Mayes, E., Scrace, G., Totty, N., Stockwell, P., Ullrich, A., Schlessinger, J., and Waterfield, M. D., 1984b, Close similarity of epidermal growth factor receptor and v-erb-B oncogene protein sequences, *Nature (Lond.)* **307**:521–527.

Dunn, W. A., Connolly, T. P., and Hubbard, A. L., 1986, Receptor-mediated endocytosis of epidermal growth factor by rat hepatocytes: Receptor pathway, *J. Cell Biol.* **102**:24–36.

Elder, J. B., Ganguli, P. C., Gillespie, I. E., Gerring, E. L., and Gregory, H., 1975, Effect of urogastrone on gastric secretion and plasma gastrin levels in normal subjects, *Gut* **16**:887–893.

Fitzpatrick, S. L., LaChance, M. P., and Schultz, G. S., 1984, Characterization of epidermal growth factor receptor and action on human breast cancer cells in culture, *Cancer Res.* **44**:3442–3447.

Flock, J. I., Fotheringham, I., Light, J., Bell, L., and Derbyshire, R., 1984, Expression in *Bacillus subtilis* of the gene for human urogastrone using synthetic ribosome binding sites, *MGG* **195**:246–251.

Freemark, J., 1986, Epidermal growth factor stimulates glycogen synthesis in fetal rat hepatocytes: Comparison with the glycogenic effects of insulin-like growth factor I and insulin, *Endocrinology* **119**:522–526.

Gray, J. S., Wieczorowski, E., and Ivy, A. C., 1939, Inhibition of gastric secretion by extracts of normal male urine, *Science* **89**:489–490.

Gray, J. S., Culmer, C. U., Wieczorowski, E., and Adkison, J. L., 1940, Preparation of a pyrogen-free urogastrone, *Proc. Soc. Exp. Biol. and Med.* **43**:225–228.

Green, M. R., and Couchman, J. R., 1984, Distribution of epidermal growth factor receptors in rat tissues during embryonic skin development, hair formation, and adult hair growth cycle, *J. Invest. Dermatol.* **83**:118–123.

Gregory, H., 1975, Isolation and structure of urogastrone and its relationship to epidermal growth factor, *Nature (Lond.)* **257**:325–327.

Gregory, H., 1985, *In vivo* aspects of urogastrone-epidermal growth factor, *J. Cell Sci.* **3**(Suppl.):11–17.

Gregory, H., and Preston, B. M., 1977, The primary structure of human urogastrone, *Int. J. Peptide Protein Res.* **9**:107–119.

Gresik, E. W., van der Noen, H., and Barka, T., 1984, Transport of 1251-EGF into milk and effect of sialoadenectomy on milk EGF in mice, *Am. J. Physiol.* **247**:E349–E354.

Gross, I., Dynia, D. W., Rooney, S. A., Smart, D. A., Warshaw, J. B., Sisson, J. F., and Hoath, S. B., 1986, Influence of epidermal growth factor on fetal rat lung development in vitro, *Pediatr. Res.* **20**:473–477.

Gullick, W. J., Marsden, J. J., Whittle, N., Ward, B., and Bobrow, L., 1986a, Expression of epidermal growth factor receptors on human cervical, ovarian, and vulval carcinomas, *Cancer Res.* **46**:285–292.

Gullick, W. J., Downward, J., Foulkes, J. G., and Waterfield, M. D., 1986b, Antibodies to the ATP-binding site of the human epidermal growth factor (EGF) receptor as specific inhibitors of EGF-stimulated protein-tyrosine kinase activity, *Eur. J. Biochem.* **158**:245–253.

Gusterson, B., Cowley, G., McIlhinney, J., Ozanne, B., and Fisher, C., 1985, Evidence for increased epidermal growth factor receptors in human sarcomas, *Int. J. Cancer* **36:**689–693.

Hayashida, H., and Miyata, T., 1985, Sequence similarity between epidermal growth factor precursor and atrial natriuretic factor precursor, *FEBS Lett.* **185:**125–128.

Hintz, R. L., and Liu, F., 1977, Demonstration of specific plasma protein binding sites for somatomedin, *J. Clin. Endocrinol. Metab.* **45:**988–995.

Hiramatsu, M., Hatakeyama, K., Kumegawa, M., and Minami, N., 1982, Plasminogen activator activity in the subunits of mouse submandibular gland nerve-growth factor and epidermal growth factor, *Arch. Oral Biol.* **27:**517–518.

Hunter, T., 1984, The epidermal growth factor receptor gene and its product, *Nature (Lond.)* **311:**477–480.

Ikeda, H., Mitsuhashi, T., Kubota, K., Kuzuya, N., and Uchimura, H., 1984, Epidermal growth factor stimulates growth hormone secretion from superfused rat adenohypophyseal fragments, *Endocrinology* **115:**556–558.

Ito, F., Ito, S., and Shimizu, N., 1984, Transmembrane delivery of polypeptide growth factors bypassing the intrinsic cell surface receptors: synthesis and biological activity of a conjugate of epidermal growth factor with alpha 2-macroglobulin, *Cell Struct. Funct.* **9:**105–115.

Jansson, L., Karlson, F. A., and Westermark, B., 1985, Mitogenic activity and epidermal growth factor content in human milk, *Acta Paediatr. Scand.* **74:**250–253.

Kasselberg, A. G., Orth, D. N., Gray, M. E., and Stahlman, M. T., 1985, Immunocytochemical localization of human epidermal growth factor/urogastrone in several human tissues, *J. Histochem. Cytochem.* **33:**315–322.

King, L. E., Jr., 1985, What does epidermal growth factor do and how does it do it? *J. Invest. Dermatol.* **84:**165–167.

Koffman, C. G., Elder, J. B., Ganguli, P. C., Gregory, H., and Geary, C. G., 1982, Effect of urogastrone on gastric secretion and serum gastrin concentration in patients with duodenal ulceration, *Gut* **23:**951–956.

Konturek, S. J., Cieszkowski, M., Jaworek, J., Konturek, J., Brzozowski, T., and Gregory, H., 1984, Effects of epidermal growth factor on gastrointestinal secretions, *Am. J. Physiol.* **246:**G580–G586.

Kurobe, M., Furukawa, S., and Hayashi, K., 1986, Molecular nature of human epidermal growth factor (hEGF)-like immunoreactivity in human plasma, *Biochem. Int.* **12:**677–683.

Laato, M., Niinikoski, J., Lebel, L., and Gerdin, B., 1986, Stimulation of wound healing by epidermal growth factor, *Ann. Surg.* **203:**379–381.

Libermann, T. A., Razon, A. D., Bartal, A. D., Yarden, Y., Schlessinger, J., and Soreq, H., 1984, Expression of epidermal growth factor receptors in human brain tumors, *Cancer Res.* **44:**753–760.

Lim, R. W., and Hauschka, S. D., 1984, A rapid decrease in epidermal growth factor-binding capacity accompanies the terminal differentiation of mouse myoblasts in vitro, *J. Cell Biol.* **98:**739–747.

Lundgren, S., Ronne, H., Rask, L., and Peterson, P. A., 1984, Sequence of an epidermal growth factor-binding protein, *J. Biol. Chem.* **259:**7780–7784.

McAuslan, B. R., Bender, V., Reilly, W., and Moss, B. A., 1985, New functions of epidermal growth factor: Stimulation of capillary endothelial cell migration and matrix dependent proliferation, *Cell Biol. Int. Rep.* **9:**175–182.

Matrisian, L. M., Planck, S. R., and Magun, B. E., 1984, Intracellular processing of epidermal growth factor in intracellular organelles, *J. Biol. Chem.* **259:**3047–3052.

Mattila, A. L., Perheentupa, J., Personen, K., and Viinikka, L., 1976, Epidermal growth factor in human urine from birth to puberty, *J. Clin. Endocrinol. Metab.* **61:**997–1000.

Mayo, K. H., 1985, Epidermal growth factor from the mouse. Physical evidence for a tiered beta-sheet domain: Two-dimensional NMR correlated spectroscopy and nuclear Overhauser experiments on backbone amide protons, *Biochemistry* **24:**3783–3794.

Moolenaar, W. H., Tertoolen, L. G., and de Laat, S. W., 1984, Growth factors immediately raise cytoplasmic free Ca^{2+} in human fibroblasts, *J. Biol. Chem.* **259:**8066–8069.

Moseley, J. M., and Suva, L. J., 1986, Molecular characterization of the EGF receptor and involvement of glycosyl moieties in the binding of EGF to its receptor on a clonal osteosarcoma cell line, UMR 106-06, *Calif. Tissue Int.* **38**:109–114.

Mroczkowski, B., Mosig, G., and Cohen, S., 1984, ATP-stimulated interaction between epidermal growth factor receptor and supercoiled DNA, *Nature (Lond.)* **309**:270–273.

Murthy, U., Basu, M., Sen-Majumdar, A., and Das, M., 1986, Perinuclear location and recycling of epidermal growth factor receptor kinase: Immunofluorescent visualization using antibodies directed to kinase and extracellular domains, *J. Cell Biol.* **103**:333–342.

Nakagawa, S., Yoshida, S., Hirao, Y., Kasuga, S., and Fuwa, T., 1985, Biological effects of biosynthetic human EGF on the growth of mammalian cells in vitro, *Differentiation* **29**:284–288.

Nanney, L. B., Magid, M., Stoscheck, C. M., and King, L. E., Jr., 1984, Comparison of epidermal growth factor binding and receptor distribution in normal human epidermis and epidermal appendages, *J. Invest. Dermatol.* **83**:385–393.

Nichols, R. A., and Shooter, E. M., 1985, Subunit interactions of the nerve and epidermal growth factor complexes: Protection of the biological subunit from proteolytic modification, *Dev. Neurosci.* **7**:216–229.

Oka, Y., Ghishan, F. K., Greene, H. L., and Orth, D. N., 1983, Effect of mouse epidermal growth factor/urogastrone on the functional maturation of rat intestine, *Endocrinology* **112**:940–944.

Oka, T., Sakamoto, S., Miyoshi, K., Fuwa, T., Yoda, K., Yamasaki, M., Tamura, G., and Miyake, T., 1985, Synthesis and secretion of human epidermal growth factor by *Escherichia coli, Proc. Natl. Acad. Sci. USA* **21**:7212–7216.

Olsen, P. S., Poulsen, S. S., Kirkegaard, P., and Nexo, E., 1984, Role of submandibular saliva and epidermal growth factor in gastric cytoprotection, *Gastroenterology* **87**:103–108.

Olsen, P. S., Poulsen, S. S., and Kirkegaard, P., 1985, Adrenergic effects on secretion of epidermal growth factor from Brunner's glands, *Gut* **26**:920–927.

Olsen, P. S., Poulsen, S. S., Therkelsen, K., and Nexo, E., 1986, Oral administration of synthetic human urogastrone promotes healing of chronic duodenal ulcers in rats, *Gastroenterology* **90**:911–917.

Petrides, P. E., Hosang, M., Shooter, E., Esch, F. S., and Bohlen, P., 1985, Isolation and characterization of epidermal growth factor from human milk, *FEBS Lett.* **187**:89–95.

Pfeffer, S., and Ullrich, A., 1985, Epidermal growth factor. Is the precursor a receptor? (news), *Nature (Lond.)* **313**:184.

Planck, S. R., Finch, J. S., and Magun, B. E., 1984, Intracellular processing of epidermal growth factor. II. Intracellular cleavage of the COOH-terminal region of ^{125}I-epidermal growth factor, *J. Biol. Chem.* **259**:3053–3057.

Rakowicz-Szulczynska, E. M., Rodeck, U., Herlyn, M., and Koprowski. H., 1986, Chromatin binding of epidermal growth factor, nerve growth factor, and platelet-derived growth factor in cells bearing the appropriate surface receptors, *Proc. Natl. Acad. Sci. USA* **83**:3728–3732.

Reisner, A. H., 1985, Similarity between the vaccinia virus 19K early protein and epidermal growth factor, *Nature (Lond.)* **383**:801–803.

Richman, R. A., Benedict, M. R., Florini, J. R., and Toly, B. A., 1985, Hormonal regulation of somatomedin secretion by fetal rat hepatocytes in primary culture, *Endocrinology* **116**:180–188.

Savage, C. R., and Cohen, S., 1972, Epidermal growth factor and a new derivative, *J. Biol. Chem.* **247**:7609–7611.

Scott, J., Urdea, M., Quiroga, M., Sanchez-Pescador, R., Fong, N., Selby, M., Rutter, W. J., and Bell, G. I., 1983, Structure of a mouse submaxillary messenger RNA encoding epidermal growth factor and seven related proteins, *Science* **221**:236–240.

Scott, J., Patterson, S., Rall, L., Bell, G. I., Crawford, R., Penschow, J., Niall, H., and Coghlan, J., 1985, The structure and biosynthesis of epidermal growth factor precursor, *J. Cell Sci.* **3**(Suppl.):19–28.

Singh-asa, P., Waters, M. J., and Wilce, P. A., 1985, A mechanism for the in vitro stimulation of adrenal cortisol biosynthesis by epidermal growth factor, *Int. J. Biochem.* **17**:857–862.

Smith, J., Cook, E., Fotheringham, I., Pheby, S., Derbyshire, R., Eaton, M. A. W., Doel, M., Lilley, D. M. J., Pardon, J. F., Lewis, H., and Bell, L. D., 1982, Chemical synthesis and cloning of a gene for human, b-urogastrone, *Nucleic Acid Res.* **10**:4467–4482.

Stanulis-Praeger, B. M., and Gilchrest, B. A., 1986, Growth factor responsiveness declines during adulthood for human skin-derived cells, Mech. Aging Dev. **35**:185–198.

Stoscheck, C. M., and King, L. E., Jr., 1986, Functional and structural characteristics of EGF and its receptor and their relationship to transforming proteins, J. Cell Biochem. **31**:135–152.

Sudhof, T. C., Russell, D. W., Goldstein, J. L., Brown, M. S., Sanchez-Pescador, R., and Bell, G. I., 1985, Cassette of eight exons shared by genes for LDL receptor and EGF precursor, Science **228**:893–895.

Sundell, H. W., Gray, M. E., Serenius, F. S., Escobedo, M. B., and Stahlman, M. T., 1980, Effects of epidermal growth factor on lung maturation in fetal lambs, Am. J. Pathol. **100**:707–726.

Taylor, J. M., Mitchell, W. M., and Cohen, S., 1972, Epidermal growth factor. Physical and chemical properties, J. Biol. Chem. **247**:5928–5934.

Taylor, J. M., Mitchell, W. M., and Cohen, S., 1974, Characterization of the high molecular weight form of epidermal growth factor, J. Biol. Chem. **249**:3198–3203.

Thornburg, W., Matrisian, L., Magun, B., and Koldovsk'y, O., 1984, Gastrointestinal absorption of epidermal growth factor in suckling rats, Am. J. Physiol. **246**:G80–G85.

Toyoda, S., Lee, P. C., and Lebenthal, E., 1986, Interaction of epidermal growth factor with specific binding sites of enterocytes isolated from rat small intestine during development, Biochim. Biophys. Acta **886**:295–301.

Tsutsumi, O., Kurachi, H., and Oka, T., 1986, A physiological role of epidermal growth factor in male reproductive function, Science **233**:975–977.

Twardzik, D. R., Brown, J. P., Ranchalis, J. E., Todaro, G. H., and Moss, B., 1985, Vaccinia virus-infected cells release a novel polypeptide functionally related to transforming and epidermal growth factors, Proc. Natl. Acad. Sci. USA **82**:5300–5304.

Ullrich, A., Coussens, L., Hayflick, J. S., Dull, T. J., Gray, A., Tam, A. W., Lee, J., Yarden, Y., Libermann, T. A., Schlessinger, J., Downward, J., Mayes, E. L. V., Whittle, N., Waterfield, M. D., and Seeburg, P. H., 1984, Human epidermal growth factor receptor cDNA sequence and aberrant expression of the amplified gene in A431 epidermoid carcinoma cells, Nature (Lond.) **309**:418–425.

Urdea, M. S., Merryweather, J. P., Mullenbach, G. T., Colt, D., Heberlein, U., Valenzuela, P., and Barr, P. J., 1983, Chemical synthesis of a gene for human epidermal growth factor urogastrone and its expression in yeast, Proc. Natl. Acad. Sci. USA **80**:7461–7465.

Wiley, H. S., VanNostrand, W., McKinley, D. N., and Cunningham, D. D., 1985, Intracellular processing of epidermal growth factor and its effect on ligand–receptor interactions, Cancer Res. **45**:1934–1939.

Woost, P. G., Brightwell, J., Eiferman, R. A., and Schultz, G. S., 1985, Effect of growth factors with dexamethasone on healing of rabbit corneal stromal incisions, Exp. Eye Res. **40**:47–60.

Yip, T. T., Tam, Y. Y., Keung, W. M., Xin, J. X., and King, Y. C., 1986, Studies on shrew (Suncus murinus) epidermal growth factor, Acta Endocrinol. (Copenh.) **111**:424–432.

Zabel, B. U., Eddy, R. L., Lally, P. A., Scott, J., Bell, G. E., and Shows, T. B., 1985, Chromosomal locations of the human and mouse genes for precursors of epidermal growth factor and the beta subunit of nerve growth factor, Proc. Natl. Acad. Sci. USA **82**:469–473.

Zapf, J., Waldvogel, M., and Froesch, E. R., 1975, Binding of nonsuppressible insulin-like activity to human serum: Evidence for a carrier protein, Arch. Biochem. Biophys. **168**:638–645.

Zidovetzki, R., Yarden, Y., Schelssinger, J., and Jovin, T. M., 1986, Microaggregation of hormone-occupied epidermal growth factor receptors on plasma membrane preparations, EMBO J. **5**:247–250.

Chapter 11

The Role of Growth Factors in Tissue Repair III
Fibroblast Growth Factor

GARY M. FOX

1. Introduction

Fibroblast growth factor (FGF) was first described by Gospodarowicz and co-workers as an activity derived from bovine brain or pituitary tissue (Gospodarowicz, 1974). As the name suggests, FGF was found to be mitogenic for fibroblasts in culture as well as endothelial cells and several other types of mesoderm-derived cells. It was first believed that FGF resulted from the degradation of myelin basic protein (Westall et al., 1978), but this was later found not to be the case (Thomas et al., 1980). Further characterization of the activity revealed that the primary mitogen from brain was different than that isolated from pituitary. These two factors were named acidic and basic FGF because they had similar if not identical biologic activities but differed in their isoelectric points.

Subsequently, other workers have isolated endothelial cell mitogens similar or identical to basic FGF from a number of tissues, tumors, and cell lines. These include hepatoma-derived growth factor (Klagsbrun et al., 1986; Lobb et al., 1986), chondrosarcoma-derived growth factor (Shing et al., 1984), β-retina-derived growth factor (Baird et al., 1985a), cartilage-derived growth factor (Sullivan and Klagsbrun, 1985), astroglial growth factor 2 (Pettmann et al., 1985), eye-derived growth factor I (Courty et al., 1985), cationic hypothalamus-derived growth factor (Klagsbrun and Shing, 1985), class 2 and β-heparin-binding growth factors (Lobb and Fett, 1984; Lobb et al., 1985,a,b, 1986), and a component of macrophage-derived growth factor (Baird et al., 1985b). All these factors share the basic property with FGF of binding tightly to heparin. A similar group of heparin-binding factors typified by acidic FGF has also been found. Among these are retina-derived growth factor (D'Amore and Klagsbrun, 1984), eye-derived growth factor II (Courty et al., 1985), endothelial cell growth factor, and α-heparin-binding growth factor (Maciag et al., 1979). Acidic FGF molecules elute from heparin at a lower NaCl concentration than does basic FGF. The heparin-binding property of acidic and basic FGF has facilitated their purifica-

---

GARY M. FOX • Amgen, Inc., Thousand Oaks, California 91320.

tion, permitting isolation of enough FGF for amino acid sequence analysis in several cases. For those of the basic FGF class, all that have been sequenced are identical to basic FGF or differ only in length at the N-terminus. The same type of N-terminal heterogeneity seems to be the only difference among members of the acidic FGF class.

2. Molecular Biology and Biochemistry

Acidic and basic FGF are probably derived from the same ancestral gene; they are 55% homologous in amino acid sequence and have the same intron/exon structure. Southern blotting experiments suggest that there is only one gene each for acidic and basic FGF (Abraham et al., 1976a,b); differences between the molecules isolated from different tissues are probably due to post-translational processing. The range of biologic activities of the two classes appears to be identical, although basic FGF is about 10 times more potent than acidic FGF in most bioassay systems. The two factors apparently bind to the same receptor. Recent reports suggest that addition of heparin to acidic FGF is able to enhance its activity, so that it is comparable to that of basic FGF.

Basic FGF as isolated from pituitary tissue is a single chain, nonglycosylated protein of 16,500 M_r. It contains four cysteine residues, two of which are believed to be involved in a disulfide bridge, while two are free sulfhydryls. The first sequence data for basic FGF was published by Bohlen et al. (1984), who determined the N-terminal 15 amino acids of material purified from bovine pituitary tissue. In a later publication, Esch et al. (1985) reported the complete sequence of basic FGF from bovine pituitary and at the same time compared it with the amino-terminal sequence from acidic FGF. A primary translation product of 155 amino acids has been proposed, but the translation initiation site is not well established; the true primary translate could be much larger. The major form found in pituitary tissue is 146 amino acids in length, but the 9 amino acids that are removed have none of the characteristics of a leader sequence in the usual sense. Currently, there is no conclusive evidence regarding the mechanism by which FGF is released from cells in vivo, although the presence of FGF receptors on the surface of some cells argues that it must somehow be released. It seems that the several molecular-weight-forms that have been isolated from different tissues may be the product of tissue-specific proteolytic cleavages rather than a product of the processing involved with secretion. All these forms, which differ only in their N-terminus, appear to retain full biologic activity. FGF is an extremely basic protein, with a pI of 9.6. It binds avidly to heparin, eluting from heparin sepharose columns at around 1.6 M NaCl. The biologic activity of FGF is destroyed by heat (70°C) or by detergents. The protein appears to be stable at 37°C for fairly long periods. Cloning of the gene for bovine basic FGF was first reported by Abraham et al. (1986a), and a later paper by the same group described the nucleotide sequence and genomic organization of human basic FGF (Abraham et al., 1986b). In the genome, coding sequences for this translation product are interrupted by two introns; the first splits codon 60 and the second separates codons 94 and 95. The size of the entire genomic coding region is unknown, but it is at least 34 kilobases (kb) in length. The gene for basic FGF is located on chromosome 4.

Acidic FGF is, like basic FGF, a single-chain nonglycosylated molecule of 16,000–18,000 M_r, depending on the tissue from which it is isolated. Purification of highly active acidic FGF to apparent homogeneity was first reported by Thomas et al. (1984) using bovine brain tissue as the source. Bohlen et al. (1985) published the N-terminal amino acid sequence, and Gimenez-Gallego et al. (1985) published the complete amino acid sequence of a 140-amino acid version of acidic FGF and observed its similarity to the sequences of basic FGF and human interleukin 1. Subsequently, Burgess et al. (1986) reported the purification and amino acid sequence of two factors, which they named endothelial cell growth factors α and β (ECGF-A, ECGF-B). One of these, ECGF-B, is 154 amino acids in length, with an acetylated N-terminal, and appears to be the primary translation product, although this has not been proven. Acidic FGF is apparently subject to the same sorts of specific cleavages near the N-terminus as basic FGF, leading to the isolation of multiple forms from different tissues. Acidic FGF has only three cysteine residues in contrast to the four cysteine residues in basic FGF, so that at least one must not be involved in disulfide bond formation. Acidic FGF binds to heparin somewhat less avidly than basic FGF, eluting at about 1 M NaCl and has a pI value of 5.0. The range of biologic activities of acidic and basic FGF has so far appeared to be identical, but the recent availability of highly purified preparations of both factors may allow resolution of as yet undiscovered differences.

3. Biologic Properties

Fibroblast growth factor has been shown to have many interesting biologic properties suggesting a possible role in the healing of wounds *in vivo*. One of the first steps in the wound-repair process is the formation of granulation tissue, which involves new blood vessel formation, fibroblast proliferation, and collagen deposition. Evidence from various *in vivo* and *in vitro* model systems indicates that FGF may be able to affect all three of these processes. FGF has been shown to be angiogenic; i.e., it can induce the formation and growth of new capillaries in a previously avascular space, such as the rabbit cornea (Gospodarowicz et al., 1979). In this experiment, a carrier material is impregnated with the growth factor and implanted in rabbit cornea. A positive response is scored if blood vessel growth toward the implant is observed with no evidence of an inflammatory response. FGF is a potent angiogenic factor in this assay; i.e., amounts in the nanogram range are able to produce a positive response. While this is approximately 1000 times the amount needed to produce a mitogenic response *in vitro*, this discrepancy could be due to technical problems such as partial inactivation of the factor by the carrier or incomplete release of FGF into the eye. FGF has also been observed to induce neovascularization when applied to the chorioallantoic membrane of a 3–5-day chick embryo, another standard assay for angiogenesis (Klagsbrun et al., 1975; Auerbach et al., 1974). The angiogenic activity of FGF appears to be potentiated by heparin, at least in crude preparations. The mechanism of this effect is unknown, but Klagsbrun and Shing (Shing et al., 1984) have proposed a three-way interaction among FGF, endothelial cells, and heparin-like molecules, such as heparan sulfate. These workers propose that heparin-binding growth factors may be concentrated in the vicinity of the endothelium by binding to heparan sulfate, the major glycosaminoglycan on the endothelial cell surface. The interaction of FGF with heparan sulfate could also play a role in transport to the extracellular matrix and possible release from the cell.

Fibroblast growth factor is a potent mitogen for fibroblasts, endothelial cells, and a wide variety of cells of mesodermal origin. The effect of FGF on cultured cells has been studied most extensively using corneal or capillary endothelial cells. The addition of FGF to cultures of these cell types results in shorter doubling times, stabilization of phenotype permitting longer-term culture, extension of the culture lifespan, and stimulation of cell migration (Duthu and Smith, 1980; Gospodarowicz, 1979; Gospodarowicz et al., 1978; 1981; Vlodavsky et al., 1976; Simonian et al., 1979; Simonian and Gill, 1979; Gospodarowicz and Bialecki, 1978). Other types of cells for which the mitogenic effect of FGF has been verified are granulosa cells, adrenal cortex cells, vascular smooth muscle cells, chondrocytes, and mouse fibroblasts (Gospodarowicz et al., 1985; Davidson et al., 1985). It was recently reported that FGF possesses neurotrophic activity for fetal rat hippocampal neurons in culture (Walicke et al., 1986).

In vivo, the formation of an extracellular matrix is a necessary event in the regeneration of lost or damaged tissue. Gospodarowicz and co-workers have examined the ability of extracellular matrix to support cell proliferation in culture (Gospodarowicz and Tauber, 1980; Gospodarowicz et al., 1982). When grown on plastic dishes, many cell types (vascular smooth muscle, corneal endothelium, fibroblasts, vascular endothelium, granulosa, adrenal cortex, and lens epithelium) require either serum or FGF or both to proliferate. However, if the cells are maintained on an extracellular matrix and exposed to plasma, they no longer require FGF. One possible explanation for this effect is that FGF could induce the synthesis of extracellular matrix by these cells. This hypothesis is supported by the observation that FGF can control the production of fibronectin and some collagen types by vascular endothelial cells (Gospodarowicz, 1984).

4. Wound-Healing Studies

Within the past few years, some direct evidence that FGF may be useful in accelerating the healing of wounds has been published. Fourtanier et al. (1986) reported that a preparation derived from bovine retina (probably a mixture of basic and acidic FGF) was able to stimulate neovascularization and re-epithelialization and to promote the healing of wounds in a guinea pig blister model. Suction was used in this model to separate the epidermis from underlying dermis, and the roof of the resulting blister was removed resulting in a pure epidermal wound. After 18 or 24 hr, the animals were sacrificed and the wound excised for examination and measurement of the area. Results indicated a significant acceleration of healing at doses around 5 pM. Davidson et al. (1985) examined the effect on wound repair of a bovine cartilage-derived factor (probably identical to basic FGF) in a rat wound model system. In this model, polyvinyl alcohol sponges were implanted subcutaneously and injected with growth factor 6 days later. At 48 or 72 hr postinjection, the sponges were removed and assayed for collagen, protein, and DNA content. The cartilage-derived factor was able to induce increases over controls in all three parameters. Since the increase in DNA content was greater than could be accounted for by increased DNA synthesis, it was concluded that an important part of the observed effects were due to migration of new mesenchymal cells to the site of injection. The factor was also observed to produce an increase in vascularization without any evident inflammatory response. Buntrock et al. (1982a,b) also reported increases in granulation tissue and neovascularization along with stimulation of wound healing in rats, using an extract of bovine brain tissue displaying FGF activity.

5. Conclusion

Although originally isolated from pituitary tissue, it is now clear that FGF (or a post-translationally modified form) is present in a wide variety of tissues. The effect of FGF on the growth of blood vessels and various cell types as well as its possible effects on the synthesis of extracellular matrix components suggest that it may be important in the healing of wounds in vivo. The recent availability of more highly purified FGF, including that from recombinant sources, should provide the means to more fully characterize the biologic and biochemical properties of this important factor.

References

Abraham, J., Mergia, A., Whang, J. L., Tumolo, A., Friedman, J., Hjerrild, K. A., Gospodarowicz, D., and Fiddes, J. C., 1986a, Nucleotide sequence of a bovine clone encoding the angiogenic protein, basic fibroblast growth factor, Science 233:545–548.

Abraham, J., Whang, J., Tumolo, A., Mergia, A., Friedman, J., Gospodarowicz, D., and Fiddes, J., 1986b, Human basic fibroblast growth factor: Nucleotide sequence and genomic organization, EMBO J. 5:2523–2528.

Auerbach, R., Kubai, L., Knighton, D., and Folkman, J., 1974, A simple procedure for the long-term cultivation of chicken embryos, Dev. Biol. 41:391–394.

Baird, A., Esch, F., Gospodarowicz, D., and Guillemin, R., 1985a, Retina- and eye-derived endothelial cell growth factors: Partial molecular characterization and identity with acidic and basic fibroblast growth factors, Biochemistry 24:7855–7860.

Baird, A., Mormede, P., and Bohlen, P., 1985b, Immunoreactive fibroblast growth factor in cells of peritoneal exudate suggests its identity with macrophage-derived growth factor, Biochem. Biophys. Res. Commun. 126:358–364.

Bohlen, P., Baird, A., Esch, R., Ling, N., and Gospodarowicz, D., 1984, Isolation and partial molecular characterization of pituitary fibroblast growth factor, *Proc. Natl. Acad. Sci. USA* **81**:5364–5368.

Bohlen, P., Esch, F., Baird, A., and Gospodarowicz, D., 1985, Acidic fibroblast growth factor (FGF) from bovine brain: Amino-terminal sequence and comparison with basic FGF, *EMBO J.* **4**:1951–1956.

Buntrock, P., Jentzsch, K. D., and Heder, G., 1982a, Stimulation of wound healing, using brain extract with fibroblast growth factor (FGF) activity. I. Quantitative and biochemical studies into formation of granulation tissue, *Exp. Pathol.* **21**:46–53.

Buntrock, P., Jentzsch, K. D., and Heder, G., 1982b, Stimulation of wound healing, using brain extract with fibroblast growth factor (FGF) activity. II. Histological and morphometric examination of cells and capillaries, *Exp. Pathol.* **21**:62–67.

Burgess, W., Mehlman, T., Marshak, D., Fraser, B., and Maciag, T., 1986, Structural evidence that endothelial cell growth factor beta is the precursor of both endothelial cell growth factor alpha and acidic fibroblast growth factor, *Proc. Natl. Acad. Sci. USA* **83**:7216–7220.

Courty, J., Loret, C., Moenner, M., Chevallier, B., Lagente, O., Courtois, Y., and Barritault, D., 1985, Bovine retina contains three growth factor activities with different affinity to heparin: Eye derived growth factor I, II, III, *Biochimie* **67**:265–269.

D'Amore, P., and Klagsbrun, M., 1984, Endothelial cell mitogens derived from retina and hypothalamus: Biochemical and biological similarities, *J. Cell. Biol.* **99**:1545–1549.

Davidson, J., Klagsbrun, M., Hills, K., Buckley, A., Sullivan, R., Brewer, P., and Woodward, S., 1985, Accelerated wound repair, cell proliferation, and collagen accumulation are produced by a cartilage-derived growth factor, *J. Cell. Biol.* **100**:1219–1227.

Duthu, G. S., and Smith, J. R., 1980, In vitro proliferation and lifespan of bovine aorta endothelial cells: Effect of culture conditions and fibroblast growth factor, *J. Cell Physiol.* **103**:385–392.

Esch, F., Baird, A., Ling, N., Ueno, N., Hill, F., Denoroy, L., Klepper, R., Gospodarowicz, D., Bohlen, P., and Guillemin, R., 1985, Primary structure of bovine pituitary basic fibroblast growth factor (FGF) and comparison with the amino-terminal sequence of bovine brain acidic FGF, *Proc. Natl. Acad. Sci. USA* **82**:6507–6511.

Fourtanier, A., Courty, J., Muller, E., Courtois, Y., Prunieras, M., and Barritault, D., 1986, Eye-derived growth factor isolated from bovine retina and used for epidermal wound healing *in vivo, J. Invest. Dermatol.* **87**:76–80.

Gimenez-Gallego, G., Rodkey, J., Bennett, C., Rios-Candelore, M., DiSalvo, J., and Thomas, K., 1985, Brain-derived acidic fibroblast growth factor: Complete amino acid sequence and homologies, *Science* **130**:1385–1388.

Gospodarowicz, D., 1974, Localization of a fibroblast growth factor and its effect alone and with hydrocortisone on 3T3 cell growth, *Nature (London)* **249**:123–127.

Gospodarowicz, D., 1979, Fibroblast and epidermal growth factors: their uses in vivo and in vitro in studies on cell functions and cell transplantation, *Mol. Cell Biochem.* **25**:79–110.

Gospodarowicz, D., 1984, in: *Hormonal Proteins and Peptides,* Vol. XII (C. H. Li, ed.), pp. 205–230, Academic, New York.

Gospodarowcz, D., and Bialecki, H., 1978, The effects of epidermal and fibroblast growth factors on the replicative lifespan of cultured bovine granulosa cells, *Endocrinology* **103**:854–858.

Gospodarowicz, D., and Tauber, J.-P., 1980, Growth factors and the extracellular matrix, *Endocr. Rev.* **1**:201–227.

Gospodarowicz, D., Greenberg, G., Bialecki, H., and Zetter, B., 1978, Factors involved in the modulation of cell proliferation in vivo and in vitro: The role of fibroblast and epidermal growth factors in the proliferative response of mammalian cells, *In Vitro* **14**:85–118.

Gospodarowicz, D., Bialecki, H., and Thakral, T. K., 1979, The angiogenic activity of the fibroblast and epidermal growth factor, *Exp. Eye Res.* **28**:501–514.

Gospodarowicz, D., Vlodavsky, I., and Savion, N., 1981, The role of fibroblast growth factor and the extracellular matrix in the control of proliferation and differentiation of corneal endothelial cells, *Vision Res.* **21**:87–103.

Gospodarowicz, D., Cohen, D. C., and Fujii, D. K., 1982, Regulation of cell growth by the basal lamina and plasma factors: relevance to embryonic control of cell proliferation and differentiation, Cold Spring Harbor Conferences on Cell Proliferation, Vol. 9. Growth of Cells in Hormonally Defined Media, Part A and B. pp. 95–124.

Gospodarowicz, D., Massoglia, S., Cheng, J., Lui, G-M, and Bohlen, P., 1985, Isolation of pituitary fibroblast growth factor by fast protein liquid chromatography (FPLC): partial chemical and biological characterization, *J. Cell. Physiol.* **122**:323–332.

Klagsbrun, M., Knighton, D., and Folkman, J., 1975, Tumor angiogenesis in cells grown in tissue culture, *Cancer Res.* **36**:110–114.

Klagsbrun, M., and Shing, Y., 1985, Heparin affinity of anionic and cationic capillary endothelial cell growth factors: Analysis of hypothalamus-derived growth factors and fibroblast growth factors, *Proc. Natl. Acad. Sci. USA* **82**:805–809.

Klagsbrun, M., Sasse, J., Sullivan, R., and Smith, J. A., 1986, Human tumor cells synthesize an endothelial cell growth factor that is structurally related to basic fibroblast growth factor, *Proc. Natl. Acad. Sci. USA* **83**:2448–2452.

Lobb, R. R., and Fett, J. W., 1984, Purification of two distinct growth factors from bovine neural tissue by heparin affinity chromatography, *Biochemistry* **23**:6295–6299.

Lobb, R. R., Alderman, E. M., and Fett, J. W., 1985a, Induction of angiogenesis by bovine brain derived class I heparin-binding growth factor, *Biochemistry* **24**:4969–4973.

Lobb, R. R., Strydom, D. J., and Fett, J. W., 1985b, Comparison of human and bovine brain derived heparin-binding growth factors, *Biochem. Biophys. Res. Commun.* **131**:586–592.

Lobb, R. R., Sasse, J., Sullivan, R., Shing, Y., D'Amore, P., Jacobs, J., and Klagsbrun, M., 1986, Purification and characterization of heparin-binding endothelial cell growth factors, *J. Biol. Chem.* **261**:1924–1928.

Maciag, T., Cerundolo, J., Ilsley, S., Kelley, P., and Forand, P., 1979, An endothelial cell growth factor from bovine hypothalamus: Identification and partial characterization, *Proc. Natl. Acad. Sci. USA* **76**:5674–5678.

Pettmann, B., Weibel, M., Sensenbrenner, M., and Labourdette, G., 1985, Purification of two astroglial growth factors from bovine brain, *FEBS Lett.* **189**:102–108.

Shing, Y., Folkmann, J., Sullivan, R., Butterfeld, C., Murray, J., and Klagsbrun, M., 1984, Heparin affinity: Purification of a tumor-derived capillry endothelial cell growth factor, *Science* **223**:1296–1299.

Simonian, M. H., and Gill, G. N., 1979, Regulation of deoxyribonucleic acid synthesis in bovine adrenocortical cells in culture, *Endocrinology* **104**:588–600.

Simonian, M. H., Hornsby, P. J., Ill, C. R., O'Hare, M. J., and Gill, G. N., 1979, Characterization of cultured bovine adrenocortical cells and derived clonal lines: Regulation of steroidogenesis and culture lifespan, *Endocrinology* **105**:99–108.

Sullivan, R., and Klagsbrun, M., 1985, Purification of cartilage-derived growth factor by heparin affinity, *J. Biol. Chem.* **260**:2399–2403.

Thomas, K. A., Rios-Candelore, M., and Fitzpatrick, S., 1984, Purification and characterization of acidic fibroblast growth factor from bovine brain, *Proc. Natl. Acad. Sci. USA* **81**:357–361.

Thomas, K. A., Riley, M. C., Lemmon, S. K., Baglan, N. C., and Bradshaw, R. A., 1980, Brain fibroblast growth factor: Nonidentity with myelin basic protein fragments, *J. Biol. Chem.* **255**:5517–5520.

Vlodavsky, I., Johnson, L. K., Greenburg, G., and Gospodarowicz, D., 1976, Vascular endothelial cells maintained in the absence of fibroblast growth factor undergo structural and functional alterations that are incompatible with their *in vivo* differentiated properties, *J. Cell. Biol.* **83**:468–486.

Walicke, P., Cowan, W. M., Ueno, N., Baird, A., and Guillemin, R., 1986, Fibroblast growth factor promotes survival of dissociated hippocampal neurons and enhances neurite extension, *Proc. Natl. Acad. Sci. USA* **83**:3012–3016.

Westall, F. C., Lennon, V. A., and Gospodarowicz, D., 1978, Brain-derived fibroblast growth factor: Identity with a fragment of basic protein of myelin, *Proc. Natl. Acad. Sci. USA* **75**:4675–4678.

Chapter 12

The Role of Growth Factors in Tissue Repair IV

Type β-Transforming Growth Factor and Stimulation of Fibrosis

RCHARD K. ASSOIAN

1. Introduction

Type β-transforming growth factor (TGF-β) is a low-molecular-weight protein with a broad array of biologic effects, including the ability both to stimulate and inhibit the proliferation of cells in culture (Tucker et al., 1984; Roberts et al., 1985; Sporn et al., 1986). This chapter focuses on a single aspect of TGF-β action: its ability to induce a striking wound-healing response in several whole-animal and cell-culture model systems. These results, considered with experiments showing storage of TGF-β in platelets and release of TGF-β during platelet degranulation, strongly suggest that this growth factor has an important physiologic role as an endogenous mediator of wound repair and fibrosis.

2. Identification of TGF-β

The history of transforming growth factors (type α and type β) is inextricably linked to the autocrine hypothesis of transformation (Sporn and Todaro, 1980). This hypothesis, which suggests that transformed cells secrete growth factors for their own use, was based on studies demonstrating that chemically and virally transformed cells in culture released a growth factor activity that was undetectable in untransformed cellular counterparts (DeLarco and Todaro, 1978). Moreover, the growth factor activity appeared to be unique in its ability to transform cultures of non-neoplastic indicator cells, e.g., normal rat kidney fibroblasts, phenotypically as assessed by loss of contact inhibition and induction of anchorage-independent growth. Considering these results, the name transforming growth factor seemed only appropriate for this activity.

RICHARD K. ASSOIAN • Department of Biochemistry and Molecular Biophysics, Center for Reproductive Sciences, College of Physicians and Surgeons, Columbia University, New York, New York 10032.

Although transforming growth factor was originally envisioned as a single species, careful analysis showed that the activity was due to the concerted action of two resolvable proteins (Anzano et al., 1982, 1983). These two proteins, called TGF-α and TGF-β on the basis of their synergistic actions on normal rat kidney fibroblasts (Roberts et al., 1983b), have now been purified and analyzed biochemically (Marquardt et al., 1983; Massagué, 1983, 1984; Assoian et al., 1983; Frolik et al., 1983; Roberts et al., 1983a). Their cDNAs have been cloned and sequenced (Derynck et al. 1984, 1985, 1986; Lee et al., 1985b). The results from these structural studies clearly show that TGF-α and -β are structurally unrelated. TGF-α, a single-chain polypeptide (6000 M_r), is structurally related to epidermal growth factor (EGF), binds to the EGF receptor, and elicits EGF-like effects (see Chapter 9, Section 2). There is no compelling evidence for a unique TGF-α receptor. By contrast, TGF-β (25,000 M_r) is a dimer of two apparently identical subunits (12,500 M_r, 112-amino acid residues) held together by disulfide bonds. There is no significant sequence homology between TGF-β and TGF-α (or EGF), although recent studies have established that a family of TGF-β-like molecules do exist (Cate et al., 1986; Mason et al., 1985; Seyedin et al., 1985, 1986). TGF-β binds to a plasma-membrane receptor that is distinct from the EGF receptor (Frolik et al., 1984; Massagué, 1985).

3. TGF-β in Non-Neoplastic Tissues and Cells

Perhaps the most striking difference between type α- and β-transforming growth factors lies in the distribution of these peptides in normal and neoplastic tissue. TGF-α or its messenger RNA (mRNA), has been detected in fetal and embryonic tissue (Nexø et al., 1980; Twardzik et al., 1982; Lee et al., 1985a), but a definitive identification of TGF-α in normal adult tissue has yet to be reported. Human platelets contain an EGF-like peptide with some structural characteristics of TGF-α; however, identity to authentic TGF-α has not been established (Assoian et al., 1984). By contrast, TGF-β has been detected in a wide variety of normal adult tissue (Roberts et al., 1982), and it has been purified from non-neoplastic sources (Assoian et al., 1983; Frolik et al., 1983; Roberts et al., 1983a). In fact, the structure of TGF-β at the protein level has been elucidated largely with growth factor purified from normal tissue and cells.

4. TGF-β and Wound Repair

4.1. Sources of TGF-β

The concept that TGF-β might play a role in wound repair arose after repeated detection in non-neoplastic tissue. Especially striking were results that showed that TGF-β activity was present in serum and derived from platelets (Childs *et al.*, 1982). Direct examination of platelets showed that they contain particularly high concentrations of the growth factor (Assoian *et al.*, 1983; Assoian and Sporn, 1986). The TGF-β concentration in fresh human platelets (1200–2400 molecules per platelet or approx 1 part per million wet weight) is 10–1000-fold higher than that of the other non-neoplastic sources examined to date. Other studies have shown that TGF-β is released from human platelets which have been degranulated by exposure to thrombin; the concentrations of thrombin required to release TGF-β are identical to those concentrations that release the α-granule marker, β-thromboglobulin (Assoian and Sporn, 1986). These data suggest fundamental similarities between TGF-β and platelet-derived growth factor (PDGF) with regard to (1) approximate concentrations in human platelets, (2) storage in α-granules, and (3) release during platelet degranulation at sites of injury (Kaplan *et al.*, 1979a,b; Ross and Vogel, 1978). It is important to note that other cell types with established roles in inflammation and repair can be sources of TGF-β. In particular, activation of lymphocytes induces transcription of the TGF-β gene and secretion of the growth factor (Kehrl *et al.*, 1986).

4.2. Latent TGF-β

Recent evidence suggests that TGF-β is released from many cells in a high-molecular-weight form that is apparently due to an association between the growth factor and a binding protein (Pircher *et al.*, 1984; Lawrence *et al.*, 1985). The biochemical properties of this binding protein have not been analyzed, but it is clear that the TGF-β/binding protein complex is biologically inactive and that the free-binding protein can actively compete with TGF-β plasma membrane receptors for ligand binding. These experiments have also shown that the binding protein is acid labile; brief exposure of a TGF-β/binding protein complex to mild acid (pH 2) results in denaturation of the binding protein and liberation of active growth factor (TGF-β is a stable to mild acid). Although the state of TGF-β, stored and released from platelets, has yet to be established biochemically, it is possible that such a growth factor/binding protein complex exists in platelets (Pircher *et al.*, 1986). It will be important to determine whether the role of this binding protein is to clear excess TGF-β from the circulation or to act as a reservoir for TGF-β. Experiments documenting physiologic equilibrium between free and bound forms of the growth factor would do much to resolve these questions.

4.3. Actions of TGF-β *in Vivo*

The wound-healing actions of TGF-β have been studied primarily in the Schilling-Hunt wound chamber model system (Sporn *et al.*, 1983; Lawrence *et al.*, 1986). In this protocol, small wire-mesh chambers are implanted subcutaneously into the back of rats. The animals respond to the presence of these chambers by encapsulating them in connective tissue. A few days after insertion, the encapsulated chambers define an enclosed space into which sterile solutions of growth factors can be injected in an attempt to induce a wound-healing response. The chambers are usually removed 1–2 weeks after insertion; connective tissue on the outside of the chambers is removed, and the contents of the chambers are analyzed for the extent of fibroblast infiltration (by measuring total protein and DNA levels) and collagen deposition (by measuring hydroxyproline levels). Initial studies in this system (Sporn et al., 1983) used partially purified TGF-β but nevertheless showed a statistically significant increase in fibroblast proliferation and collagen deposition both biochemically and histologically. These experiments were the first to document an in vivo effect of TGF-β.

A more recent study (Lawrence et al., 1986) documented striking effects of TGF-β on the wound healing response in vivo. In these experiments, the protocol described was modified by incorporating a type I collagen gel (containing the growth factor of interest) into Schilling-Hunt chambers prior to implantation. This procedure minimized diffusion of growth factors from the chamber and obviated the need for daily injection. The contents of the chambers were analyzed in the usual manner, with total collagen levels minus the amount added to the chambers initially. A second modification was the use of Adriamycin-treated rats; this drug impairs the basal rate of wound healing and growth factor reversal of the impaired rate can be measured. (Basal wound repair in untreated rats is used as a positive control.) Third, all growth factors in this study were purified to homogeneity.

The following results, as reported by Lawrence et al. (1986), confirmed and extended the likelihood that TGF-β has a crucial role in wound repair in vivo. First, a single dose of purified TGF-β (100 ng/ml) reversed most of the Adriamycin-induced wound-healing impairment, as judged by collagen content, protein content, cellular proliferation rate, and histology. Second, of the growth factors tested (PDGF, EGF, and TGF-β), TGF-β most effectively reversed the Adriamycin-induced impairment. Third, the effect of TGF-β could be potentiated by the presence of PDGF and EGF; together, these three peptides reversed almost 90% of the Adriamycin-induced impairment. Since PDGF, TGF-β, and an EGF-like peptide are all present in human platelets (Assoian et al., 1984), the concerted action of these growth factors is feasible in vivo.

In a related study, Roberts et al. (1986) injected purified TGF-β (< 1 µg) subcutaneously into newborn mice. After 2–3 days of daily injection, granulation tissue formed at the site of injection. Morphologic analysis of this tissue showed that angiogenesis and collagen deposition were induced by injection of TGF-β. Fibroblasts, macrophages, and granulocytes were present. Injections of EGF or saline did not induce the response. Taken with the studies already described, it is apparent that in vivo administration of TGF-β is closely associated with a wound-healing response. Nevertheless, these studies with whole animals cannot be used to determine which cell types respond directly to TGF-β during the overall process of wound repair.

4.4. Effects of TGF-β on Matrix Protein Formation *in Vitro*

Although a complete review of TGF-β action in cell culture is beyond the scope of this chapter, certain effects of TGF-β on isolated cells have important implications for the potential role of this growth factor in fibrosis. Of particular interest are recent studies that have examined the effect of TGF-β on matrix protein production by cultured fibroblasts. Two reports (Roberts *et al.*, 1986; Ignotz and Massagué, 1986) have shown that TGF-β efficiently stimulates collagen and fibronectin formation in a variety of fibroblastic cell lines. The effect is selective and specific for these extracellular matrix proteins. Thus, the specificity and action of TGF-β in whole-animal models for wound repair can be reproduced in a cell-culture system with isolated fibroblasts. Taken together, these studies suggest that the increased collagen deposition observed in whole-animal wound-healing model systems, in response to TGF-β, probably results from a direct effect of this growth factor on matrix protein formation by fibroblasts.

4.5. Effects of TGF-β on Fibroblast Proliferation *in Vitro*

TGF-β was identified on the basis of its ability to synergize with EGF and stimulate proliferation of normal rat kidney fibroblasts in soft agar (conditions of anchorage-independent growth). Although the relevance of this assay to wound repair has yet to be established, recent studies by Ignotz and Massagué (1986) have shown that normal rat kidney cells grow in soft agar when cultured in the presence of serum, EGF, and fibronectin; fibronectin replaced (at least in part) the requirement for TGF-β. These intriguing results suggest that TGF-β may induce three-dimensional growth of normal rat kidney cells in an anchorage-dependent manner, and not anchorage-independent growth as usually thought. If this interpretation is correct, the biologic principles of TGF-β action established in soft agar assays may be much more relevant to its *in vivo* role in wound repair. For example, the positive interaction among TGF-β, PDGF, and EGF, as reported in the Lawrence study (1986), has also been observed for colony formation of normal rat kidney fibroblasts; efficient proliferation of these cells in soft agar is stimulated by the concerted action of TGF-β, PDGF, and EGF (Assoian *et al.*, 1984). It is essential to realize, however, that the growth factors required to induce colony formation of normal rat kidney cells (serum, EGF, and TGF-β) are not necessarily required by other fibroblastic cell lines. For example, rat-1 fibroblasts grow in soft agar in response to serum and EGF (Kaplan and Ozanne, 1983), whereas AKR-2B fibroblasts and primary dermal fibroblasts require serum and TGF-β (Tucker *et al.*, 1983; Moses *et al.*, 1985). Other fibroblast lines are inhibited by TGF-β in culture (Anzano *et al.*, 1986). Clearly, the interpretation of these cell culture data is complicated by the widespread use of serum (a source of PDGF, TGF-β, and EGF) and by the possibility that different quantitative requirements for growth factors may mask qualitatively similar needs. The appropriate culture system to examine the effect of TGF-β on fibroblast proliferation *in vivo* and its physiologic interactions with other growth factors remains elusive.

5. Conclusion

Although it was first envisioned as a secretory product of transformed cells, it is now clear that TGF-β is a protein widely distributed in normal tissue. The identification of TGF-β in platelets and lymphocytes, considered with the evidence for TGF-β enhancement of wound repair *in vivo*, and fibroblast proliferation and matrix protein formation *in vitro*, strongly argue that this growth factor has an important physiologic role in wound repair. The development of an appropriate culture system to examine these actions in greater detail would do much to advance our understanding of the biology of TGF-β.

References

Anzano, M. A., Roberts, A. B., Meyers, C. A., Komoriya, A., Lamb, L. C., Smith, J. M., and Sporn, M. B., 1982, Synergistic interaction of two classes of transforming growth factors from murine sarcoma cells, *Cancer Res.* **42:**4776–4778.

Anzano, M. A., Roberts, A. B., Smith, J. M., Sporn, M. B., and DeLarco, J. E., 1983, Sarcoma growth factor from conditioned medium of virally transformed cells is composed of both type alpha and type beta transforming growth factors, *Proc. Natl. Acad. Sci. USA* **80:**6264–6269.

Anzano, M. A., Roberts, A. B., and Sporn, M. B., 1986, Anchorage-independent growth of primary rat embryo cells is induced by platelet-derived growth factor and inhibited by type-beta transforming growth factor, *J. Cell. Physiol.* **126:**312–318.

Assoian, R. K., and Sporn, M. B., 1986, Type beta transforming growth factor in human platelets: Release during platelet degranulation and action on vascular smooth muscle cells, *J. Cell Biol.* **102:**1217–1223.

Assoian, R. K., Komoriya, A., Meyers, C. A., Miller, D. M., and Sporn, M. B., 1983, Transforming growth factor-beta in human platelets: Identification of a major storage site, purification, and characterization, *J. Biol. Chem.* **258:**7155–7160.

Assoian, R. K., Grotendorst, G. R., Miller, D. M., and Sporn, M. B., 1984, Cellular transformation by coordinated action of three peptide growth factors from human platelets, *Nature (Lond.)* **309:**804–806.

Cate, R. L., Mattaliano, R. J., Hession, C., Tizard, R., Farber, N. M., Cheung, A., Ninfa, E. G., Frey, A. Z., Gash, D. J., Chow, E. P., Fisher, R. A., Bertonis, J. M., Torres, G., Wallner, B. P., Ramachandran, K. L., Ragin, R. C., Manganaro, T. F., MacLaughlin, D. T., and Donahoe, P. K., 1986, Isolation of the bovine and human genes for Mullerian Inhibiting Substance and expression of the human gene in animal cells, *Cell* **45:**5312–5316.

Childs, C. B., Proper, J. A., Tucker, R. F., and Moses, H. L., 1982, Serum contains a platelet-derived transforming growth factor-alpha: Precursor structure and expression in *E. coli, Cell* **38:**287–297.

DeLarco, J. E., and Todaro, G. J., 1978, Growth factors from murine sarcoma virus-transformed cells, *Proc. Natl. Acad. Sci. USA* **75:**4001–4005.

Derynck, Roberts, A. B., Winkler, M. E., Chen, E. Y., and Goeddel, D. V., 1984, Human transforming growth factor-alpha: precursor structure and expression in *E. coli, Cell* **38:**287–297.

Derynck, R., Jarrett, J. A., Chen, E. Y., Eaton, D. H., Bell, J. R., Assoian, R. K., Roberts, A. B., Sporn, M. B., and Goeddel, D. V., 1985, Human transforming growth factor-beta complementary DNA sequence and expression in normal and transformed cells, *Nature (Lond.)* **316:**701–705.

Derynck, R., Jarrett, J. A., Chen, E. Y., and Goeddel, D. V., 1986, The murine transforming growth factor-beta precursor, *J. Biol. Chem.* **261**:4377–4379.

Frolik, C. A., Dart, L. L., Meyers, C. A., Smith, D. M., and Sporn, M. B., 1983, Purification and initial characterization of type beta transforming growth factor from human placenta, *Proc. Natl. Acad. Sci. USA* **80**:3676–3680.

Frolik, C. A., Wakefield, L. M., Smith, D. M., and Sporn, M. B., 1984, Characterization of a membrane receptor for transforming growth factor-beta in normal rat kidney fibroblasts, *J. Biol. Chem.* **259**:10995–11000.

Ignotz, R. A., and Massagué, J., 1986, Transforming growth factor-beta stimulates the expression of fibronectin and collagen and their incorporation into the extracellular matrix, *J. Biol. Chem.* **261**:4337–4345.

Kaplan, P. L., and Ozanne, B., 1983, Cellular responsiveness to growth factors correlates with a cell's ability to express the transformed phenotype, *Cell* **33**:931–938.

Kaplan, D. R., Chao, F. C., Stiles, C. D., Antoniades, H. N., and Scher, C. D., 1979a, Platelet alpha granules contain a growth factor for fibroblasts, *Blood* **53**:1043–1052.

Kaplan, K. L., Brockman, M. J., Chernoff, A., Lesznik, G. R., and Drillings, M., 1979b, Platelet alpha granule proteins: Studies on release and subcellular localization, *Blood* **53**:604–618.

Kehrl, J. H., Wakefield, L. M., Roberts, A. B., Jakowlew, S., Alvarez-Mon, M., Derynck, R., Sporn, M. B., and Fauci, A. S., 1986, Production of transforming growth factor-beta by human T lymphocytes and its potential role in the regulation of T cell growth, *J. Exp. Med.* **163**:1037–1050.

Lawrence, D. A., Pircher, R., and Jullien, P., 1985, Conversion of a high molecular weight latent beta-TGF from chicken embryo fibroblasts into a low molecular weight active beta-TGF under acidic conditions, *Biochem. Biophys. Res. Commun.* **133**:1026–1034.

Lawrence, W. T., Sporn, M. B., Gorschboth, C., Norton, J. A., and Grotendorst, G. R., 1986, The reversal of an adriamycin induced healing impairment with chemoattractants and growth factors, *Ann. Surg.* **203**:142–147.

Lee, D. C., Rochford, R., Todaro, G. J., and Villarreal, L. P., 1985a, Developmental expression of rat transforming growth factor-alpha mRNA, *Mol. Cell. Biol.* **5**:3644–3646.

Lee, D. C., Rose, T. M., Webb, N. R., and Todaro, G. J., 1985b, Cloning and sequence analysis of a cDNA for rat transforming growth factor-alpha, *Nature (Lond.)* **313**:489–491.

Marquardt, H., Hunkapiller, M. W., Hood, L. E., Twardzik, D. R., DeLarco, J. E., Stephenson, J. R., and Todaro, G. J., 1983, Transforming growth factors produced by retrovirus-transformed rodent fibroblasts and human melanoma cells: Amino acid sequence homology with epidermal growth factor, *Proc. Natl. Acad. Sci. USA* **80**:4684–4688.

Mason, A. J., Hayflick, J. S., Ling, N., Esch, F., Ueno, N., Ying, S., Guillemin, R., Niall, H., and Seeburg, P. H., 1985, Complementary DNA sequences of ovarian follicular fluid inhibin show precursor structure and homology with transforming growth factor-beta, *Nature (Lond.)* **318**:659–663.

Massagué, J., 1983, Epidermal growth factor-like transforming growth factor: Isolation, chemical characterization, and potentiation by other transforming factors from feline sarcoma virus-transformed rat cells, *J. Biol. Chem.* **258**:13606–13613.

Massagué, J., 1984, Type beta transforming growth factor from feline sarcoma virus-transformed rat cells, *J. Biol. Chem.* **259**:9756–9761.

Massagué, J., 1985, Subunit structure of a high-affinity receptor for type beta transforming growth factor: Evidence for a disulfide-linked glycosylated receptor complex, *J. Biol. Chem.* **260**:7059–7066.

Moses, H. L., Tucker, R. F., Leof, E. B., Coffey, R. J., Halper, J., and Shipley, G. D., 1985, Type-beta transforming growth factor is a growth stimulator and a growth inhibitor, *Cold Spring Harbor Conf. Cancer Cells* **3**:65–71.

Nexø, E., Hollenberg, M. D., Figueroa, A. A., and Pratt, R. M., 1980, Detection of epidermal growth factor-urogastrone and its receptor during fetal mouse development, *Proc. Natl. Acad. Sci. USA* **77**:2782–2785.

Pircher, R., Lawrence, D. A., and Jullien, P., 1984, Latent beta-transforming growth factor in nontransformed and Kirsten sarcoma virus-transformed normal rat kidney cells, clone 49F, *Cancer Res.* **44**:5538–5543.

Pircher, R., Jullien, P., and Lawrence, D. A., 1986, Beta-transforming growth factor is stored in human blood platelets as a latent high molecular weight complex, *Biochem. Biophys. Res. Commun.* **136**:30–37.

Roberts, A. B., Anzano, M. A., Frolik, C. A., and Sporn, M. B., 1982, Transforming growth factors: Characterization of two classes of factors from neoplastic and nonneoplastic tissues, *Cold Spring Harbor Conf. Cell Prolif.* **9**:319–332.

Roberts, A. B., Anzano, M. A., Meyers, C. A., Wideman, J., Blacher, R., Pan, Y.-C., Stein, S., Lehrman, R., Smith, J. M., Lamb, L. C., and Sporn, M. B., 1983a, Purification and properties of a type beta transforming growth factor from bovine kidney, *Biochemistry* **22**:5692–5698.

Roberts, A. B., Frolik, C. A., Anzano, M. A., and Sporn, M. B., 1983b, Transforming growth factors from neoplastic and nonneoplastic tissues, *Fed. Proc.* **42**:2621–2626.

Roberts, A. B., Anzano, M. A., Lamb, L. C., Smith, J. M., and Sporn, M. B., 1985, Type beta transforming growth factor: A bifunctional regulator of cellular growth, *Proc. Natl. Acad. Sci. USA* **82**:119–123.

Roberts, A. B., Sporn, M. B., Assoian, R. K., Smith, J. M., Roche, N. S., Wakefield, L. M., Heine, U. I., Liotta, L. A., Falanga, V., Kehrl, J. H., and Fauci, A. S., 1986, Transforming growth factor type beta: Rapid induction of fibrosis and angiogenesis *in vivo* and stimulation of collagen formation *in vitro*, *Proc. Natl. Acad. Sci. USA* **83**:4167–4171.

Ross, R., and Vogel, A., 1978, The platelet-derived growth factor, *Cell* **14**:203–210.

Seyedin, S. M., Thomas, T. C., Thompson, A. Y., Rosen, D. M., and Piez, K. A., 1985, Purification and characterization of two cartilage-inducing factors from bovine demineralized bone, *Proc. Natl. Acad. Sci. USA* **82**:2267–2271.

Seyedin, S. M., Thompson, A. Y., Bentz, H., Rosen, D. M., McPherson, J. M., Conti, A., Siegel, N. R., Galluppi, G. R., and Piez, K. A., 1986, Cartilage-inducing factor-A: Apparent identity to transforming growth factor-beta, *J. Biol. Chem.* **261**:5693–5695.

Sporn, M. B., and Todaro, G. J., 1980, Autocrine secretion and malignant transformation of cells, *N. Engl. J. Med.* **303**:878–880.

Sporn, M. B., Roberts, A. B., Shull, J. H., Smith, J. M., Ward, J. M., and Sodek, J., 1983, Polypeptide transforming growth factor isolated from bovine sources and used for wound healing *in vivo*, *Science* **219**:1329–1331.

Sporn, M. B., Roberts, A. B., Wakefield, L. M., and Assoian, R. K., 1986, Transforming growth factor-beta: Biological function and chemical structure, *Science* **233**:532–534.

Tucker, R. F., Volkenant, M. E., Branum, E. L., and Moses, H. L., 1983, Comparison of intra- and extracellular transforming growth factors from nontransformed and chemically transformed mouse embryo cells, *Cancer Res.* **43**:1581–1586.

Tucker, R. F., Shipley, G. D., Moses, H. L., and Holley, R. W., 1984, Growth inhibitor from BSC-1 cells closely related to platelet type beta transforming growth factor, *Science* **226**:705–707.

Twardzik, D. R., Ranchalis, J. E., and Todaro, G. J., 1982, Mouse embryonic transforming growth factors related to those isolated from tumor cells, *Cancer Res.* **42**:590–593.

Chapter 13

Mechanisms of Parenchymal Cell Migration into Wounds

JAMES B. McCARTHY, DARYL F. SAS, and LEO T. FURCHT

1. Introduction

Successful wound repair is highly dependent on the orderly influx of specific cell populations into the lesion. The sequence of morphologic events that ensues after a wound occurs is well understood in general terms. However, despite the long interest in wound healing, it is only recently that specific factors that might regulate cell motility into wounded tissues have been identified. The number of factors recognized is increasing as techniques of isolation and characterization become more sophisticated, and undoubtedly the list is far from complete. This chapter is designed to describe cell motility within the context of a continuously changing environment such as occurs within a healing wound. The nature of the stimuli and the responding cells vary somewhat depending on the structure of the tissue and the type of lesion. Although the thrust of this chapter is on parenchymal cell movement, leukocyte migration is briefly outlined for contrast and comparison. Cell proliferation, the other important component of parenchymal cell repopulation of injured tissue, is covered in Chapters 9–12 and 16.

2. Mechanisms of Directing Cell Motility

Various mechanisms have been advanced to explain the phenomenon of directed cell motility, a property of cells that is basic not only to wound healing but to many aspects of development and metastatic spread of malignant neoplasms as well (Trinkaus, 1984; Thiery, 1984; LeDouarin, 1984; Singer, 1986). Clearly, motility per se is a phenomenon of cell behavior subject to the control of highly interrelated and complex biochemical/biophysical processes; obviously, a detailed treatment of this topic is beyond the scope of this chapter. Although distinctions may be made in vitro concerning the different mechanisms of directing motility, they all share several qualities. Regardless of the

JAMES B. McCARTHY, DARYL F. SAS, and LEO T. FURCHT • Department of Laboratory Medicine and Pathology, University of Minnesota, Minneapolis, Minnesota 55455. Present address for D. F. S.: Gastrointestinal Research Unit, Mayo Clinic, Rochester, Minnesota 55905.

mechanism, cells must become asymmetric in order to move, forming thrusting protrusions, and must establish an active dominant leading edge. The leading edge must in turn establish adherence to the substratum, and ultimately, through contractile forces, pull the rear edge of the cell forward. Directional influences *in vivo* must persist long enough to establish a net direction for the motility of entire cell populations. The stimulus for directional movement can be a soluble attractant (chemotaxis), a substratum-bound gradient of a particular matrix constituent (haptotaxis), or the three-dimensional array of extracellular matrix within the tissue (contact guidance). The directional movement of epithelial cell sheets presents a special biologic problem. For cells within the sheet, directionality results from marginal cells extending lamellipodia away from the sheet. This phenomenon has been termed the free edge effect. Mechanisms must also exist *in vivo* acting to open up spaces within the extracellular matrix as cells migrate into a given area. With these principles in mind, the following account reviews the major mechanisms that might coordinate the ordered migration of specific cell populations that debride and heal the wound.

2.1. Chemotaxis

Defined as the directed migration of cells in response to a concentration gradient of a soluble attractant, chemotaxis is the most often reported (and least rigorously proven) mechanism of directed cell motility. The biologic effect of a chemoattractant is regulated by diffusion of the attractant from its source into an attractant-poor environment. Much of the knowledge about chemotaxis in higher organisms stems from extensive research on the migration of neutrophils and monocytes in response to attractants generated during inflammation. These studies are briefly reviewed, since principles learned from inflammatory cell chemotaxis may apply to connective tissue cell chemotaxis.

When circulating neutrophils and monocytes are exposed to chemotactic agents released at sites of inflammation, the cells change their adherent properties (Schiffman and Gallin, 1979; Snyderman and Goetzl, 1981; Wilkinson, 1982), marginate in the postcapillary venules, and emigrate into the extravascular space. Several such chemotactic agents have been shown capable of stimulating leukocyte migration *in vitro*. A partial list of these attractants includes complement-derived factors, such as C5a (Snyderman *et al.*, 1968); bacterial factors (presumably mimicked by the synthetic attractant formyl-methionyl-leucyl-phenylalanine, FMLP, and related analogues) (Showell *et al.*, 1976); certain clotting factors, such as platelet factor 4 (Deuel *et al.*, 1981) and thrombin (Bar-Shivat *et al.*, 1983); and cleavage products of elastin (Senior *et al.*, 1980), collagen (Postlethwaite and Kang, 1976), and plasma fibronectin (Norris *et al.*, 1982). Cell-derived factors have also been reported to promote leukocyte migration. Leukotriene B_4 and a neutrophil-derived chemoattractant released upon monosodium urate ingestion have been reported to attract leukocytes (Spilberg *et al.*, 1976; Ford-Hutchinson *et al.*, 1980). Fibroblasts and lymphocytes, through the production of chemotactic factors, can also stimulate leukocyte migration in delayed-type hypersensitivity reactions (Wahl, 1981). Leukocyte migration has been studied *in vitro* using several assay systems, including in Boyden chambers (Zigmond and Hirsch, 1973), under agarose (Nelson *et al.*, 1978), and in special orientation chambers (Zigmond, 1977).

In studies using Boyden chambers, stimulated neutrophil migration was demonstrated to be composed of two components: (1) directional migration, in which cells moved up a positive concentration gradient of attractant called chemotaxis, and (2) increased random migration, in which cells moved independent of a concentration gradient termed chemokinesis (Zigmond and Hirsch, 1973). Later studies by Zigmond used a special orientation chamber in order to visualize cells directly that are put into a concentration gradient of attractant (Zigmond, 1977). Zigmond observed that cells structurally orient in response to gradients of chemotactic substances, with a leading lamellipodium extending toward the source of the attractant and with a trailing uropod. Cells could orient in gradients as small as 1% across the cell surface (Zigmond, 1977). Other investigators have shown that this cytologic polarization is accompanied by asymmetry in the distribution of receptors and membrane activities. Concanavalin A (Con A) and Fc receptors, coated pits, and pinocytotic vesicles have been shown to concentrate in the trailing uropod of an oriented cell (Davis *et al.*, 1982). This location of membrane receptors is dependent on metabolic activity, since cells incubated at 4°C show a preferential receptor expression (e.g., Fc receptors) at the lamellipodium (Davis *et al.*, 1982). These studies suggest that new receptors are first inserted anteriorly during migration and are then swept to the trailing edge as the cell moves forward. It has been hypothesized that the anterior/posterior sweeping of receptor–ligand complexes on the cell surface could serve to amplify even relatively shallow attractant gradients across the cell (Zigmond *et al.*, 1981; Davis *et al.*, 1982), helping maintain directional motility during chemotaxis.

Many studies have addressed the nature of neutrophil chemoattractant receptors (reviewed in Snyderman and Pike, 1984). In general, these receptors have high to moderately high affinity for their respective ligands, with dissociation constants ranging from 10^{-9} to 10^{-8} M. Detailed work on the FMLP receptor has indicated that there are two classes of receptors for this peptide on the cell surface of neutrophils that can be distinguished by differing affinities (Koo *et al.*, 1982; Mackin *et al.*, 1982). It is believed that the neutrophil/monocyte receptor interaction with a particular chemoattractant is a specific event. Preincubating cells with an attractant desensitizes the response to that attractant but does not affect the responsiveness of the cells to a different attractant (Ward and Becker, 1968; Becker, 1972). The mechanism of signal transduction is still poorly understood, but it is thought to involve changes in membrane potential (Gallin and Gallin, 1977) and ion influx (Gallin and Rosenthal, 1974; Naccache *et al.*, 1977). Transmethylation reactions, mediated by S-adenosyl-methionine, have also been implicated in signal transduction (Hirata *et al.*, 1979; Pike *et al.*, 1978). Methylation reactions activate phospholipase, which releases membrane phospholipids. The phospholipids then activate protein kinase C, which mediates certain chemoattractant-induced responses (McPhail et al., 1984).

Importantly, chemoattractants also exert a variety of effects on leukocyte function in addition to motility. Attractants stimulate bursts of oxidative metabolism (Klebanoff and Clark, 1978) and exocytosis of a variety of lysosomal enzymes (Goldstein et al., 1973). Thus, during inflammation, chemoattractants can enhance bactericidal properties of leukocytes as well as facilitate the invasion of these inflammatory cells through the subendothelial basement membrane and other connective tissues (see Chapter 6). Parenchymal cells also can respond to chemotactic signals in vitro (Section 5) but in vivo are often constrained by strong interactions with matrix substratum (Section 4) or interactions with other cells (Section 2.4).

2.2. Haptotaxis

A second mechanism of promoting directional single-cell migration is along an adhesion gradient; this is termed haptotaxis. On the basis of time-lapse (Harris, 1973) and other studies (reviewed in Trinkaus, 1984), haptotaxis may be distinguished in vitro from chemotaxis. The directional information during migration by haptotaxis comes from the substratum as opposed to fluids surrounding the cell. Directional haptotactic motility does not result from the stimulation of protrusions at the leading edge of the cell, as occurs in chemotaxis. By contrast, cells migrating by haptotaxis extend lamellipodia more or less randomly, and each of these protruding lamellipodia competes for a finite amount of membrane, such that when one lamellipodium adheres, spreads, and becomes dominant, tension on the remainder of the cell inhibits further protrusive activity. Thus, the increasing adhesion gradients on the substratum appear to influence directional movement by favoring stabilization of a leading edge on one side of a motile cell. After the cell becomes asymmetric, with a trailing and leading edge, the cell advances and the trailing edge is pulled forward forming retraction fibers, which are created by the residual adherence of mature focal adhesion plaques. As the cell lunges forward and breaks old adhesions, the excess membrane at the trailing edge becomes available for incorporation at the leading edge, hence motility continues. Chen (1981) observed that mechanically lifting the trailing edge of a migrating cell off the substratum accelerated the advance of the leading edge of the cell, a phenomenon that he termed retraction-induced spreading. Again, detachment of the trailing edge probably provides excess membrane for the leading lamellipodium, consistent with the observations of Harris (1973). There is also evidence that new membrane from the Golgi apparatus may be inserted selectively at the leading edge of the cell (Bergmann et al., 1983).

The concept of haptotaxis for regulating directional cell movement was originally suggested by Carter (1967a,b, 1970). In these early studies, substrata of varying adhesiveness were used to manipulate directional cell migration in vitro. Briefly, hydrophilic palladium was evaporated in a gradient fashion across a hydrophobic cellulose acetate substratum. L cells plated onto such substrata accumulated in areas of greater adhesivity (i.e., hydrophilic palladium). Similar results could be demonstrated using haptotactic islands, created by shadowing palladium onto cellulose acetate strips protected by electron microscope grids (Carter, 1967b). As with gradient shadowing, cells localized preferentially to the areas of increasing adhesion (i.e., the squares of palladium).

Harris (1973) extended these findings by demonstrating that the direction of adhesion-mediated migration was related to the *relative* hydrophilicity of substrates used. For example, chicken fibroblasts would localize on palladium squares when coated onto a nonwettable background, such as underivatized polystyrene; however, the same cells would localize on the highly hydrophilic polystyrene derivatized for tissue culture when it was used as a background for palladium shadowing. Cells therefore discriminate between two substrata of differing hydrophilicity and segregate according to this hierarchy toward more hydrophilic substrata. In a follow-up study, Rich and Harris (1981) demonstrated that not all cell types seek out an increasingly hydrophilic substratum. Macrophages were observed to localize onto increasingly hydrophobic substrata when presented with a choice, indicating that haptotactic motility is a function not only of the hydrophilic gradient but of cell-specific membrane properties as well.

Letourneau (1975), using embryonic chick neurons *in vitro*, showed that developing neurites will extend along adhesion gradients in a manner analogous to non-nerve cell haptotaxis. The extending microspikes from the growth cones discriminated between substrata of variable hydrophilicity and formed firm adhesions according to a hierarchy. Furthermore, works by Rogers *et al.* (1983) and others (Akers *et al.*, 1981; Baron von Evercooren *et al.*, 1982) suggested a role for matrix adhesion molecules such as fibronectin and laminin in supporting neuronal adhesion and haptotactic neurite outgrowth. A recent report by Hammarback *et al.* (1985) demonstrated that developing neurites *in vitro* can be guided by biopathways of laminin. These observations suggest that axonal development *in vivo*, such as would happen following crush injuries to nerves, could rely in part on haptotactic cues provided by the sheath proteins produced by glial cells and fibroblasts (Palm and Furcht, 1982; Cornbrooks *et al.*, 1983).

2.3. Contact Guidance

Contact guidance, initially proposed by Weiss as a mechanism for directing cell movements (Weiss, 1945, 1958) is probably closely related to haptotaxis. Briefly, contact guidance simply refers to the tendency of cells to align along discontinuities in substrata to which they are attached. As an example, cells migrating on scratched substrata *in vitro* tend to align with and move along the scratches. In addition, cells implanted at two discrete foci in a plasma clot soon begin to orient and migrate toward each other, a phenomenon that Weiss termed the two-center effect (Trinkaus, 1984). The mutually opposing contractile forces created by the cells exert tension on the clot matrix, reorganizing random fibrin strands into colinear fibrils along which the cells then migrate. Presumably, the reason for orientation in contact guidance is similar to that proposed for haptotaxis. In contact guidance, however, competition of lamellipodia for a finite amount of membrane is subject to the added influence of the three-dimensional orientation (as well as adhesive quality) of the substratum, accentuating orientation. This mechanism of orientation may in fact account for the highly oriented appearance of infiltrating fibroblasts as these cells enter the granulation tissue (Peacock and Van Winkle, 1976; Bryant, 1977).

The orientation of fibrils within resolving granulation tissue can also have dramatic effects on wound contraction, hence wound closure. The contractile forces of the myofibroblasts, which are enriched in more mature granulation tissue, can effectively operate along the lines of stress which contact guidance forces have set up (see Chapter 17). As the wound heals, lines of stress and patterns of orientation develop along axes parallel to the wound surface (Repesh et al., 1982). Wound contraction along these stress lines efficiently closes the wound and can reduce the diameter of the original defect by 75% (Peacock and Van Winkle, 1976). Recent work from our laboratory (Sas et al., 1985) (see Section 5.1) as well as others (Stopak and Harris, 1982; Stopak et al., 1985) has demonstrated a role for cell motility in organizing the architecture of connective tissue not only in wound healing but in certain phases of development as well.

2.4. Migration of Cell Sheets

The epithelial cells lining the body's surface, cavities, and circulatory system all live in extremely close apposition to one another. It is well established that these cell types are joined to each other by some or all of the following cell-to-cell junctions: zonulae occludens and adherens, macula adherens (desmosome), and nexus (gap junction) (Trinkaus, 1984). In addition, epithelial cells have specialized adhesion structures on substrata, as exemplified by hemidesmosomes (Gipson et al., 1983a; Trinkaus-Randall and Gipson, 1984). Therefore, motility of epithelial cells in a wound poses special mechanistic problems not encountered by other cells that spend most of their time as isolated components within connective tissue.

Essentially two mechanisms have been proposed to explain epidermal cell migration during wound closure. In the first model, it has been proposed that as cells proximal to the wound contact the substratum, they cease moving, and distal cells migrate over them until the defect is completely closed. This model for epithelial migration, termed the leapfrog model, was supported by the observations of Krawczyk (1971) and Repesh and Oberpriller (1980). In contrast to this model, it has been proposed that cells of an epithelial sheet might move forward much as a caterpillar moves forward; i.e., the proximal cell advances, freeing a small space in front of the immediate submarginal cell, which in turn extends a leading lamellipodium, and so on (Radice, 1980a,b; Mahan and Donaldson, 1985). In the latter model, the cells near the defect contribute in a coordinated manner to the motility of the sheet as a whole without changing relative positions (see Chapter 11). In general, stratified epithelium like the epidermis tends to migrate in a manner similar to the leapfrog model, while simple epithelium like corneal epithelium or endothelium migrates in a caterpillar fashion.

Directionality of movement in migrating epithelial sheets seems to be regulated by the sheet itself, a property termed the free-edge effect (Trinkaus, 1984). When an epithelial defect is created, the marginal cells extend lamellipodia into the defect, in some cases within seconds (Trinkaus, 1984). Interestingly, isolated epithelial cells, while able to move in a random manner, are not as able as fibroblasts to orient and move in a persistent direction. Epithelial cells also exhibit more blebbing than fibroblasts, implying that cells present in a sheet somehow impart directionality of movement to one another (Dipasquale, 1975). It is now appreciated that the submarginal cells appear to inhibit the formation of lamellipodia at the trailing edge of marginal cells by a contact-inhibition mechanism (Vaughn and Trinkaus, 1966; Abercrombie, 1967; Dipasquale, 1975). This effectively stabilizes asymmetry of the leading cells and regulated directional movement away from the sheet toward the defect. The motility rate varies greatly with cell type and species of origin. It can range from 5 μM/hr in rat epidermis to almost 700 μM/hr in *Xenopus* tailfin epidermis (Krawczyk, 1971; Pang et al., 1978).

2.5 *In Vivo* Cell Movement

Whether each parenchymal cell type uses one or all of the mechanisms of motility stated in Sections 2.1–2.4 *in vivo* is unknown. Certainly, fibroblasts *in vitro* demonstrate the ability to translocate by either chemotaxis, haptotaxis, or contact guidance. Likewise, *in vitro* studies with endothelial cells suggest that they may use all these mechanisms of motility plus the caterpillar model of short motility (see Chapter 15). Thus, during wound repair, a given parenchymal cell may migrate into the wound space by multiple mechanisms occurring concurrently or in succession, depending on the nature of the stimulus and surrounding environment (see Sections 5.1–5.3 for specifics on fibroblast, endothelial cell, and keratinocyte movement, respectively).

3. Extracellular Matrices

The extracellular space in both normal and wounded tissue is occupied by matrix and plasma transudate. It is now appreciated that certain components of the extracellular matrix can serve to promote the migration of cells directly, while other constituents might actually impede it. In fact, recent experiments have demonstrated that for certain cell types, such as the basal cells of a healing epidermis, components of extracellular matrices probably provide the primary mechanism for promoting epithelial sheet movement, while other matrix components actually impede motility of this cell type. The importance of the extracellular matrix to wound healing dictates that a brief description of the better understood constituents that have been studied with regard to cell movement be given here.

Normal human skin is composed of a stratified squamous epithelium and an underlying connective tissue stroma that constitute the epidermis and dermis, respectively. As with all surface linings, the epithelium is separated from the underlying issue by a basal lamina and reticular lamina, representing the dermal–epidermal junction. Several components of this junction have recently been elucidated and include type IV collagen, laminin, bullous pemphigoid antigen, and heparan sulfate proteoglycan (see reviews by Hay, 1982; Yamada, 1983; Piez and Reddi, 1984; McCarthy et al., 1985) (see Chapters 22 and 23). The basal lamina is anchored to the underlying papillary dermis with anchoring fibrils. The dermis, which for the most part constitutes dense irregular connective tissue, is enriched in types I and III collagen (see Chapter 17), dermatan, chondroitin, and probably heparan sulfate proteoglycans (Pringle et al., 1985) (see Chapter 19) and fibronectin associated with either collagen fibers or existing as independent fibrils within the ground substance (Fleischmajer and Timpl, 1984) (see Chapter 18).

When normal dermis is wounded, the composition of the extracellular matrix changes drastically (Grinnell et al., 1981; Repesh, 1982). As a result of the vascular response following injury, a transudate of plasma escapes into the extravascular space and coagulates within the lesion forming a clot. The fibrin within the clot is decorated with fibronectin originating from plasma (Kurkinen et al., 1980; Grinnell et al., 1981). As the wound matures and granulation tissue is formed, the composition of the extracellular matrix changes. Fibroblast infiltration into the region coincides with an increase in the appearance of reticular (type III) collagen fibers and hyaluronate (Grinnell et al., 1981; Repesh et al., 1982). Fibronectin is also prominent in granulation tissue, and experiments have demonstrated that this fibronectin is also largely derived from the infiltrating fibroblasts (Kurkinen et al., 1980; Grinnell et al., 1981; Repesh et al., 1982). Evidence has also been presented that keratinocytes migrating in from the margins can synthesize fibronectin as well (Clark et al., 1983; Clark et al., 1985). As the granulation tissue resolves, fibrillar (type I) collagen begins to predominate, and the wound undergoes remodeling.

The adhesive noncollagenous proteins of the extracellular matrix are of primary importance when considering the migration of connective tissue cells into the wound. In addition to fibronectin and laminin (Kleinman et al., 1985), other adhesive proteins important to consider in the context of wound repair are serum-spreading factor or vitronectin (Barnes et al., 1981; Hayman et al., 1983), thrombospondin (Raugi et al., 1982) and specific epithelial adhesion proteins, such as epinectin (Enenstein and Furcht, 1984), entactin (Bender et al., 1981), and bullous pemphigoid antigen (Stanley et al., 1981). Most is known about fibronectin, so a brief description of its properties is discussed here. More detailed discussions about the structure and function of fibronectin,

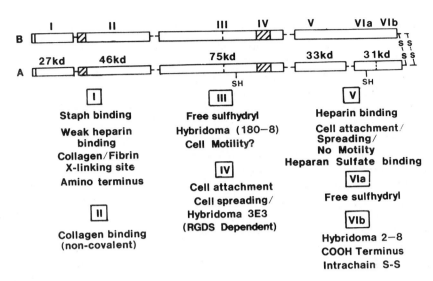

Figure 1. Model of human plasma fibronectin. The domain organization of plasma fibronectin is shown. Selected domains of the molecule are indicated by Roman numerals I–VI. Circulating fibronectin is a disulfide-bonded dimer composed of two similar but not identical (Schwarzbauer *et al.*, 1983; Kornblihtt *et al.*, 1984) chains termed the A and B chains (Yamada, 1983). These chains differ in primary structure with respect to inserts in the A chain, between domains V and VI, that are lacking in the B chain. The apparent molecular weights shown in the diagram refer to specific tryptic or tryptic/catheptic fragments characterized in our laboratory (McCarthy *et al.*, 1985) or others (Hayashi and Yamada, 1983). The 75,000-M_r tryptic fragment causes cells to adhere and exhibit haptotactic motility (McCarthy *et al.*, 1985). This fragment contains an RGDS adhesion sequence in domain IV, and possibly an additional adhesion/motility sequence in domain III (McCarthy *et al.*, 1985). The 33,000-M_r tryptic/catheptic fragment, which originates from the A chain, promotes cell adhesion and spreading but not motility (McCarthy *et al.*, 1985). This fragment probably contains some or all of the inserted sequence characteristic of the A chain of the molecule (Schwarzbauer *et al.*, 1983; Kornblihtt *et al.*, 1984). Hatched marks reflect the best estimate of the location of domains II and IV.

laminin, and the other matrix proteins in this class may be found in several reviews (Hay, 1982; Piez and Reddi, 1984; McCarthy *et al.*, 1985) (see Chapters 18, 22, and 23).

Fibronectin is a high-molecular-weight adhesive glycoprotein found in a soluble form in plasma and in an insoluble fibrillar form in many adult tissues (reviewed by Furcht, 1983; Mosher, 1984; Grinnell, 1984; Yamada *et al.*, 1985; Hynes, 1985). In plasma, fibronectin exists as a 440,000-M_r protein composed of two similar but not identical disulfide bonded subunits of approximately 220,000 M_r. The protein has multiple ligand-binding activities, which are responsible for the remarkable biologic activities of this molecule (Fig. 1). This listing of binding activities, which has grown to considerable length at this point, can be simplified for the purposes of this discussion. First fibronectin binds to other scaffolding constituents of the extracellular matrix. This list includes type I–IV collagens, fibrin, thrombospondin (a high-molecular-weight adhesion protein released by platelets and endothelial cells) (Lahav *et al.*,

1984), and chondroitin/dermatan sulfate and heparin/heparan sulfate proteoglycans (Yamada *et al.*, 1980; Ruoslahti *et al.*, 1981). Cell (fibroblast) fibronectin has also been shown to bind hyaluronic acid (Yamada *et al.*, 1980),
whereas plasma fibronectin fails to bind this ligand (Stamatoglou and Keller,
1982), even when the fibronectin is aggregated (Laterra and Culp, 1982).

In addition to binding both fibrous and ground substance constituents of the
matrix, fibronectin has also been shown to bind to the surface of a variety of
connective tissue cells, including fibroblasts, macrophages, and vascular endothelial cells (see reviews by Hynes and Yamada, 1982; Furcht, 1983; Yamada *et
al.*, 1985). It is now known that the binding of fibronectin to cells is a relatively
low-affinity interaction (Akiyama, 1985; Yamada *et al.*, 1985; Pierschbacher *et
al.*, 1985). As a consequence, most early studies have relied on observing cell
adhesion and spreading on fibronectin-coated surfaces to demonstrate cell interactions. Fibronectin-coated latex (Schwarz and Juliano, 1984) or gelatin (Saba
and Jaffe, 1980) particles have also been used to visualize cell interaction with
fibronectin. Recently, with the identification of a tetrapeptide sequence within
the molecule that promotes cell adhesion, direct binding studies have also been
done on certain cell types (reviewed by Yamada *et al.*, 1985; Pierschbacher *et al.*,
1985) (see also Section 4.3). The consequences of fibronectin–cell interactions
on cell behavior are dramatic. Fibronectin has been shown to affect the growth,
motility, and differentiation of a variety of cell types *in vitro*, and it is known that
fibronectin is an important factor in matrix assembly (see Chapter 18).

Since it is relatively easy to isolate large amounts of fibronectin, a tremen-
dous amount of information has been learned on the structure, function, and
molecular biology of fibronectin during the past 10 years. The binding activities of fibronectin are now known to exist in discrete domains within the
molecule (Fig. 1). The illustrated arrangement of binding activities is generally
agreed on; however, a specific structure has so far only been elucidated for one
of the domains, a major cell-binding domain (Yamada *et al.*, 1985;
Pierschbacher *et al.*, 1985). The entire sequence of fibronectin has been established using a combination of protein sequencing (Petersen *et al.*, 1983) and
recombinant DNA technologies (Schwarzbauer *et al.*, 1983; Kornblihtt *et al.*,
1984). The protein contains three types of internal repeating structural homologies, designated types I, II, and III, and the different biologic activities seem to
segregate to different homologies (Petersen *et al.*, 1983; Schwarzbauer *et al.*,
1983; Kornblihtt *et al.*, 1984). For example, fibrin binding is associated with
type I homologies, collagen binding with type II, and cell and heparin binding
with type III homologies (reviewed by Yamada *et al.*, 1985) (see Chapter 18).
Recent molecular biology data have shown conclusively that fibronectin is
actually a structurally heterogeneous group of proteins (Schwarzbauer *et al.*,
1983; Kornblihtt *et al.*, 1984). Extra peptide sequences have been found to be
inserted in some fibronectin chains yet absent in others (Schwarzbauer *et al.*,
1983; Kornblihtt *et al.*, 1984). Since there appears to be only one gene for
fibronectin (Kornblihtt *et al.*, 1983; Tamkun *et al.*, 1984), the structural heterogeneity appears to occur at the level of RNA splicing. Recent evidence from our

laboratory suggests that this structural heterogeneity may have some importance for regulating cell adhesion to this protein (McCarthy et al., 1986) (see Section 4.3); as such, these different forms of the molecule may play different roles in wound healing.

Like fibronectin, other cell-adhesion proteins of the matrix also seem to have multivalent binding capabilities. For example, laminin, the major adhesion protein of basement membranes, binds to type IV collagen (Rao et al., 1982; Charonis et al, 1985), heparan sulfate/heparin (Sakashita et al., 1980) and to the surfaces of many cell types, including both epithelial cells and cells derived from embryonic mesenchyme (reviewed by Yamada et al., 1983; Kleinman et al., 1985). Similarly, serum-spreading factor has been shown to bind to heparin (Barnes et al., 1985), and thrombospondin can bind to both fibronectin and fibrinogen (Lahav et al., 1984). The in vitro binding data support the concept that these proteins serve as linking components between fibrous and ground substance components of the extracellular matrix and the cell surface.

Even though these proteins all participate in cell to substratum adhesion in vitro, further studies are needed to establish the precise biologic role they play in wound healing. These studies will have to include immunolocalizing these proteins within healing wound tissue as well as performing detailed in vitro studies on cell motility, growth, and differentiation in response to each protein. For example, laminin has been shown to promote the migration of a variety of transformed cells including tumors of neuroectodermal origin (McCarthy et al., 1983; McCarthy and Furcht, 1984) as well as tumors of mesenchymal origin (Fligiel et al., 1985). The role of laminin in promoting the active translocation of normal nonneuronal cells is less clear. Migrating basal cells of amphibian epidermis that move on fibronectin (Donaldson and Mahan, 1983) do not migrate well over laminin-coated surfaces (Donaldson and Mahan, 1984) despite the fact that cells of these histologic types will adhere to laminin. Furthermore, in certain epithelial wound models such as healing cornea, laminin does not appear beneath the migrating epithelium until re-epithelialization is completed and basement membranes are being regenerated (Fujikawa et al., 1984). This suggests that laminin may not be as important as fibronectin in promoting the influx of cells into a healing wound and may be involved instead in cellular differentiation later in the process. Further work is needed on the molecular basis of cell adhesion to laminin as well as other adhesion promoting constituents of the wound extracellular matrix to fully understand the biology of these proteins in repair.

4. Molecular Basis of Cell–Substratum Adhesion

The cell surface is involved in regulating a number of important biologic phenomena, including cell motility, cell recognition, growth control, and differentiation. The outer cell membrane is also the site of final assembly of both fibrous and ground substance constituents for the extracellular matrix. The importance of adhesion to movement, while intuitively obvious, cannot be overemphasized when considering mechanisms of cell motility. Clearly, cells must adhere sufficiently to the substrata to generate the traction force required for motility yet not be so adherent that they are incapable of breaking adhesions and translocating. It has become increasingly clear that cell adhesion to extracellular matrices is a complex phenomenon mediated by multiple distinct cell-surface constituents. Certain cell–matrix interactions are involved in promoting motility, while others may be involved in apparently unrelated processes such as the assembly of the extracellular matrix (see Chapter 18). There are also adhesions between the surface and extracellular matrix (e.g., cell adhesion via cell surface heparan sulfate), for which the biologic significance has not yet been established (see Section 4.3). It is quite possible that these interactions could be involved in regulating cell growth or differentiation (see Chapter 19).

Several recent advances have been made in understanding cell to substratum adhesions, from both structural and biochemical points of view. A detailed discussion of this topic is clearly beyond the scope of the current chapter and additional reviews are offered for the interested reader (Kleinman et al., 1981; Hay, 1982; Trinkhaus, 1984; Vasiliev, 1985; Singer, 1986). This discussion focuses on three aspects of the problem and is restricted to connective tissue (fibroblast) cell adhesion. First, the structural organization and cytoskeletal involvement in adhesions are presented. Second, the biochemical nature of cell membrane receptors involved in cell–matrix adhesion are discussed. Finally, the molecular characterization of extracellular matrix adhesion domains is summarized. While the following account deals primarily with adhesion to fibronectin, in vivo cell adhesion to other constituents occurs as well. For example, cells have been shown to adhere to type I and IV collagen directly (Kurkinen et al., 1984; Nagata et al., 1985) and to have receptors for both heparan sulfate proteoglycan (Kjellen et al., 1981) as well as hyaluronate (Underhill and Toole, 1981). In fact, adhesion mutant cells unable to attach to fibronectin but adherent to other molecules have been described (Brown and Juliano, 1985). Laminin has been shown to interact with cell surfaces via a high-affinity ($K_d = 2 \times 10^{-9}$ M) 70,000-M_r receptor that is distinct from the receptor for fibronectin (Rao et al., 1983; Malinoff and Wicha, 1983).

Even though it is simplistic relative to the in vivo situation, a discussion of fibronectin-mediated adhesion is an extremely useful model to consider for several reasons. First, fibronectin is certainly of major influence in wound repair—it is a major adhesion protein of the clot (Kurkinen et al., 1980; Grinnell et al., 1981) and of granulation tissue (Grinnell et al., 1981; Repesh et al., 1982; Clark et al., 1983). Second, numerous studies both in vivo and in vitro relate fibronectin and cell motility; thus, a detailed knowledge of fibronectin-mediated adhesion may lead to the understanding of the molecular basis of this motility. Finally, knowledge of the multiple interactions that cells have with fibronectin may contribute to our understanding of the ways in which matrices affect not only cell motility, but also growth control, differentiation, and assembly of the extracellular matrix.

4.1. Structural and Cytoskeletal Aspects of Cell Adhesion

The in vitro cell adhesion of fibroblasts to components of extracellular matrices can be divided into two discrete phases: an initial energy-independent attachment phase in which rounded up cells interact with the matrix, and a subsequent energy-dependent spreading phase, during which cytoskeletal reorganization occurs. As cells initially spread, they extend pseudopodial projections in all directions, forming thin ruffling lamellipodia which exclude cellular organelles. Cytoplasmic projections may be classified morphologically as one of several distinct types, including ruffles, hemispheric projections or blebs, and elongated projections such as filopodia or microspikes (Trinkaus, 1984). Although most cytoplasmic extensions may be associated with the action of actin (Singer, 1986), it is probable that other forces (e.g. turgor) act within cells to contribute in a specific fashion to the regulation of these strikingly different protrusions (Trinkaus, 1984). Microtubules progressively polymerize as these cytoplasmic projections extend. Microtubule polymerization begins perinuclearly (near the satellites of the centrioles), radiating peripherally to the cytoplasm in the extending lamellae (Brinkley et al., 1981). It has been proposed that microtubules exert a stabilizing influence on fibroblast morphology, permitting the cell to establish asymmetry important in sustaining directional motility (Vasiliev et al., 1970; Trinkhaus, 1984).

The edges of the lamellipodia contain extensive meshworks of interconnected microfilaments (Small, 1981; Suitlana et al., 1984; Singer, 1986). Presumably, contractile activity involves actin–myosin interactions; however, myosin does not appear to be concentrated at the active edge of an advancing lamellipodium (Heggeness et al., 1977; Willingham et al., 1981; Singer, 1986). The extensive ruffles of lamellipodia can sometimes be seen to move in a centripetal fashion. Indeed, surface-attached particles on spread cells can be observed to move toward the perinuclear region (Dembo and Harris, 1981). The traction force from this membrane movement has been shown to wrinkle distensible substrata, e.g., silicone sheets (Harris et al., 1980). Recent work in our laboratory has demonstrated that fibroblasts adhering to passively adsorbed matrix constituents, e.g., fibronectin, on glass coverslips can move this matrix protein from the ruffling edge of the cell into a perinuclear distribution (see Section 5.1). The centripetal movement of membrane constituents is probably indicative of the forces that eventually cause retraction of the advancing pseudopod. Recent evidence obtained from injecting fluorescently tagged actin into fibroblasts and photobleaching the cell during spreading suggests that F-actin is assembled from G-actin at the plasma membrane and the assembled structure subsequently treadmills toward the nucleus (Wang, 1985). This treadmilling effect, most likely caused by asymmetric polymerization of actin filaments, may contribute to the traction force observed in actively spreading and moving cells (Harris et al., 1980).

Interference reflection microscopy has been used to visualize the different type of adhesion structures of attached cells in vitro (Izzard and Lochner, 1980). Using this technique, two types of adhesion structures, distinguished on the basis of the distance from the cell surface to the substratum, have been identified. One type of adhesion, termed a close contact, is seen as gray by interference reflection microscopy, and is characterized by a distance of 20–30 nm from the membrane to the substratum (Izzard and Lochner, 1980). By contrast, focal contacts, which appear black by interference reflection microscopy, represent tighter adhesions than close contacts, with a cell–substratum distance of 10–15 nm. The focal adhesions apparently represent actin nucleation centers for actin bundle (stress fiber) formation. Focal adhesions are also enriched in the cytoskeletal components vinculin (Singer, 1982), α-actinin (Lazarides and Burridge, 1975), fimbrin (Bretscher and Weber, 1980), and talin (Burridge and Connell, 1983), which are involved in anchoring and packing these bundles of microfilaments originating from the extending microspikes. Importantly, detailed studies of these adhesion plaques demonstrate that they do not pre-exist on the surface, but rather form as the result of interactions of the cell surface with adhesion proteins, such as fibronectin (Izzard, 1985). The formation of close contacts may precede the formation of focal contacts *in vitro*, and as focal contacts mature, fibronectin is excluded from beneath these adhesion plaques and localizes to neighboring close-contact regions. Although the biologic significance of these different classes of adhesions is not yet established *in vivo*, correlations to cell migration have been observed *in vitro*. As the number of focal adhesions and stress fibers increases, the motility rate decreases, suggesting that close contacts might be involved in promoting cell movement (Kolega *et al.*, 1982).

4.2. Membrane Receptors for Fibronectin

The most straightforward approach toward demonstrating direct interaction of fibronectin with the cell surface would be to characterize the binding of soluble fibronectin to cells. Early efforts to do so were frustrated, however, by the fact that cell interactions with soluble fibronectin are of a weak to moderate affinity. Indeed, early studies attempting to block fibronectin-mediated attachment by preincubating cells with soluble fibronectin failed, and the results were used to conclude that soluble fibronectin interacted poorly, or not at all, with cells in suspension (Grinnell, 1980; Carter *et al.*, 1981). Despite initial failures to demonstrate binding, the incontrovertible observation was that fibronectin, bound on plastic surfaces, collagen, or fibrin, actively promoted cell adhesion, spreading, and motility. It was suggested that fibronectin undergoes conformational changes when binding to substrata that enhance the interaction of the protein with cell surfaces. A number of membrane constituents, including proteoglycans, glycoproteins, and glycolipids, have been implicated as participants in fibronectin-mediated adhesion. While each individual association is apparently of low to moderate affinity, collectively these interactions may cooperate to form cell–fibronectin bonds of considerably high avidity.

Recently there has been increasing evidence for the role of integral membrane glycoproteins in mediating cell adhesion to fibronectin. Adhesion-disrupting monoclonal antibodies have been used to isolate and identify a membrane-associated complex of glycoproteins, with an apparent molecular weight of 140,000 M_r, which is apparently involved in mediating cell adhesion to fibronectin (Wylie et al., 1979; Chen et al., 1985b; Damsky et al., 1985). Importantly, these antibodies do not inhibit the adhesion of all cells to fibronectin (Decker et al., 1984), suggesting that the molecular basis of cell adhesion to fibronectin varies in a cell-specific fashion. A 140,000-M_r cell-surface-associated glycoprotein has also been isolated by direct affinity chromatography on fibronectin affinity columns (Pytela et al., 1985a). These investigators eluted the putative 140,000-M_r receptor from fibronectin-affinity columns by the addition of the tetrapeptide adhesion sequence RGDS present in fibronectin (see Section 4.3). The primary structure of one subunit of this complex has recently been predicted from the sequencing of cDNA clones (Tamkun, 1986). This subunit, which has a molecular weight of 89,000 M_r, has three domains evident from the primary structure—an N-terminal extracellular domain with an uncommonly high degree of cystine residues, a single transmembrane (hydrophobic) segment, and a C-terminal cytoplasmic domain that contains a potential acceptor site for tyrosine kinases. These results present the first definitive evidence for a direct transmembrane link between fibronectin and the cell interior. These investigators proposed the name integrin for this complex, to denote its role as a direct transmembrane link between the extracellular matrix and the cytoskeleton. Despite the recent popularity of this theory, it must be emphasized that integrin is not the only membrane glycoprotein that has been implicated in fibronectin-mediated cell adhesion. Early studies using crosslinking reagents on cells adherent to fibronectin demonstrated a 49,000-M_r cell-surface protein in close apposition to fibronectin (Aplin, 1981). Recent studies by Urushihara and Yamada (1986) used polyclonal antibodies to demonstrate a glycoprotein of similar molecular weight (47,000 M_r) involved in fibronectin-mediated adhesion of some (but not all) cell types. Thus, the molecular basis of cell adhesion to fibronectin (or any other extracellular matrix component) must be considered in a cell-specific fashion.

Several approaches have also suggested a role for membrane-associated glycosaminoglycans and proteoglycans in mediating cell adhesion to fibronectin. Treatment of cells adherent on fibronectin with crosslinking reagents suggests that proteoglycans are in close proximity to adhesion sites (Perkins et al., 1979). Adherent cells can also be detached by using chelating agents, leaving substratum-attached material (SAM) behind (Culp, 1974). Studies have shown that SAM represents remnants of old focal adhesion plaques as well as subsets of close contacts (Lark et al., 1985). Biochemical studies on SAM have identified heparan sulfate and chondroitin sulfate proteoglycans as well as hyaluronic acid as components of adhesion plaques. Platelet factor 4 (PF4) (Laterra et al., 1983a) and more recently isolated heparin-binding fragments of fibronectin (Laterra et al., 1983b) (see Section 4.3) have been used as a model for heparin/heparan sulfate-mediated cell adhesion. In addition, Schwartz and Juliano (1985) used fibronectin-coated beads to suggest a role for cell-surface-associated glycosaminoglycans in cell adhesion to fibronectin. Binding of these beads represents one of the earliest events in adhesion, as it is independent of metabolic and cytoskeletal activity (Schwartz and Juliano, 1984). Using beads of different charge to adsorb fibronectin, these workers demonstrated differential effects of exogenous heparin on the inhibition of bead binding to cell surfaces. It was concluded that the bead surface charge changed the conformation of bound fibronectin and exposed alternative cell-binding sites within fibronectin, at least one of which was inhibited by heparin (Schwarz and Juliano, 1985).

There is also evidence that glycolipids (gangliosides) are involved in fibronectin-mediated cell adhesion. Kleinman et al. (1981) originally demonstrated that gangliosides and associated oligosaccharides can inhibit the adhesion of Chinese hamster ovary (CHO) cells to fibronectin. Gangliosides have also been shown to inhibit fibronectin-mediated hemagglutination, baby hamster kidney cell spreading, and to restore normal morphology of transformed cells (Yamada et al., 1981). Direct binding of fibronectin and gangliosides has also been demonstrated (Perkins et al., 1982). Adherent cells have been shown to incorporate exogenously added gangliosides into the membrane (Spiegel et al., 1984). Recently, this approach has been used to demonstrate a positive functional correlation between the addition of gangliosides to the culture medium of transformed cells and cell membrane binding of fibronectin (Spiegel et al., 1985). Although the identification of gangliosides as fibronectin receptors remains controversial (Carter et al., 1981; Perkins et al., 1982), it seems clear that these membrane constituents are most likely involved in the interaction.

4.3. Cell-Adhesion Domains of Fibronectin

The other approach to developing an understanding of the molecular basis of cell and fibronectin interactions has been to isolate proteolytic fragments of fibronectin that contain biological activity. Clearly, intact fibronectin has been shown to interact (albeit in some cases weakly) with most of the candidates mentioned above as fibronectin receptors. Gangliosides, glycosaminoglycans, as well as integrin have all been reported to bind fibronectin directly (see Section 4.2). Limited proteolysis of fibronectin yields several proteolytic fragments with biologically active domains. Affinity chromatography using natural ligands (e.g., heparin, gelatin) or constructed ligands (e.g., monoclonal antibodies) have been used to purify and characterize such fragments. The amino acid sequence responsible for a given biologic activity within the fragment can be determined, chemically synthesized, and the synthetic peptides used to characterize cell-adhesion receptors.

Pierschbacher et al. (1981) were the first to use this approach in isolating and characterizing a major cell-adhesion determinant on the fibronectin molecule. The initial studies used a monoclonal antibody, which inhibited cell adhesion to fibronectin, to isolate an 11,500-M_r cell-attachment promoting fragment from a pepsin digest of the molecule. This fragment was sequenced, overlapping peptides were synthesized from the region, and a minimal cell-adhesion structure was determined (Pierschbacher and Ruoslahti, 1984a). The minimal structure found to promote adhesion was a tetrapeptide sequence of arginyl-glycyl-aspartyl-serine (RGDS, using the single-letter amino acid code). In addition to promoting attachment directly, high levels of RGDS in solution have been shown to inhibit cell adhesion in a competitive manner to substratum-bound fibronectin (Yamada and Kennedy, 1984; Pierschbacher and Ruoslahti, 1984b; McCarthy et al., 1986). Consistent with the early studies with plasma fibronectin, the interaction of fragments containing this sequence with cell surfaces is of moderate affinity, with a dissociation constant 0.89 μM (Akiyama et al., 1985). Structural/functional studies with various amino acid substitutions of RGDS have shown that RGD is the minimal sequence required for adhesion activity, and the fourth position residue can modulate this activity. Conservative substitution for any of the three amino acids in the sequence causes a loss in biologic activity (Pierschbacher and Ruoslahti, 1984b). The reverse sequence, SDGR, has been reported to exhibit biologic activity (Yamada and Kennedy, 1985). Importantly, Pytela et al. (1985a) have used the RGDS tetrapeptide to elute a fibronectin 140,000-M_r receptor from a fibronectin-affinity column. Curiously, when serum-spreading factor (vitronectin) was used to isolate receptors from cell surfaces, a 125,000-/115,000-M_r protein was isolated, despite the fact that serum-spreading factor contains RGD in its sequence (Pytela et al., 1985b) and soluble RGDS inhibits cell adhesion to this protein (Silnutzer and Barnes, 1985). This suggests that regions which flank RGD sequences in adhesion promoting proteins may play an important role in determining the specificity of binding to cell surface receptors. In addition, RGDS has been shown to inhibit cells from attaching to substratum-bound laminin (Silnutzer and Barnes, 1985) despite the previous observations that laminin and fibronectin interact with cells via distinct receptors (Johansson et al., 1981; Carlsson et al., 1981). It is quite possible that cells exhibit a multiplicity of adhesion promoting receptors for different proteins (Decker et al., 1984) and that RGDS is a basic component of many of these adhesion structures, although alternative explanations exist as well. Clearly, this field is rapidly evolving and promises to be an area of active investigation in the next several years.

We have also used proteolytic fragments of fibronectin to determine the relationship between their adhesion promoting activities and their stimulation of haptotactic migration (McCarthy et al., 1986). The system used for these studies uses a modified Boyden chamber with a porous polycarbonate filter having a surface that is poorly adherent for cells. Fibronectin added to the lower well diffuses through the filter, binds to it, and sets up haptotactic gradients on the filter surface reminiscent of those initially set up by Carter (reviewed by McCarthy et al., 1985). Cells migrate directionally to the lower surface and are counted manually through a microscope or automatically with the aid of an image analyzer. Using this approach, the minimum proteolytic fragment that we have observed that can stimulate cell migration is a 75,000-M_r tryptic fragment derived from the central portion of the molecule (Fig. 1) (McCarthy et al., 1986). This fragment, which represents the 75,000-M_r cell-adhesion fragment described by Hayashi and Yamada (1983) includes the RGDS cell-adhesion sequence (Yamada and Kennedy, 1984). Importantly, we have been unable to stimulate migration with the pepsin-derived 11,500-M_r cell adhesion fragment, and RGDS is only partially effective at inhibiting adhesion to the 75,000-M_r fragment (Yamada and Kennedy, 1984; McCarthy et al., 1986). These studies suggest that an additional motility/adhesion domain may be present in the 75,000-M_r fragment that is distinct from the RGDS domain.

The studies conducted in our laboratory also clearly demonstrate the presence of a cell-adhesion site in a carboxy-terminal heparin-binding region of fibronectin distinct from RGDS. This region of fibronectin presumably promotes adhesion via cell-surface-associated proteoglycan (McCarthy et al., 1986). In contrast to adhesion on the 75,000-M_r fragment, cell adhesion to this heparin-binding fragment is resistant to the presence of high levels of exogenous soluble RGDS. While cell adhesion to this carboxy-terminal heparin-binding domain results in cell spreading, haptotactic motility is not observed in response to this fragment (McCarthy et al., 1986). The results imply that distinct cell surface constituents are involved in cell binding to the carboxy-terminal heparin-binding fragment and the motility-promoting 75,000-M_r fragment.

The work of Culp and associates has been instrumental in establishing the role of proteoglycans in mediating cell adhesion to fibronectin. Biochemical analysis of SAM (see Section 4.2) demonstrates the presence of hyaluronate, heparan sulfate, and chondroitin sulfate within focal adhesions (Lark et al., 1985). Early studies using the heparin-binding protein PF4 demonstrated that cells adhered to and spread on it (Laterra et al., 1983a,b) and formed close but not focal contacts on this protein. Furthermore, cells adherent on fragments of fibronectin that contain RGDS but lack heparin-binding activity also exhibit only close contacts (Beyth and Culp, 1984; Lark et al., 1985). By contrast, these cells formed both focal and close contact sites when adherent on intact fibronectin. These studies have also shown that cells adherent on surfaces coated with both PF4- and RGDS-containing domains of fibronectin do exhibit the full adhesion phenotype (i.e., both focal and close contacts), indicating that strong adhesion to intact fibronectin results from the collective influence of several distinct but weak interactions.

The biologic significance of proteoglycan-mediated adhesion is not yet understood. It has been suggested that cell-associated chondroitin sulfate might compete with cell-associated heparan sulfate for binding to fibronectin and promote cell de-adherence, which could be important for promoting motility (Brennan et al., 1983). Studies by Lark and Culp (1983, 1984a,b) have shown that heparan sulfate does turnover within focal adhesions as they mature, indicating another possible mechanism of mediating de-adhesion or cell detachment. Heparin/heparan sulfate proteoglycans have been implicated by some investigators in regulating cell growth (Fritze et al., 1985) and differentiation (Majack and Bornstein, 1984, 1985), Heparin-binding fragments of fibronectin (Rogers et al., 1985) and laminin (Edgar et al., 1984) will support neuronal attachment and neurite extension in vitro.

Finally, domain(s) of fibronectin that participate in matrix assembly have been isolated that exclude both the RGDS-containing and heparin-binding fragments mentioned above. Intact fibronectin has been shown to be associated with collagen fibrils both in vitro (Furcht et al., 1980a,b) and in vivo (Grinnell et al., 1981; Fleischmajer and Timpl, 1984), and antibodies against the collagen-binding domain of fibronectin can inhibit collagen fibril deposition in vitro (McDonald et al., 1982). McKeown-Longo and Mosher (1983) directly measured the incorporation of fibronectin into extracellular matrices and demonstrated that it occurs in two distinct but temporally related phases, including an early detergent-sensitive phase and a later detergent-resistant phase. The initial binding of fibronectin to cells and their matrices is saturable and reversible (McKeown-Longo and Mosher, 1983); binding is sensitive to reduction and alkylation of intrachain disulfide bonds of fibronectin (McKeown-Longo and Mosher, 1984). Proteolytic fragments of fibronectin have been used to determine the molecular basis for activity; it has been shown that this domain is in the amino-terminal one-third of the molecule (McKeown-Longo and Mosher, 1985). Despite the lack of cell-adhesion activity in this fragment (McKeown-Longo and Mosher, 1984), it apparently can bind to the cell surface and serves to further illustrate the complexity of fibronectin cell interactions. Pytela et al. (1985a) suggested that the 49,000-M_r fibronectin receptor of Aplin et al. (1981) may be involved in fibril formation, although this remains to be proved. Since the processes of motility and fibril formation involve distinct domains of fibronectin, matrix assembly can apparently occur concomitantly with cell motility, a feat that might facilitate the orientation of developing fibrils in granulation tissue as fibroblasts infiltrate during the onset of repair (see Section 5.1).

5. Migration of Specific Cell Populations into Wounds

This section addresses what is known about factors and influences that determine the migration of specific cell populations into the wound environment. Although several cell types participate in wound healing, three types are discussed: fibroblasts, endothelial cells, and keratinocytes. It should be appreciated that the entry of these cells involves not only migration but proliferative responses and differentiation of newly arriving cell populations as well. Space limitations preclude a detailed presentation of these activities; however, these topics are covered in Chapters 14–17 as well as in a number of recent reviews (Wahl, 1981; Gospodarowicz, 1985; Ross et al., 1981).

5.1. Fibroblasts

The recruitment of fibroblasts into the wound initiates the reparative phase of wound healing. The fibroblasts that emigrate into wounds arise from the undifferentiated mesenchymal cells in the surrounding tissue. These cells undergo phenotypic changes as they enter the wound to synthesize elevated levels of type I and III collagens. They also give rise to the highly contractile and biosynthetically active myofibroblasts of granulation tissue that contract the wound (Gabbiani, 1981) (see Chapter 17). The migration of fibroblasts is subject to the control of a variety of processes that are related in a complex manner. These processes include chemoattractants, haptotactic influences, and contact guidance mechanisms. In addition, the extracellular matrix must open up to provide space for the penetration of cells. The processes inducing migration act in a coordinated manner to attract fibroblasts that contract the wound to a more manageable size, which then produce and replace granulation tissue with normal (or scar) tissue.

A variety of substances have been shown to promote the migration of fibroblasts *in vitro* and may contribute to the reparative phase of healing *in vivo*. Components of the early wound implicated in this process include a serum-derived chemoattractant produced by complement activation. This factor, apparently derived from the complement component C5a, does not attract monocytes or neutrophils as C5a does (Postlethwaite *et al.*, 1979). In addition, platelet-derived growth factor (PDGF), which is released by platelets upon aggregation, has been shown to stimulate fibroblasts and smooth muscle cell chemotaxis *in vitro* (Grotendorst *et al.*, 1981; Seppa *et al.*, 1982). In studies testing a variety of growth factors that have mitogenic properties for fibroblasts, only PDGF was observed to stimulate fibroblast migration (Seppa *et al.*, 1982). Thus, it has been suggested that PDGF (and perhaps other growth factors as well) may act as a wound-healing hormone by stimulating both migration and growth of fibroblasts (Seppa *et al.*, 1982) (see also Chapter 9). Fibronectin may also play a role in initiating fibroblast migration into the early wound. As clots form, a high percentage of plasma fibronectin can become incorporated into the fibrin strands by both noncovalent and covalent associations via factor XIIIa (Mosher, 1975, 1976). Interaction of fibroblasts with fibrin has been shown to be dependent on the presence of fibronectin associated with either the cell surface (Mosher, 1976) or with fibrin itself (Grinnell *et al.*, 1980).

As the wound tissue evolves, additional factors play a role in stimulating fibroblast motility. Macrophages, through production of fibronectin (Alitalo *et al.*, 1980; Tsukamoto *et al.*, 1981) or other mediators may stimulate fibroblast migration (Ali and Hynes, 1978; Postlethwaite *et al.*, 1981; Mensing *et al.*, 1983; Albini *et al.*, 1983) and growth (Bitterman *et al.*, 1983; Wahl *et al.*, 1979). Macrophage collagenase, which can be produced by nonspecific (Wahl *et al.*, 1974; 1979; Werb and Gordon, 1975) or lymphocyte- (immune) mediated mechanisms (Wahl *et al.*, 1975) could degrade collagen into fragments that have also been shown to promote fibroblast motility *in vitro* (Postlethwaite *et al.*, 1978). In addition, lymphocytes can also directly stimulate fibroblast motility by the production of a chemoattractant for these cells (Postlethwaite *et al.*, 1976; Postlethwaite and Kang, 1980).

Cells must have the capacity to penetrate the extracellular matrix. A variety of enzymes, both macrophage and fibroblast derived, are potential candidates for this task, including plasmin, plasminogen activator, and collagenases (reviewed by Reich *et al.*, 1976) (see Chapter 18). Fibroblasts and macrophages can also clear spaces by actively phagocytosing the extracellular matrix, and fibronectin may potentiate the phagocytic process (Saba and Jaffe, 1980). Mechanical forces can also play a role in opening spaces within the matrix of the healing wound. Granulation tissue is rich in hyaluronate produced by fibroblasts (Repesh et al., 1982; Toole, 1981); the pressure exerted by the extraordinarily large radius of hydration of this glycosaminoglycan could serve to open up the tissue. The water held in place by hyaluronate could also produce an environment that stabilizes chemotactic gradients within a wound, thereby ensuring a continued net movement of cells into the lesion (see Chapter 19).

The orientation of the fibrous component of the wound matrix also changes as a wound heals; this reorientation can have importance to the healing process. The early wound clot contains fibrils arranged more or less randomly, and newly deposited collagen at the wound periphery is deposited in more or less a random manner. As fibroblasts invade the wound, however, there is a progressive change from this random orientation to a more orderly array of fibrils that often run parallel to the surface of the wound (Repesh et al., 1982). Ultimately, the granulation tissue becomes rich in modified fibroblasts with characteristics similar to those of smooth muscle cells—these are called myofibroblasts (Gabbiani, 1981) (see Chapter 17). These cells, which apparently originate from mesenchymal cells or pericytes, are rich in actin and myosin, gap junctions, and adherence junctions; they act in a concerted manner to contract the wound along the lines of stress that have developed within the extracellular matrix (Gabbiani, 1981; Baur and Parks, 1983). These highly

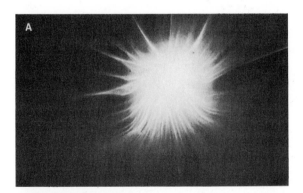

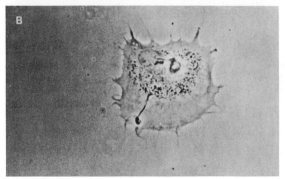

Figure 2. Fibril formation by adherent cells on adsorbed fibronectin. Fibroblasts were allowed to adhere for 4 hr on glass coverslips to which fibronectin had been adsorbed and labeled with rhodamine isothiocyanate. The initiation of fibril formation appeared to occur at the edge of these spreading cells. (a) Fluorescence. (b) Phase contrast. (×1000)

specialized cells have been shown to interact with the wound matrix via fibrils rich in fibronectin (Baur and Parks, 1983; Singer *et al.*, 1984).

We recently performed a series of experiments designed to examine the role of cell motility in rearranging the three-dimensional organization of the wound extracellular matrix (Sas *et al.*, 1985). These experiments used coverslips to which fibronectin had been weakly adsorbed and then labeled with fluorescent rhodamine. Cells adhered to the fibronectin substratum, removed the fibronectin from the surface of the coverslips, and developed it into substratum-associated fibrils (Fig. 2). The production of these fibrils appears to initially involve the capping of fibronectin receptors into a perinuclear distribution (Fig. 3), a phenomenon long associated with cell spreading and locomotion (Harris *et al.*, 1980). By scanning electron microscopy (SEM), these fibronectin fibrils appear to extend from the top (or dorsal) surface of the cell (Fig. 4). This capping of peripherally associated fibronectin to a perinuclear distribution is reminiscent of the treadmilling of actin and cell-surface receptors from the periphery to the interior (Harris *et al.*, 1980; Wang, 1985) (see Section 4.1). Additional support for the relationship between fibril formation and motility comes from the observation of fibrils extending from the leading and trailing edges of highly polarized motile cells (Fig. 5). The orientation of the fibrils to the cell body gives the distinct impression that the force being applied to the fibrils is in a direction coincident with the direction of motility. Furthermore, the addition of cytochalasin B to these cultures prevents micro-

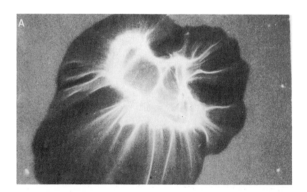

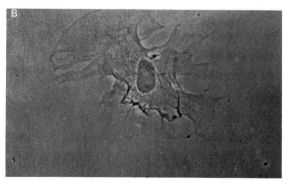

Figure 3. Perinuclear distribution of reorganized fibronectin. Fibroblasts adherent for 8 hr on fluorescently labeled fibronectin substrata displayed prominent perinuclear staining in addition to well-developed fibrillar projections extending far past the edge of the cell. (A) Fluorescence. (B) Phase-contrast photomicrographs. (×1000)

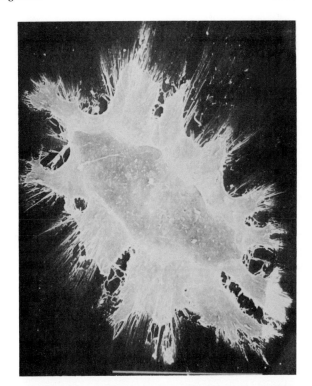

Figure 4. Scanning electron microscopy (SEM) of substrate fibrils. Cells adherent on fibronectin-coated surfaces were prepared for SEM. Fibrils can be seen clearly extending from an area on the dorsal surface to regions past the cell periphery. A perinuclear accumulation of material, reminiscent of that seen by fluorescence microscopy (see Fig. 3) can be seen. Bar, 50 μM.

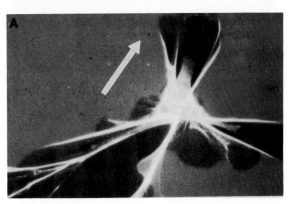

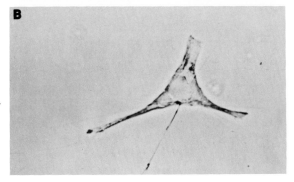

Figure 5. Motile fibroblast on fluorescently labeled fibronectin. Extensive fibrils composed of fluorescent fibronectin were formed by this motile fibroblast. Note the orientation of the fibrils as they flare away from the trailing edge of the cell. Fibronectin can be observed to be capped at the trailing edge of the cell. Arrow indicates direction of motility. (A) Fluorescence. (B) Phase-contrast photomicrograph. (×1000)

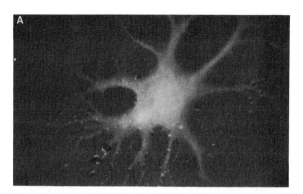

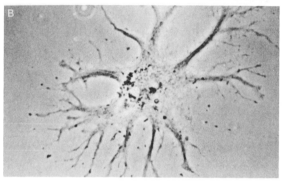

Figure 6. Effect of cytochalasin B on fibril formation. Cells were plated on fluorescently labeled fibronectin as before in the presence of 10 μg/ml cytochalasin B and examined for fibril formation. Cytochalasin B inhibits polymerization of actin and cell motility and creates the striking arborized morphology shown in the photographs. Fibril formation by these cells is totally inhibited (compare fluorescence pattern in Figs. 2 and 3. (A) By contrast, 10 μg/ml of vinblastine, an inhibitor of tubulin polymerization, has no effect on fibril formation (not shown). (B) Phase-contrast photomicrograph. (×1000)

filament assembly (and cell motility) and also inhibits the production of these substratum-associated fibrils (Fig. 6).

Orientation of the fibrous component of granulation tissue matrix can influence the entry of cells into a lesion. As fibroblasts migrate into such oriented matrices, they tend to align in a fashion parallel to the arrangement of the matrix fibers (Bryant, 1977; Repesh et al., 1982). In this way, contact guidance forces exerted by the fibers contribute directly to sustaining the next influx of fibroblasts into the lesions (see Section 2.3). Indirect effects of the matrix on guiding cell motility have also been demonstrated. For example, neutrophils migrating along oriented fibrin strands migrate better in response to chemotactic gradients of FMLP when these gradients are presented in a direction parallel to the axis of fiber orientation than when applied perpendicular to this axis (Wilkinson and Lackie, 1983). Thus, matrix fibers can provide directional information to cell populations migrating by chemotaxis.

5.2. Endothelial Cells

Resolving granulation tissue is characterized in part by the abundant anastomosing capillary beds found within it. These capillary beds form by the influx of microvessel buds originating in the vasculature of the surrounding tissue. Angiogenesis is also important to a variety of other pathologic conditions. For example, an adequate vascular supply is thought to be a limiting factor in tumor growth, survival, and progression (Folkman et al., 1983). In addition, wound-healing problems encountered by diabetics, although complicated in etiology, may be directly related to the abnormalities (i.e., thickening or altered composition) of microvessel basement membranes, which may inhibit neovascularization (Joyner et al., 1981).

The development of techniques to isolate and grow microvessel endothelial cells has been crucial to understanding angiogenesis. Angiogenesis can be measured in vivo in a variety of experimental model systems, including the cornea of the rabbit eye (Gimbrone et al., 1974), and implantation of specialized viewing chambers in rabbit ears (Knighton et al., 1981). It has become clear that angiogenesis in situ is a complicated process involving several factors, including endothelial cell migration, growth, and capillary tubule formation (see Chapter 15). There is evidence that each of these activities is controlled by many separate but overlapping influences that occur within the resolving wound.

Several factors are reported to be capable of promoting capillary endothelial cell migration in vitro. Wound-healing fluid has been shown to contain a factor that stimulates angiogenesis and capillary cell migration in vitro (Banda et al., 1982). Preliminary characterization of this factor suggests it is a low-molecular-weight (2,000–14,000-M_r) factor probably produced by macrophages within the wound (Banda et al., 1982). There is also evidence that macrophages are activated by factors within the wound to produce this factor by biologic activators (e.g., bacterial endotoxin) as well as physico/chemical stimuli (e.g., hypoxia) that occur in healing wounds (Ausprunk and Folkman, 1977; Knighton et al., 1981, 1983, 1984; Banda et al., 1982). Heparin, a major product of degranulating mast cells, has also been shown to promote capillary endothelial cell migration in vivo, and this effect can be blocked with protamine sulfate (Azizkhan et al., 1980). Despite the fact that mast cells alone cannot induce angiogenesis (Kessler et al., 1976), these studies suggest a role for mast cell heparin in vessel formation and suggest that heparin might act in vivo in concert with other factors to promote vascularization. In addition to these wound-derived factors, tumor-derived factors have been described that promote angiogenesis and endothelial cell migration in vitro (Zetter, 1980). Enzymes elaborated by endothelial cells may also be important in angiogenesis. For example, type IV and V collagenases have been shown to be associated with migrating endothelial cells in vitro (Kalebic et al., 1983). Penetration of the subendothelial basement membrane and connective tissues may be an important step during the early phases of angiogenesis.

The extracellular matrix has multiple affects on angiogenesis. Fibronectin-rich matrices have been associated with capillary ingrowth during development of the kidney (Sariola et al., 1984) and in healing wounds (Clark et al., 1982). Madri and Williams (1983) showed that extracellular matrix can modulate the phenotype of capillary endothelial cells (see Chapter 15). In these studies, cells grown on interstitial collagens proliferated, became confluent, and eventually formed tubelike structures. By contrast, cells plated on basement membrane proteins did not grow but rather went on directly to form tubelike structures. These tubelike structures, which form from anastomosing vacuoles that originate from within the endothelial cytoplasm (Folleman *et al.*, 1979), presumably represent efforts on the part of the endothelial cells to form a lumen. The extracellular matrix also affects the proliferation and rate of protein synthesis by microvascular endothelium (Madri and Williams, 1983). Intact hyaluronic acid, a prominent component of granulation tissue, has been shown to inhibit angiogenesis, whereas fragments of this glycosaminoglycan have been reported to be a potent angiogenic stimulus (West *et al.*, 1985). As with fibroblast infiltration, contact guidance forces exerted by the extracellular matrix of the contracting wound may also serve to orient and promote endothelial cell migration into the healing wound.

Wounds of confluent large-vessel endothelium *in vitro* or *in vivo* have been used by several laboratories for studying the healing of defects on the lumenal surface; these studies have demonstrated a role for endothelial cell migration in this type of healing (Haudenschild and Harris-Hooker, 1984; Young and Herman, 1985; Pederson and Bowyer, 1985) (see Chapter 16). Rapid healing is imperative to prevent exposure of a subendothelial thrombogenic surface and to discourage the possible initiation of atherosclerotic lesions (Schwartz *et al.*, 1978; Haudenschild and Harris-Hooker, 1984). The orientation of the subendothelial matrix has been shown to affect the rate of endothelial cell migration into a defect (Jackman, 1982). Furthermore, isolated components of the extracellular matrix have been shown to influence the cytoskeletal organization and migration rate of endothelial cells *in vitro* by different assay systems (Young and Herman, 1985; Bowersox and Sorgente, 1982). Cells grown on interstitial collagens exhibit faster migration rates than do cells grown on basement membrane collagen; this difference was correlated to the presence of stress fibers in nonmigrating cells (Young and Herman, 1985). Detailed studies have shown that once confluent, large-vessel endothelial cells continue to move past each other at a much reduced albeit detectable rate (Haudenschild and Harris-Hooker, 1984). The dynamic nature of the endothelium may account for its ability to migrate into and repair vascular defects created by normal cell death without exposing the subendothelial connective tissue (Hanson and Schwartz, 1983) (see Chapter 16).

5.3. Movement of Keratinocytes and Other Epithelial Cells

The re-epithelialization of a wound is a crucial aspect of wound closure, since the epidermis is needed to re-establish a permeability barrier for the underlying tissue. These cells migrate directionally as sheets, with the marginal cells exhibiting advancing lamellipodia into the region of the defect and the submarginal cells following along as space permits (the so-called free-edge effect). Epithelial cells can also dissect the border between the scab and the underlying granulation tissue by phagocytosing extracellular debris (Repesh *et al.*, 1982). Following re-epithelialization, the cells proliferate, deposit a new basement membrane, and restratify to restore the original epidermis (Mackenzie and Fusenig, 1983).

The basal cell layer of stratified epithelium appears to be the only layer capable of exhibiting a motile response. The upper layers of epidermis, which are joined to the basal cell layer through desmosomes, are apparently pulled passively along as the basal layer spreads (Trinkaus, 1984). Gipson et al. (1983b) used lectin binding to probe characteristics of migrating corneal epithelial cells. These investigators found that the carbohydrates of the apical surface of migrating cells differed from those of the apical surface of normal epithelium. Importantly, these studies demonstrated that lectin binding of migrating cells more closely resembled that of the basal layer of normal epithelium (Gipson and Anderson, 1980). The addition of lectins to a migrating epithelium has been shown to slow or completely block cell movement in corneal wounds (Gipson and Anderson, 1980). Previous work by Stenn et al. (1979) suggests that protein synthesis is required for epithelial cell movement on mouse skins, although this is not a universal finding for all animals (Stenn et al., 1983). Cells of wounded rat corneas do synthesize increased amounts of protein during healing, and recent evidence suggests that migrating epithelia in this system synthesize a 110,000-M_r protein that disappears upon cessation of migration (Zieske and Gipson, 1986). Stenn and Milstone (1984) presented evidence demonstrating a two-step mechanism for keratinocyte-mediated wound closure based on protein-synthesis mechanisms. It was concluded that migration was initially dependent on substratum-bound proteins, whereas later migration depended on protein synthesis of the migrating epithelium. Perhaps the protein synthesis-dependent late stage of epidermal spreading represents the formation of new matrix by the regenerating epithelium (Stenn and Milstone, 1984). These studies suggest that the basal layer provides the motile force for sheet movement and argue strongly for examination of the effect of the composition of the underlying matrix on epithelial sheet movement.

Several types of substrata have been shown in a variety of systems to be compatible with epithelial sheet movement. In healing amphibian epidermis, substrata coated with extracellular matrix proteins such as collagen, fibrin(ogen), and fibronectin have all been shown to be compatible with wound closure (Donaldson and Mahan, 1983, 1984; Donaldson et al., 1985). Recent work by Donaldson et al. (1985) showed that proteolytic fragments of fibronectin containing the RGDS tetrapeptide sequence can promote epithelialization when coated onto nitrocellulose sheets and implanted in wounds. Laminin was reported to be a relatively poor substratum for epithelial cell sheet movement, and in fact, laminin-coated type IV collagen substrata caused decreased epithelial cell migration relative to that observed on type IV collagen alone (Donaldson and Mahan, 1984). The importance of fibronectin in other epithelialization models has also been studied. Fibronectin has been reported to participate in a provisional matrix beneath rat epidermal (Clark et al., 1983) and rabbit corneal (Suda et al., 1981) migrating epithelia. The main source of fibronectin for early wounds is plasma (Grinnell et al., 1981; Clark et al., 1983). Cells that invade the granulation tissue (macrophages, fibroblasts), as well as epithelial cells in the later stages of wound repair (Clark et al., 1983; Kubo et al., 1984) also serve as a source of fibronectin during later stages of healing and repair.

There is evidence to suggest that fibronectin may play an opsonic role for migrating keratinocytes (Takashima and Grinnell, 1984). Direct topical application of fibronectin to healing rabbit (Nishida *et al.*, 1983*a*) or human (Nishida *et al.*, 1983*b*) corneas has been reported to accelerate epithelialization. Basement membrane constituents (laminin, type IV; collagen and bullous pemphigoid antigen) appear in histologic sections only after the completion of wound closure (Fujikawa *et al.*, 1984), suggesting that an intact basement membrane is not absolutely necessary to epithelial cell migration and may instead represent a differentiation marker once closure is completed.

6. Concluding Remarks

Despite the fact that wound healing has long been a subject of interest, it is only recently that the molecular basis of cell migration into wounds has begun to be elucidated. A variety of factors present in clots, inflamed tissue, and granulation tissue have been identified that could promote cell migration. These factors are cell-derived or are part of the extracellular matrix itself. Advances in this field in the future will undoubtedly apply principles that are learned from these efforts to healing wounds that are potentially clinical problems (e.g., corneal ulcerations), as well as to aid healing in patients with chronic wound-healing disorders (e.g., diabetics or the aged). Better methods of preparing artificial skin for burn patients and blood vessels as well are also likely to evolve. In addition, an understanding of the molecular basis of collagen deposition during wound healing potentially leads to therapeutic strategies that could decrease the severity of fibrotic reactions commonly associated with many chronic inflammatory disorders, such as rheumatoid arthritis or scleroderma. Principles learned from these studies may also prove useful in treatment of other pathologic lesions in which cell motility plays a role, such as in tumor growth, progression, and metastatic spread of malignancies.

References

Abercrombie, M., 1967, Contact inhibition: The phenomenon and its biological implications, *Natl. Cancer Inst. Monog.* **26:**249–277.

Abercrombie, M., and Heaysman, J. E. M., 1954, Observations on the social behavior of cells in tissue culture. II. Monolayering of fibroblasts, *Exp. Cell Res.* **6:**293–306.

Akers, R. M., Mosher, D. L., and Lilien, J. E., 1981, Promotion of retinal neurite outgrowth by substratum-bound fibronectin, *Dev. Biol.* **86:**179–188.

Akiyama, S. K., Hasegawa, E., Hasegawa, T., and Yamada, K. M., 1985, The interaction of fibronectin fragments with fibroblastic cells, *J. Biol. Chem.* **260:**13256–13260.

Albini, A., Richter, H., and Ponte, B. F., 1983, Localization of the chemotactic domain in fibronectin, *FEBS Lett.* **156:**222–226.

Ali, I. V., and Hynes, R. O., 1978, Effects of LETS glycoprotein on cell motility, *Cell* **14:**439–446.

Alitalo, K., Hovi, T., and Vaheri, A., 1980, Fibronectin is produced by human macrophages, *J. Exp. Med.* **151:**602–613.

Aplin, J. D., Hughes, R. C., Jaffe, C. L., and Sharon, N., 1981, Reversible cross-linking of cellular components of adherent fibroblasts to fibronectin and lectin-coated substrata, *Exp. Cell Res.* **134:**488–494.

Mechanisms of Parenchymal Cell Migration **309**

Ausprunk, D., and Folkman, J., 1977, Migration and proliferation of endothelial cells in preformed and newly formed blood vessels during tumor angiogenesis, *Microvasc. Res.* **14**:53–65.

Azizkhan, R. G., Azizkhan, J., Letter, B. R., and Folkman, J., 1980, Mast cell heparin stimulates migration of capillary endothelial cells *in vitro*, *J. Exp. Med.* **152**:931–944.

Banda, M. J., Knighton, D. R., Hunt, T. K., and Werb, Z., 1982, Isolation of a non-mitogenic angiogenesis factor from wound fluid, *Proc. Natl. Acad. Sci. USA* **79**:7773–7777.

Barnes, D. W., Reing, J. E., and Amos, E., 1985, Heparin-binding properties of human serum spreading factor, *J. Biol. Chem.* **260**:9117–9122.

Barnes, D. W., Silnutzer, J., See, C., and Shaffer, M., 1981, Characterization of human serum spreading factor with monoclonal antibody, *Proc. Natl. Acad. Sci. USA* **78**:196–201.

Baron Von Evercooren, A., Kleinman, H. K., Ohno, S., Marangoes, P., Schartz, J. P., and Dubois-Dalcq, M. E., 1982, Nerve growth factor, laminin, and fibronectin promote neurite growth in human fetal sensory ganglia cultures, *J. Neurosci. Res.* **8**:179–193.

Bar-Shivat, R., Kahn, A., Fenton, J. W., and Wilner, G. D., 1983, Chemotactic response of monocytes to thrombin, *J. Cell Biol.* **96**:282–285.

Baur, P. S., and Parks, D. H., 1983, The myofibroblast anchoring strand—the fibronectin connection in wound healing and the possible loci of collagen fibril assembly, *J. Trauma* **23**:853–862.

Becker, E. L., 1972, The relationship of the chemotactic behavior of the complement-derived factors, C3a, C5a, and C567, and a bacterial chemotactic factor to their ability to activate the proesterase I of rabbit polymorphonuclear leukocytes, *J. Exp. Med.* **135**:376–387.

Bender, B. L., Jaffe, R., Carlin, B., and Chung, A. E., 1981, Immunolocalization of entactin, a sulfated basement membrane component in rodent tissues and comparison with GP-2 (laminin), *Am. J. Pathol.* **103**:419–425.

Bergmann, J. E., Kupfer, A., and Singer, S. J., 1983, Membrane insertion at the leading edge of motile fibroblasts, *Proc. Natl. Acad. Sci. USA* **80**:1367–1371.

Beyth, R. J., and Culp, L. A., 1984, Complementary adhesive responses of human skin fibroblasts to the cell binding domain of fibronectin and the heparan sulfate-binding protein, platelet factor 4, *Exp. Cell Res.* **155**:537–548.

Bitterman, P. B., Rennard, S. I., Adelberg, S., and Crystal, R. G., 1983, Role of fibronectin as a growth factor for fibroblasts, *J. Cell Biol.* **97**:1925–1932.

Bowersox, J. C., and Sorgente, N., 1982, Chemotaxis of aortic endothelial cells in response to fibronectin, *Cancer Res.* **42**:2547–2551.

Brennan, M. J., Oldberg, A., Hayman, E. G., and Ruoslahti, E., 1983, Effect of a proteoglycan produced by rat tumor cells on their adhesion to fibronectin-collagen substrata, *Cancer Res.* **43**:4302–4307.

Bretscher, A., and Weber, K., 1980, Fimbrin, a new microfilament-associated protein present in microvilli and other cell surface structures, *J. Cell Biol.* **86**:335–340.

Brinkley, B. R., Cox, S. M., Pepper, D. A., Wible, L., Brenner, S. L., and Pardue, R. I., 1981, Tubulin assembly sites and the organization of cytoplasmic microtubules in cultured mammalian cells, *J. Cell Biol.* **90**:554–562.

Brown, P. J., and Juliano, R. L., 1985, Selective inhibition of fibronectin-mediated cell adhesion by monoclonal antibodies to a cell-surface glycoprotein, *Science* **228**:1448–1451.

Bryant, W. M., 1977, Wound healing, *CIBA Clin. Symp.* **29**:1–36.

Burridge, K., and Connell, L., 1983, A new protein of adhesion plaques and ruffling membranes, *J. Cell Biol.* **97**:359–367.

Carlsson, R., Engvall, E., Freeman, A., and Ruoslahti, E., 1981, Laminin and fibronectin in cell adhesion: Enhanced adhesion of cells from regenerating liver to laminin, *Proc. Natl. Acad. Sci. USA* **78**:2403–2406.

Carter, S. B., 1967a, Haptotaxis and the mechanism of cell motility, *Nature (Lond.)* **213**:256–260.

Carter, S. B., 1967b, Haptotactic islands. A method of confining single cells to study individual cell reactions and clone fermentation, *Exp. Cell Res.* **48**:188–193.

Carter, S. B., 1970, Cell movement and cell spreading: A passive or an active process?, *Nature (Lond.)* **255**:858–859.

Carter, W. G., Rauvala, H., and Hakomori, S-I, 1981, Studies on cell adhesion and recognition. II. The kinetics of cell adhesion and cell spreading on surface coated with carbohydrate-reactive proteins, (glycosidases and lectins) and fibronectin, *J. Cell Biol.* **88**:138–148.

Charonis, A. S., Tsilibary, E. C., Yuchenco, P. E., and Furthmayr, H., 1985, Binding of laminin to type IV collagen: A morphological study, *J. Cell Biol.* **100**:1848–1853.

Chen, W.-T., 1981, Mechanism of retraction of the trailing edge during fibroblast movement, *J. Cell Biol.* **90**:187–200.

Chen, W.-T., Greve, J. M., Gottlieb, D. I., and Singer, S. J., 1985a, Immunocytochemical localization of 140 kd cell adhesion molecules in cultured chicken fibroblasts, and in chicken smooth muscle and intestinal epithelial tissues, *J. Histochem. Cytochem.* **33**:576–586.

Chen, W.-T., Hasegawa, E., Hasegawa, T., Weinstock, C., and Yamada, K. M., 1985b, Development of cell surface linkage complexes in cultured fibroblasts, *J. Cell Biol.* **100**:1103–1114.

Clark, R. A. F., DellaPelle, P., Manseau, E., Lanigan, J. M., Dvorak, H. F., and Colvin, R. B., 1982, Blood vessel fibronectin increases in conjunction with endothelial cell proliferation and capillary ingrowth during wound healing, *J. Invest. Dermatol.* **79**:269–276.

Clark, R. A. F., Winn, H. J., Dvorak, H. F., and Colvin, R. B., 1983, Fibronectin beneath reepithelializing epidermis *in vivo*: Sources and significance, *J. Invest. Dermatol.* **80**(Suppl):26s–30s.

Clark, R. A. F., Nielsen, L. D., Howell, S. E., and Folkvord, J. M., 1985, Human keratinocytes that have not terminally differentiated synthesize laminin and fibronectin by deposit on fibronectin in the pericellular matrix, *J. Cell Biochem.* **28**:127–141.

Colvin, R. B., 1983, Fibrinogen-fibrin interactions with fibroblasts and macrophages, *Ann. N.Y. Acad. Sci.* **408**:621–633.

Cornbrooks, C. J., Carey, D. J., McDonald, J. A., Timpl, R., and Bunge, R. P., 1983, In vivo and in vitro observations on myelin production by Schwann cells, *Proc. Natl. Acad. Sci. USA* **80**:3850–3854.

Culp, L. A., 1974, Substrate-attached glycoproteins mediating adhesion of normal and virus-transformed mouse fibroblasts, *J. Cell Biol.* **63**:71–83.

Damsky, C. H., Knudsen, K. A., Bradley, D., Buck, C. A., and Horwitz, A. F., 1985, Distribution of the cell substratum attachment (CSAT) antigen on myogenic and fibroblastic cells in culture, *J. Cell Biol.* **100**:1528–1539.

Davis, B. H., Walter, R. J., Pearson, C. B., Becker, E. L., and Oliver, J. M., 1982, Membrane activity and topography of f-Met-Leu-Phe-treated polymorphonuclear leukocytes, *Am. J. Pathol.* **108**:206–213.

Decker, C., Greggs, R., Duggan, K., Stubs, J., and Horwitz, A., 1984, Adhesive multiplicity in the interaction of embryonic fibroblasts and myoblasts with extracellular matrices, *J. Cell Biol.* **99**:1398–1404.

Dembo, M., and Harris, A. K., 1981, Motion of particles adhering to the leading lamela of crawling cells, *J. Cell Biol.* **91**:528–536.

Deuel, T. F., Senoir, R. M., Chang, D., Griffin, G. L., Heinrikson, R. L., and Kaiser, E. T., 1981, Platelet factor 4 is chemotactic for neutrophils and monocytes, *Proc. Natl. Acad. Sci. USA* **78**:4584–4581.

Dipasquale, A., 1975, Locomotory activity of epithelial cells in culture, *Exp. Cell Res.* **94**:191–215.

Donaldson, D. J., and Mahan, J. T., 1983, Fibrinogen and fibronectin as substrates for epidermal cell migration during wound closure, *J. Cell Sci.* **62**:117–127.

Donaldson, D. J., and Mahan, J. T., 1984, Epidermal cell migration on laminin-coated substrates. Comparison with other extracellular matrix and non-matrix proteins, *Cell Tissue Res.* **235**:221–224.

Donaldson, D. J., Smith, G. N., and Kang, A. H., 1982, Epidermal cell migration on collagen and collagen-derived peptides, *J. Cell Sci.* **57**:15–23.

Donaldson, D. J., Mahan, J. T., Hasty, D. L., McCarthy, J. B., and Furcht, L. T., 1985, Location of a fibronectin domain involved in newt epidermal cell migration, *J. Cell Biol.* **101**:73–78.

Edgar, D., Timpl, R., and Thoenen, H., 1984, The heparin binding domain of laminin is responsible for its effects on neurite outgrowth and neuronal survival, *EMBO J.* **3**:1463–1468.

Enenstein, J., and Furcht, L. T., 1984, Isolation and characterization of epinectin, a novel adhesion protein for epithelial cells, *J. Cell Biol.* **99**:464–470.

Fleischmajer, R., and Timpl, R., 1984, Ultrastructural localization of fibronectin to different anatomic structures of human skin, *J. Histochem. Cytochem.* **32**:315–321.

Fligiel, S. E. G., Rodriguez, A. F., Knibbs, R. N., McCoy, J. P., and Varani, J., 1985, Characterization of laminin-stimulated adherence and motility in tumor cells, *Oncology* **42**:265–271.

Folkman, J., Haudenschild, C. C., and Zetter, B. R., 1979, Long term culture of capillary endothelial cells, *Proc. Natl. Acad. Sci. USA* **76**:5217–5221.

Folkman, J., Langer, R., Linhardt, R. J., Haudenschild, C., and Taylor, S., 1983, Angiogenesis inhibition and tumor regression caused by a heparin or a heparin fragment in the presence of cortisone, *Science* **221**:719–725.

Ford-Hutchinson, A. W., Bray, M. A., Doig, M. V., Shipley, M. E., and Smith, M. J. H., 1980, Leukotriene B, a potent chemokinetic and aggregating substance released from polymorphonuclear leukocytes, *Nature (Lond.)* **286**:264–265.

Fritze, L. M. S., Reilly, C. F., and Rosenberg, R. D., 1985, An antiproliferative heparan sulfate species produced by postconfluent smooth muscle cells, *J. Cell Biol.* **160**:1041–1049.

Fujikawa, L. S., Foster, S., Gipson, I. K., and Colvin, R. B., 1984, Basement membrane components in healing rabbit corneal epithelial wounds: Immunofluorescence and ultrastructural studies, *J. Cell Biol.* **98**:128–138.

Furcht, L. T., 1983, Structure and function of the adhesive glycoprotein fibronectin, *Mod. Cell Biol.* **1**:53–117.

Furcht, L. T., Smith, D., Wendelschafer-Crabb, G., Mosher, D. F., and Foidart, J. M., 1980a, Fibronectin presence in native collagen fibrils of human fibroblasts, *J. Histochem. Cytochem.* **28**:1319–1333.

Furcht, L. T., Wendelschafer-Crabb, G., Mosher, D. F., and Foidart, J. M., 1980b, An axial periodic fibrillar arrangement of antigenic determinants for fibronectin and procollagen on ascorbate treated human fibroblasts, *J. Supramol. Struct.* **13**:15–33.

Furthmayr, H., and von der Mark, K., 1982, The use of antibodies to connective tissue proteins in studies on their localization issues, in: *Immunochemistry of the Extracellular Matrix*, Vol. II (H. Furthmayr, ed.), pp. 89–118, CRC Press, Boca Raton, Florida.

Gabbiani, G., 1981, The myofibroblast: A key cell for wound healing and fibrocontractive disease, in: *Connective Tissue Research: Chemistry, Biology, and Physiology* (M. Adam, ed.), pp. 183–194, Alan R. Liss, New York.

Gallin, E. K., and Gallin, J. I., 1977, Interaction of chemotactic factors with human macrophages: Induction of transmembrane potential changes, *J. Cell Biol.* **75**:277–289.

Gallin, J. I., and Rosenthal, A. S., 1974, The regulatory role of divalent cations in human granulocyte chemotaxis: Evidence for an association between calcium exchanges and microtubule assembly, *J. Cell Biol.* **62**:594–609.

Gimbrone, M. A., Cotran, R. S., Leapman, S. B., and Folkman, J., 1974, Tumor growth and neovascularization: An experimental model using the rabbit cornea, *J. Natl. Cancer Inst.* **52**:413–427.

Gipson, I. K., and Anderson, R. A., 1980, Effect of lectins on migraton of the corneal epithelium, *Invest. Ophthalmol. Vis. Sci.* **19**:341–349.

Gipson, I. K., Grill, S. M., Spurr, S. J., and Brennan, S. J., 1983a, Hemidesmosome formation in vitro, *J. Cell Biol.* **97**:849–857.

Gipson, I. K., Riddle, C. V., Kiorpes, T. C., and Spurr, S. J., 1983b, Lectin binding to cell surfaces: Comparisons between normal and migrating corneal epithelium, *Dev. Biol.* **96**:337–345.

Gospodarowicz, D., 1983, Growth factors and their action in vivo and in vitro, *J. Pathol.* **141**:201–233.

Goldstein, I., Hoffstein, S., Gallin, J., and Weissman, G., 1973, Mechanisms of lysosomal enzyme release from human leukocytes: Microtubule assembly and membrane fusion induced by a component of complement, *Proc. Natl. Acad. Sci. USA* **70**:2916–2920.

Grinnell, F., 1980, Fibroblast receptor for cell-substratum adhesion: Studies on the interaction of baby hamster kidney cells with latex beads coated by cold insoluble globulin (plasma fibronectin), *J. Cell Biol.* **86**:104–112.

Grinnell, F., 1984, Fibronectin and wound healing, *J. Cell Biochem.* **26**:107–116.

Grinnell, F., Feld, M., and Minter, D., 1980, Fibroblast adhesion to fibrinogen and fibrin substrata: Requirement for cold-insoluble globulin (plasma fibronectin), *Cell* **19**:517–525.

Grinnell, F., Billingham, R. E., and Burgess, L., 1981, Distribution of fibronectin during wound healing in vivo, *J. Invest. Dermatol.* **76**:181–189.

Grotendorst, G. R., Seppa, H. E. J., Kleinman, H. K., and Martin, G. R., 1981, Attachment of smooth muscle cells to collagen and their migration toward platelet-derived growth factor, *Proc. Natl. Acad. Sci. USA* **78**:3669–3672.

Hammarback, J. A., Palm, S. L., Furcht, L. T., and Letourneau, P. C., 1985, Guidance of neurite outgrowth by pathways of substratum-adsorbed laminin, *J. Neurol. Res.* **13**:213–220.

Hanson, G. K., and Schwartz, S. M., 1983, Evidence for cell death in the vascular endothelium *in vivo* and *in vitro*, *Am. J. Pathol.* **112**:278–286.

Harris, A. K., 1973, The behavior of cultured cells on substrata of variable adhesiveness, *Exp. Cell Res.* **77**:285–297.

Harris, A. K., Wild, P., and Stopak, S., 1980, Silicone rubber substrata: A new wrinkle in the study of cell locomotion, *Science* **208**:177–179.

Haudenschild, C. C., and Harris-Hooker, S., 1984, Endothelial cell motility, in: *Biology of Endothelial Cells* (E. A. Jaffe, ed), pp. 74–78, Martinus Nijhoff, Boston.

Hay, E. D., 1982, *Cell Biology of Extracellular Matrix*, Plenum, New York.

Hayashi, M., and Yamada, K. M., 1983, Domain structure of the carboxyl-terminal half of human plasma fibronectin, *J. Biol. Chem.* **258**:3332–3340.

Hayman, E. G., Pierschbacher, M. D., Ohgren, Y., and Ruoslahti, E., 1983, Serum spreading factor (vitronectin) is present at the cell surface and in tissues, *Proc. Natl. Acad. Sci. USA* **80**:4003–4007.

Heggeness, M. H., Wang, K., and Singer, S. J., 1977, Intracellular distributions of mechanochemical proteins in cultured fibroblasts, *Proc. Natl. Acad. Sci. USA* **74**:3883–3887.

Hirata, F., Corcoran, B. A., Venkatasubramanian, K., Schiffman, E., and Axelrod, J., 1979, Chemoattractants stimulate degradation of methylated phospholipids and release of arachidonic acid in neutrophils, *Proc. Natl. Acad. Sci. USA* **76**:2640–2643.

Hynes, R. O., 1985, The molecular biology of fibronectin, *Annu. Rev. Cell Biol.* **1**:67–90.

Hynes, R. O., and Yamada, K. M., 1982, Fibronectins: Multifunctional modular glycoproteins, *J. Cell Biol.* **95**:369–377.

Izzard, C. S., and Lochner, L. R., 1980, Formation of cell-to-substrate contacts during fibroblast motility: An interference-reflexion study, *J. Cell Sci.* **42**:81–116.

Izzard, C. S., Izzard, S. L., and DePasquale, J. A., 1985, Molecular basis of cell-substrate adhesion, in: *Motility of Vertebrate Cells in Culture and in the Organism* (G. Haemmerli and P. Strauli, eds.), pp. 1–22, S. Karger, New York.

Jackman, R. W., 1982, Persistence of axial orientation cues in regenerating intima of cultured aortic explants, *Nature (Lond.)* **296**:81–83.

Johansson, S., Kjellen, L., Hook, M., and Timpl, R., 1981, Substrate adhesion of rat hepatocytes: A comparison of laminin and fibronectin as attachment proteins, *J. Cell Biol.* **90**:260–264.

Joyner, W. L., Mayhan, W. G., Johnson, R. L., and Phores, C. K., 1981, Microvascular alterations develop in Syrian hamsters after the induction of diabetes mellitus by streptozotocin, *J. Am. Diab. Assoc.* **30**:93–100.

Kalebic, T., Garbisa, S., Glaser, B., and Liotta, L. A., 1983, Basement membrane collagen: Degradation by migrating endothelial cells, *Science* **221**:281–283.

Kessler, D. A., Langer, R. S., Pless, N. A., and Folkman, J., 1976, Mast cells and tumor angiogenesis, *Int. J. Cancer* **18**:703–709.

Kjellen, L., Petersson, I., and Hook, M., 1981, Cell-surface heparan sulfate: An intercalated membrane proteoglycan, *Proc. Natl. Acad. Sci. USA* **78**:5371–5375.

Klebanoff, S. J., and Clark, R. A., 1978, *The Neutrophil: Function and Clinical Disorders*, North-Holland, New York.

Kleinman, H. K., Martin, G. R., and Fishman, P. H., 1979, Ganglioside inhibition of fibronectin-mediated cell adhesion of collagen, *Proc. Natl. Acad. Sci. USA* **74**:2909–2913.

Kleinman, H. K., Martin, G. R., and Fishman, P. H., 1979, Ganglioside inhibition of fibronectin-mediated cell adhesion on collagen, *Proc. Natl. Acad. Sci. USA* **74**:2909–2913.

Kleinman, H. K., Cannon, F. B., Laurie, G. W., Hassell, J. R., Aumailley, M., Terranova, V. P., Martin, G. R., and DuBois-Dalcq, M., 1985, Biological activities of laminin, *J. Cell Biochem.* **27**:317–325.

Knighton, D. R., Silver, I. A., and Hunt, T. K., 1981, Regulation of wound-healing angiogenesis—Effect of oxygen gradients and inspired oxygen concentration, *Surgery* **90**:262–270.

Knighton, D. R., Hunt, T. K., Scheuenstuhl, H., Halliday, B. J., Werb, Z., and Banda, M. J., 1983, Oxygen tension regulates the expression of angiogenesis factor by macrophages, *Science* **221**:1283–1285.

Knighton, D. R., Silver, I. A., and Hunt, T. K., 1984, Studies on inflammation and wound healing: Angiogenesis and collagen synthesis stimulated *in vivo* by resident and activated wound macrophages, *Surgery* **96**:48–54.

Kolega, J., Shure, M. S., Chen, W-T., and Young, N. D., 1982, Rapid cellular translocation is related to close contacts formed between various cultured cells and their substrata, *J. Cell Sci.* **54**:23–34.

Koo, C., Lefkowitz, R. J., and Snyderman, R., 1982, The oligopeptide chemotactic factor receptor on human polymorphonuclear leukocyte membrane exists in two affinity states, *Biochem. Biophys. Res. Commun.* **106**:442–449.

Kornblihtt, A. R., Vibe-Pedersen, K., and Baralle, F. E., 1983, Isolation and characterization of cDNA clones for human and bovine fibronectins, *Proc. Natl. Acad. Sci. USA* **80**:3218–3222.

Kornblihtt, A. R., Vibe-Pedersen, K., and Baralle, F. E., 1984, Human fibronectin: Molecular cloning evidence for two mRNA species differing by an internal segment coding for a structural domain, *EMBO J.* **3**:221–226.

Kornblihtt, A. R., Umezawa, K., Vibe-Pedersen, K., and Baralle, F. E., 1985, Primary structure of human fibronectin: Differential splicing may generate at least 10 polypeptides from a single gene, *EMBO J.* **4**:1755–1759.

Krawczyk, W. S., 1971, A pattern of epidermal cell migration during wound healing, *J. Cell Biol.* **49**:247–263.

Kubo, M., Norris, D. A., Howell, S. E., Ryan, S. R., and Clark, R. A. F., 1984, Human keratinocytes synthesize, secrete, and deposit fibronectin in the extracellular matrix, *J. Invest. Dermatol.* **82**:580–586.

Kurkinen, M., Vaheri, A., Roberts, D. J., and Stenman, S., 1980, Sequential appearance of fibronectin and collagen in experimental granulation tissue, *Lab. Invest.* **43**:47–51.

Kurkinen, M., Taylor, A., Garrels, J. I., and Hogan, B. L. M., 1984, Cell surface proteins which bind native type IV collagen or gelatin, *J. Biol. Chem.* **259**:5915–5922.

Lahav, J., Lawler, J., and Grimbrone, M. A., 1984, Thrombospondin interactions with fibronectin and fibrinogen, *Eur. J. Biochem.* **145**:151–156.

Lark, M. W., and Culp, L. A., 1983, Modification of proteoglycans during maturation of fibroblast substratum adhesion sites, *Biochemistry* **22**:2289–2296.

Lark, M. W., and Culp, L. A., 1984*a*, Turnover of heparan sulfate proteoglycans from substratum adhesion sites of murine fibroblasts, *J. Biol. Chem.* **259**:212–217.

Lark, M. W., and Culp, L. A., 1984*b*, Multiple classes of heparan sulfate proteoglycans from fibroblast substratum adhesion sites. Affinity fractionation on columns of platelet factor 4, plasma fibronectin, and octyl-Sepharose, *J. Biol. Chem.* **259**:6773–6782.

Lark, M. W., Laterra, J., and Culp, L. A., 1985, Close and focal contact adhesions of fibroblasts to a fibronectin-containing matrix, *Fed. Proc.* **44**:394–403.

Laterra, J., and Culp, L., 1982, Differences in hyaluronate binding to plasma and cell surface fibronectins. Requirement for aggregation, *J. Biol. Chem.* **257**:719–726.

Laterra, J., Norton, E. K., Izzard, C. S., and Culp, L. A., 1983*a*, Contact formation by fibroblasts adhering to heparan-sulfate-binding substrata (fibronectin or platelet factor 4), *Exp. Cell Res.* **146**:15–27.

Laterra, J., Silberg, J. E., and Culp, L. A., 1983*b*, Cell surface heparan sulfate mediates some adhesive responses to glycosaminoglycan-binding matrices, including fibronectin, *J. Cell Biol.* **96**:112–123.

Lazarides, E., and Burridge, K., 1975, α-actinin: Immunofluorescent localization of a muscle structural protein in nonmuscle cells, *Cell* **6**:289–298.

LeDouarin, N. M., 1984, Cell migrations in embryos, *Cell* **35**:353–360.

Letourneau, P. C., 1975, Cell-to-substratum adhesion and guidance of axonal elongation, *Dev. Biol.* **44**:92–101.

Mackenzie, I. C., and Fusenig, N. E., 1983, Regeneration of organized epithelial structure, *J. Invest. Dermatol.* **81**:1895–1945.

Mackin, W. M., Chi-Kuang, H., and Becker, E. L., 1982, The formyl peptide chemotactic receptor on rabbit peritoneal neutrophils, *J. Immunol.* **129:**1608–1611.

Madri, J. A., and Williams, K. S., 1983, Capillary endothelial cell cultures: Phenotypic modulation by matrix components, *J. Cell Biol.* **97:**153–165.

Mahan, J. T., and Donaldson, D. J., 1985, Events in the movement of newt epidermal cells across implanted substrates, *J. Exp. Zool.* **235:**35–44.

Majack, R. A., and Bornstein, P., 1984, Heparin and related glycosaminoglycans modulate the secretory phenotype of vascular smooth muscle cells, *J. Cell Biol.* **99:**1688–1695.

Majack, R. A., and Bornstein, P., 1985, Heparin regulates the collagen phenotype of vascular smooth muscle cells: Induced synthesis of a 60,000 M_r collagen, *J. Cell Biol.* **100:**613–619.

Malinoff, H. L., and Wicha, M. S., 1983, Isolation of a cell surface receptor protein for laminin from murine fibrosarcoma cells, *J. Cell Biol.* **96:**1474–1479.

McCarthy, J. B., and Furcht, L. T., 1984, Laminin and fibronectin promote the haptotactic migration of B 16 mouse melanoma cells *in vitro*, *J. Cell Biol.* **98:**1474–1480.

McCarthy, J. B., Palm, S. L., and Furcht, L. T., 1983, Migration by haptotaxis of a Schwann cell tumor line to the basement membrane glycoprotein laminin, *J. Cell Biol.* **97:**772–777.

McCarthy, J. B., Basara, M. L., Palm, S. L., Sas, D. F., and Furcht, L. T., 1985, The role of cell adhesion proteins—laminin and fibronectin—in the movement of malignant and metastatic cells, *Cancer Met. Rev.* **4:**125–152.

McCarthy, J. B., Hagen, S. T., and Furcht, L. T., 1986, Human fibronectin contains distinct adhesion- and motility-promoting domains for metastatic melanoma cells, *J. Cell Biol.* **102:**179–188.

McDonald, J. A., Kelley, D. G., and Broekelmann, T. J., 1982, Role of fibronectin in collagen deposition: Fab' to the gelatin-binding domain of fibronectin inhibits both fibronectin and collagen organization in fibroblast extracellular matrix, *J. Cell Biol.* **92:**485–492.

McKeown-Longo, P. J., and Mosher, D. F., 1983, Binding of plasma fibronectin to cell layers of human skin fibroblasts, *J. Cell Biol.* **97:**466–472.

McKeown-Longo, P. J., and Mosher, D. F., 1984, Mechanism of formation of disulfide-bonded multimers of plasma fibronectin in cell layers of cultured human fibroblasts, *J. Biol. Chem.* **259:**12210–12215.

McKeown-Longo, P. J., and Mosher, D. F., 1985, Interaction of the 70,000-mol. wt. amino terminal fragment of fibronectin with the matrix-assembly receptor of fibroblasts, *J. Cell Biol.* **100:**364–374.

McPhail, L. C., Clayton, C. C., and Snyderman, R., 1984, A potential second messenger role for unsaturated fatty acids: Activation and modulation of Ca^{++} dependent protein kinase, *Science* **224:**622–625.

Mensing, H., Ponte, B. P., Muller, D. K., and Gauss-Muller, V., 1983, A study on fibroblast chemotaxis using fibronectin and conditioned medium as chemoattractants, *Eur. J. Cell Biol.* **29:**268–273.

Mosher, D. F., 1975, Cross-linking of cold-insoluble globulin by fibrin-stabilizing factor, *J. Biol. Chem.* **250:**6614–6621.

Mosher, D. F., 1976, Action of fibrin-stabilizing factor on cold-insoluble globulin and α_2-macroglobulin in clotting plasma, *J. Biol. Chem.* **251:**1639–1645.

Mosher, D. F., 1984, Physiology of fibronectin, *Annu. Rev. Med.* **35:**564–575.

Naccache, P. H., Showell, H. J., Becker, E. L., and Shaa'fr, R. I., 1977, Transport of sodium, potassium, and calcium across rabbit polymorphonuclear leukocyte membranes: Effect of chemotactic factor, *J. Cell Biol.* **73:**428–444.

Nagata, K., Humphries, M. J., Olden, K., and Yamada, K. M., 1985, Collagen can modulate cell interactions with fibronectin, *J. Cell Biol.* **101:**386–394.

Nelson, R. D., McCormack, R. T., and Fiegel, V. D., 1978, Chemotaxis of human leukocytes under agarose, in: *Leukocyte Chemotaxis* (J. I. Gallin and P. C. Quie, eds.), pp. 25–42, Raven, New York.

Nishida, T., Nakagawa, S., Awata, T., Ohashi, Y., Watanabe, K., and Manabe, R., 1983a, Fibronectin promotes epithelial migration of cultured rabbit cornea in situ, *J. Cell Biol.* **97:**1653–1657.

Nishida, T., Ohashi, Y., Awata, T., and Manabe, R., 1983b, Fibronectin: A new treatment for corneal trophic ulcer, *Arch. Ophthalmol.* **101:**1046–1048.

Norris, D. A., Clark, R. A. F., Swigart, L. M., Huff, J. C., Weston, W. L., and Howell, S. E., 1982, Fibronectin fragments are chemotactic for human peripheral blood monocytes, *J. Immunol.* **129:**1612–1618.

Odland, G., and Ross, R., 1968, Human wound repair. I. Epidermal regeneration, *J. Cell Biol.* **39:**135–151.

Palm, S. L., and Furcht, L. T., 1982, Production of laminin and fibronectin by Schwannoma cells: Cell–protein interactions *in vitro* and protein localization in peripheral nerve *in vivo, J. Cell Biol.* **96:**1218–1226.

Pang, S. C., Daniels, W. H., and Buck, R. C., 1978, Epidermal migration during the healing of suction blisters in rat skin: A scanning and transmission electron microscopic study, *Am. J. Anat.* **153:**177–192.

Peacock, E. E., and Van Winkle, W., 1976, *Wound Repair,* WB Saunders, Philadelphia.

Pederson, D. C., and Bowyer, D. E., 1985, Endothelial injury and healing *in vitro.* Studies using an organ culture system, *Am. J. Pathol.* **119:**264–272.

Perkins, M. E., Ji, H. T., and Hynes, R. O., 1979, Crosslinking of fibronectin to proteoglycans at the cell surface, *Cell* **16:**944–952.

Perkins, R. M., Kellie, S., Patel, B., and Critchley, D. R., 1982, Gangliosides as receptors for fibronectin, *Exp. Cell Res.* **141:**231–243.

Petersen, T. E., Thorgersen, H. C., Skorstengaard, K., Vibe-Petersen, K., Sahl, P., Sottrup-Jensen, L., and Magnusson, S., 1983, Partial primary structure of bovine plasma fibronectin: Three types of internal homology, *Proc. Natl. Acad. Sci. USA* **80:**137–141.

Pierschbacher, M. D., and Ruoslahti, E., 1984a, Cell attachment activity of fibronectin can be duplicated by small synthetic fragments of the molecule, *Nature (Lond.)* **309:**30–33.

Pierschbacher, M. D., and Ruoslahti, E., 1984b, Variants of the cell recognition site of fibronectin that retain attachment-promoting activity, *Proc. Natl. Acad. Sci. USA* **81:**5985–5988.

Pierschbacher, M. D., Hayman, E. G., and Ruoslahti, E., 1981, Location of the cell attachment site in fibronectin with monoclonal antibodies and proteolytic fragments of the molecule, *Cell* **26:**259–267.

Pierschbacher, M. D., Hayman, E. G., and Ruoslahti, E., 1985, The cell attachment determinant in fibronectin, *J. Cell Biochem.* **28:**115–126.

Piez, K. A., and Reddi, A. H., 1984, *Extracellular Matrix Biochemistry,* Elsevier, New York.

Pike, M. C., Kredich, N. M., and Snyderman, R., 1978, Requirement of S-adenosyl-L-methionine mediated methylation for human monocyte chemotaxis, *Proc. Natl. Acad. Sci. USA* **75:**3928–3932.

Postlethwaite, A. E., and Kang, A. H., 1976, Collagen and collagen peptide-induced chemotaxis of human blood monocytes, *J. Exp. Med.* **143:**1299–1307.

Postlethwaite, A. E., and Kang, A. H., 1980, Characterization of guinea pig lymphocyte-derived chemotactic factor for fibroblasts, *J. Immunol.* **124:**1462–1466.

Postlethwaite, A. E., Snyderman, R., and Kang, A. H., 1976, The chemotactic attration of human fibroblasts to a lymphocyte-derived factor, *J. Exp. Med.* **144:**1188–1203.

Postlethwaite, A. E., Seyer, J. M., and Kang, A. H., 1978, Chemotactic attraction of human fibroblasts to type I, II, and III collagens and collagen-derived peptides, *Proc. Natl. Acad. Sci. USA* **75:**871–875.

Postlethwaite, A. E., Keski-Oja, J., Bahan, G., and Kang, A. H., 1981, Induction of fibroblast chemotaxis by fibronectin. Localization of the chemotactic region to a 140,000-molecular weight non-gelatin-binding fragment, *J. Exp. Med.* **153:**494–499.

Postlethwaite, A. E., Snyderman, R., and Kang, A. H., 1979, Generation of a fibroblast chemotactic factor in serum by activation of complement, *J. Clin. Invest.* **64:**1379–1385.

Pringle, G. A., Dodd, C. M., Osborn, J. W., Pearson, C. H., and Mosmann, T. R., 1985, Production and characterization of monoclonal antibodies to bovine skin proteodermatan sulfate, *Collagen Rel. Res.* **5:**23–29.

Pytela, R., Pierschbacher, M. D., and Ruoslahti, E., 1985a, Identification and isolation of a 140 kd cell surface glycoprotein with properties expected of a fibronectin receptor, *Cell* **40:**191–198.

Pytela, R., Pierschbacher, M. D., and Ruoslahti, E., 1985b, A 125/115 kD cell surface receptor for vitronectin interacts with the Arg-Gly-Asp adhesion sequence derived from fibronectin, *Proc. Natl. Acad. Sci. USA* **82:**5766–5770.

Radice, G. P., 1980a, The spreading of epithelial cells during wound closure in Xenopus laevis, *Dev. Biol.* **76**:26–46.

Radice, G. P., 1980b, Locomotion and cell-substratum contacts of *Xenopus* epidermal cells *in vitro* and *in situ*, *J. Cell Sci.* **44**:201–223.

Rao, C. N., Margulies, I. M. K., Tralka, T. S., Terranova, V. P., Machi, J. A., and Liotta, L. A., 1982, Isolation of a subunit of laminin and its role in molecular structure and tumor cell attachment, *J. Biol. Chem.* **257**:9740–9744.

Rao, C. N., Barsky, J. H., Terranova, V. P., and Liotta, L. A., 1983, Isolation of a tumor cell laminin receptor, *Biochem. Biophys. Res. Commun.* **111**:804–808.

Raugi, G. J., Mumby, S. M., Abbott-Brown, D., and Bornstein, P., 1982, Thrombospondin: Synthesis and secretion by cells in culture, *J. Cell Biol.* **95**:351–354.

Reich, E., Rifkin, D. B., and Shaw, E. (eds.), 1976, *Proteases and Biological Control*, Cold Spring Harbor Conference on Cell Proliferation.

Repesh, L. A., Fitzgerald, T. J., and Furcht, L. T., 1982, Fibronectin involvement in granulation tissue and wound healing in rabbits, *J. Histochem. Cytochem.* **30**:351–358.

Repesh, L. A., and Oberpriller, J. C., 1980, Ultrastructural studies on migrating epidermal cells during the wound healing stage of regeneration in the adult newt, *Notophthalmus visidescens*, *Am. J. Anat.* **159**:187–208.

Rich, A. M., and Harris, A. K., 1981, Anomalous preference of cultured macrophages for hydrophobic and roughened substrata, *J. Cell Sci.* **50**:1–7.

Rich, A. M., Pearlstein, E., Weissman, G., and Hoffstein, S. T., 1981, Cartilage proteoglycans inhibit fibronectin-mediated adhesion, *Nature (Lond.)* **293**:224–226.

Rogers, S. L., Letourneau, P. C., Palm, S. L., McCarthy, J., and Furcht, L. T., 1983, Neurite extension by peripheral and central nervous system neurons in response to substratum-bound fibronectin and laminin, *Dev. Biol.* **98**:212–220.

Rogers, S. L., McCarthy, J. B., Palm, S. L., Furcht, L. T., and Letourneau, P. C., 1985, Neuron-specific interactions with two neurite-promoting fragments of fibronectin, *J. Neurosci.* **5**:369–378.

Ross, R., Raines, E., Glenn, K., DiCorleto, P., and Vogel, A., 1981, Growth factors from the platelet, the monocyte/macrophage, and the endothelial cell: Their potential role in biology, in: *Cellular Responses to Molecular Modulators*, Miami Winter Symposia, Vol. 18, pp. 169–182, (L. W. Mozes, ed.), Academic, New York.

Ruoslahti, E., Hayman, E. G., Engvall, E., Cothran, W. C., and Butler, W. T., 1981, Alignment of biologically active domains in the fibronectin molecule, *J. Biol. Chem.* **256**:7277–7281.

Saba, T. M., and Jaffe, E., 1980, Plasma fibronectin (opsonic glycoprotein): Its synthesis by endothelial cells and role in cardiopulmonary integrity after trauma as related to reticuloendothelial function, *Am. J. Med.* **68**:577–594.

Sakishita, S., Engvall, E., and Ruoslahti, E., 1980, Basement membrane glycoprotein laminin binds to heparin, *FEBS Lett.* **116**:243–246.

Sariola, H., Peault, B., LeDourarin, N., Buch, C., Dieterlen-Lievre, F., and Saxen, L., 1984, Extracellular matrix and capillary ingrowth in interspecies chimeric kidneys, *Cell Diff.* **15**:43–51.

Sas, D. F., Herbst, T. J., and Furcht, L. T., 1985, Cell locomotion and formation of fibronectin substrate fibrils, submitted for publication.

Schiffman, E., and Gallin, J. J., 1979, Biochemistry of phagocyte chemotaxis, *Curr. Top. Cell Regul.* **15**:203–261.

Schwartz, S. M., Haudenschild, C. C., and Eddy, M., 1978, Endothelial regeneration. I. Quantitative analysis of initial stages of endothelial regeneration in rat aortic intima, *Lab. Invest.* **38**:568–580.

Schwarz, M. A., and Juliano, R. L., 1984a, Interaction of fibronectin coated beads with CHO cells, *Exp. Cell Res.* **152**:302–312.

Schwarz, M. A., and Juliano, R. L., 1984b, Surface activation of the cell adhesion fragment of fibronectin, *Exp. Cell Res.* **153**:550–555.

Schwarz, M. A., and Juliano, R. L., 1985, Two distinct mechanisms for the interaction of cells with fibronectin substrata, *J. Cell Physiol.* **124**:113–119.

Schwarzbauer, J. E., Tamkun, J. W., Lemischka, J. R., and Hynes, R. O., 1983, Three different fibronectin mRNAs arise by alternative splicing within the coding region, *Cell* **135**:421–431.

Senior, R. M., Griffin, G. L., and Mecham, R. P., 1980, Chemotactic activity of elastin derived peptides, *J. Clin. Invest.* **66**:859–862.

Seppa, H., Grotendorst, G., Seppa, S., Schiffman, E., and Martin, G. R., 1982, Platelet-derived growth factor is chemotactic for fibroblasts, *J. Cell Biol.* **92**:584–588.

Showell, H. J., Freer, R. J., Zigmond, S. H., Shiffman, E., Aswanikumar, S., Corcoran, B. A., and Becker, E. L., 1976, The structure-activity relations of synthetic peptides as chemotactic factors and inducers of lysosomal enzyme secretion for neutrophils, *J. Exp. Med.* **143**:1154–1169.

Silnutzer, J. E., and Barnes, D. W., 1985, Effects of fibronectin-related peptides on cell spreading, *In Vitro* **21**:73–78.

Singer, I. I., 1982, Association of fibronectin and vinculin with focal contacts and stress fibers in stationary hamster fibroblasts, *J. Cell Biol.* **92**:398–408.

Singer, S. J., and Kupfer, A., 1986, The directed migration of eukaryotic cells, *Annu. Rev. Cell Biol.* **2**:337–365.

Singer, I. I., Kawka, D. W., Kazazis, D. M., and Clark, R. A. F., 1984, In vivo co-distribution of fibronectin and actin fibers in granulation tissue: Immunofluorescence and electron microscope studies of the fibronexus of the myofibroblast surface, *J. Cell Biol.* **98**:2091–2106.

Small, J. V., 1981, Organization of actin in the leading edge of cultured cells: Influence of osmium tetroxide and dehydration on the ultrastructure of actin meshworks, *J. Cell Biol.* **91**:695–705.

Snyderman, R., and Goetzl, E. J., 1981, Molecular and cellular mechanisms of leukocyte chemotaxis, *Science* **213**:830–837.

Snyderman, R., and Pike, M. C., 1984, Chemoattractant receptors on phagocytic cells, *Annu. Rev. Immunol.* **2**:257–281.

Snyderman, R., Gewurz, H., and Mergenhagen, C. E., 1968, Interactions of the complement system with endotoxin lipopolysaccharide. Generation of a factor chemotactic for polymorphonuclear leukocytes, *J. Exp. Med.* **128**:259–275.

Spiegel, S., Schlessinger, J., and Fishman, P. H., 1984, Incorporation of fluorescent gangliosides into human fibroblasts: Mobility, fate, and interaction with fibronectin, *J. Cell Biol.* **99**:699–704.

Spiegel, S., Yamada, K. M., Hom, B. E., Moss, J., and Fishman, P. H., 1985, Fluorescent gangliosides as probes for the retention and organization of fibronectin by ganglioside-deficient mouse cells, *J. Cell Biol.* **100**:721–726.

Spilberg, I., Gallacher, A., Mehta, J., and Mandell, B., 1976, Urate crystal induced chemotactic factor, isolation and partial characterization, *J. Clin. Invest.* **58**:815–819.

Stamatoglou, S. C., and Keller, J. M., 1982, Interactions of cellular glycosaminoglycans with plasma fibronectin and collagen, *Biochim. Biophys. Acta* **719**:90–97.

Stanley, J. R., Hawley-Nelson, P., Yaspa, S. H., Shevach, E. M., and Katz, S. I., 1981, Characterization of bullous pemphigoid antigen: A unique basement membrane protein of stratified squamous epithelium, *Cell* **24**:897–903.

Stenn, K. S., and Milstone, L. M., 1984, Epidermal cell confluence and implications for a two-step mechanism of wound closure, *J. Invest. Dermatol.* **83**:445–447.

Stenn, K. S., Madri, J. A., and Roll, F. J., 1979, Migrating epidermis produces AB_2 collagen and requires continual collagen synthesis for movement, *Nature (Lond.)* **277**:229–232.

Stenn, K. S., Madri, J. A., Tinghitella, T., and Terranova, V. P., 1983, Multiple mechanisms of dissociated epidermal cell spreading, *J. Cell Biol.* **96**:63–67.

Stopak, D., and Harris, A. K., 1982, Connective tissue morphogenesis by fibroblast traction, *Dev. Biol.* **90**:383–392.

Stopak, D., Wessells, N. K., and Harris, A. K., 1985, Morphogenetic rearrangement of injected collagen in developing chicken limb buds, *Proc. Natl. Acad. Sci. USA* **82**:2804–2808.

Suda, T., Nishida, T., Ohashi, Y., Nakagawa, S., and Manabe, R., 1981, Fibronectin appears at the site of stromal wound in rabbits, *Curr. Eye Res.* **1**:553–556.

Suitlana, T. M., Shevelev, A. A., Bershadsky, A. D., and Gelfand, U. I., 1984, Cytoskeleton of mouse embryo fibroblasts. Electron microscopy of platinum replicas, *Eur. J. Cell Biol.* **34**:64–74.

Takashima, A., and Grinnell, F., 1984, Human keratinocyte adhesion and phagocytosis promoted by fibronectin, *J. Invest. Dermatol.* **83**:352–358.

Tamkun, J. W., Schwarzbauer, J. E., and Hynes, R. O., 1984, A single rat fibronectin gene generates three different mRNAs by alternative splicing of a complex exon, *Proc. Natl. Acad. Sci. USA* **81**:5140–5144.

Tamkun, J. W., DeSimone, D. W., Fonda, D., Patel, R. S., Buck, C., Horwitz, A. F., and Hynes, R. O., 1986, Structure of integrin, a glycoprotein involved in the transmembrane linkage between fibronectin and actin, *Cell* **46**:271–282.

Thiery, J. P., 1984, Mechanisms of cell migration in the vertebrate embryo, *Differentiation* **15**:1–15.

Toole, B. D., 1981, Glycosaminoglycans in morphogenesis, in: *Cell Biology of the Extracellular Matrix* (E. D. Hay, ed.), pp. 259–294, Plenum, New York.

Trinkaus, J. P., 1984, *Cells Into Organs. The Forces that Shape the Embryo*, Prentice-Hall, Englewood Cliffs, New Jersey.

Trinkaus-Randall, V., and Gipson, I. K., 1984, Role of calcium and calmodulin in hemidesmosome formation *in vitro*, *J. Cell Biol.* **98**:1565–1571.

Tsukamoto, Y., Helsel, W. E., and Wahl, S. M., 1981, Macrophage production of fibronectin, a chemoattractant for fibroblasts, *J. Immunol.* **127**:673–678.

Underhill, C. B., and Toole, B. P., 1981, Receptors for hyaluronate on the surface of parent and virus transformed cell lines, *Exp. Cell Res.* **131**:419–423.

Urushihara, H., and K. M. Yamada, 1986, Evidence for involvement of more than one class of glycoprotein in cell interactions with fibronectin, *J. Cell. Physiol.* **126**:323–332.

Vasiliev, J. M., 1985, Spreading of non-transformed and transformed cells, *Biochim. Biophys. Acta* **780**:21–65.

Vasiliev, J. M., Cefand, I. M., Domnina, L. U., Ivanova, O. Y., Komm, S. G., and Olshevskaja, L. V., 1970, Effect of colcemid on the locomotory behavior of fibroblasts, *J. Embryol. Exp. Morphol.* **24**:625–640.

Vaughn, R. B., and Trinkaus, J. P., 1966, Movements of epithelial cell sheets *in vitro*, *J. Cell Sci.* **1**:407–413.

Wahl, S. M., 1981, Inflammation and wound healing, in: *Cellular Functions in Immunity and Inflammation* (J. J. Oppenhein, D. L. Rosenstrich, and M. Potter, eds.), pp. 453–466, Elsevier/North-Holland, New York.

Wahl, L. M., Wahl, S. M., Mergenhagen, S. E., and Martin, G. R., 1974, Collagenase production by endotoxin-activated macrophages, *Proc. Natl. Acad. Sci. USA* **71**:3598–3601.

Wahl, L. M., Wahl, S. M., Mergenhagen, S. E., and Martin, G. R., 1975, Collagenase production by lymphokine-activated macrophages, *Science* **187**:261–263.

Wahl, S. M., Altman, L. C., Oppenheim, J. J., and Mergenhagen, S. E., 1974, In vitro studies of a chemotactic lymphokine in the guinea pig, *Int. Arch. Allergy Appl. Immunol.* **46**:768–784.

Wahl, S. M., Wahl, L. M., McCarthy, J. B., Chedid, L., and Mergenhagen, S. E., 1979, Macrophage activation by mycobacterial water soluble compounds and synthetic muramyl dipeptide, *J. Immunol.* **122**:2226–2231.

Wang, Y-L., 1985, Exchange of actin subunits at the leading edge of living fibroblasts: Possible role of treadmilling, *J. Cell Biol.* **101**:597–602.

Ward, P. A., and Becker, E. L., 1968, The deactivation of rabbit neutrophils by chemotactic factor and the nature of the activatable esterase, *J. Exp. Med.* **127**:693–709.

Weiss, P., 1945, The problem of specificity in growth and development, *Yale J. Biol. Med.* **19**:239–278.

Weiss, P., 1958, Cell contact, *Int. Rev. Cytol.* **7**:391–423.

Werb, Z., and Gordon, S., 1975, Secretion of a specific collagenase by stimulated macrophages, *J. Exp. Med.* **142**:346–360.

West, D. C., Hampson, I. N., Arnold, F., and Kumar, S., 1985, Angiogenesis induced by degradation products of hyaluronic acid, *Science* **228**:1324–1326.

Wilkinson, P. C., 1982, The measurement of leukocyte chemotaxis, *J. Immunol. Methods* **31**:133–148.

Wilkinson, P. C., and Lackie, J. M., 1983, The influence of contact guidance on chemotaxis of human neutrophil leukocytes, *Exp. Cell Res.* **145**:255–264.

Willingham, M. C., Yamada, S. S., Bechtel, P. J., Rutherford, A. V., and Pastan, I. H., 1981, Ultrastructural immunocytochemical localization of myosin in cultured fibroblastic cells, *J. Histochem. Cytochem.* **29**:1289–1301.

Wylie, D. E., Damsky, C. H., and Buck, C. A., 1979, Studies on the function of cell surface glycoproteins. I. Use of antisera to surface membranes in the identification of membrane components relevant to cell-substrate adhesion, *J. Cell Biol.* **80**:385–402.

Yamada, K. M., 1983, Cell surface interaction with extracellular matrix materials, *Ann. Rev. Biochem.* **52**:761–799.

Yamada, K. M., and Kennedy, D. W., 1984, Dualistic nature of adhesive protein function: Fibronectin and its biologically active peptide fragments can autoinhibit fibronectin function, *J. Cell Biol.* **99**:29–36.

Yamada, K. M., and Kennedy, D. W., 1985, Amino acid sequence specificities of an adhesive recognition signal, *J. Cell Biochem.* **28**:99–104.

Yamada, K. M., Kennedy, D. W., Kimata, K., and Pratt, R. M., 1980, Characterization of fibronectin interactions with glycosaminoglycans and identification of active proteolytic fragments, *J. Biol. Chem.* **255**:6055–6063.

Yamada, K. M., Kennedy, D. W., Grotendorst, G. R., and Mormoi, T., 1981, Glycolipids: Receptors for fibronectin?, *J. Cell Physiol.* **109**:343–351.

Yamada, K. M., Akiyama, S. K., Hasegawa, T., Hasegawa, E., Humphries, M. J., Kennedy, D. W., Naguta, K., Urushihara, H., Olden, K., and Chen, W-T., 1985, Recent advances in research on fibronectin and other cell attachment proteins, *J. Cell Biochem.* **28**:79–97.

Young, W. C., and Herman, I. M., 1985, Extracellular matrix modulation of endothelial cell shape and motility following injury *in vitro*, *J. Cell Sci.* **73**:19–32.

Zetter, B. R., 1980, Migration of capillary endothelial cells stimulated by tumor-derived factors, *Nature (Lond.)* **285**:41–43.

Zieske, J. D., and Gipson, I. K., 1986, Protein synthesis during corneal epithelial wound healing, *Invest. Ophthalmol. Vis. Sci.* **27**:1–7.

Zigmond, S. H., 1977, Ability of polymorphonuclear leukocytes to orient in gradients of chemotactic factors, *J. Cell Biol.* **75**:606–616.

Zigmond, S. H., and Hirsch, J. G., 1973, Leukocyte locomotion and chemotaxis. New methods for evaluation and demonstration of a cell derived chemotactic factor, *J. Exp. Med.* **137**:387–410.

Zigmond, S. H., Levitsky, H. I., and Kreel, B. J., 1981, Cell polarity: An examination of its behavior expression and its consequences for polymorphonuclear leukocyte chemotaxis, *J. Cell Biol.* **89**:585–592.

Chapter 14

Re-epithelialization

KURT S. STENN and LOUIS DEPALMA

1. Introduction

Central to the survival of each living organism is the protective outer layer separating the organism from the environment. In all but the simplest forms of life, the barrier is made up of cells that adhere tightly to one another. Such cells, referred to as epithelium or epidermis, generally form single-layered coverings in invertebrates and multilayered coverings in vertebrates. Wounding of this outer barrier layer is potentially lethal to the organism, as body fluids are lost to the environment or destructive environmental elements (chemicals or microorganisms) gain access into the organism. It is to the advantage of a wounded organism to close the rent rapidly, even before underlying tissue repair begins.

Wound closure is effected by two mechanisms. First, there is a temporary cover of the wound by an insoluble protein exudate, which staunches the flow of body fluid; second, there is rapid movement of the adjacent epithelium (epidermis) over the rent. It is the purpose of this chapter to review the latter, that is, epithelial cell movement—its structure and its dependence on substrate, milieu, and cellular processes.

This chapter focuses on the movement of epidermis (i.e., epithelial sheets) in particular but also considers, where relevant, the spreading of single dissociated epithelial cells. In this discussion, the phenomena of single-cell adhesion, spreading, and movement are considered related and essential to epithelial sheet movement. This is not a discussion of cell motility in general (for reviews, see Middleton and Sharp, 1984; Trinkaus, 1984) or of basement membrane physiology (Katz, 1984) (see Chapter 22) or of cell–cell interactions specifically (see Chapter 16). Although an attempt has been made to address current concepts, all studies pertinent to this area could not be included because of space limitations. Since liberal reference to the literature has been made, it is hoped the interested reader will be able to pursue specific topics with ease.

KURT S. STENN • Department of Dermatology, Yale University, New Haven, Connecticut 06510.   LOUIS DEPALMA • Department of Pathology and Laboratory Medicine, Yale University, New Haven, Connecticul 06510.

2. Morphology of Epithelial Migration in Wounds

A skin wound that destroys the epidermis results in a localized escape of body fluids and penetration of environmental elements. The resultant blood clot, which dries to become a scab, covers the wound effectively, though tenuously. Repair begins soon after clot formation with the migration of residual epithelium over the moist viable tissue and below the protective cover of the scab. A variable lag period occurs before migration begins. Subsequently, the rate of wound closure depends on the animal species, the wound site, substrate, and size. The rate of re-epithelialization is enhanced if the wound is only superficial and the basal lamina is left intact (Krawczyk, 1971; Pfister and Burnstein, 1976) and if the wound environment is kept moist (Croft and Tarin, 1970; Krawczyk, 1971; Winter, 1972; Martinez, 1972; Miller, 1980).

The migrating epithelium arises from the wound periphery in deep wounds; when dermis is retained in the wound, however, most comes from the residual dermal epithelial appendages (i.e., hair, eccrine) (Gillman et al., 1963; Hinshaw and Miller, 1965; Pang et al., 1978). To restore surface integrity of the wound, the migrating epithelium consists not of dissociated cells, but of a unified sheet, preserving its protective features as it moves. Epithelium covers the rent by a process of active horizontally directed movement, and not by growth pressure, as demonstrated many times in various epithelial systems (Arey, 1936; Marks and Nishikawa, 1973; Kuwabara et al., 1976; Pang et al., 1978).

There appears to be an inverse relationship between cell movement and mitosis. In incisional wounds, for example, cell division is found a distance from the wound margin but not at the wound margin, where most of the motile activity is found. Even under conditions that block cell division, epithelial cell and sheet motility persists (DiPasquale, 1975; Dunlap and Donaldson, 1978; Gipson et al., 1982).

Initial migration of epithelial cells starts from the lowest cell layers of the stratum spinosum or basale. These marginal cells flatten out in the direction of the rent, forming lamellipodial and ruffling cytoplasmic projections (Odland and Ross, 1968; Fejerskov, 1972). As the greatest motile activity of the epithelial sheet occurs at the wound margin, dramatic cytologic changes occur in these cells (Gabbiani and Ryan, 1974; Krawczyk, 1971; Gibbins, 1968; Andersen and Fejerskov, 1974). The marginal cells lose desmosomal and hemidesmosomal contacts, the basement membrane zone loses definition, and cells appear more loosely attached. Tonofilament bundles retract from their peripheral desmosomal attachments to a perinuclear location. The distal portion of the lamellipodia stain for actin and the proximal portion for α-actinin (Bereiter-Hahn et al., 1981). Peripherally positioned microfilament bundles appear and the cytoplasm of the marginal cells stain with antiactin and antimyosin. Concomitantly, an increase in the proportion of epidermal cell surface occupied by gap junctions is observed (Gabbiani et al., 1978). The direct correlation between gap-junction density and contractile protein concentration suggests a mechanism of synchronized locomotion of cells in the sheet. Indeed, wounding alters the normal voltage found across regions of amphibian and mammalian skins (Barker et al., 1982). The voltage gradient may help guide the cellular movements in wound closure. At the same time, the cells at the leading edge of the migrating epidermis become actively phagocytic and thus can be marked with fluorescein (Betchaku and Trinkaus, 1978), Thorotrast (Gibbins, 1968) or erythrocytes (Fejerskov, 1972). Phagocytosis may facilitate migration by permitting the cells to ingest the plasma clot and debris along the migratory path. Evidence that fibronectin enhances epidermal cell phagocytosis has been presented (Takashima and Grinnell, 1984).

The sheets continue to spread until microvillus processes of cells from opposing epithelial sheets contact and form attachments. This response is interpreted as an example of contact inhibition of movement. With the wound covered, epithelial cells now quickly reassume the cytologic properties of stationary cells: cell processes become inapparent, cytoplasmic actin and myosin are less easily stained, phagocytic vacuoles become scarce, desmosomes and hemidesmosomes increase in number, tonofilament bundles reattach to the cell periphery, and the basement membrane zone re-forms. Of these processes, it is desmosome formation that appears to be necessary for the end of migration (Martinez, 1972). Little is known about the control of desmosome or hemidesmosome formation, although they can form rapidly (2–6 hr). Recently, it has been shown that the appearance of both structures is calcium-dependent (Trinkaus-Randall and Gipson, 1984; Hennings et al., 1980). Moreover, where hemidesmosomes form is predictable. On an intact basal lamina, they arise above the area of dermal anchoring fibrils (Gipson et al., 1983a).

The cellular mechanism of epithelial sheet movement appears to vary with the system studied. In tissue culture, it is well established that monolayered epithelial sheets (Vaughan and Trinkaus, 1966) spread by the pulling force of their marginal cells and that the sheets adhere to the substratum entirely by these same marginal cells. If the marginal cells are perturbed, the whole sheet retracts, a response that illustrates that the tension generated the motile cells at the leading edge of these sheets. Likewise, when cells are plucked from the double-layered epidermis of tadpoles (basement membrane remains intact), broad lamellipodia extend out from neighboring basal cells and across the wound surface within seconds (Radice, 1980). The lamellipodia plasma membrane surface adheres evenly to the substrate, and actin microfilaments within the lamellipodia initiate a contractile process that pulls the marginal cell into and over the wounded space. Thus, the whole sheet is set in motion. The first migrating cell on retracting leaves a trailing edge behind, which forms a gap and stimulates the formation of lamellipodia in the adjacent cell. These in turn spread and retract and so forth. Contact inhibition is demonstrated, since lamellipodia do not form unless there is a free margin. The overlying epithelial cells adhere tightly to the basal cells and are pulled along by the underlying moving basal cells.

The mechanism of epidermal sheet movement suggested by direct studies of the epithelial sheet in vitro and from amphibian epidermal wound closure in vivo supports the model set forth by Weiss (1961) that asserts that the marginal cells lead the sheet and pull it along. This *sliding model* assumes that the order of cells in the sheet is fairly well established and retained throughout wound closure. The sliding model is believed accurate, even though it is recognized that (1) epithelial cells in a sheet may change neighbors and thus break and reform attachments (Keller, 1978) while retaining the mechanical and physiologic integrity of the sheet; and (2) new cells must be added to a sheet of cells moving outward from an original finite source of cells. Since marginal cells do not appear to divide, cells added to the sheet must arise from submarginal populations and thus must enhance the extent to which the sheet can extend. Evidence for the sliding model has been presented for epithelial cells in culture (Vaughan and Trinkaus, 1966), for embryonic epiboly (Bellairs, 1963), for amphibian wound closure (Radice, 1980), and for corneal wound closure (Buck, 1979).

In mammalian skin, the pattern of epithelial wound closure appears somewhat different. Here, too, wound closure is effected by cell movement, the most motile cells are at the wound margin, and significant mitotic activity may not be observed until sometime after the restoration of epidermal continuity (Krawczyk, 1971). One important difference from the other systems, however, is that the moving epithelial sheet is multilayered. Morphologically, mammalian epidermis appears to move across a wound by the rolling of marginal cells over one another. This leapfrog model (Winter, 1964) gleaned from indirect structural data proposes that a suprabasal cell rolls over an attached basal cell, contacts the basal lamina and attaches itself firmly by hemidesmosomes to form a new basal cell. Successive submarginal cells crawl over the newly adherent basal cell in turn. This model has many proponents (Krawczyk, 1971; Winter, 1972; Beerens *et al.*, 1975; Sciubba *et al.*, 1977; Gibbins, 1978).

Recent evidence has been presented by Ortonne *et al.* (1981) in support of the rolling model for mammalian wound closure, as opposed to the sliding model. First, if the epidermis were migrating as a sheet, these investigators argue, melanocytes would presumably be within the migrating cell mass. However, in contrast to intact epidermis, newly re-epithelialized epidermis lacks melanocytes. Second, by antigen staining, it is found that the basal cells of quiescent epidermis lack a 67,000-M_r keratin contained by the suprabasal cells, while the basal cells at a wound margin contain that 67,000-M_r keratin. Thus, suprabasal cells appear to move onto the basement membrane to form new basal cells, as predicted by the rolling model. However, the evidence from immunostaining keratin may be more difficult to interpret, since keratin expression alters with keratinocyte differentiation (Fuchs and Green, 1980); that is, wounded basal cells may express the 67,000-M_r keratin.

The sliding model of epithelial sheet movement is well documented because the systems to which it applies are simple and amenable to direct analytic methods. By contrast, the morphologic data of mammalian epidermal wound repair are adequately and convincingly explained by the rolling model, even though unequivocal direct evidence has not been presented. It may be that the rolling mechanism is better suited for more complex stratified epithelia and the sliding mechanism for single epithelia. Thus, in higher organisms, either or both mechanisms may contribute to wound closure, depending on the type of epithelium wounded.

3. Substrate and Epithelial Migration in Wounds

In referring to epithelial sheet movements, Trinkaus writes "Any epithelium artificially provided with a free edge . . . as in wounding, will spread if provided with the proper substratum" (Trinkaus, 1984). In recent years, considerable attention has been given to this issue of the proper substratum (reviewed recently by Woodley et al., 1985a). Although much has been learned concerning the structure and constituents of the basement membrane zone, we still do not know exactly upon what molecules the intact epidermis rests, even though we do know that within the basement membrane zone are glycoproteins (e.g., laminin, bullous pemphigoid antigen), collagen (types IV and V), and proteoglycans (heparan sulfate).

Direct and indirect studies of epidermis, dissociated or in sheets, indicate that the epidermis is capable of reexpressing the basement membrane into its typical ultrastructural form (Briggaman et al., 1971; Marks et al., 1975). Bullous pemphigoid antigen, now recognized to be a component of the cytoplasmic hemidesmosome (Westgate et al., 1985), is synthesized in cell or organ cultures (Stanley et al., 1980; Woodley et al., 1980b). Type V collagen is observed around the basal epidermal cells (Stenn et al., 1979; Smith et al., 1986). The production of laminin, a constituent of the lamina lucida, and type IV collagen, a constituent of the lamina densa, have been documented in cultures (Hintner et al., 1980; Woodley et al., 1980a; Stanley et al., 1981; Oikarinen et al., 1982; Alitalo et al., 1982), as has epidermolysis bullosa aquisita antigen, a component of the subbasal lamina area (Woodley et al., 1985c). The presence of fibronectin in the basement membrane zone (BMZ) remains problematic (Katz, 1984). Some studies have reported the presence of fibronectin in this region (Couchman et al., 1979; Foidart and Yaar, 1981; Fyrand, 1979), and others have not (Stenman and Vaheri, 1978). Ultrastructurally, when it is found, fibronectin is present in only scant amounts in two regions—the basal cell plasmalemma-upper lamina lucida region and the subbasal lamina area. Since fibronectin sticks to many surfaces and has been shown to adhere specifically to some basement membrane constituents (Woodley et al., 1985b), it is particularly difficult to interpret these studies.

Knowing some elements of the BMZ, the significance of these constituents in epidermal cell adhesion and spreading was analyzed. Early studies suggested that epidermal cells show relative substrate specificities for adhesion and spreading. It was observed that epidermal cells attach preferentially to type IV collagen compared with types I–III collagen (Murray et al., 1979) and that epithelial cells in general attach to collagen by means of an intermediate molecule, laminin (Terranova *et al.*, 1980) similar to fibroblast adhesion to collagen via fibronectin. In these studies, however, fibronectin did not enhance epidermal cell adhesion to collagen.

Although conceptually the linkage of epidermal cells to type IV collagen via laminin is attractive because of their spatial location in the BMZ, when these interactions were examined more closely, the specificity of the interactions was less clear. In culturing epidermal cells, it was observed that a greater number of cells attached if the plates were fibronectin coated (Gilchrest, 1980). Moreover, corneal epithelium spread better in the presence of fibronectin (Nishida *et al.*, 1983). On testing the spread of dissociated epidermal cells on multiple substrates it was observed that the cells spread about as well on serum as type IV collagen, laminin, and epibolin (Stenn *et al.*, 1983). Recently, several laboratories (Clark *et al.*, 1985; O'Keefe *et al.*, 1985; Donaldson and Mahan, 1983; Donaldson *et al.*, 1982) found that epidermal cells adhere and spread as well on fibronectin as on type I, III, and IV collagen and laminin. One fibronectin domain important to epidermal cell movement has been identified as the RGDS cell-binding domain (Donaldson *et al.*, 1985). The conclusion one can draw from these studies is that dissociated epidermal cells, just as hepatocytes (Rubin *et al.*, 1981) and lens epithelial cells (Hughes *et al.*, 1979), have multiple modes of adhesion and spreading. The above studies do not exclude an adhesion protein common to all sticking and spreading cells. However, when the latter possibility is tested by measuring epidermal cell adhesion in the absence of protein synthesis or in the presence of substrate antibodies (Stenn *et al.*, 1983; O'Keefe *et al.*, 1985; Clark *et al.*, 1985), no support for it can be gleaned. Current studies show that no one of these substrate proteins is absolutely necessary and that each supports adhesion and spreading to about the same degree.

In the above studies, dissociated epidermal cells were added to media *in vitro* containing various purified basement membrane proteins. If the experiment is done inversely, with the cells added to the dish first, permitted to adhere nonspecifically in defined medium, and then exposed to the various attachment proteins, the results are strikingly different (Federgreen and Stenn, 1980; Stenn *et al.*, 1983). In that case, the cells are fastidious and do not spread unless serum or the serum protein epibolin (Stenn, 1981) is added to the media: fibronectin, collagen, and laminin are ineffective substrates for cell spreading. Thus, the order in which the cells are exposed to basement membrane proteins is critical to the cell response. This observation begs the question whether epidermal cells actually reside on basement membrane components that support spreading. If so, the release of contact inhibition alone will lead to cell movement. By contrast, if they reside on a surface that does not support spreading, the release of contact inhibition alone is not adequate to initiate movement. In the latter case, cell spreading is initiated either after exposure to the plasma protein epibolin or after the cell begins synthesizing its own suitable spreading substratum.

When re-epithelializing epidermis has been examined *in vivo* and *in vitro*, the BMZ proteins reappear sequentially (Hintner *et al.*, 1980; Clark *et al.*, 1982; Stanley *et al.*, 1981). Appearing first at the advancing tip of the migrating epithelium is bullous pemphigoid antigen and later type IV collagen and laminin, in that order. By electron microscopy, the formation of the lamina densa accompanies the appearance of type IV collagen and laminin. So it appears from these studies that the repairing epidermis simply reassembles the basement membrane constituents in the proper structure, as it re-epithelializes the surface of viable tissue.

Past studies had shown that the migrating marginal epidermal cells do not move over a defined basal lamina (Krawczyk, 1971; Martinez, 1972; Marks *et al.*, 1975). More recent studies indicate that migrating epidermis probably needs and uses a different substratum than stationary epidermis. When epidermal explants were placed on BMZ substrates (laminin, heparan sulfate, proteoglycan, collagens IV and V) few of the explants spread out, but explants in contact with non-BMZ proteins, collagens I and III or fibronectin, exhibited superior migration (Woodley *et al.*, 1985a). Studies have found that the substrate of early migrating epithelium is rich in fibronectin and fibrin (Clark *et al.*, 1982; Fujikawa, 1981). At first, the epithelium transits over serum-derived fibronectin, but later the fibronectin is produced by the migrating cells themselves (Clark *et al.*, 1983). That epidermal cells in culture can also produce fibronectin has been demonstrated both directly (O'Keefe *et al.*, 1984; Kariniemi *et al.*, 1982; Kubo *et al.*, 1984) and indirectly (Alitalo *et al.*, 1982). In a recent study, Stenn and Milstone (1984) found that keratinocytes arising from confluent cultures are unable to spread in defined medium. Cells arising from subconfluent cultures, however, acquire a property sensitive to cycloheximide, which enables them to spread in defined media. These studies and those of Clark *et al.* (1983) suggest that there are two phases to epidermal cell wound healing. In the first phase, cell movement is dependent on the substrate of the wound environment; in the second phase, after the break of confluence (the release of confluent block), the cells produce their own substrate and become relatively autonomous of the wound environment.

While wound closure undoubtedly requires some protein synthesis by the migrating cells, it also requires protein resorption. Although the marginal cells of the epithelial sheet move over a fibrin–fibronectin provisional matrix, once the rent is covered the provisional matrix disappears and is replaced by a mature BMZ. Early studies have described the fragmentation and dissolution of the underlying collagen (Hinshaw and Miller, 1965). Such a transformation implies the release of proteolytic enzymes. In the culture system of Freeman *et al.* (1976), as epithelial cells migrate over the dermal collagen substrate, the substrate becomes transparent. In related studies, migrating epithelial cells have been shown to release collagenase (Grillo and Gross, 1967; Donoff, 1970; Woodley *et al.*, 1982) and plasminogen activator (Morioka *et al.*, 1985). The role of proteases in epithelial cell movement has not been elucidated. A process whereby migrating cells simultaneously form and restructure their own substrate would appear to be a plausible mechanism.

4. Metabolic Requirements and Epithelial Migration

4.1. Protein Synthesis

Epithelial sheets appear to require protein synthesis in order to move (Gibbins, 1973; Stenn et al., 1979; Rocha et al., 1986). In a study of mouse skin epiboly (Stenn et al., 1979), epidermal sheet movement was blocked by low concentrations of the protein synthesis inhibitor, cycloheximide. The proline analogue, L-azetidine-2-carboxylic acid, also reversibly blocked migration implicating the synthesis and importance of a proline-rich protein in the migratory process. Since similar epidermal preparations were found to synthesize type V collagen, the conclusion was drawn that type V collagen production is necessary for mouse epidermal sheet movement. This conclusion contrasts first, with the movement of wounded newt epidermal sheets accelerated by cycloheximide (Donaldson and Mason, 1978), and second, with the spreading properties of dissociated mammalian epidermal cells (Stenn et al., 1983; Clark et al., 1985) that spread in the absence of protein synthesis if the substrate is appropriate. Thus, protein synthesis may be necessary for epidermal movement in some situations but not others.

Synthesis of cell-surface glycoproteins appears to be necessary for epithelial sheet migration. Early workers reported that the cell surface blood groups on membranes of migrating reparative epithelium were different from those on membranes of stationary cells (Anderson and Fejerskov, 1974). If asparagine-linked glycosylation is blocked with tunicamycin, corneal epidermal sheet migration is inhibited (Gipson and Anderson, 1980). That glycosylation may be relevant to membrane changes was reported by Gipson et al. (1982, 1983b, 1984), who found that there are more lectin- (concanavalin A, wheat germ agglutinin) binding sites on migratory epithelial membranes than on quiescent epithelial cells and that migrating epithelium synthesizes glycoprotein at a rate 12 times that of quiescent epithelium. The actual mechanism of membrane protein glycosylation in facilitating motility (Gipson and Anderson, 1980; Donaldson and Mason, 1977) remains to be established.

4.2. cAMP

Although the level of cyclic adenosine monophosphate (cAMP) in migrating epithelium is higher than in resting epithelium (Dunlap, 1980), the relationship between elevated cAMP and motility has not been resolved. Indeed, elevated cAMP levels are not necessarily associated with cell movement. Appropriate doses of theophylline, which blocks phosphodiesterase, an enzyme that cleaves cAMP, not only block migration but lead to cAMP levels higher than that of migrating epithelium.

All three of the catecholamines, isoproterenol, epinephrine, and norepinephrine, studied by Donaldson and Mahan (1984) inhibited epidermal sheet migration. Since the isoproterenol effect is blocked by the β-antagonist, propranolol, these workers concluded that epidermal cell migration occurs through a β_2-adrenergic receptor on the cell surface, implicating the second messenger cAMP in the chain of events. Although such studies do not establish a causal relationship between cAMP and motility, the studies suggest that cAMP at specific concentrations may modify cell movement.

4.3. Cytoskeleton

Microtubule formation appears to play a minimal role in epithelial cell or sheet movement. Blocking microtubule formation in epithelial cells with colchicine or colcemid does not block movement (DiPasquale, 1975; Dunlap and Donaldson, 1978; Gipson et al., 1982). By contrast, actin filament formation appears to be crucial to the movement of these cells. Blocking microfilament formation with cytochalasin reversibly prevents migration in dissociated epidermal cells (DiPasquale, 1975) or corneal epithelial sheets (Gipson et al., 1982). Tonofilament formation has not been ascribed a role in epithelial cell motility.

4.4. Energy

In various systems, epidermal sheet movement is blocked by inhibitors of glycolytic and sulfhydryl enzymes, such as parahydroxymercuribenzoate or iodoacetate (Kuwabara et al., 1976; Gibbins, 1972), and not blocked by inhibitors of respiration (Kuwabara et al., 1976), Krebs (tricarboxyl acid, or TCA) cycle, oxidative phosphorylation, and gluconeogenesis (Gibbins, 1972). Migrating cells are thought to consume glycogen as a primary energy source. Thus, epithelial migration appears to be dependent on an intact glycolytic pathway but not on the more efficient TCA cycle, respiratory pathway, or oxidative phosphorylation.

4.5. Divalent Cations

The cation dependence of epithelial sheet movement has not been studied. For adhesion and spreading, dissociated epidermal cells show a highly specific divalent cation dependence. In reviewing a series of cations, Fritsch et al (1979) and Stenn and Core (1986) found that only three cations (Mg^{2+}, Ca^{2+}, Mn^{2+}) support adhesion and spreading of isolated epithelial cells but that the crucial ion in usual growth media is Mg^{2+}. Ca^{2+} alone is much less active. Both Mg^{2+} and Ca^{2+} support spreading only in the presence of serum. By contrast, Mn^{2+} supports spreading in the absence of serum but in the presence of serum albumin, a protein usually inactive in adhesion or spreading assays (Stenn and Core, 1986). The mechanism of Mn^{2+}-induced cell spreading appears to be different from Mg^{2+}-induced spreading because of its serum independence, its kinetics of spreading (more rapid than Mg^{2+} induced), its reversibility by Ca^{2+}, and its toxicity to cells after 24 hr of exposure. Because of its toxicity, the Mn^{2+} effect on epithelial cell spreading is considered a laboratory artifact; nevertheless, it is considered an important experimental model with which to dissect the mechanism of epidermal cell spreading.

4.6. Serum Protein

It has long been recognized that serum (or plasma) is necessary to support epidermal cell spreading *in vitro*. Early attempts (Levine, 1972; Mitrani and Marks, 1978) were made to isolate that serum fraction responsible for supporting epidermal spreading because it was assumed such a fraction could be used to accelerate wound closure. Although pure fibronectin has been shown to support epidermal cell adhesion and spreading (Gilchrest et al., 1980), a second serum fraction was identified that also had these properties (Stenn, 1978; Stenn and Dvoretzky, 1979). Using standard procedures of protein purification, the nonfibronectin activity was isolated and ascribed to a single-chain glycoprotein species of 65,000 M_r that travels electrophoretically as an $\alpha_1-\alpha_2$ globulin. In contrast to fibronectin, this purified protein, named epibolin, supports the spreading of dissociated epidermal cells whether exposed to epibolin before or after plating (Stenn, 1981; Stenn et al., 1983). It has become apparent that other serum-derived cell spreading proteins are related, if not identical to epibolin. These preparations have been referred to as serum-spreading factor (Barnes and Silnutzer, 1984), 70 K-spreading factor (Whatley and Knox, 1980), vitronectin (Suzuki et al., 1984), and S protein (Dahlbäck and Podack, 1985). Serum-spreading factor is maximally active on a variety of cell types in defined media in culture. By contrast, although epibolin is active in supporting epidermal cell spreading in a purified state, its activity is potentiated 10–60 times by the addition of serum albumin, a protein that alone does not support cell spreading (Stenn, 1987). It is not clear how albumin potentiates the action of epibolin or why such a cofactor is needed for epidermal cells. Recently, we found that tumor-promoting phorbol esters at low concentrations exhibit cofactor activity but do not support epidermal cell spreading alone (Stenn et al., 1987). Such an association may implicate the protein kinase C system in cofactor-enhanced epibolin-supported cell spreading.

5. Perspectives

The studies outlined describe a great deal of largely phenomenologic work that helps elucidate the processes of wound closure and epithelial cell movement. The time is ripe to address some important molecular questions: What initiates cell movement? What does the release of contact inhibition mean in terms of the constituent molecules of the cytoplasm and membrane? What are the signals that initiate the formation of cell attachments (e.g., desmosomes, hemidesmosomes, gap junctions)? In molecular terms, what are the membrane changes that occur in a motile cell? What are the molecular mechanisms of epithelial cell movement? Upon what elements of the basement membrane zone do epidermal cells actually rest? What controls the production of protease release and substrate protein production by motile cells? By answering these questions, it is hoped mechanistic insight will lead to effective therapeutic controls.

ACKNOWLEDGMENTS. This work was supported in part by grant CA34470-01 from the U.S. Public Health Service, awarded to K.K.S. by the National Cancer Institute, Department of Health and Human Services. The authors express appreciation to Dr. D. J. Donaldson, Dr. E. J. O'Keefe, and Dr. L. T. Smith, who provided unpublished material for use in this chapter.

References

Alitalo, K., Kuismanen, E., Myllyla, R., Kiistala, U., Askoseljavaara, S., and Vaheri, A., 1982, Extracellular matrix proteins of humanepidermal keratinocytes and feeder 3T3 cells, *J. Cell. Biol.* **94:**497–505.

Andersen, L., and Fejerskov, O., 1974, Ultrastructure of initial epithelial cell migration in palatal wounds of guinea pigs, *J. Ultrastruct. Res.* **48:**313–324.

Arey, L. B., 1936, Wound healing, *Physiol. Rev.* **16:**327–406.

Barker, A. T., Jaffe, L. F., and Vanable, J. W., Jr., 1982, The glabrous epidermis of cavies contains a powerful battery, *Am. J. Physiol.* **242:**R358–R366.

Beerens, E. G. T., Slot, T. W., and Van der Leun, J. C., 1975, Rapid regeneration of the dermal–epidermal junction after partial separation by vacuum. An electron microscopic study, *J. Invest. Dermatol.* **65:**513–521.

Bellairs, R., 1963, Differentiation of the yolk sac of the chick studied by electron microscopy, *J. Embryol. Exp. Morphol.* **11:**201–225.

Bereiter-Hahn, J., Strohmeier, R., Kunzenbacher, I., Beck, K., and Voth, M., 1981, Locomotion of xenopus epidermis cells in primary culture, *J. Cell. Sci.* **52:**289–311.

Betchaku, T., and Trinkaus, J. P., 1978, Contact relations, surface activity and cortical microfilaments of marginal cells of the enveloping layer and of the yolk synctial and yolk cytoplasmic layers of fundulus before and during epiboly, *J. Exp. Zool.* **206:**381–426.

Briggaman, R. A., Dalldorf, F. G., and Wheeler, C. E., 1971, Formation and origin of basal lamina and anchoring fibrils in adult human skin, *J. Cell. Biol.* **51:**384–395.

Buck, R. C., 1979, Cell migration in repair of mouse corneal epithelium, *Invest. Ophthalmol. Vis. Sci.* **18:**767–784.

Clark, R. A. F., Lanigan, J. M., DellaPelle, P., Manseau, E., Dvorak, H. F., and Colvin, R. B., 1982, Fibronectin and fibrin provide a provisional matrix for epidermal cell migration during wound reepithelialization, *J. Invest. Dermatol.* **79:**264–269.

Clark, R. A. F., Winn, H. J., Dvorak, H. F., and Colvin, R. B., 1983, Fibronectin beneath reepithelialization epidermis in vivo: Sources and significance, *J. Invest. Dermatol.* (Suppl.)**80:**26S–30S.

Clark, R. A. F., Folkvord, J. M., and Wertz, R. L., 1985, Fibronectin, as well as other extracellular matrix proteins, mediate human keratinocyte adherence, *J. Invest. Dermatol.* **85:**378–373.

Couchman, J. R., Gibson, W. T., Thorn, D., Weaver, A. C., Rees, D. A., and Parish, W. E., 1979, Fibronectin distribution in epithelial and associated tissues of the rat, *Arch. Dermatol. Res.* **266:**295–310.

Croft, C. B., and Tarin, D., 1970, Ultrastructural studies on wound healing in mouse skin. I. Epithelial behavior, *J. Anat.* **106:**63–77.

Dahlback, B., and Podack, E. R., 1985, Characterization of human S protein, an inhibitor of the membrane attack complex of complement. Denaturation of a free reactive thiol group, *Biochemistry* **24**:2368–2374.

DiPasquale, A., 1975, Locomotion of epithelial cells, *Exp. Cell Res.* **95**:425–439.

Donaldson, D. J., and Mahan, J. T., 1983, Fibrinogen and fibronectin on substrates from epidermal cell migration during wound closure, *J. Cell Sci.* **62**:117–123.

Donaldson, D. J., and Mahan, J. T., 1984, Influence of catecholamines on epidermal cell migration during wound closure in adult newts, *Comp. Biochem. Physiol.* **78C**:267–270.

Donaldson, D. J., and Mason, J. M., 1977, Inhibition of epidermal cell migration by concanavalin A in skin wounds on the adult newt, *J. Exp. Zool.* **200**:55–64.

Donaldson, D. J., and Mason, J. M., 1978, Inhibition of protein synthesis in newt. Epidermal cells: Effects on cell migration and concanavalin A-mediated inhibition of migration *in vivo*, *Growth* **42**:243–252.

Donaldson, D. J., Smith, G. N., and Kang, A. H., 1982, Epidermal cell migration on collagen and collagen-derived peptides, *J. Cell Sci.* **57**:15–23.

Donaldson, D. J., Mahan, J. T., Hasty, D. L., McCarthy, J. B., and Furcht, L. T., 1985, Location of a fibronectin domain involved in newt epidermal cell migration, *J. Cell Biol.* **101**:73–78.

Donoff, R. B., 1970, Wound healing biochemical events and potential role of collagenase, *J. Oral Surg.* **28**:356–363.

Dunlap, M. K., 1980, Cyclic AMP levels in migrating and non-migrating newt epidermal cells. *J. Cell Physiol.* **104**:367–373.

Dunlap, M. K., and Donaldson, D. J., 1978, Inability of colchicine to inhibit newt epidermal cell migration or prevent concanavalin A-mediated inhibition of migration studies *in vivo*, *Exp. Cell Res.* **116**:15–19.

Federgreen, W. R., and Stenn, K. S., 1980, Fibronectin does not support epithelial cell spreading, *J. Invest. Dermatol.* **75**:261–263.

Fejerskov, O., 1972, Excision wounds in palatal epithelium in guinea pigs, *Scand. J. Dent. Res.* **80**:139–154.

Foidart, J. M., and Yaar, M., 1981, Type IV collagen, laminin and fibronectin at the dermo-epidermal junction, *Front. Matrix Biol.* **9**:175–188.

Freeman, A. E., Eigel, H. J., Herman, B. J., Kleinfeld, K. L., 1976, Growth and characterization of human skin epithelial cell cultures, *In Vitro* **12**:352–358.

Fritsch, P., Tappeiner, G., and Huspek, G., 1979, Keratinocyte substrate adhesion is magnesium-dependent and calcium independent, *Cell Biol. Int. Rep.* **3**:593–598.

Fuchs, E., and Green, H., 1980, Changes in keratin gene expression during terminal differentiation of the keratinocyte, *Cell* **19**:1033–1042.

Fujikawa, L. S., Foster, S., Harrist, T. J., Lanigan, J. M., and Colvin, R. B., 1981, Fibronectin in healing rabbit corneal wounds, *Lab. Invest.* **45**:120–129.

Fyrand, O., 1979, Studies on fibronectin in the skin, *Br. J. Dermatol.* **101**:263–269.

Gabbiani, G., and Ryan, G. B., 1974, Development of a contractile apparatus in epithelial cells during epidermal and liver regeneration, *J. Submicrisc. Cytol.* **6**:143–157.

Gabbiani, G., Chaponnier, C., and Huttner, I., 1978, Cytoplasmic filament and gap functions in epithelial cells and myofibroblasts during wound healing, *J. Cell Biol.* **76**:561–568.

Ginnins, J. R., 1968, Migration of stratified squamous epithelium *in vivo*, *Am. J. Pathol.* **53**:929–941.

Gibbins, J. R., 1972, Metabolic requirements for epithelial migration as defined by the use of metabolic inhibitors in organ culture, *Exp. Cell Res.* **71**:329–337.

Gibbins, J. R., 1973, Epithelial migration in organ culture. Role of protein synthesis as determined by metabolic inhibitors, *Exp. Cell Res.* **80**:281–290.

Gibbins, J. R., 1978, Epithelial migration in organ culture. A morphological and time lapse cinematographic analysis of migrating stratified squamous epithelium, *Pathology* **10**:207–218.

Gilchrest, B. A., Nemore, R. E., and Maciag, T., 1980, Growth of human keratinocytes on fibronectin-coated plates, *Cell Biol. Int. Rep.* **4**:1009–1016.

Gillman, T., Penn, J., Brooks, D., and Roux, M., 1963, Reactions of healing wounds and granulation tissue in man to auto-thiersch, autodermal and homodermal grafts, *Br. J. Plast. Surg.* **6**:153–223.

Gipson, I. K., and Anderson, R. A., 1980, Effect of lectin on migration of the corneal epithelium, *Invest. Ophthalmol Vis. Sci.* **19**:341–349.

Gipson, I. K., and Kiorpes, T. C., 1982, Epithelial sheet movement: Protein and glycoprotein synthesis, *Dev. Biol.* **92**:259–262.

Gipson, I. K., Westcott, M. J., and Brooksby, N. G., 1982, Effects of cytochalasins B and D and colchicine on migration of the corneal epithelium, *Invest. Ophthal. Vis. Sci.* **22**:633–642.

Gipson, I. K., Grill, S. M., Spurr, S. J., and Brennan, S. J., 1983a, Hemidesmosome formation *in vitro, J. Cell Biol.* **97**:849–857.

Gipson, I. K., Riddle, C. V., Kiorpes, T. C., and Spurr, S. J., 1983b, Lectin binding to cell surfaces: Comparisons between normal and migrating corneal epithelium, *Dev. Biol.* **96**:337–345.

Gipson, I. K., Kiorpes, T. C., and Brennan, S. J., 1984, Epithelial sheet movement: Effects of tunicamycin on migration and glycoprutein synthesis, *Dev. Biol.* **101**:212–220.

Grillo, H. C., and Gross, J., 1968, Collagenolytic activity during mammalian wound repair, *Dev. Biol.* **15**:300–317.

Hennings, H. R., Michael, D., Cheng, C., Steinert, P., Holbrook, K., and Yuspa, S. H., 1980, Calcium regulation of growth and differentiation of mouse epidermal cells in culture, *Cell* **19**:245–254.

Hinshaw, J. R., and Miller, E. R., 1965, Histology of healing split-thickness, full thickness autogenous skin grafts and donor sites, *Arch. Surg.* **91**:658–670.

Hintner, H., Fritsch, P. O., Foidart, T. M., Stingl, G., Schuler, G., and Katz, S. I., 1980, Expression of basement membrane zone antigens at the dermo-epibolic junction in organ cultures of human skin, *J. Invest. Dermatol.* **74**:200–204.

Hughes, R. C., Mills, G., and Courtois, Y., 1979, Role of fibronectin in the adhesiveness of bovine lens epithelial cells, *Biol. Cell.* **36**:321–330.

Kariniemi, A. L., Lehto, V. P., Vartio, T., and Virtanen, I., 1982, Cytoskeleton and pericellular matrix organization of pure adult human keratinocytes cultured from suction-blister roof epidermis, *J. Cell Sci.* **58**:49–61.

Katz, S. I., 1984, The epidermal basement membrane, *Ciba Found. Symp.* **108**:243–259.

Keller, R. E., 1978, Time lapse cinemicrographic analysis of superficial cell behavior during and prior to gastrolation, *J. Morphol.* **157**:223–248.

Krawczyk, W. S., 1971, A pattern of epidermal cell migration during wound healing, *J. Cell Biol.* **49**:247–263.

Kubo, M., Norris, D. A., Howell, S. A., Ryan, S. R., and Clark, R. A. F., 1984, Human keratinocytes synthesize, recreate and deposit fibronectin in the pericellular matrix, *J. Invest. Dermatol.* **82**:580–586.

Kuwabara, T., Perkins, D. G., and Cogan, D. G., 1976, Sliding of the epithelium in experimental corneal wounds, *Invest. Ophthalmol.* **15**:4–14.

Levine, M., 1972, The growth of adult human skin *in vitro, Br. J. Dermatol.* **86**:481–490.

Marks, R., and Nishikawa, T., 1973, Active epidermal movement in human skin *in vitro, Br. J. Dermatol.* **88**:245–248.

Marks, R., Abell, E., and Nishikawa, T., 1975, The junctional zone beneath migrating epidermis, *Br. J. Dermatol.* **92**:311–319.

Martinez, I. R., 1972, Fine structural studies of migrating epidermal cells following incision wound, in: *Epidermal wound Healing* (H. I. Maibach and D. T. Rovee, eds.), pp. 323–342, Year Book, Chicago.

Middleton, C. A., and Sharp, J. A., 1984, *Cell Locomotion In Vitro. Techniques and Observations,* Croom and Helm, London.

Miller, T. A., 1980, The healing of partial thickness skin injuries, in: *Wound Healing and Wound Infection* (T. K. Hunt, ed.), pp. 81–96, Appleton-Century-Crofts, New York.

Mitrani, E., and Marks, R., 1978, Towards characterization of epidermal cell migration promoting activity in serum, *Br. J. Dermatol.* **99**:513–518.

Morioka, S., Jensen, P. J., and Lazarus, G. S., 1985, Association of plasminogen activator with epidermal cell differentiation and migration, *J. Invest. Dermatol.* **84**:305 (abst).

Murray, J. C., Stingl, G., Kleinman, H., Martin, G. R., and Katz, S. I., 1979, Epidermal cells adhere preferentially to type IV collagen, *J. Cell Biol.* **80**:197–202.

Nishida, T., Nakagawa, S., Awata, T., Ohashi, Y., Watanabe, K., and Manabe, R., 1983, Fibronectin promotes epithelial migration of cultured rabbit cornea in situ, *J. Cell Biol.* **97**:1653–1657.

Odland, G., and Ross, R., 1968, Human wound repair. I. Epidermal regeneration, *J. Cell Biol.* **39**:135–151.

Oikarinen, A., Savolainen, E.-R., Tryggvasum, K., Foidart, J. M., and Kiistala, U., 1982, Basement membrane components and galactosylhydroxylysyl glucosyltransferase in suction blisters of human skin, *Br. J. Dermatol.* **106**:257–266.

O'Keefe, E. J., Woodley, D., Castillo, G., Russell, N., and Payne, R. E., 1984, Production of soluble and cell associated fibronectin by cultured keratinocytes, *J. Invest. Dermatol.* **82**:150–155.

O'Keefe, E. J., Payne, R. E., Russell, N., and Woodley, D. T., 1985, Spreading and enhanced motility of human keratinocytes on fibronectin, *J. Invest. Dermatol.* **85**:125–130.

Ortonne, J. P., Loning, T., Schmitt, D., and Thivolet, J., 1981, Immunomorphological and ultrastructural aspects of keratinocyte migration in epidermal wound healing, *Virchows Arch. [A]* **392**:217–230.

Pfister, R. R., and Burnstein, N., 1976. The alkali burned cornea. I. Epithelial and stromal repair, *Exp. Eye Res.* **23**:519–535.

Pang, S. C., Daniels, W. H., and Buck, R. C., 1978, Epidermal migration during the healing of suction blisters in rat skin: A scanning and transmission electron microscopic study, *Am. J. Anat.* **153**:177–191.

Radice, G., 1980, The spreading of epithelial cells during wound closure in xenopus larvae, *Dev. Biol.* **76**:26–46.

Rocha, V., Hom, Y. K., and Marinkovich, M. P., 1986, Basal lamina inhibition suppresses synthesis of calcium-dependent proteins associated with mammary epithelial cell spreading, *Exp. Cell Res.* **165**:450–460.

Rubin, K. M., Hook, B., Obrik, B., and Timpl, R., 1981, Substrate adhesion of rat hepatocytes: Mechanism of attachment to collagen substrates, *Cell* **24**:463–470.

Sciubba, J. J., 1977, Regeneration of the basal lamina complex during epithelial wound healing, *J. Periodont. Res.* **12**:204–217.

Silnutzer, T., and Barnes, D. W., 1984, Human serum spreading factor: Assay, preparation and use in serum-free cell culture, *Cell Cult. Methods Mol. Cell Biol.* **1**:245–268.

Smith, L. T., Holbrook, K. A., and Madri, J. A., 1986, Collagen types I, III, and V in human embryonic and fetal skin, *Am. J. Anat.* **175**:507–521.

Stanley, J. R., Hawley-Nelson, P., Poirer, M., Katz, S. I., and Yuspa, S., 1980, Detection of pemphigoid antigen, pemphigus antigen and keratin filaments by indirect immunofluorescence in cultured human epidermal cells, *J. Invest. Dermatol.* **75**:183–186.

Stanley, J. R., Alvarez, O. M., Bere, E. W., Eaglestein, W. H., and Katz, S. I., 1981, Detection of membrane zone antigens during epidermal wound healing in pigs, *J. Invest. Dermatol.* **7**:240–243.

Stenman, S., and Vaheri, A., 1978, Distribution of a major connective tissue protein, fibronectin, in human tissues, *J. Exp. Med.* **147**:1054–1063.

Stenn, K. S., 1978, The role of serum in the epithelial outgrowth of mouse skin explants, *Br. J. Dermatol.* **98**:411–416.

Stenn, K. S., 1981, Epibolin: A protein of human plasma which supports epithelial cell movement, *Proc. Natl. Acad. Sci. USA* **78**:6907–6911.

Stenn, K. S., 1987, Coephibolin, the activity of human serum that enhances the cell-spreading properties of epibolin, associates with albumin, *J. Invest. Dermatol.* **89**:59–63.

Stenn, K. S., and Core, N. G., 1986, Cation dependence of guinea pig epidermal cell spreading, *In Vitro Cell. Dev. Biol.* **22**:217–222.

Stenn, K. S., and Dvoretzky, I., 1979, Human serum and epithelial spread in tissue culture, *Arch. Dermatol. Res.* **246**:3–15.

Stenn, K. S., and Milstone, L. M., 1984, Epidermal cell confluence and implications for a two step mechanism of wound closure, *J. Invest. Dermatol.* **83**:445–447.

Stenn, K. S., Madri, J. A., and Roll, F. J., 1979, Migrating epidermis produces AB_2 collagen and requires continual collagen synthesis for movement, *Nature (Lond.)* **277**:229–232.

Stenn, K. S., Madri, J. A., Tinghitella, T., and Teranova, V., 1983, Multiple mechanism of dissociated epidermal cell spreading, J. Cell Biol. 96:63–67.

Stenn, K. S., Core, N. G., and Halaban, R., 1987, Phorbol ester serves as a coepibolin in the spreading of primary guinea pig epidermal cells, J. Invest. Dermatol. 87:754–757.

Suzuki, S., Pierschbacher, M. D., Hayman. E. G., Nguyen, K., Ohgren, Y., and Ryoslahti, E., 1984, Domain structure of vitronectin, J. Biol. Chem. 259:15307–15314.

Takashima, A., and Grinnell, F., 1984, Human keratinocyte adhesion and phagocytosis promoted by fibronectin, J. Invest. Dermatol. 83:352–358.

Terranova, V., Rohrbach, D. H., and Martin, G. R., 1980, Role of laminin in the attachments of PAM 12 cells to basement membrane collagen, Cell 22:719–726.

Trinkaus, J. P., 1984, Cells into Organs. The Forces That Shape the Embryo, 2nd ed., Prentice-Hall, Englewood Cliffs, New Jersey.

Trinkaus-Randall, V., and Gipson, L. K., 1984, Role of calcium and calmodulin in hemidesmosome formation in vitro, J. Cell Biol. 98:1565–1571.

Vaughan, R. B., and Trinkaus, J. P., 1966, Movements of epithelial cell sheets in vitro. J. Cell. Sci. 1:407–413.

Weiss, P., 1961, The biological foundations of wound repair, Harvey Lecture 55:13–42.

Westgate, G. E., Weaver, A. C., and Couchman, J. R., 1985, Bullous pemphigoid antigen localization suggests an intracellular association with hemidesmosomes, J. Invest. Dermatol. 84:218–224.

Whatley, T. G., and Knox, P., 1980, Isolation of a serum component that stimulates the spreading of cells in culture, Biochem. J. 185:349–354.

Winter, G. D., 1964, Movement of epidermal cells over the wound surface, Adv. Biol. Skin 5:113–127.

Winter, G. D., 1972, Epidermal regeneration studied in the domestic pig, in: Epidermal Wound Healing (H. I. Maibach and D. T. Rovee, eds.), pp. 71–112, Year Book, Chicago.

Woodley, D. T., Regnier, M., and Prunieras, M., 1980a, In vitro basal lamina formations may require non-epidermal cell living substrate, Br. J. Dermatol. 103:397–404.

Woodley, D. T., Didierjean, L., Regnier, M., Saurat, J., and Prunieras, M., 1980b, Bullous pemphigoid antigen synthesized in vitro by human epidermal cells, J. Invest. Dermatol. 75:148–151.

Woodley, D. T., Liotta, L. A., and Brundage, R., 1982, Adult human epidermal cells migrating on nonviable matrix produce a Type IV collagenase, Clin. Res. 30:266 (abst.).

Woodley, D. T., O'Keefe, E. J., and Prunieras, M., 1985a, Cutaneous wound healing: A model for cell–matrix interactions, J. Am. Acad. Dermatol. 12:420–433.

Woodley, D. T., O'Keefe, E. J., Briggaman, R. A., Reese, M. J., and Gammon, W. R., 1985b, Specific binding of fibronectin to epidermolysis bullosa acquisita antigen, J. Invest. Dermatol. 84:356 (abs.).

Woodley, D. T., Briggaman, R. A., Gammon, W. R., and O'Keefe, E. J., 1985c, Epidermolysis bullosa acquisita antigen is synthesized by human keratinocytes cultured in serum-free medium, Biochem. Biophys. Res. Commun. 130:1267–1272.

Chapter 15

Angiogenesis

JOSEPH A. MADRI and BRUCE M. PRATT

1. Introduction

The response of vascularized tissue to injury depends in part upon complex and diverse microvascular endothelial cell activities. Although various aspects of the inflammatory response have been known and written about for approximately 4000 years, the central importance of the vascular endothelial cell in this phenomenon has only recently been appreciated (Folkman and Haudenschild, 1980; Folkman, 1984; Macleod, 1971; Ryan and Majino, 1977). Since Cohnheim's landmark paper (1889) describing the changes in microvasculature during the acute phases of inflammation, a large research effort has been directed at elucidating the roles of plasma, serum, and cellular and tissue factors involved in the inflammatory response (Macleod, 1971; Ryan and Majino, 1977). However, specific endothelial cell responses to acute and chronic inflammation have only recently been appreciated and are thus less well studied and documented. The great disparity in information is largely due to the absence, until relatively recently, of appropriate methodologies (e.g., electron microscopy, cell culture systems, and modern cell physiology and biochemistry) with which to study the microvascular endothelial cell and its complex metabolism (Madri and Williams, 1983; Folkman and Haudenschild, 1980; Kramer et al., 1984).

This chapter does not attempt an exhaustive review of the endothelial cell literature, but instead refers the reader to several extensive general reviews of endothelial cell biology (Folkman and Cotran, 1976; Folkman and Haudenschild, 1980; Fishman, 1982; Robbins et al., 1984). Here we consider selected aspects of the neovascular response of microvascular endothelial cells to soft tissue injury, sufficient to elicit granulation tissue. We have divided our discussion into six main sections: (1) stimulation, (2) migration, (3) proliferation, (4) tube formation, (5) stabilization/differentiation, and (6) regression/downregulation. Within each section, the roles, responses, and behavior of the microvascular endothelial cell are reviewed and discussed. In addition, the importance of cell–matrix interactions in the neovascularization response and

JOSEPH A. MADRI and BRUCE M. PRATT • Department of Pathology, Yale University School of Medicine, New Haven, Connecticut 06510.

the concepts of matrix composition, organization, and dimensionality as modulators of endothelial cell behavior are emphasized.

2. Stimulation

Normally, microvascular endothelial cells have complex cell–cell junctions and are surrounded by a basement membrane (Rhodin, 1974). Following soft tissue injury, a variety of cellular and tissue factors are released from the damaged tissue. Two of these compounds, histamine and serotonin, are potent vasoactive agents that bind to specific membrane-bound receptor molecules on the luminal surface of postcapillary venule endothelial cells (N. Simionescu et al., 1982; M. Simionescu et al., 1982). When bound to the cell surface, these vasoactive compounds cause both the separation of the cell–cell junctions and retraction of the endothelial cells, permitting increased flow of fluids and cells from the vessel lumen into the surrounding interstitium. Vasoactive mediator effects on the microvasculature is discussed at length in Chapter 5.

Stimulated microvascular endothelial cells also appear to permit leukocyte sticking and diapedesis (Robbins et al., 1984; Macleod, 1971; Ryan and Majino, 1977). This is a poorly understood phenomenon; however, several investigators have proposed that leukocyte–endothelial cell adhesion is partially caused by injury-mediated changes in the luminal surface of the endothelial cell, that is, the upregulation of leukocyte-specific receptors (Pober and Gimbrone, 1982; Montesano et al., 1984; Pober et al., 1983). The concept of specialized endothelial cell-surface molecules that recognize leukocyte cell surface moieties is supported by several groups who have adduced evidence consistent with the existence of such proteins in the high endothelium of lymph node postcapillary venules for lymphocytes and in cultured endothelial cells for monocytes and neutrophils (McConnell, 1983; Gallatin et al., 1983; Stamper and Woodruff, 1976; Kuttner and Woodruff, 1979; Bevilacqua et al., 1985; DiCorleto and de la Motte, 1985; Chin et al., 1985). Neutrophil–endothelial cell interactions are discussed in more detail in Chapter 5.

In order for neovascularization to occur, the endothelial cells must be freed from the constraints of their investing basement membranes. Since activated, migrating leukocytes are known to produce and secrete collagenases capable of degrading the vascular basement membrane, and it is possible that collagenase and other enzymes released during leukocyte emigration could free the endothelial cells from their basement membranes (Mainardi et al., 1980; Horowitz et al., 1977; Russo et al., 1981; Sholley et al., 1978). However, extensive fragmentation of the microvascular basement membrane is not observed during leukocyte emigration. Alternatively, the microvascular basement membrane may be breached by inducible secreted endothelial cell enzymes. Several investigators have shown that when induced to migrate, cultured endothelial cells produce several enzymes, specifically plasminogen activator, plasmin, and collagenases, all of which are capable of digesting basal lamina components (Gross et al., 1983; Gross et al., 1982; Kalebic et al., 1983). The existence of these inducible endothelial cell proteases provides an attractive explanation for the loss of investing basement membrane that precedes endothelial cell migration and proliferation during neovascularization.

In addition to stimulation by factors present in the inflammatory exudate, including matrix-degradation products and autocrine stimulation by endothelial cell-derived factors, the microvascular endothelial cells may also be stimulated by the drastic changes in the surrounding matrix, from basement membrane to interstitial connective tissue. As demonstrated in a number of *in vitro* experimental systems, and as discussed in Section 5, intact basement membranes and purified basement membrane components, such as type IV collagen, appear to promote the development and maintenance of a mitotically inactive, nonmigratory, highly differentiated phenotype. Alternatively, intact interstitial connective tissue and purified interstitial components, types I and III collagen, promote elevated rates of mitosis and cell migration (Madri and Williams, 1983; Folkman and Haudenschild, 1980; Schor *et al.*, 1979; Madri and Pratt, 1986). Thus, the endothelial cell stimulation that occurs during the early phases of inflammation and neovascularization is complex, in part derived from resident mast cells and macrophages, recently emigrated leukocytes, endothelial cells themselves, and the matrix components in the immediate extracellular environment.

3. Migration

A prominent aspect of the formation of granulation tissue is the migration of microvascular endothelial cells into the injured area (Bryant, 1977; Robbins *et al.*, 1984; Macleod, 1971; Ryan and Majno, 1977). One or more environmental factors may be responsible for this migration, such as (1) chemotactic factors secreted by leukocytes; (2) degradation products of various matrix components; (3) release from investing basement membrane constraints; (4) change in matrix composition from a basement membrane to interstitial connective tissue; and (5) change from a polarized two-dimensional to a relatively nonpolarized three-dimensional extracellular environment. In this section, we discuss these potential stimuli in detail.

Microvascular endothelial cells are metabolically active, mitotically quiescent cells invested by a morphologically identifiable basement membrane, which provides the overlying endothelial cells with an organized substratum for attachment and expression of a differentiated phenotype (Denekamp and Hobson, 1984; Folkman and Cotran, 1976) and which does not permit any appreciable migration.

Acute inflammatory cells (leukocytes) are a major cell type observed in the inflammatory response and are noted to precede vascular ingrowth into injured areas. It is widely accepted that leukocytes contain chemotactic factors and release them when stimulated during inflammation (Ryan and Majno, 1977). Such factors could act on surrounding microvascular endothelial cells, eliciting a migratory response. However, leukocytic infiltration and release of chem-

otactic factors are unnecessary for the initiation of angiogenesis and endothelial migration, as significant neovascularization does occur in the face of
leukocyte depletion (Sholley et al., 1978). This finding is consistent with the
concept that during angiogenesis many factors are available that can act as
stimulators of the migratory response.

During an angiogenic response in inflammation, there is significant connective tissue destruction. Matrix component fragments generated by such a
process are known to have chemotactic activity for a number of mesenchymal
cells (Chiang et al., 1978; Postlethwaite and Kang, 1976; Postlethwaite et al.,
1978; McCarthy and Furcht, 1984), and microvascular endothelial cells should
prove to be no exception. Several studies have demonstrated that matrix components dramatically effect endothelial cell attachment and migration (Folkman and Haudenschild, 1980; Madri and Stenn, 1982). Thus, matrix components and breakdown fragments appear to provide stimuli for endothelial cell
migration during the angiogenic response.

Since physical constraints imposed on cells by surrounding supporting
structures (matrices) have been shown to be powerful modulators of cell function, release from this organization/orientation by partial destruction of the
basement membrane may be sufficient to stimulate and initiate endothelial cell
migration (Ingber and Jamieson, 1985). In the resting state, microvascular endothelial cells exist in a polarized environment, having a luminal surface in
contact with a fluid phase and an abluminal surface in intimate contact with
the basement membrane. Preliminary evidence has been adduced supporting
the presence of cell–surface matrix binding proteins (specifically for type IV
collagen and laminin) on large and microvascular endothelial cells (Yannariello-Brown et al., 1985a,b; Madri et al., 1987). Thus, it is possible that the
asymmetric, polarized cell contact with the basement membrane may be reflected in a polarized distribution of cell-surface matrix-binding proteins. Such
an asymmetric localization of cell-surface matrix-binding proteins may have
significant effects on the organization of the cell cytoskeleton, which in turn
may permit the expression of a particular cell phenotype (nonmigrating,
mitotically quiescent, metabolically active, and differentiated). By contrast, in
response to an angiogenic stimulus, microvascular endothelial cells undergo a
transition to a comparatively less polar environment of interstitial connective
tissue in which all surfaces of the cell are surrounded by similar extracellular
components. This change of microenvironment, and the probable subsequent
changes in type and distribution of cell-surface matrix-binding proteins and
cytoskeleton may permit the expression of an alternative phenotype, namely, a
migrating, mitotically active cell type (Martin et al., 1984; Terranova et al.,
1984; Madri et al., 1987). This concept of extracellular matrix-mediated
changes in cellular phenotype is supported by in vitro studies of vascular
endothelial and glandular epithelial cells, in which investigators have noted
dramatic changes in cell morphology, cell function, and multicellular organization when the cells were placed in or migrated into a three-dimensional environment (Fig. 1) (Madri and Williams, 1983; Madri and Pratt, 1986; Hall et
al., 1982; Bissell et al., 1982; Lwebuga-Mukasa et al., 1984; Ingber et al., 1986a).

Just as organization of cell substratum (basement membrane versus in-

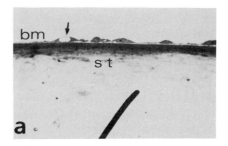

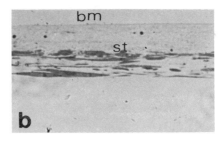

Figure 1. Comparison of microvascular endothelial cells isolated from rat epididymal fat pads plated and grown on (a) the basement membrane vs. (b) the stromal aspect of the human amnion for one week. The cells plated on the basement membrane surface (bm) are apparently constrained by the basal lamina and are observed to form tubelike structures with lumina (arrow). In contrast, cells plated on the stromal surface (st) are observed to migrate into the interstitial connective tissue as single cells. (×100)

terstitial connective tissue) appears to be an important determinant of cell function, so too is composition of the surrounding extracellular matrix. Following release from the constraints of their investing basement membranes (containing predominantly type IV collagen and laminin), microvascular endothelial cells come into contact with the interstitial matrix components, consisting mainly of types I and III collagen (Stenn *et al.*, 1979). The change in matrix composition has been implicated in influencing subsequent cell behavior. Specifically, microvascular endothelial cells cultured *in vitro* form confluent monolayers when plated on native or denatured interstitial collagens (types I or III collagen), while the same cells form multicellular tubelike structures when plated on selected basement membrane components (type IV collagen or laminin) (Madri and Williams, 1983; Madri and Pratt, 1986). This apparent relationship between matrix composition and cell behavior has also been documented in other vascular endothelial cells. Specifically, bovine aortic endothelial cells (BAEC) cultured on purified interstitial collagens have (1) the archetypal *in vitro* "cobblestone" morphology, (2) a relatively high mitotic index (34%) in subconfluent cultures, and (3) a high rate of sheet migration in confluent cultures. By contrast, BAEC cultured on purified fibronectin (1) shows a highly spread and flattened morphology, (2) have a relatively low mitotic index (23%) in subconfluent cultures, and (3) have a low rate of sheet migration in confluent cultures (Pratt *et al.*, 1984; Madri and Pratt, 1986; Leto *et al.*, 1986; Form *et al.*, 1986).

In addition to the change in matrix composition experienced by the migrating microvascular endothelial cells during the early stages of neovascularization, local changes in matrix composition may be caused by endogenous endothelial cell-matrix biosynthesis during this period. Studies have shown that cultured microvascular endothelial cells modulate their collagen biosynthesis profiles according to the substratum on which they are grown (Madri and Williams, 1983; Madri and Pratt, 1985). Specifically, in comparison with microvascular endothelial cells grown on tissue-culture plastic, cells cultured on any collagenous substrate show increased levels of type IV and V collagen synthesis. Furthermore, cells cultured on interstitial collagen substrates synthesize types IV and V collagen in a 1 : 2 ratio, while cells cultured on basement membrane collagen substrates alter their type IV–type V ratio to 1 : 1. Thus, it is quite possible that as microvascular endothelial cells migrate through an interstitial matrix, they continually alter their matrix biosynthesis, which in turn further modulates their behavior during this period (a phenomenon labeled dynamic reciprocity by Bornstein) (Bissell *et al.*, 1982; Bornstein *et al.*, 1982). Indeed, previous experiments with large-vessel and microvascular endothelial cells and epithelial cells demonstrate a definite staggered appearance of *de novo* synthesized matrix components during migration. At the leading edge of migration, type V collagen and laminin and, in the case of epithelium, bullous pemphigoid antigen are the first matrix molecules to appear in close apposition to the migrating cells. Later, at some distance from the migrating edge, laminin and then type IV collagen are deposited beneath the cells and become part of the structurally identifiable basement membrane (Madri and Stenn, 1982; Stenn *et al.*, 1979; Stanley *et al.*, 1981; Hintner *et al.*, 1980; Form *et al.*, 1986).

4. Proliferation

During the early phases of angiogenesis, closely following the migratory phenomenon, there is a dramatic proliferative response in the neovascular endothelial cells. Evidence suggests that the leading migratory cells are not proliferating; rather, the cells immediately behind them make up the actively proliferating cell region (Ausprunk and Folkman, 1977; Burger and Klintworth, 1981). Similar to the migratory stimuli discussed above, proliferative stimuli are diverse and complex, including (1) proteases acting on cell surfaces, (2) mitogenic factors secreted by leukocytes (see Chapters 9–12 and 3) and degradation products of matrix components, (4) release from the constraints of the basement membrane, (5) changes in matrix composition, (6) changes from a two-dimensional to a three-dimensional cell environment, and (7) migration. The following section discusses selected aspects of these phenomena in detail.

Following injury, there is release and activation of a number of proteases (Ryan and Majno, 1977). One enzyme known to interact with endothelial cells is thrombin, which enhances the mitogenic potential of fibroblast growth factor (Isaacs *et al.*, 1981). A possible effect of thrombin is the stimulation of endothelial cell proliferation and tube formation noted when rat aortic rings are placed in fibrin-clot cultures (Nicosia *et al.*, 1982). Thus, following injury in which there is activation of the clotting cascade, active thrombin may play a role in triggering endothelial cell proliferation by direct interaction with the endothelial cell surface as well as catalyzing the formation of a fibrin network that may provide a framework for the neovasculature to grow into (Nicosia and Madri, 1987).

In addition to the various proteases that may stimulate endothelial cells to proliferate, several other mechanisms exist for stimulating endothelial cell proliferation during angiogenesis. During the past several years, a multitude of endothelial cell growth factors have been identified and characterized (Lobb *et al.*, 1986). From these studies, it has become clear that although a diverse number of molecules exhibit this acLivity, they seem to share some common features, one of which is an affinity for heparin and an increase in activity when given in conjunction with heparin. The role of heparin in modulating the activity of endothelial cell growth factors is further complicated by the finding that it also enhances the suppressive effects that certain steroids have on angiogenesis (Crum *et al.*, 1986). Much more work is necessary before a clear understanding of the roles of growth factors in angiogenesis is attained.

Previous studies in several *in vitro* and *in vivo* models have demonstrated the interrelationships between cell migration and proliferation (Sholley *et al.*, 1977). During angiogenesis, migration always precedes proliferation by approximately 24 hr (Ausprunk and Folkman, 1977; Burger and Klintworth, 1981; Sholley *et al.*, 1984). Thus, the loss of cell–cell and cell–substratum contact and subsequent migration (triggered, in part, by loss of basement membrane structural, organizational, and compositional integrity) may act as stimuli of the endothelial cell proliferation. The stimulus may be the result of complex changes in the way the cells interact with the matrix. Since it is generally accepted that matrices contain information (resident in their organization and/or composition), it is reasonable to assume that microvascular endothelial cells perceive this information via cell-surface matrix-binding proteins (receptors) (Madri, 1982; Lesot *et al.*, 1983; Madri and Williams, 1983; Malinoff and Wicha, 1983; Rao *et al.*, 1983; Terranova *et al.*, 1983; Madri *et al.*, 1984, 1987; Brown *et al.*, 1983; Yannariello-Brown *et al.*, 1983, 1985a,b). Information may then be transduced via cellular cortical membrane proteins, such as spectrin and protein 4.1, and the filamentous cytoskeletal network to the nucleus, eliciting changes in cell behavior including proliferative rate (Folkman and Moscona, 1978; Pratt *et al.*, 1984; Leto *et al.*, 1986; Madri *et al.*, 1987). Cell shape may be an observable end result of complex, incompletely understood, matrix-driven, cytoskeletal reorganizations that modulate many aspects of cell behavior. Data accrued from several studies support this concept. For example, Folkman *et al.* (1979) and Schor *et al.* (1979) found that a gelatin substratum was necessary for the continual culture of capillary endothelial cells, consistent with a permissive effect on matrix growth suggested by Gospodarowicz *et al.* (1980, 1983). In later studies, microvascular endothelial cells cultured on different matrix components were observed to exhibit different rates of proliferation, which roughly correlated with differences noted in cytoskeletal organizations, interaction with matrix, and cell shape (Madri and Williams, 1983; Kramer *et al.*, 1984; Nicosia *et al.*, 1982) (Fig. 2). Thus, once released from the constraints of the investing basement membrane, endothelial cells experience a microenvironment that allows for (or causes) an increased proliferation rate.

Microvascular endothelial cells respond to their microenvironment by altering their matrix biosynthetic profiles and then may respond to the changed matrix in a variety of ways (Madri and Williams, 1983; Kramer *et al.*, 1984).

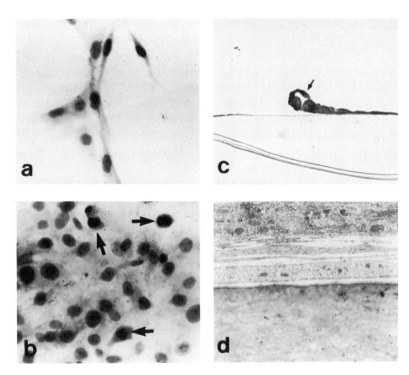

Figure 2. Comparison of the morphology, proliferation rate, and multicellular organization of microvascular endothelial cells cultured on coatings of purified basement membrane collagens types IV and V (a, c) vs. purified interstitial collagens types I and II (b, d). (From Madri and Williams, 1983, with permission. Representative micrographs of (a) cells grown on types IV and V collagens illustrating string- or tubelike structures having no mitotic figures vs. (b) cells grown on types I and III collagens revealing many more cells with several mitotic figures per high power field (arrows). (×400) Representative micrographs of cross-sections of (c) microvascular endothelial cells grown on types IV and V collagens for 96 hr illustrating a tubelike structure with a lumen (arrow). (×1,100) In contrast, cells grown on types I and III collagens for 96 hr. (d) appear as a multilayer of flattened, spread cells. (×8,000)

Preliminary experiments have shown that during angiogenesis endothelial cells may exhibit a temporal and staggered synthesis of matrix components, as has been shown for migrating aortic endothelial cells and epithelial cells (Madri and Stenn, 1982; Stenn *et al.*, 1979). In these studies, it was found that cultured migrating aortic endothelial cells synthesize and secrete laminin early during the migratory response, while the appearance of type IV collagen is detected later. In addition, during angiogenesis the selective appearance of particular matrix components appears to have a regulatory effect on proliferation rate *in vitro* (Form and Madri, 1985; Form *et al.*, 1986). Specifically, cultured microvascular endothelial cells grown on a laminin substratum (a matrix component noted early in the response to injury) exhibit a high proliferation rate, while cells grown on type IV collagen (a component observed later in the response) exhibit a much lower rate. Furthermore, mixing type IV collagen with laminin elicited a lower proliferation rate, further suggesting specific matrix modulation of proliferation (Form et al., 1986).

Another process that should be considered as a potential modulator of proliferation during angiogenesis is the change in dimensionality experienced by the endothelial cells. Namely, the change from a two-dimensional environment (luminal and abluminal) to a three-dimensional one in which the cells are completely surrounded by matrix (with resultant changes in types of and organization of cell surface matrix-binding molecules and cytoskeleton) may profoundly affect cell proliferation. While invested by a basement membrane, microvascular endothelial cells are known to exhibit a very low mitotic index, in contrast to cells in the interstitium near the migrating tip in an angiogenic response (Burger and Klintworth, 1981). As the angiogenic response progresses, tube formation occurs concurrently with the appearance of morphologically identifiable basal lamina-like material. Mitotic index is noted to drop in these areas, suggesting that changing from a three-dimensional to a polarized two-dimensional environment influences proliferation rate.

5. Tube Formation and Stabilization

In the later stages of angiogenesis, tube formation is observed in areas proximal to the migrating and proliferating cells. Our understanding of this complex phenomenon and of the factors that influence it is incomplete. A multitude of studies have demonstrated the importance of various cell and tissue factors, matrix composition, organization and dimensionality, and cell–cell interactions in the process of tube formation (Madri and Williams, 1983; Madri and Pratt, 1986; Folkman and Haudenschild, 1980; Wagner, 1980; Bryant, 1977; Montesano et al., 1983; Folkman, 1982). In this section, we discuss the importance of cell–matrix and cell–cell interactions in the development and maintenance of tubes in the process of angiogenesis.

During the angiogenic process following migration and proliferation, the microvascular endothelial cells form highly organized three-dimensional structures with lumina. Lumen formation is thought to occur via intercellular and intracellular mechanisms (Wagner, 1980). One theory for lumen formation involves the development of spaces between the plasma membranes of adjacent cells or the joining of plasma membrane processes of individual cells and/or adjacent cells. For instance, Montesano et al. (1983) demonstrated in vitro lumen formation by two and more contiguous endothelial cells in collagen gels, and we and others have demonstrated the presence of tubelike structures composed of endothelial cell plasma membrane processes joined by organized junctional complexes (Madri and Williams, 1983; Pratt et al., 1985; Williams et al., 1980; Maciag et al., 1982) (Fig. 3). By contrast, a second mechanism of lumen formation involves extensive intracellular vacuolization followed by intracellular vacuolar fusion, and ultimately cell–cell plasma membrane fusion, forming seamless endothelia. In vivo and in vitro data from several labora-

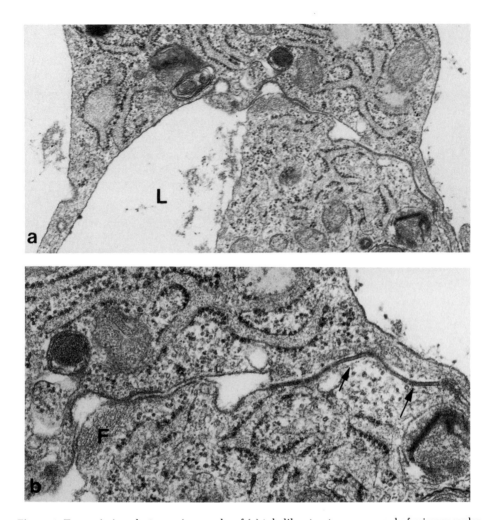

Figure 3. Transmission electron micrographs of (a) tubelike structure composed of microvascular endothelial cells cultured on a coating of types IV/V collagen illustrating a lumen (L) containing amorphous, electron-dense material; (b) cell processes that are joined by highly-organized junctional complexes suggestive of gap junctions (arrows); and organized cytoplasmic filamentous (F) arrays adjacent to these junctional complexes. (a) ×9,700; (b) ×19,500. (From Madri and Williams, 1983.)

tories support this hypothesis as well, namely, the finding of ring cells, which have no apparent junctions and form a continuous cytoplasmic ring, in cultures of microvascular endothelial cells (Folkman and Haudenschild, 1980) (Fig. 4). Extensively vacuolated cells in culture have amorphous material in the lumina and typical lumina plasmalemmal membrane microdomain specializations including plasmalemmal vesicles with and without diaphragms, coated pits, and fenestralike structures, consistent with the second mechanism of tube forma-

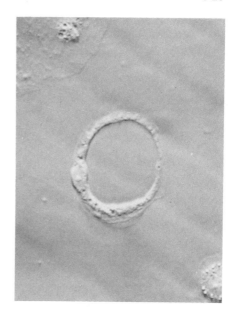

Figure 4. Hoffmann interference photomicrograph of typical "ring" form of a microvascular endothelial cell isolated from rat epididymal fat pad and plated on a coating of types I and III collagen. Note the "signet ring" morphology with an apparently continuous cytoplasmic ring surrounding a central lumen. (×200)

tion (Folkman and Haudenschild, 1980; Madri and Williams, 1983). The two mechanisms need not be mutually exclusive as investigators have found evidence suggestive of both in several *in vitro* culture systems.

The signals or stimuli for tube formation are also poorly understood. Various conditioned media and endothelial cell growth factor preparations appear to be necessary for the expression of tubes *in vitro*, consistent with the notion that a variety of cell- and tissue-derived factors may be involved in the *in vivo* process (Madri and Williams, 1983; Folkman and Haudenschild, 1980; Maciag *et al.*, 1982; Zetter, 1980; Folkman *et al.*, 1979; Fenselau *et al.*, 1981; Alessandri *et al.*, 1983). Another factor that appears to play an important role in tube formation is the surrounding substratum. Matrix composition, organization, and integrity have been implicated as controlling factors in various stages of the angiogenesis process (Madri and Williams, 1983; Folkman and Haudenschild, 1980; Schor *et al.*, 1979; Montesano *et al.*, 1983; Madri and Pratt, 1986). Specifically, Folkman and Haudenschild (1980) noted that a gelatin coating was necessary for tube formation by cultured capillary endothelial cells. Madri and Williams (1983) noted more specific matrix effects using individual matrix components as coatings. In this study, capillary endothelial cells formed tubes rapidly when plated on the basement membrane components types IV and V collagen, as compared with the interstitial collagen types I and III (Fig. 5). In other experiments, the basement membrane aspect of the amnion supported rapid tube formation relative to its stromal aspect (Fig. 6) (Madri and Williams, 1983; Madri and Pratt, 1986). Studies also demonstrated the appearance of amorphous electron-dense basal lamina-like material surrounding the abluminal surfaces of the endothelial cells following tube formation (Montesano *et al.*, 1983). These data are consistent with the concept that specific matrix

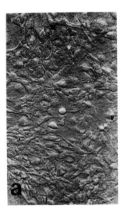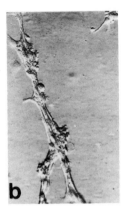

Figure 5. Hoffman Interference photomicrographs of microvascular endothelial cells cultured on (a) coatings of types I and III collagen vs. (b) IV and V for 96 hr. (a) Cells cultured on the interstitial collagens form a continuous multilayer while (b) cells cultured on the basement membrane collagens have organized into tubelike structures having lumina and highly-organized junctional complexes. (×100) (From Madri and Williams, 1983.)

components have significant influences in directing endothelial cell behavior during angiogenesis.

Although evidence suggests that the appearance, accumulation, and organization of basement membrane components promotes rapid tube formation, the role of the surrounding interstitial tissue should not be minimized. Possible roles for the surrounding interstitial tissue may include (1) trapping and stabilizing secreted basal lamina components in areas immediately adjacent to the endothelial cells, providing the desired cell–matrix interactions for tube formation; and (2) eliciting a change in endothelial cell connective tissue biosynthesis, causing an increase in basement membrane component synthesis. The finding that cultured microvascular endothelial cells change their collagen synthetic profiles in response to changes in underlying substratum supports the second role (Madri and Williams, 1983; Madri and Pratt, 1986). Furthermore, capillary endothelial cells cultured on interstitial or basement membrane components synthesize less interstitial and more basement membrane collagenous components than the same cells grown on a plastic substratum.

Once formed, the new capillary structures must be stabilized and maintained if they are to become functional. One way these delicate new vessels may be stabilized is by envelopment in a continuous basal lamina synthesized by the capillary endothelial cells themselves. The highly organized basal lamina structure provides a stable attachment surface for the two-dimensional polarized configuration. The basal lamina may also provide the capillary with a reasonable degree of strength against the forces of distention that may otherwise destroy the cell–cell junctional complexes that exist in the capillary bed. A second way in which the matrix may maintain the newly formed capillary network may be through the information resident in its organization/composition. By specifically ordering or structuring the biosynthetic machinery of the endothelial cells via cytoskeletal organization, the matrix may direct luminal and abluminal secretion of specific functional and structural cell products that allow for the maintenance and proper physiologic function of the capillary network (Bissell *et al.*, 1982). Support for this concept stems from observations in several *in vitro* model systems, including (1) cultured MDCK cells form tubelike structures with apical microvilli and cultured mammary gland epithelial cells form acinar-like structures and secrete *de novo* synthesized milk-specific proteins into luminal spaces when cultured in collagen gels (Sholley *et al.*, 1977; Lesot *et al.*, 1983; Lee *et al.*, 1984); (2) type II pneumocytes cultured on amnion basement membrane maintain their polarized cuboidal morphology and apical microvilli and secrete lamellar bodies into the medium—the same cells cultured on the interstitial surface of the amnion take on a flattened morphology and become devoid of microvilli and lamellar bodies (Lweubuga-Mukasa *et al.*, 1984); and (3) rat pancreatic adenocarcinoma cells cultured on amnion basement membrane exhibit polarized distribution of zymogen granules, Golgi complexes, and nuclei and lipid droplets (from apex to base). When these cells are cultured on the interstitial aspect of the amnion, the cells attach poorly and remain rounded and unpolarized (Ingber *et al.*, 1986a).

Although the ability to form tubes appears to be resident in the endothelial cell, the microvascular vessel has other cell types closely associated with it, namely, the pericyte (Joyce *et al.*, 1985a,b). It is therefore reasonable to assume that this cell type may have a role in the maturation, stability, and functioning of the newly formed capillaries. The roles of the pericyte are only incompletely known: (1) it is considered to function as a contractile cell that may regulate the tone of the microvasculature; and (2) since it is in intimate contact with the vascular basement membrane, it may contribute to the synthesis and maintenance of this structure. Further *in vivo* and *in vitro* experimentation is necessary before the roles of this cell type in the angiogenic response can be further elucidated.

6. Capillary Regression

Following capillary ingrowth and the resultant increase in blood flow to the injured area, the repair process continues with the reconstitution of parenchyma or replacement with new connective tissue (Bryant, 1977; Robbins *et al.*, 1984). Once this is completed, there is no longer a need for a rich continuous vascular supply and the recently formed capillary network regresses. The regression of the vascular network includes the selective loss of endothelial cells and possibly pericytes as well as the dissolution of their basement membranes. Folkman and co-workers have studied the regression phase of the angiogenic process using a corneal pocket assay (Folkman, 1982; Ausprunk *et al.*, 1978). When angiogenic stimuli were withdrawn, endothelial cells of the newly forming capillary network showed several changes, namely, endothelial cells at the migrating tip underwent mitochondrial swelling. Platelets adhered to the endothelial cell surfaces and vascular stasis ensued, followed by endothelial cell death and digestion of cell debris by local macrophages. Thus, it appears that the loss of a specific angiogenic signal may be sufficient to trigger regression, suggesting that continuous positive stimuli are required for sustained angiogenesis. This does not necessarily exclude a requirement for negative or suppressive stimuli such as those observed in inhibition of tumor-

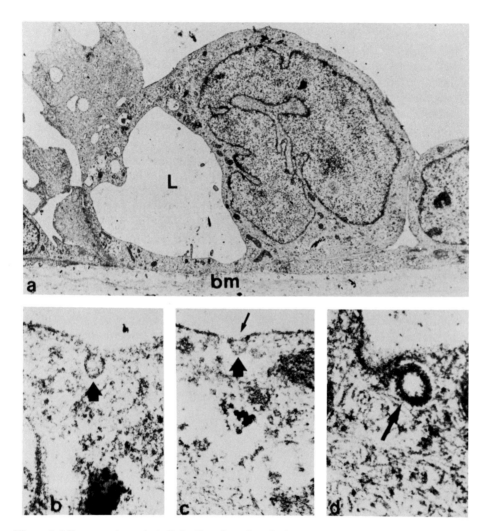

Figure 6. Microvascular endothelial cells cultured on the basement membrane aspect of the human amnion. Cells adhere to the basal lamina and form tubelike structures with lumina (L) early in the culture period (5 days). (a) Low power electron micrograph of a cell forming a tubelike structure having a lumen (L), and adherent to the underlying basal lamina (bm). (×3,100) (b to f) Higher power electron micrographs revealing details of luminal and abluminal structures including: (b) luminal plasmalemmal vesicles (arrow); (c) luminal plasmalemmal vesicles (large arrow) with stomatal diaphragms (small arrow); (d) luminal coated pits and vesicles (arrow); (e) multiple abluminal focal adhesion attachment sites (small arrows) in close contact (10–20 nm) with the underlying basal lamina and organized filamentous arrays (large arrow) running in a plane parallel to the plasma membrane; and (f) occasional intermittent contacts with the basal lamina (arrowhead and small arrow) and associated organized filamentous arrays. (×24,000) (From Madri and Williams, 1983.)

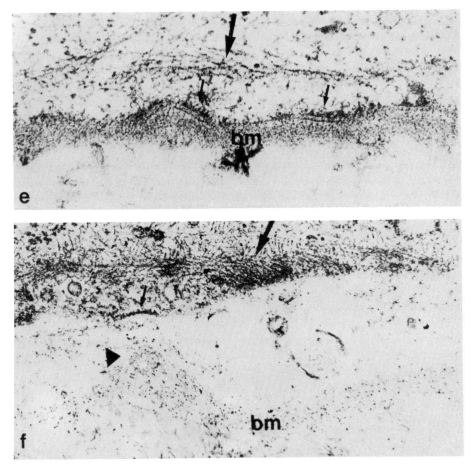

Figure 6. (*Continued*)

induced angiogenesis by heparin, particular steroids, and selected tissue factors, and the downregulation of smooth muscle proliferation by endothelial cell products (Azmi and O'Shea, 1984; Folkman *et al.*, 1983; Langer *et al.*, 1980; Castellot *et al.*, 1981, 1982, 1984; Karnovsky, 1981; Crum *et al.*, 1986; Ingber *et al.*, 1986b).

The signals for initiation of capillary regression phase in the wound-repair process are likewise ill understood at this time. Potential signals could include (1) containment of the injury and subsequent downregulation of the acute inflammatory response, leading to a marked decrease in the production of various inflammatory cell and tissue derived stimulatory factors; (2) changes in the tone of the affected vasculature, resulting in stasis and thrombosis, followed by endothelial cell death and dissolution of the capillary network structure; (3) specific immune cell-mediated modulation of the neovascular endothelial cells and pericytes, leading to downregulation and death of the vascular cells and dissolution of their connective tissue scaffolding; and (4) epithelial and/or mesenchymal cell factors or products that downregulate neovascular cells, such as transforming growth factor-β (TGF-β) (Ignotz and Massague, 1986; Frater-Schroder et al., 1986).

7. Conclusions and Speculations

Angiogenesis (neovascularization) is an important component of several processes, including wound healing, recanalization of thrombi, tumor growth and metastasis, and normal growth and development. After wounding, the formation of a rich vascular bed is essential for optimal reconstitution of parenchyma and repair. It is also apparent that this process is dynamic—usually transient in nature during the repair process. The up- and downregulation of the microvascular endothelial cell during the process of wound repair has been the subject of intensive study over the past several years. In addition, the observations that the metastatic spread of a variety of neoplasms is dependent on angiogenesis have stimulated work in the area of tumor-induced angiogenesis and its control (Langer et al., 1980; Crum et al., 1986; Ingber et al., 1986b). While much has been learned, there still remains a number of unanswered questions.

In particular, the areas of matrix organization and extracellular matrix and of cell membrane–cytoskeleton interactions as they pertain to the endothelial cell repair response are under intense investigation (Madri et al., 1984; Pratt et al., 1984; Leto et al., 1985; Yurchenco and Furthmayr, 1984; Wong et al., 1983). During the past several years, many investigators have shown that matrix composition and organization profoundly influences cell behavior (Hay, 1981; Madri and Williams, 1983; Madri, 1982; Bissell et al., 1982). The mechanisms by which information residing in the matrix is transduced to the cell have been speculated on, and evidence supports the existence of cell-surface matrix-binding proteins in many cell types (Lesot et al., 1983; Rao et al., 1983; Malinoff and Wicha, 1983; Terranova et al., 1983, 1984; Brown et al., 1983. Furthermore, investigators have speculated on the existence of a cell-surface matrix receptor–integral membrane protein–cortical protein–cytoskeleton–nuclear transduction network capable of signal transduction to cytoplasmic compartments and nucleus (Bissell et al., 1982; Hay, 1981). Preliminary data support the existence of such receptors and a transducing network responsive to changes in matrix in endothelial cells (Pratt et al., 1984; Madri and Pratt, 1986; Madri et al., 1987). A more complete understanding of the organization of extracellular matrices and of how microvascular endothelial cells and pericytes perceive and interact with the extracellular matrix will undoubtedly afford a better appreciation of angiogenesis and insight into how to favorably manipulate this process to effect optimal repair (Fig. 7).

Another area of importance is that of neovascular downregulation and capillary regression. As more is learned regarding this aspect of the repair

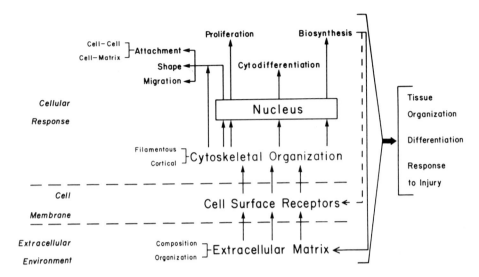

Figure 7. General schematic representation for cell–matrix interactions illustrating how information resident in the composition and/or organization of the extracellular matrix (ECM) may be transduced to the interior of the cell. In this scheme, cell surface matrix receptors are organized by the ECM, and they themselves or in concert with as yet undefined membrane proteins organize the cortical filamentous cytoskeleton of the cell. Organization of cortical membrane proteins such as spectrin, ankyrin, vinculin, and band 4.1 leads to unique interactions, assemblies, and organizations of the filamentous cytoskeleton, i.e., microfilaments, intermediate filaments, and microtubules. This, in turn, permits/directs a coordinated cell response which may include: (1) cytoskeletal rearrangements which directly cause changes in cell attachment, shape, and migration, and (2) cytoskeletal-mediated transduction of information to the nucleus resulting in cell proliferation, cytodifferentiation, and the biosynthesis and expression of new matrix receptors and ECM components. The ability of the cell to continually respond to and modify the ECM allows for a flexible, dynamic cellular response resulting in complex tissue organization, differentiation, and appropriate response to injury.

process, strategies may be devised that will permit us to reduce the incidence and amount of scarring following some injuries.

References

Alessandri, G., Raju, K., and Gullino, P. M., 1983, Mobilization of capillary endothelium *in vitro* induced by effectors of angiogenesis *in vivo, Cancer Res.* **43**:1790–1797.

Ausprunk, D. H., and Folkman, J., 1977, Migration and proliferation of endothelial cells in preformed and newly formed blood vessels during tumor angiogenesis, *Microvasc. Res.* **14**:53–65.

Ausprunk, D. H., Falterman, K., and Folkman, J., 1978, The sequence of events in the regression of corneal capillaries, *Lab. Invest.* **38**:284–294.

Azmi. T. I., and O'Shea, J. D., 1984, Mechanism of deletion of endothelial cells during regression of the corpus luteum, *Lab. Invest.* **51**:206–217.

Bevilacqua, M. P., Pober, J. S., Wheeler, M. E., Mendrick, D., Cotran, R. S., and Gimbrone, M. A., 1985, Interleukin 1 (IL-1) acts on vascular endothelial cells to increase their adhesivity for leukocytes, *Fed. Proc.* **44**:1494.

Bissell, M. L., Hall, H. G., and Parry, G., 1982, How does the extracellular matrix direct gene expression? *J. Theoret. Biol.* **99**:31–68.

Bornstein, P., McPherson, J., and Sage, H., 1982, Synthesis and secretion of thrombospondin and fibronectin by cultured human endothelial cells, in: *Pathobiology of the Endothelial Cell*, P and S Biomedical Sciences Symposia Series, Vol. 6 (H. Nossel and H. Vogel, eds.), pp. 215–228, Academic, New York.

Brown, S. S., Malinoff, H. L., and Wicha, M. S., 1983, Connectin: Cell surface protein that binds both laminin and actin, *Proc. Natl. Acad. Sci. USA* **80**:5927–5930.

Bryant, W. M., 1977, Mound healing, in: *Clinical Symposia*, Vol. 29 (B. Bekiesz, ed.), pp. 1–36, CIBA Pharmaceuticals Co., Summit, New Jersey.

Burger, P. C., and Klintworth, G. K., 1981, Autoradiographic study of corneal neovascularization induced by chemical cautery, *Lab. Invest.* **45**:328–335.

Castellot, J. J., Addonnizio, M. L., Rosenberg, R., and Karnovsky, M. J., 1981, Cultured endothelial cells produce a heparin-like inhibitor of smooth muscle growth, *J. Cell Biol.* **90**:372–279.

Castellot, J. J., Favreau, L. V., Karnovsky, M. J., and Rosenberg, R. D., 1982, Inhibition of vascular smooth muscle cell growth by endothelial cell-derived heparin. Possible role of a platelet endoglycosidase, *J. Biol. Chem.* **257**:1256–1260.

Castellot, J. J., Beeler, D. L., Rosenberg, R. D., and Karnovsky, M. J., 1984, Structural determinants of the capacity of heparin to inhibit the proliferation of vascular smooth muscle cells, *J. Cell Physiol.* **120**:315–320.

Chiang, T. M., Postlethwaite, A. E., Beachey, E. H., Seyer, J. M., and Kang, A. H., 1978, Binding of chemotactic collagen-derived peptides to fibroblasts, *J. Clin. Invest.* **62**:916–922.

Chin, Y. H., Rasmussen, R. A., and Woodruff, J. J., 1985, Lymphocyte adhesion molecules for Peyer's patch high endothelium, *Fed. Proc.* **44**:1495.

Cohnheim, J. F., 1889, The pathology of circulation. Section I, in: *Lectures on General Pathology: A Handbook for Practitioners and Students*, transl. from the German by A. B. McKee, ed.), pp. xvii–528, New Sydenham Society, London.

Crum, R., Szabo, S., and Folkman, J., 1986, A new class of steroids inhibits angiogenisis in the presence of heparin or a heparin fragment, *Science* **230**:1375–1378.

DiCorleto, P. E., and de la Motte, C. A., 1985, Serum stimulation causes expression of monocyte binding sites on cultured endothelial cells, *Fed. Proc.* **44**:1494.

Fenselau, A. P., Watt, S., and Mello, R. J., 1981, Tumor angiogenic factor. Purification from the Walker 256 rat tumor, *J. Biol. Chem.* **256**:9605–9611.

Fishman, A. P. (ed.), 1982, *Endothelium*, Vol. 401, New York Academy of Sciences, New York.

Folkman, J., 1983, Angiogenesis: Initiation and control, *Ann. NY Acad. Sci.* **401**:212–227.

Folkman, J., 1984, What is the role of endothelial cells in angiogenesis? *Lab. Invest.* **51**:601–604.

Folkman, J., and Cotran, R., 1976, Regulation of vascular proliferation to tumor growth, in: *Intl. Rev. Exp. Pathol.* Vol. 16 (G. W. Richter and M. A. Epstein, eds.), pp. 297–248, Academic, New York.

Folkman, J., and Haudenschild, C. C., 1980, Angiogenesis *in vitro*, *Nature (Lond.)* **288**:551–556.

Folkman, J., and Moscona, A., 1978, Role of cell shape in growth control, *Nature (Lond.)* **273**:345–349.

Folkman, J., Haudenschild, C. C., and Zetter, B. R., 1979, Long-term culture of capillary endothelial cells, *Proc. Natl. Acad. Sci. USA* **76**:5217–5221.

Folkman, J., Langer, R., Linhardt, R. J., Haudenschild, C., and Taylor, S., 1983, Angiogenesis inhibition and tumor regression caused by heparin or a heparin fragment in the presence of cortisone, *Science* **221**:719–725.

Form, D. M., and Madri, J. A., 1985, Proliferation of microvascular endothelial cells *in vitro*: Modulation by extracellular matrix, *Fed. Proc.* **44**:1660.

Form, D. M., Pratt, B. M., and Madri, J. A., 1986, Endothelial cell proliferation during angiogenesis: *In vitro* modulation by basement membrane components, *Lab. Invest.* **55**:521–530.

Frater-Schroder, M., Muller, G., Birchmeier, W., and Bohlen, P., 1986, Transforming growth factor-beta, inhibits endothelial cell proliferation, *Biochem. Biophys. Res. Commun.* **137**:295–302.

Gallatin, W. G., Weissman, I. L., and Butcher, E. C., 1983, A cell-surface molecule involved in organ-specific homing of lymphocytes, *Nature (Lond.)* **304**:30–34.

Gospodarowicz, D., Delgado, D., and Vlodavsky, I., 1980, Permissive effect of the extracellular matrix on cell proliferation *in vitro*, *Proc. Natl. Acad. Sci. USA* **77**:4094–4098.

Gospodarowicz, D., Ganzales, R., and Fujii, D. K., 1983, Are factors originating from serum, plasma, or cultured cells involved in the growth-promoting effect of the extracellular matrix produced by cultured bovine corneal endothelial cells?, *J. Cell Physiol.* **114**:191–202.

Gross, J. L., Moscatelli, D., Jaffe, E. A., and Rifkin, D. B., 1982, Plasminogen activator and collagenase production by cultured capillary endothelial cells, *J. Cell Biol.* **95**:974–981.

Gross, J. L., Moscatelli, D., and Rifkin, D. B., 1983, Increased capillary endothelial cell protease activity in response to angiogenic stimuli *in vitro*, *Proc. Natl. Acad. Sci. USA* **880**:2623–2627.

Hall, H. G., Farson, D. A., and Bissell, M. J., 1982, Lumen formation by epithelial cell lines in response to collagen overlay: A morphogenetic model in culture *Proc. Natl. Acad. Sci. USA* **79**:4672–4676.

Hay, E. D., 1981, Collagen and embryonic development, in: *Cell Biology of the Extracellular Matrix* (E. D. Hay, ed.), pp. 379–409, Plenum, New York.

Hintner, H., Fritsch, P. O., Foidart, J.-M., Stingl, G., Schuler, G., and Katz, S. I., 1980, Expression of basement membrane zone antigens at the demo-epibolic junction on organ cultures of human skin, *J. Invest. Dermatol.* **74**:200–204.

Hobson, B., and Denekamp, J., 1984, Endothelial proliferation in tumors and normal tissues: Continuous labelling studies, *Br. J. Cancer* **49**:405–413.

Horowitz, A. L., Hance, A. J., and Crystal, R. G., 1977, Granulocyte, collagenase: Selective digestion of type I relative to type III collagen, *Proc. Natl. Acad. Sci. USA* **74**:87–901.

Ignotz, R. A., and Massague, J., 1986, Transforming growth factor-β stimulates the expression of fibronectin and collagen and their incorporation into the extracellular matrix, *J. Biol. Chem.* **261**:4337–4345.

Ingber, D. E., and Jamieson, J. D., 1985, Cell as tensegrity structures: Architectural regulation of histodifferentiation by physical forces transduced over basement membrane, in: *Gene Expression During Normal and Malignant Differentiation* (L. C. Anderson, C. G. Gahmber, and P. Ekblom, eds.)., pp. 13–82, Academic, New York.

Ingber, D. E., Madri, J. A., and Jamieson, J. D., 1986a, Basement membrane as a spatial organizer of polarized epithelia: Exogenous basement membrane reorients pancreatic epithelial tumor cells *in vitro*, *Am. J. Pathol.* **122**:129–139.

Ingber, D. E., Madri, J. A., Folkman, J., 1986b, Angiostatic steroids induce capillary basement membrane dissolution and inhibit angiogenesis, *Endocrinology* **119**:1768–1775.

Isaacs, J., Savion, N., Gospodarowicz, D., and Shuman, M. A., 1981, Effect of cell density on thrombin binding to a specific site on bovine vascular endothelial cells, *J. Cell Biol.* **90**:670–674.

Joyce, N. C., Haire, M. F., and Palade, G. E., 1985, Contractile proteins in pericytes. II. Immunocytochemical evidence for the presence of two isomysoins in graded concentrations, *J. Cell Biol.* **100**:1387–1395.

Joyce, N. C., Haire, M. F., and Palade, G. E., 1985a, Contractile proteins in pericytes. I. Immunolocalization of tropamysoin, *J. Cell Biol.* **100**:1379–1386.

Kalebic, T., Garbisa, S., Glaser, B., and Liotta, L., 1983, Basement membrane collagen: Degradation by migrating endothelial cells, *Science* **221**:281–283.

Karnovsky, M. J., 1981, Endothelial-vascular smooth muscle cell interactions, *Am. J. Pathol.* **105**:200–206.

Kramer, R. J., Bensch, K. G., Davison, P. M., and Karasek, M. A., 1984, Basal lamina formation by cultured microvascular endothelial cells, *J. Cell Biol.* **99**:692–698.

Kuttner, B. J., and Woodruff, J. J., 1979, Adherence of recirculating T and B lymphocytes to high endothelium of lymph nodes *in vitro*, *J. Immunol.* **123**:1421–1422.

Langer, R. R., Conn, H. M., Vacanti, J., Haudenschild, C., and Folkman, J., 1980, Control of tumor growth in animals by infusion of an angiogenesis inhibitor, *Proc. Natl. Acad. Sci. USA* **77**:4331–4335.

Lee, E. Y. H., Parry, G., and Bissell, M. J., 1984, Modulation of secreted proteins of mouse mammary epithelial cells by the collagenous substrata, *J. Cell Biol.* **98**:146–155.

Lesot, H., Kuhl, U., and von der Mark, K., 1983, Isolation of a laminin-binding protein from muscle membranes, *EMBO J.* **2**:861–865.

Leto, T. L., Pratt, B. M., and Madri, J. A., 1985, Mechanisms of cytoskeletal regulation: Modulation of aortic endothelial cell band 4.1 by the extracellular matrix, *Fed. Proc.* **44:**1660.

Leto, T. L., Pratt, B. M., and Madri, J. A., 1986, Mechanisms of cytoskeletal regulation: Modulation of aortic endothelial cell band protein 4.1 by the extracellular matrix, *J. Cell Physiol.* **127:**423–431.

Lobb, R., Sasse, J., Sullivan, R., Shing, Y., D'Amore, P., Jacobs, J., and Klagsburn, M., 1986, Purification and characterization of heparin-binding endothelial cell growth factors, *J. Biol. Chem.* **261:**1924–1928.

Lwebuga-Mukasa, J., Thulin, G., Madri, J. A., Barrett, C., and Warshaw, J., 1984, An acellular human amnionic membrane model for *in vitro* culture of type II pneumocytes: The role of the basement membrane on cell morphology and function, *J. Cell Physiol.* **121:**215–225.

Maciag, T., Kadish, J., Wilkins, L., Stemerman, M. B., and Weinstein, R., 1982, Organizational behavior of human umbilical vein endothelial cells, *J. Cell Biol.* **94:**511–520.

Macleod, A. G., 1971, *Aspects of Acute Inflammation,* Upjohn Co., Kalamazoo, Michigan.

Madri, J. A., 1982, Endothelial cell–matrix interactions in hemostasis; in: *Progress in Hemostasis and Thrombosis,* Vol. 6 (T. H. Spaet, ed.), pp. 1–24, Grune & Stratton, New York.

Madri, J. A., and Pratt, B. P., 1986, Endothelial cell–matrix interactions: *In vitro* models of angiogenesis, *J. Histochem. Cytochem.* **34:**85–91.

Madri, J. A., and Stenn, K. S., 1982, Aortic endothelial cell migration. I. Matrix requirements and composition, *Am. J. Pathol.* **106:**180–186.

Madri, J. A., and Williams, S. K., 1983, Capillary endothelial cell cultures: Phenotypic modulation by matrix components, *J. Cell Biol.* **97:**153–165.

Madri, J. A., Pratt, B. M., Yurchenco, P. D., and Furthmayr, H., 1984, The ultrastructural organization and architecture of basement membranes, *Ciba Found. Symp.* **108:**6–24.

Madri, J. A., Pratt, B. M., and Yannariello-Brown, J., 1987, Endothelial cell extracellular matrix interactions: Matrix as a modulator of cell function, in: *Endothelial Cell Biology* (N. Simionescu and M. Simionescu, eds.), Plenum, New York, in press.

Mainardi, C. L., Dixit, S. N., and Kang, A. H., 1980, Degradation of type IV (basement membrane) collagen by a proteinase isolated from human polymorphonuclear leukocyte granules, *J. Biol. Chem.* **255:**5435–5441.

Malinoff, H. L., and Wicha, M. S., 1983, Isolation of a cell surface receptor protein for laminin from murine fibrosarcoma cells, *J. Cell Biol.* **96:**1475–1479.

Martin, G. R., Kleinman, K. H., Terranova, V. P., Ledbetter, S., and Hassell, J. R., 1984, The regulation of basement membrane formation and cell–matrix interactions by defined supramolecular components. in: *Basement Membranes and Cell Movement,* Vol. 108, (R. Porter and J. Whelan eds.), pp. 197–209, Pitman, London.

McCarthy, J. B., and Furcht, L. T., 1984, Laminin and fibronectin promote the haptotactic migration of B16 mouse melanoma cells in vitro, *J. Cell Biol.* **98:**1474–1480.

McConnell, I., 1983, Roving lymphocytes. *Nature (Lond.)* **304:**17.

Montesano, R., Orci, L., and Vassali, P., 1983, *In vitro* rapid organization of endothelial cells into capillary-like networks is promoted by collagen matrices, *J. Cell Biol.* **97:**1648–1652.

Montesano, R., Mossaz, A., Ryser, J.-E., Orci, L., and Vassalli, P., 1984, Leukocyte interleukins induce cultured endothelial cells to produce a highly organized glycosaminoglycan-rich pericellular matrix, *J. Cell Biol.* **99:**1706–1715.

Nicosia, R. F., and Madri, J. A., 1987, The microvascular extracellular matrix: Developmental changes during angiogenesis in the aortic ring-plasma clot model, 1987, *Amer. J. Pathol.* **128:**78–90.

Nicosia, R. F., Tchao, T., and Leighton, J., 1982, Histotypic angiogenesis *in vitro:* Light microscopic, ultrastructural, and radioautographic studies, *In Vitro* **18:**538–549.

Pober, J. S., and Gimbrone, M. A., 1982, Expression of Ia-like antigens by human vascular endothelial cells is inducible *in vitro:* Demonstration by monoclonal antibody binding and immunoprecipitation, *Proc. Natl. Acad. Sci. USA* **79:**6641–6445.

Pober, J. S., Gimbrone, M. A., Cotran, R. S., Reiss, C. S., Burakoff, S. J., Fiers, W., and Ault, K. A., 1983, Ia expression by vascular endothelial is inducible by activated T cells and by human gamma interferon, *J. Exp. Med.* **157:**1339–1353.

Postlethwaite, A. E., and Kang, A. H., 1976. Collagen and collagen peptide-induced chemotaxis of human blood monocytes, *J. Exp. Med.* **143**:1299–1307.

Postlethwaite, A. E., Seyer, J. M., and Kang, A. H., 1978, Chemotactic attraction of human fibroblasts to type I, II, III collagens and collagen-derived peptides, *Proc. Natl. Acad. Sci. USA* **75**:871–875.

Pratt, B. M., Form, D., and Madri, J. A., 1985, Endothelial cell–extracellular matrix interactions, *Ann. NY Acad. Sci.* **460**:274–288.

Pratt, B. M., Harris, A. S., Morrow, J. S., and Madri, J. A., 1984, Mechanisms of cytoskeletal regulation. Modulation of aortic endothelial cell spectrin by the extracellular matrix, *Am. J. Pathol.* **117**:349–354.

Rao, N. C., Barsky, S. H., Terranova, V. P., and Liotta, L. A., 1983, Isolation of a tumor cell laminin receptor, *Biochem. Biophys. Res. Comm.* **111**:804–808.

Rhodin, J. A. G., 1974, *Histology*, Oxford University Press, New York.

Robbins, S. L., Cotran, R. S., and Kumar, V., 1984, *Pathologic Basis of Disease*, W. B. Saunders, Philadelphia.

Russo, R. G., Liotta, L. A., Thorgiersson, U., Brundage, R., and Schiffmann, E., 1981, Polymorphonuclear leukocyte migration through human amnion membrane, *J. Cell Biol.* **91**:459–467.

Ryan, G. B., and Majno, G., 1977, *Inflammation*, Upjohn Co., Kalamazoo, Michigan.

Schor, A. M., Schor, S. L., and Kumar, S., 1979, Importance of a collagen substratum for stimulation of capillary endothelial cell proliferation by tumour angiogenesis factor, *Int. J. Cancer* **24**:225–234.

Sholley, M. M., Gimbrone, M. A., and Cotran, R. S., 1977, Cellular migration and replication in endothelial regeneration—A study using irradiated endothelial cultures, *Lab Invest.* **36**:18–25.

Sholley, M. M., Gimbrone, M. A., and Cotran, R. S., 1978, The effects of leukocyte depletion on corneal neovascularization, *Lab. Invest.* **38**:32–40.

Sholley, M. M., Ferguson, G. P., Seibel, H. R., Montour, J. L., and Wilson, J. D., 1984, Mechanisms of neovascularization. Vascular sprouting can occur without proliferation of endothelial cells, *Lab. Invest.* **51**:624–634.

Simionescu, M., Simionescu, N., and Palade, G. E., 1982, Biochemically differentiated microdomains of the cell surface of capillary endothelium, in: *Endothelium*, Vol. 401 (A. P. Fishman, ed.). pp. 9–23, New York Academy of Science, New York.

Simionescu, N., Heltianu, C., Antohe, F., and Simionescu, M., 1982, Endothelial receptors for histamine, in: *Endothelium*, Vol. 401 (A. P. Fishman, ed.), pp. 132–148, New York Academy of Science, New York.

Stamper, H. B., Jr., and Woodruff, J. J., 1976, Lymphocyte homing into lymph nodes: *In vitro* demonstration of the selective affinity of recirculating lymphocytes for high-endothelial venules, *J. Exp. Med.* **144**:828–833.

Stanley, J. R., Alvarez, O. M., Bere, E. W., Eaglestein, W. H., and Katz, S. I., 1981, Detection of basement membrane zone antigens during epidermal wound healing in pigs, *J. Invest. Dermatol.* **77**:240–243.

Stenn, K. S., Madri, J. A., and Roll, F. J., 1979, Migrating epidermis produces AB$_2$ collagen and requires continual collagen synthesis for movement, *Nature (Lond.)* **277**:229–232.

Terranova, V. P., Rao, C. N., Kalebic, T., Margulies, I. M., and Liotta, L. A., 1983, Laminin receptor on human breast carcinoma cells. *Proc. Natl. Acad. Sci. USA* **80**:444–448.

Terranova, V. P., Williams, J. E., Liotta, L. A., and Martin, G. R., 1984, Modulation of the metastatic activity of melanoma cells by laminin and fibronectin, *Science* **226**:982–985.

Wagner, R. C., 1980, Endothelial cell embryology and growth, *Adv. Microcirc.* **9**:45–75.

Williams, S. K., Gillis, J. F., Mathews, M. A., Wagner, R. C., and Bitensky, M. W., 1980, Isolation and characterization of brain endothelial cell: Morphology and enzyme activity, *J. Neurochem.* **35**:374–381.

Wong, A. J., Pollard, T. D., and Herman, I. M., 1983, Actin filament stress fibers in vascular endothelial cells *in vivo*, *Science* **219**:867–869.

Yannariello-Brown, J., and Madri, J. A., 1985, Aortic endothelial cells synthesize specific binding proteins for laminin and type IV collagen, *J. Cell Biol.* **101**:333 (abst).

Yannariello-Brown, J., Tchao, N. K., Liotta, L. A., and Madri, J. A., 1985, Co-distribution of the laminin receptor with actin microfiliments in permeabilized aortic and microvascular endothelial cells, *J. Cell Biol.* **101**:333 (abst).

Yurchenco, P. D., and Furthmayr, H., 1984, Self-assembly of basement membrane collagen, *Biochemistry* **23**:1839–1850.

Zetter, B. R., 1980, Migration of capillary endothelial cells in stimulated by tumour-derived factors, *Nature (Lond.)* **285**:41–43.

Chapter 16

The Role of Cell–Cell Interaction in the Regulation of Endothelial Cell Growth

RONALD L. HEIMARK and STEPHEN M. SCHWARTZ

1. Introduction: The Quiescent Cell

Studies of growth control have focused on the role of low-molecular-weight proteins that stimulate growth. Like other hormones or cytokines, these small proteins, including platelet-derived growth factor (PDGF) and epidermal growth factor (EGF), bind to receptors in target cell membranes and initiate a set of events leading to DNA synthesis. The existence of these growth factors is consistent with the usual view of growth stimulus and response, which occurs when a tissue proliferates during wound repair. That is, we usually think of a wound as disrupting a resting environment. Cytokines and lymphokines released at sites of injury might be thought of as wound-repair hormones, initiating margination of leukocytes, chemotaxis, release of proteases, hemostasis, and so on. In a similar manner, it is reasonable to imagine that growth factors released at a wound site would stimulate cells in the wounded tissue to begin replicating. This idea is well supported by studies showing that many of the blood cells responding to a wound can release mitogens (Ross *et al.*, 1974) and by more recent studies showing that these agents can be effective when released in a wound chamber *in vivo* (Sporn *et al.*, 1983; Assoian *et al.*, 1984) (see Chapter 9–12).

The emphasis of current scientific reports on growth stimulants begs the question of the nature of the quiescent cell. Growth factors may simply release cells from a quiescent state by a positive signal input. However, the critical importance of quiescence and the probability that growth factors are present in the absence of injury suggest that quiescence might be actively maintained. Examples of this sort of negative feedback or active maintenance of a system in a resting state range from repressor signals in the genome, to negative feedback loops in the control of blood pressure and blood coagulation (see Chapters 3 and 4).

RONALD L. HEIMARK and STEPHEN M. SCHWARTZ • Department of Pathology, University of Washington, Seattle, Washington 98195.

To go beyond philosophy, we need to identify a mechanism of growth inhibition at a molecular level. Unfortunately, attempts to isolate most growth inhibitors have failed until recently. There could be many reasons for the difficulties. For instance, one possibility is that incorrect assays have been chosen. Culture systems have been optimized to stimulate cell growth rather than to maintain quiescence. Furthermore, there is reason to doubt whether most culture systems ever become truly quiescent, even when optimal growth conditions are removed. Smith and Martin (1973), for example, have argued that cells in culture show a defined probability of dividing given specific culture conditions. When that probability is low, we say the cells are quiescent, or in G_0. Their analysis, however, says that the cells are still in the growth fraction with random entry into the cell cycle. This idea is consistent with the thymidine index values typically described for quiescent cultured cells. Values as high as 5% are often described for the thymidine index of confluent, quiescent cultures. If this is a single pulse of [^{3}H]thymidine in a typical culture system, with 8 hr required for DNA synthesis and a cell cycle time of 24 hr, it may reflect a daily replication rate as high as 10–15%. That is hardly quiescent by comparison with endothelial cells *in vivo*, for which replication rates may be as low as 1×10^{-3} per day (Schwartz and Benditt, 1977). Indeed, replication rates as high as 10–15% per day *in vivo* are more typical of proliferation in response to injury (Schwartz and Benditt, 1977). Nevertheless, even in states of relative *in vivo* quiescence, it seems likely that cells making up a majority of the tissues of the body do not have states of absolute quiescence.

2. Endothelium as a Model System of Quiescence

2.1. *In Vivo* Studies

It remains to be seen whether quiescent cells *in vitro* are comparable to uninjured adult cells *in vivo*. Among the best examples of an *in vivo* tissue showing quiescence is the arterial endothelium. Because these cells exist as a simple flat surface, it is possible to label all the cells with [^{3}H]thymidine and count all cells making DNA (Schwartz *et al.*, 1980). When this is done in a normal adult animal, daily frequencies of replication range from 10^{-3} to 10^{-4} replications per day. By contrast, regenerating endothelium reaches peak values as high as 30% of the cells simultaneously in S phase, and values of a few percentages (10^{-2}–10^{-1}) are typical of hypertension and atherosclerosis (Schwartz and Benditt, 1977; Hansson and Bondjers, 1980). It seems reasonable to believe that this cell type has a true G_0 quiescent state.

It is important to point out that unless serum factors are adsorbed onto the exposed wound surface, stimulation of endothelial replication occurs in plasma with only those growth factors that are always available to the endothelium. While plasma factors may be required for growth, it seems unlikely that endothelial regeneration *in vivo* is initiated by plasma or serum growth factors. More likely, growth starts when the cell senses injury to, or loss of, a neighboring cell. It also seems unlikely that the factors controlling quiescence are present in serum or plasma. Regeneration occurs for a certain distance; cell movement and replication then cease before regenerating cells meet each other (Reidy et al., 1983). This process probably does not occur as a result of cells having a limited replicative life-span, since growth can be restimulated by a wound at right angles to the regenerated edge of the regenerated sheet (Reidy et al., 1983). It is intriguing to speculate whether this also represents some sort of inhibition of growth by cell–cell interaction or synthesis of some growth inhibitor by the healed vessel wall.

2.2. *In Vitro* Studies

Cultured endothelium mimics some of the behavior of endothelium *in vivo* (Fig. 1a). Typically, confluent cells have a low-replication frequency with approximately 1–2% of the cells being in the S phase at any one time. While this is considerably higher than replication rates *in vivo*, it is independent of serum concentration or the presence of known growth factors (Schwartz et al., 1979). Furthermore, both endothelium derived from bovine aorta (BAE) and human umbilical vein (HUVE) will grow to a maximum density that is independent of the concentration of serum in the medium used (Haudenschild et al., 1976; Schwartz et al., 1979). This might reflect the ability of the regenerating endothelium to synthesize mitogens, including PDGF (DiCorleto and Bowen-Pope, 1983; Barrett et al., 1984). However, there is no evidence that these self-derived mitogens or the mitogens present in serum, generally used to culture cells, are required for growth. In addition, there is no evidence that they are consumed by the growing cells to the point of depletion.

2.3. Cell–Cell Interaction and Quiescence

Once endothelial cells have reached saturation density, further increases in replication only occur when continuity of the monolayer is disrupted. This can be done by overlaying the cells with collagen (Delvos et al., 1982), wounding the cell layer with a razorblade or causing the cells to retract with colchicine (Selden et al., 1981). Conversely, even when the cells are wounded or stimulated to replicate by colchicine (Selden et al., 1981), cytochalasin B inhibits proliferation, perhaps by inhibiting the ability of the cells to move away from their resting quiescent locations. These observations led us to suggest that quiescence of the cultured endothelium is controlled by some sort of cell–cell interaction (Schwartz et al., 1980).

3. The Contact-Inhibition Controversy

The idea that growth of cell sheets is controlled by cell–cell interaction is not new. Evidence for this mechanism in culture, however, has been controversial, perhaps because of the particular cell lines chosen for study. Most of the

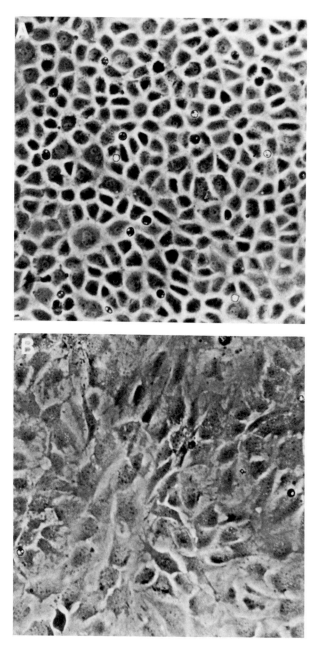

Figure 1. Phase-contact micrograph of a confluent culture of bovine aortic endothelial cells (A) and of Swiss 3T3 cells (B).

work has been done with established immortal cell lines that provide a model for the strict confinement of simple squamous epithelia *in vivo* to a monolayer. The most popular model system has been the mouse 3T3 cell (Todaro and Green, 1963) (Fig. 1b), which was originally a mixed culture of embryonic cells. The cells were regularly passaged at relatively low density and limited serum concentration. Once established, the 3T3 cells appeared to have adapted to these conditions in such a way that their cell-culture density is serum dependent (Todaro and Green, 1963). That is, 3T3 cells at low serum concentration have low-culture densities with limited cell overlap; however, if the serum concentration is raised, the cells overgrow each other to high-culture densities. Thus, the cells are density inhibited, but density inhibition in this system is as dependent on the availability of soluble medium factors as on direct cell–cell interaction.

Nevertheless, some studies have suggested that growth of 3T3 cells is controlled by some form of cell–cell interaction (Lieberman and Glaser, 1981); however, most of the evidence has been indirect. For example, like endothelial cells, 3T3 cells respond to a wound by growing into the wound area without requiring additional mitogens (Dulbecco, 1970). The growth response has been explained by a release from cell contact or by the greater access of cells at the wound edge to diffusible growth factors or nutrients in the surrounding medium. In addition, studies of cell movement support the idea that 3T3 cells do respond to cell contact (Albrecht-Buehler, 1977). As growing cells encounter each other, microcinephotography studies clearly show either that cell movement stops or that cells reverse direction. Since 3T3 cells are somewhat confined to a monolayer, contact inhibition of movement may account for failure of cells to grow on top of one another. Unless we expect cells to grow into tall grasslike structures, it seems reasonable to imagine that restriction to a monolayer would also require some contact-dependent mechanism to inhibit cell replication.

Unfortunately, other attempts at testing the contact inhibition of growth hypothesis for 3T3 cells have not been convincing. In one study, cells were filmed as they grew (Martz and Steinberg, 1972). No correlation could be found between nearest-neighbor frequency or other measures of contact and the probability of an individual cell entering mitosis. Since we know that some sort of density-dependent mechanism must be present to control growth, three conclusions may be drawn: either (1) control of growth depends on soluble factors, while restriction to monolayer morphology is regulated by cell–cell interactions; (2) the time required for cell contact to inhibit cell growth is longer than the interval of one to two cell cycles observed in this study; or (3) cell contact maintains quiescent cells in a nondividing state but plays no role in the transition from the dividing state to a quiescent state. The importance of the experiment conducted by Martz and Steinberg (1972) lies in its failure to provide convincing evidence for contact inhibition. We simply do not have any direct evidence from time-lapse studies for cell contact as an inhibitor of growth.

Better evidence in support of contact inhibition of growth comes from studies with growth inhibitors isolated from 3T3 cell-surface membranes

(Natraj and Datta, 1978; Whittenberger and Glaser, 1977). An enriched 3T3 plasma membrane fraction from confluent cells provided 50% inhibition of 3T3 cell replication. The addition of the plasma membrane fraction increases the proportion of cells in G_1, implying a physiologic G_0 block or prolonged G_1 interval. The effect of membrane is not absolute, since it can be overcome by addition of increasing concentrations of serum. The inhibition is not due, however, to depletion of the mitogen from the media because preincubation of media with membranes did not alter its ability to support growth. In addition, this is unlikely, since similar studies using membranes from a variant 3T3 cell line lacking EGF receptors showed inhibition of EGF-induced DNA synthesis in normal 3T3 cells (Vale et al., 1984). The inhibitory activity appears to be due to an intrinsic membrane protein that can be solubilized with octylglucoside (Whittenberger et al., 1978). One possibility is that the added plasma membranes have overloaded the cell with growth factor receptors that act in some way to inhibit growth. A similar activity from 3T3 cells, which inhibited DNA synthesis by 50%, was extracted from quiescent cells by a low concentration of urea and ascribed to a glycoprotein(s) (Natraj and Datta, 1978). Analysis of the molecular weight by gel filtration chromatography gave a value of 540,000 M_r and sodium dodecyl sulfate-polyacrylamide gel electrophoresis (SDS-PAGE) showed that several proteins were present. These 3T3 cell fractions, as yet unpurified, share a number of important properties. First, the growth inhibitory agent or agents seem to be glycoproteins. Second, the growth inhibitory proteins (GIPs) appear to be an integral component of the cell membrane. Third, GIPs are readily extracted from the cell by mild treatment with urea, suggesting that they exist in a specialized region of the cell membrane.

In contrast to these intramembranous growth inhibitory proteins, other soluble growth inhibitory fractions have been identified in culture that are not associated with the cell membrane. These include transforming growth factor-β (TGF-β), the interferons, and other factors isolated from conditioned media of density-inhibited cells. Soluble growth inhibitors from conditioned media have been purified and have molecular weights of 25,000 M_r from BSC-1 cells (Holley et al., 1983) and 10,000 and 13,000 M_r from 3T3 cells (Steck et al., 1982). Monoclonal antibodies have identified the active peptide from 3T3 cells as the 13,000-M_r component (Hsu et al., 1984). One monoclonal antibody not only neutralized the soluble 13,000-M_r growth inhibitor activity but bound to the surface of 3T3 cells, raising the possibilities that the soluble protein could be a fragment of a membrane protein or may bind to a membrane receptor. In addition, this antibody appeared to stimulate [³H]thymidine incorporation into DNA. The relationship between the cell-surface bound and soluble molecules has yet to be determined. It is possible that soluble inhibitors are either parts of membrane proteins or are themselves bound to critical membrane proteins.

Holley and co-workers (Tucker et al., 1984) noted a striking similarity in the molecular weight of a growth inhibitor for BSC-1 cells and TGF-β. Both proteins display nearly identical activity in stimulation of colony formation in soft agar and inhibition of [³H]thymidine incorporation in monolayer cultures of mouse embryo AKR.2B cells. However, the growth inhibitor from BSC-1 cells does not inhibit 3T3 cells, while TGF-β does (Holley et al., 1983). The purification of TGF-β has been described from several sources, including bovine kidney (Roberts et al., 1983), human placenta (Frolik et al., 1983), and human platelets (Assoian et al., 1983). This peptide presents an interesting dilemma. Not only does TGF-β act as a growth inhibitor of certain cells grown in monolayer, but it is required, along with EGF, for growth of the same cells in soft agar (Tucker et al., 1984; Assoian et al., 1983). Thus, we return to the issues raised by the Martz and Steinberg experiment. We need to distinguish the controls of monolayer formation; that is, morphogenic controls from growth stimulation itself. In this view, TGF-β may be a morphogenic agent permitting growth in the absence of substrate but restricting growth on solid growth surfaces.

4. Endothelial Cell Growth Inhibitory Protein(s)

Our approach to endothelium is also based on the concept of growth inhibitory proteins. The biology of endothelial cells suggests that cell–cell interactions may regulate endothelial cell growth control and formation of the monolayer. It seemed reasonable then that endothelial cell membranes would contain a GIP that is an endothelial growth inhibitory protein (EGIP) similar to that described for 3T3 cells. Moreover, given the lack of evidence for control of endothelial growth by soluble growth factors, it is reasonable to postulate that EGIP(s) would constitute the major agent or agents controlling endothelial growth. We prepared a cell-surface fraction from confluent endothelial cells by treatment with a low concentration of urea (Heimark and Schwartz, 1985). Addition of the cell-surface membrane fraction to growing cells inhibits DNA synthesis approximately 60% in a concentration-dependent manner. Both migration and replication are blocked by the cell-surface membrane fraction in a wound-edge assay. The inhibition is transient when added to growing cells, 48 hr after the addition, the rate of growth returns to that of the control. The activity is labile to proteases, heat treatment, and reduction, suggesting that it is a protein. This fraction is enriched in enzyme markers for the plasma membrane and endoplasmic reticulum, in addition to the density-dependent 60,000-M_r cell surface protein, CSP-60 (Vlodavsky et al., 1979). The inhibitor is solubilized from membrane vesicles by octylglucoside but is not dissociated from the vesicles by sodium carbonate treatment, which removes extrinsic membrane proteins. This extends the result of Whittenberger and Glaser (1977) on the ability of membrane fraction to mimic the inhibitory effect of density in a normal cell of defined origin. In summary, endothelial cell membranes have protein(s) with the following properties: (1) ability to inhibit motility at a wound edge, (2) ability to prevent initiation of growth in a wound, and (3) ability to inhibit growth in sparsely plated cells.

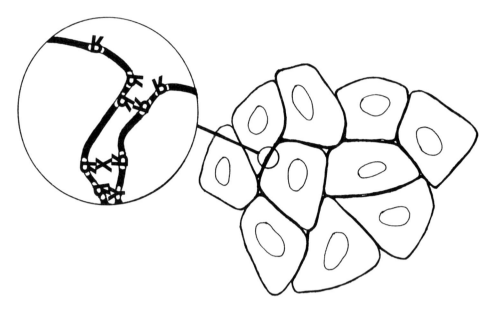

Figure 2. Types of interactions predicted for an endothelial growth-inhibitory protein (EGIP), represented as the integral membrane protein (R). The following types of interactions could provide positional information between cells. EGIP could interact with an identical molecule in a neighboring cell (R–R), or there could be an intermediate, such as calcium, linking the two molecules of EGIP (R–X–R). Alternatively, EGIP could interact with a dissimilar molecule, such as in a glycoprotein—lectin interaction (R–Y). Occupancy of few receptors would not be enough to stop growth, but could inform interacting cells to change their direction of movement. Only when a critical number of receptors become occupied would this be expected to stop growth.

5. Location of a Growth-Inhibitory Protein

It is interesting to speculate on the possible location and identity of proteins with specific growth-inhibitory properties (Fig. 2). Upon transformation of endothelial cells, there is an alteration in structure and thrombogenicity due to an abnormal expression of fibronectin on the upper surface of the endothelial cell (Zetter *et al.*, 1978). Following the proposal of Margolis *et al.* (1979), this suggests that the limitation of growth to a monolayer and the nonthrombogenicity of endothelial cell monolayers might depend on the restriction of specific sets of proteins to the upper and lower cell membranes. Vlodavsky *et al.* (1979) speculated about the role of a 60,000-M_r endothelial cell surface protein, CSP-60, in this process. CSP-60 is present in the urea-extracted surface fraction. It is one of the major iodinatable proteins on the upper cell surface (Heimark and Schwartz, 1985). To answer whether CSP-60 is the active agent will have to await purification and generation of specific antibodies directed at the inhibitory component.

It is also conceivable that the growth-inhibitory protein might be specifically localized to the cell junction. Both cultured bovine aortic endothelial and

3T3 cells have simple junctional complexes; tight junctions are lost and gap junctions are small and sparsely distributed (Larson and Sheridan, 1982). There are, however, extensive areas of apposition of cell membranes of adjacent cells without any specific structure. Certain well-defined junctional elements between cells have been described by morphologic criteria and a number of proteins associated with junctional structures. One example is the liver gap junction, which contains a major 27,000-M_r component (Hertzberg et al., 1982). A recent report of monoclonal antibodies of 3T3 cell surfaces is of interest (Murphy et al., 1983). One antibody was able to localize a 100,000-M_r protein to the cell junctions. Other possible candidates for growth-inhibitory proteins are cell surface proteins shown to be involved in cell–cell adhesion, either calcium-dependent cell adhesion molecules (Gallin et al., 1983; Ogou et al., 1983; Ocklind et al., 1983) or calcium-independent cell adhesion molecules (Hoffman et al., 1982). Antibodies that interfere with specific cell–cell interactions have been used to identify these cell surface proteins and, in some cases, to localize them at junction sites. A specific protein located at the junction or at the cell surface would be an obvious candidate for the agent responsible for the effect reported here.

We also need to consider the possibility that regeneration depends on interactions of endothelial membrane proteins with the substrate. The importance of the extracellular matrix in cell proliferation was recognized by Greenburg and Gospodarowicz (1982). At least for some cells, the extracellular matrix may replace the requirement for growth factors such as PDGF. This is supported by evidence that fibronectin, a major component of the extracellular matrix, acts as a competence factor that allows fibroblasts to replicate (Bitterman et al., 1983). For endothelial cells, however, it does not appear to be enough. Madri and co-workers (Pratt et al., 1984) showed that matrix component can affect the degree of migration and proliferation of endothelial cells when cultured on a fibronectin versus a type I/III collagen substrate (see Chapter 12). The substrate also showed a dramatic effect on the distribution of spectrin, a component of the membrane skeleton. These results suggest that extracellular matrix components have a role, which has yet to be clearly defined, in regulation of endothelial cell growth. One could speculate that endothelial cells at rest "sense" some stable interaction between a membrane protein and fixed extracellular structures. If the growth-inhibitory protein were to be such a sensor, cells released from contact inhibition of movement might displace enough inhibitor matrix complexes to permit stimulation of growth. Addition of exogenous membrane, if reinserted, could mimic the normal quiescent state, either by increasing the numbers of membrane–matrix receptors or by altered properties of the reinserted molecules. However, none of these hypotheses can be meaningful until the inhibitor is isolated and purified.

It is of interest to consider the possible roles of an endothelial growth inhibitor in vivo. Histologists classify endothelium as a simple squamous epithelium. This means that under normal circumstances, endothelium is strictly limited to the formation of monolayers lining tubes. The only exception is the growth of transformed endothelial cells in hemangioendotheliosarcomas. Even here, malignant growths may preserve their monolayer structure as tubes. Thus, uncontrolled growth can occur while the surface-limited topography of endothelium is maintained, which is similar to the form of endothelial growth seen in wounds or in the vascular response to tumors. Here, too, endothelial cells grow as tubes, since they preserve the type of growth seen in the fetal development of blood vessels in various forms of response called angiogenesis. This process contrasts with the regeneration that occurs when disruption of the monolayer produces endothelial regeneration. Regrowth onto a wounded surface, regeneration, occurs in all epithelia. When epithelial continuity is disrupted the cells respond by moving onto the wound surface and replicating to replace the lost cells. We would like to suggest a simple hypothesis: both processes could be controlled by cell contact somewhat as suggested by Margolis and colleagues (1979). These investigators suggested that lack of "adhesiveness" of the upper membrane of epithelial cells could account for both antithrombogenicity and contact inhibition of movement. In their model, endothelial cells fail to overgrow one another because of the absence of the same adhesive protein on the luminal surface responsible for failure of platelets to adhere. Alternatively, one might imagine that EGIP is not only inhibitory to growth but antithrombogenic or, perhaps most likely, the upper membrane contains inhibitory molecules and lacks molecules required for stimulation of reactive processes such as thrombosis and coagulation (Heimark and Schwartz, 1983; Stern et al., 1983) (see Chapter 4). Put another way, one might ask whether the inhibition of growth is an active process due to the presence of a growth inhibitor in the membrane or the absence of a molecule required for movement of one cell over another. Moreover, we need to consider the possibility that inhibition of growth is a secondary phenomenon while the primary event is inhibition of movement, with growth somehow stimulated by movement. Since we know that endothelial cells will not replicate if movement is inhibited, then one might speculate that regeneration simply represents liberation from a state where cells could not move. However, this relatively nonspecific model seems unlikely. Contact inhibition of movement is more than just a failure of cells to grow over each other. Cells coming into contact appear to stop and reverse motion, suggesting some form of specific recognition. The existence of a specific membrane fragment able to mimic contact inhibition supports the idea that this is a specific process but certainly does not distinguish between contact events controlling growth secondary to controlling movement and contact events controlling replication and movement independently.

In either case, it is not difficult to see how modulation of growth-inhibitory protein could account for angiogenesis. In angiogenesis, endothelial cells must replicate while maintaining continuity. It is interesting to note that none of the angiogenic factors has been reported to stimulate growth of endothelium at quiescent density. There have, however, been reports that angiogenic factors stimulate a remodeling of cultured endothelium from flat sheets into more vessel-like tubes. Moreover, a correlation has been found (see Chapter 18) between angiogenic activity and the ability to stimulate collagenase production

(Gross *et al.*, 1982). Perhaps angiogenic substances act by disrupting the integrity of the substrate, permitting endothelial cells to fall into a hole, creating a new growth area. If this occurs, disruption in continuity would release a region of cells from inhibition of replication. Thus, angiogenesis could be primarily a structure-dependent event, that is, a remodeling process with endothelial replication occurring as a result of the loss of continuity at remodeling sites.

6. Summary

Growth control in the endothelium is constrained by the maintenance of a cell monolayer. We have presented evidence for a membrane protein, EGIP, that is able to mimic the effects of contact inhibition. We have also proposed a model in which contact inhibition and disruption of cell contact may, in a reciprocal fashion, control the various forms of endothelial cell growth.

References

Albrecht-Buehler, G., 1977, The phagokinetic tracks of 3T3 cells, *Cell* **11**:395–404.

Assoian, R. K., Komoriya, A., Meyer, C. A., Miller, D. M., and Sporn, M. B., 1983, Transforming growth factor-beta in human platelets. *J. Biol. Chem.* **258**:7155–7160.

Assoian, R. K., Grotendorst, G. R., Miller, D. M., and Sporn, M. B., 1984, Cellular transformation by coordinated action of three peptide growth factors from human platelets, *Nature (Lond.)* **309**:804–80

Barrett, T. B., Gajdusek, C. M., Schwartz, S. M., McDougall, J. K., and Benditt, E. P., 1984, Expression of the *sis* gene by endothelial cells in culture and *in vivo*, *Proc. Natl. Acad. Sci. USA* **81**:6772–6774.

Bitterman, P. B., Rennard, S. I., Adelberg, S., and Crystal, R. G., 1983, Role of fibronectin as a growth factor for fibroblasts, *J. Cell Biol.* **97**:1925–1932.

Delvos, U., Gajdusek, C., Sage, H., Harker, L. A., and Schwartz, S. M., 1982, Interactions of vascular wall cells with collagen gels, *Lab. Invest.* **46**:61–72.

DiCorleto, P. E., and Bowen-Pope, D. F., 1983, Cultured endothelial cells produce a platelet-derived growth factor-like protein, *Proc. Natl. Acad. Sci. USA* **80**:1919–1923.

Dulbecco, R., 1970, Topoinhibition and serum requirement of transformed and untransformed cells, *Nature (Lond.)* **227**:802–806.

Frolik, C. A., Dart, L. L., Meyers, C. A., Smith, D. M., and Sporn, M. B., 1983, Purification and initial characterization of a type beta transforming growth factor from human placenta, *Proc. Natl. Acad. Sci. USA* **80**:3676–3680.

Gallin, W. J., Edelman, G. M., and Cunningham, B. A., 1983, Characterization of L-CAM, a major cell adhesion molecule from embryonic liver cells, *Proc. Natl. Acad. Sci. USA* **80**:1038–1042.

Greenburg, G., and Gospodarowicz, D., 1982, Inactivation of a basement membrane component responsible for cell proliferation but not for cell attachment, *Exp. Cell Res.* **140**:1–14.

Gross, J. L., Moscatelli, D., Jaffe, E. A., and Rifkin, D. B., 1982, Plasminogen activator and collagenase production by cultured capillary endothelial cells, *J. Cell Biol.* **95**:974–981.

Hansson, G. K., and Bondjers, G., 1980, Endothelial proliferation and atherogenesis in rabbits with moderate hypercholesterolemia, *Artery* **7**:316–329.

Haudenschild, C. C., Zahniser, D., Folkman, J., and Klagsbrun, M., 1976, Human vascular endothelial cells in culture. Lack of response to serum growth factors, *Exp. Cell Res.* **98**:175–183.

Heimark, R. L., and Schwartz, S. M., 1983, Binding of coagulation Factors IX and X to the endothelial cell surface, *Biochem. Biophys. Res. Commun.* **111**:723–731.

Heimark, R. L., and Schwartz, S. M., 1985, The role of membrane–membrane interactions in the regulation of endothelial cell growth, *J. Cell Biol.* **100**:1934–1940.

Hertzberg, E. L., Anderson, D. J., Friedlander, M., and Gilula, N. B., 1982, Comparative analysis of the major polypeptides from liver gap junctions and lens fiber junctions, *J. Cell Biol.* **92**:53–59.

Hoffman, S., Sorkin, B. C., White, P. C., Brackenbury, R., Mailhammer, R., Rutishauser, U., Cunningham, B. A., and Edelman, G. M., 1982, Chemical characterization of a neural cell adhesion molecule purified from embryonic brain membranes, *J. Biol. Chem.* **257**:7720–7729.

Holley, R. W., Armour, R., Baldwin, J. H., and Greenfield, S.. 1983, Preparation and properties of a growth inhibitor produced by kidney epithelial cells, *Cell Biol. Int. Rep.* **7**:525–526.

Hsu, Y.-M., Barry, J. M., and Wang, J. L., 1984, Growth control in cultured 3T3 fibroblasts: Neutralization and identification of a growth-inhibitory factor by a monoclonal antibody, *Proc. Natl. Acad. Sci. USA* **7**:2107–2111.

Larson, D. M., and Sheridan, J. D., 1982, Intercellular juctions and transfer of small molecules in primary vascular endothelial cultures, *J. Cell Biol.* **92**:183–191.

Lieberman, M. A., and Glaser, L., 1981, Density-dependent regulation of cell growth: An example of a cell–cell recognition phenomenon, *J. Membrane Biol.* **63**:1–11.

Margolis, L. B., Vasilieva, E. J., Vasilev, J. M., and Gelfand, I. M., 1979, Upper surface of epithelial sheels and of fluid lipid films are nonadhesive for platelets, *Proc. Natl. Acad. Sci. USA* **76**:2303–2305.

Martz, E., and Steinberg, M. S., The role of cell–cell contact in "contact" inhibition of cell division: A review and new evidence, *J. Cell. Physiol.* **79**:189–210.

Murphy, T. L., Decker, G., and August, J. T., 1983, Glycoproteins of coated pits, cell junctions, and the entire cell surface revealed by monoclonal antibodies and immunoelectron microscopy, *J. Cell Biol.* **97**:533–541.

Natraj, C. V., and Datta, P., 1978, Control of DNA synthesis in growing BALB/c 3T3 mouse cells by a fibroblast growth regulatory factor, *Proc. Natl. Acad. Sci. USA* **75**:6115–6119.

Ocklind, C., Forsum, U., and Obrink, B., 1983, Cell surface localization and tissue distribution of a hepatocyte cell–cell adhesion glycoprotein (cell-CAM 105), *J. Cell Biol.* **96**:1168–1171.

Ogou, S.-I., Yoshida-Noro, C., and Takeichi, M., 1983, Calcium-dependent cell–cell adhesion molecules common to hepatocytes and teratocarcinoma stem cells, *J. Cell Biol.* **97**:944–948.

Pratt, B. M., Harris, A. S., Morrow, J. S., and Madri, J. A., 1984, Mechanisms of cytoskeletal regulation. Modulation of aortic endothelial cell spectrin by the extracellular matrix, *Am. J. Pathol.* **117**:349–354.

Reidy, M. A., and Silver, M. A., 1985, Endothelial regeneration. VII. Lack of intimal proliferation after refined injury to rat aorta, *Am. J. Pathol.* **118**:173–178.

Roberts, A. B., Anzano, M. A., Meyers, C. A., Wideman, J., Blacher, R., Pan, Y.-C. E., Stein, S., Lehrman, S. R., Smith, J. M., Lamb, L. C., and Sporn, M. B., 1983, Purification and properties of a type beta transforming growth factor from bovine kidney, *Biochemistry* **22**:5692–5698.

Ross, R., Glomset, J., Kariya, B., and Harker, L., 1974, A platelet-dependent serum factor that stimulates the proliferation of arterial smooth muscle cells *in vitro*, *Proc. Natl. Acad. Sci. USA* **71**:1207–1210.

Schwartz, S. M., and Benditt, E. P., 1977, Aortic endothelial cell replication. I. Effects of age and hypertension in the rat, *Circ. Res.* **41**:248–255.

Schwartz, S. M., Selden, S. C. III, and Bowman, P., 1979, Growth control in aortic endothelium at wound edges, in: *Hormones and Cell Culture*, Vol. 6 (R. Ross and G. Sato, eds.), pp. 593–610, Cold Spring Harbor Laboratory, New York.

Schwartz, S. M., Gajdusek, C. M., Reidy, M. A., Selden, S. C. III, and Haudenschild, C. C., 1980, Maintenance of integrity in aortic endothelium, *Fed. Proc.* **39**:2618–2625.

Selden, S. C. III, Rabinovitch, P. S., and Schwartz, S. M., 1981, Effects of cytoskeletal disrupting agents on replication of bovine endothelium, *J. Cell. Physiol.* **108**:195–211.

Smith, J. A., and Martin, L., 1973, Do cells cycle?, *Proc. Natl. Acad. Sci. USA* **70**:1263–1267.

Sporn, M. B., Roberts, A. B., Shuli, J. H., Smith, J. M., Ward, J. M., and Sodek, J., 1983, Polypeptide transforming growth factors isolated from bovine sources and used for wound healing *in vivo*, *Science* **219**:1329–1331.

Steck, P. A., Blenis, J., Voss, P. G., and Wang, J. L., 1982, Growth control in cultured 3T3 fibroblasts.

II. Molecular properties of a fraction enriched in growth inhibitory activity, *J. Cell Biol.* **92**:523–530.

Stern, D. M., Drillings, M., Nossel, H. L., Hurlet-Jensen, A., LaGamma, K. S., and Owen, J., 1983, Binding of Factors IX and IX$_a$ to cultured vascular endothelial cells, *Proc. Natl. Acad. Sci. USA* **80**:4119–4123.

Todaro, G. J., and Green, H., 1963, Quantitative studies of the growth of mouse embryo cells in culture and their development established lines, *J. Cell Biol.* **17**:299–313.

Tucker, R. F., Shipley, G. D., Moses, H. L., and Holley, R. W., 1984, Growth inhibitor from BSC-1 cells closely related to platelet beta transforming growth factor, *Science* **226**:705–707.

Vale, R. D., Peterson, S. W., Matiuck, N. V., and Fox, C. F., 1984, Purified plasma membranes inhibit polypeptide growth factor-induced DNA synthesis in subconfluent 3T3 cells, *J. Cell Biol.* **98**:1129–1132.

Vlodavsky, I., Johnson, L. K., and Gospodarowicz, D., 1979, Appearance in confluent vascular endothelial cell monolayers of a specific cell surface protein (CSP-60) not detected in actively growing endothelial cells or in cell types growing in multiple layers, *Proc. Natl. Acad. Sci. USA* **76**:2306–2310.

Whittenberger, B., and Glaser, L., 1977, Inhibition of DNA synthesis in cultures of 3T3 cells by isolated surface membranes, *Proc. Natl. Acad. Sci. USA* **74**:2251–2255.

Whittenberger, B., Raben, D., Lieberman, M. A., and Glaser, L., 1978, Inhibition of growth of 3T3 cells by extract of surface membranes, *Proc. Natl. Acad. Sci. USA* **75**:5457–5461.

Zetter, B. R., Johnson, L. K., Shuman, M. A., and Gospodarowicz, D., 1978, The isolation of vascular endothelial cell lines with altered cell surface and platelet-binding properties, *Cell* **14**:501–509.

Chapter 17

The Biology of the Myofibroblast Relationship to Wound Contraction and Fibrocontractive Diseases

OMAR SKALLI and GIULIO GABBIANI

1. Definition and Characterization of Wound Contraction

The process of wound repair is of vital importance for animals as well as for plants (Shigo, 1985), since a wound perturbs body homeostasis and may result in infection by microorganisms. A wound may occur without or with tissue loss (Robbins et al., 1984). In both cases, but more clearly in the second case, wound healing consists schematically of acute inflammation followed by formation of granulation tissue, a transitional tissue able to retract the wound space, and finally scar formation.

Granulation tissue consists of layers of fibroblastic cells separated by a collagenous extracellular matrix containing capillary buds and inflammatory cells. During healing of a tissue defect, the edges of the wound are progressively brought together by the retraction of granulation tissue. This phenomenon, called wound contraction, is of great clinical importance in reducing the size of the wound. However, it may result in complications, which, according to the nature, extent, and site of injury, can produce disfigurement, excessive scarring and impaired function of the affected organs (Montandon et al., 1973; Peacock and Van Winkle, 1970).

Extensive investigations have been done to delineate the forces responsible for wound contraction. Carrel and Hartmann (1916) recognized that the contractive forces reside in the granulation tissue itself. Collagen was thought to be the contractile element of granulation tissue until Abercrombie et al. (1956) observed that wound contraction occurred in scorbutic guinea pigs despite defective collagen synthesis. The finding that granulation tissue fibroblasts had structural and biologic properties intermediate between those of fibroblasts and those of smooth muscle cells suggested that they might produce the force of wound contraction (Gabbiani et al., 1971a). These cells were called myofibroblasts.

OMAR SKALLI and GIULIO GABBIANI • Department of Pathology, University of Geneva, 1211 Geneva 4, Switzerland.

In vivo studies of wound contraction have been carried out on a variety of animals, including human subjects, mostly using skin lesions. Other in vivo models are the granuloma pouch produced by subcutaneous injection of air and croton oil (Selye, 1953) and the subcutaneous implantation of synthetic sponges, which become invaded by granulation tissue (Dunphy et al., 1956; Holund et al., 1979; Roberts and Hayry, 1976). An in vitro equivalent of granulation tissue contraction was set up by Bell et al. (1979), consisting of the contraction of a collagen gel by fibroblasts.

Wound contraction depends on various parameters investigated in the classic study of Carrel and Hartmann (1916) on guinea pigs, cats, and humans and then later by Billingham and Russel (1956) on rabbits. For these studies, the wound area was planimetrically measured and its log area was then plotted as a function of time. This resulted in an exponential relationship expressed by the formula:

$$A = A_0 e^{-kT}$$

where A and A_0 stand for the surface of the wound at time T and 0, respectively, and T for time after injury (Billingham and Russel, 1956). K is the slope of the straight line and was called specific rate of contracture; practically, it represents the amount by which a unit area of wound diminishes in 1 day. The specific rate of contracture K is uniform for rectangular or triangular wounds of different initial sizes but is lower for circular wounds. Other equations expressing wound healing were calculated by Du Noüy (1916a, 1919) from the curves of Carrel and Hartmann (1916) but are less easy to handle than the formula of Billingham and Russel (1956).

Other variables influencing wound healing and contraction are infection, dressing, and the age of the animal. Wounds of older animals heal more slowly than wounds in young animals (Du Noüy, 1916b; Billingham and Russel, 1956). In fact, in fetuses, healing of gaping wounds occurs without granulation tissue formation and wound contraction. This was shown in rats (Dixon, 1960; Goss, 1977), rabbits (Somasundaram and Prathap, 1970, 1972), lambs (Burrington, 1971), oppossums (Block, 1960), and humans (Rowlatt, 1979). The structure and function of myofibroblasts in wound contraction and fibrocontractive diseases are discussed in the following sections.

2. The Myofibroblast

2.1. Ultrastructure and Biochemical Features

The most striking feature of the myofibroblast cytoplasm is a well-developed actin microfilamentous system (Gabbiani et al., 1971a), different from normal fibroblasts, which have few actin microfilaments (Gabbiani and Runger-Brändle, 1981), but similar to the bundles of parallel actin microfilaments found in smooth muscle cells in vivo or in cultured fibroblasts (Fig. 1). Micro-

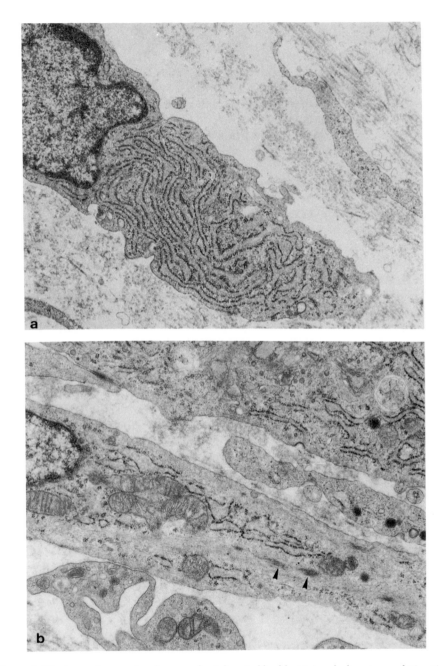

Figure 1. Electron micrographs of a normal rat dermis fibroblast (a) and of a rat granulation tissue myofibroblast 7 days after removal of a 4-cm² skin fragment (b). The main feature of the fibroblast (a) is a regularly arranged rough endoplasmic reticulum. The myofibroblast (b) shows still an abundant rough endoplasmic reticulum with dilated cisternae but in addition, bundles of micro-filaments with dense bodies scattered in between (arrows). (×14,000) (From Gabbiani and Rungger-Brändle, 1981.)

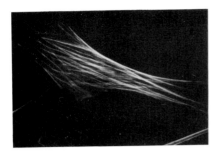

Figure 2. Stress fibers of a rat fibroblast in culture stained with antiactin antibodies. Stress fibers run mostly parallel to the long axis of the cell. (×400)

filaments are usuually arranged parallel to the long axis of the cell. Many electron-opaque areas (dense bodies), similar to the attachment site in smooth muscle or cultured fibroblasts, are scattered among the bundles or located beneath the plasma membrane.

Bundles of microfilaments in cultured fibroblasts have been called stress fibers (Buckley and Porter, 1967) (Fig. 2). They may measure up to 2 μm in diameter and may branch or radiate from focal points (Goldman, 1975). The microfilaments constituting stress fibers contain actin, as shown by decoration with heavy meromyosin (Ishikawa *et al.*, 1969) and by immunofluorescence (Fig. 2) or immunoelectron microscopy with actin antibodies (Goldman *et al.*, 1975; Willingham *et al.*, 1981). A variety of studies using indirect immunofluorescence microscopy has shown that stress fibers contain actin-associated proteins, such as myosin (Fujiwara and Pollard, 1976; Weber and Groeschel-Stuart, 1974), tropomyosin (Lazarides, 1975), α-actinin (Lazarides and Burridge, 1975), and filamin (Wang, 1977). Immunofluorescence studies of the myofibroblast in granulation tissue have shown that it is strongly stained with antiactin and antimyosin antibodies (Gabbiani *et al.*, 1978), a result consistent with the development of a microfilamentous apparatus as seen on electron microscopic examination. Thus, it appears that the myofibroblasts acquire many features of cultured fibroblasts (Gabbiani *et al.*, 1973). Up to now, the mammalian nonmuscle cells in which stress fibers have been noted are myofibroblasts (Gabbiani and Rungger-Brändle, 1981), endothelial cells of large vessels (Gabbiani *et al.*, 1983; White *et al.*, 1983; Wong *et al.*, 1983; Kocher *et al.*, 1985), perineural cells (Ross and Reith, 1969), brain pericytes (Le Beux and Willemot, 1978), and Sertoli cells (Toyama, 1976; Toyama *et al.*, 1979).

The function of stress fibers is unknown. In analogy to *in vitro* situations, stress fibers could play a role in cell–substrate adhesion, since they are well developed in greatly spread stationary cultured fibroblasts and relatively less developed in motile or transformed cells (Herman *et al.*, 1981; Hynes *et al.*, 1982).

Microtubules (for review, see Dustin, 1978) are abundant in myofibroblasts of human and pig granulation tissue and run parallel to the bundles of microfilaments (Rudolph and Woodward, 1978; Rudolph *et al.*, 1977). These investigators have also noted that in old granulation tissue myofibroblasts, microtubules are scarce, but intermediate filaments are particularly prominent.

Intermediate filaments are, along with microfilaments and microtubules, one of the cytoskeletal components of most cells. They are relatively insoluble and have a diameter of about 10 nm. With various techniques, it is possible to distinguish at least five distinct classes of proteins that constitute intermediate filaments in different cells or tissues (for review, see Steinert *et al.*, 1984) including desmin in muscular cells, vimentin in mesenchymal cells, cytokeratins in epithelial cells, neurofilament proteins in neuronal cells, and glial fibrillary acidic protein in glial cells. Intermediate filaments were identified by means of electron microscopy in myofibroblasts present in the stroma of mammary carcinomas and in fibromatoses. Immunofluorescence done with antivimentin, antidesmin, and antiprekeratin antibodies on these tissues showed that these myofibroblasts contain only vimentin (Schürch *et al.*, 1984). Similar results were obtained with myofibroblasts of rat granulation tissue (O. Skalli and G. Gabbiani, unpublished data) (Fig. 3). The meaning of these results with regards to the nature and origin of the myofibroblast is discussed in Section 2.5.

Another prominent feature of the myofibroblast cytoplasm is that it contains packed cisternae of rough endoplasmic reticulum typical of *in vivo* and *in vitro* fibroblasts (Fig. 1). Furthermore, the nuclei consistently show multiple indentations or deep folds, an appearance quite unlike that of normal fibroblasts but reminiscent of smooth muscle cells (and of any other contractile cells) *in vivo*. Nuclear folds have been correlated with cellular contraction in

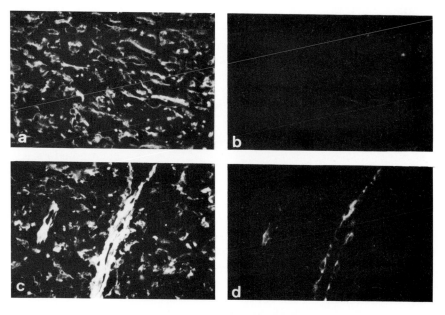

Figure 3. Immunofluorescent staining for vimentin (a,c) and desmin (b,d) of rat granulation tissue 2 weeks after removal of a 4-cm² skin fragment. (a,b) A tissue area containing only myofibroblasts; all myofibroblasts are vimentin positive and desmin negative. (c,d) In addition to the vimentin-containing myofibroblasts, there are also two blood vessels strongly stained for vimentin; some of the cells in the blood vessels wall are however also positive for desmin. (×400)

several systems: smooth muscle (Lane, 1965), myocardium (Bloom and Can-cilla, 1969), venular endothelium (Majno et al., 1969), and striated muscle (Franke and Schinko, 1969). In vitro, the contraction of a sheet of fibroblasts results in a reduction of nuclear length and breadth accompanied by an in-crease in vertical depth (Taylor, 1971).

Several gap junctions between granulation tissue myofibroblasts were found by transmission electron microscopy and freeze etching (Gabbiani et al., 1978). Gap junctions also interconnect cultured fibroblasts (Pinto da Silva and Gilula, 1972) but are not found between normal tissue fibroblasts (Gabbiani and Rungger-Brändle, 1981). In addition, part of the cell surface of the myofibro-blast is often covered by a well-defined layer of material with the structural features of a basal lamina, generally separated from the cell membrane by a translucent layer. Where it is covered by a basal lamina, the cell often shows dense zones in the fibrillar bundles immediately beneath the surface mem-brane. The resulting complex is also found in vivo among endothelial cells, pericytes, and smooth muscle cells, and their basement membranes (Gabbiani et al., 1972a). A peculiar and possibly important connection between myo-fibroblasts and the extracellular matrix, called fibronexus, was described by Singer et al. (1984). The fibronexus was first described by Singer (1979) in cultured fibroblasts and consists of an apparent continuity between intra-cellular actin fibers and extracellular matrix fibers which contain fibronectin (Heggeness et al., 1978). Thus, the fibronexus is a transmembrane complex of intracellular microfilaments and extracellular fibronectin fibers organized into a close 1 : 1 association. At the myofibroblast surface, three kinds of fibronexus observed include (1) plaquelike, (2) tracklike, and (3) tandem associations (Singer et al., 1984). Fibronexus-type complexes were also observed between the extracellular matrix and endothelial cells of embryonic and newborn rats (O. Kocher and G. Gabbiani, unpublished observations) (Fig. 4) or between the extracellular matrix and regenerating aortic endothelial cells (Hüttner et al., 1985). In both cases, endothelial cells show prominent stress fibers as com-pared with normal adult animal endothelial cells.

2.2. Pharmacologic Features

The contractile properties of granulation tissue were studied using various drugs known to act on smooth muscle contraction. Strips of granulation tissue from animal or human wounds contracted or relaxed when exposed to these drugs (Gabbiani et al., 1972a; Majno et al., 1971; Ryan et al., 1974). Control strips of connective tissues (e.g., normal skin) did not react to the various agents tested. Among the substances most active in inducing contraction are serotonin, angiotensin, vasopressin, bradykinin, epinephrine, and prostaglan-din $F_{1\alpha}$. The intensity of the response depended on the origin, age, and initial degree of contraction of the granulation tissue tested. Among the most active relaxing agents are papaverine and prostaglandin E_1 and E_2. (PGE$_1$ and PGE$_2$, respectively). Trocinate (β-diethylaminoethyldiphenylthioacetate), an-

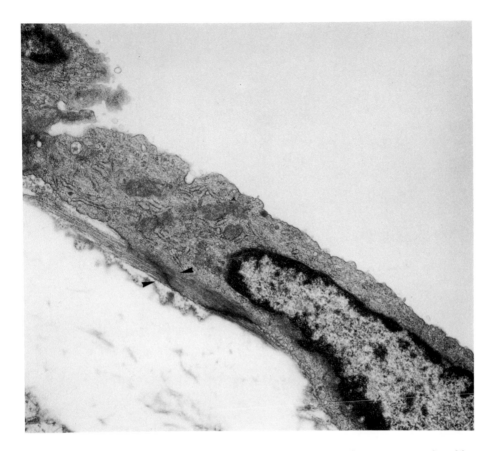

Figure 4. Fibronexus connecting an endothelial cell and the extracellular matrix in a 5-day-old rat. Microfilaments form a thick bundle lying immediately beneath the plasma membrane and in apparently continuity with extracellular fibronectin fibers (arrows). ($\times$10,800) (Courtesy of Dr. O. Kocher, Department of Pathology, University of Geneva.)

other inhibitor of smooth muscle contraction, has been reported to decrease contraction when applied topically on rabbit wounds (Madden *et al.*, 1974).

In the liver of rats with carbon tetrachloride (CCl_4) induced cirrhosis, many myofibroblasts appear, and when strips of cirrhotic liver are exposed to smooth muscle stimulating agents they develop a significant contractile response as compared with strips of normal liver (Irle *et al.*, 1980) (Fig. 5). A severe myofibroblastic fibrosis is also developed in the lungs of bleomycin injected rats and, when strips of these fibrotic lungs are exposed to acetylcholine (ACh), epinephrine, and a K^+ depolarizing solution, the force of contraction is approximately twice that of normal lung strips (Evans *et al.*, 1982).

The relative reactivity of myofibroblasts from different organs to various stimulating agents may be different; thus, ACh causes contraction of strips of fibrotic lungs, but not of granulation tissue from a skin wound or a granuloma

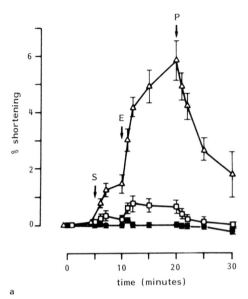

a

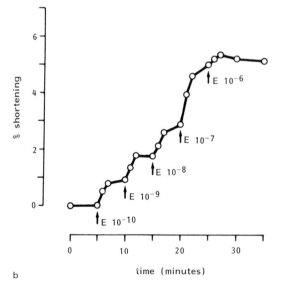

b

Figure 5. *In vitro* contraction of different liver strips in response to various pharmacologic agents. (a) Response to serotonin (S, 10^{-5} g/ml), epinephrine (E, 10^{-7} mg/ml), and papaverine (P, 2×10^{-4} mg/ml) of (1) strips of cirrhotic liver after 5 months of CCl_4 treatment ($\triangle$), (2) normal control liver ($\blacksquare$), and (3) regenerative liver 13 days after partial hepatectomy ($\square$). (b) The contraction of strips of cirrhotic livers (5 months after CCl_4 treatment) increases with increasing doses of epinephrine (10^{-10}–10^{-6} mg/ml). (From Irle *et al.*, 1980.)

pouch; serotonin causes the retraction of strips for granuloma pouch, but not strips from a skin wound (Gabbiani *et al.*, 1972a). In addition to the heterogeneity in drug response among granulation tissue strips from different origins, there are differences between the response of granulation tissue strips and that of classic smooth muscle preparations (Gabbiani *et al.*, 1972a). Thus, granulation tissue strips reach their peak of contraction slower and maintain it longer than do strips of smooth muscle. In addition, smooth muscle contracts in response to $BaCl_2$, but granulation tissue strips fail to do so.

Drugs known to interact with cytoskeletal components can influence the spontaneous or drug-induced contraction of granulation tissue. Cytochalasin B, an actin–depolymerizing drug (Korn, 1982; Wessels et al., 1971), causes a slight relaxation of granulation tissue strip and inhibits contraction due to serotonin or angiotensin (Gabbiani et al., 1972a). Ehrlich et al. (1977) reported that colchicine, a microtubule-disrupting agent (Owellen et al., 1972), inhibits wound contraction when applied topically. However, Rudolph et al. (1981) attributed the inhibition of wound contraction by colchicine to a toxic rather than a specific effect on myofibroblast structure or function.

2.3. Factors Influencing Wound Contraction and Role of Myofibroblasts in Wound Contraction

The literature on acceleration and inhibition of wound healing by topical treatments with various tissue extracts, hormones, vitamins, and drugs is far too voluminous to be discussed extensively here. Unfortunately, conflicting results have been obtained with the same agent when tested under different experimental conditions. Moreover, parameters investigated in order to assess wound healing are often different or are not sufficiently precise to be quantified.

Studies on the role of saliva in wound healing may be taken as an example of confusing results. Hutson et al. (1979) observed that the wound-contraction rate is significantly increased in mice housed in groups of five to eight, as compared with mice caged individually. Since removal of salivary glands abrogated this effect, it was suggested that mouse salivary glands produce a factor accelerating wound contraction. Li et al. (1980b) identified this factor as being nerve growth factor (HMW-NGF) and found that it stimulated the rate of wound contraction in mice. However, Leitzel et al. (1982) reported later that murine HMW-NGF has no effect on time of wound healing in hamsters.

Skin autograft is the most recognized means to inhibit wound contraction in rabbits, rats, and humans (Billingham and Russel, 1956; Rudolph and Klein, 1973). The inhibition is effective when grafting is done immediately after the wound or later when granulation tissue has already been formed (delayed skin graft). Covering of the wound by epithelial layers alone fails to prevent wound contraction, suggesting that the inhibitory effect of skin graft lay in the dermis of grafted skin. Skin grafts with complete dermis (full-thickness skin grafts) are more effective than grafts in which basal dermal layers are removed (split-thickness grafts). This effect is not dependent on the thickness of the graft but on the integrity of the dermis, since wound-contraction inhibition is higher with full-thickness grafts thinner than split thickness grafts (Rudolph, 1976). These findings suggest that there may be some special physical or biochemical features in the deep portions of the dermis compared with more superficial portions that explain these differences. Full-thickness skin autografts produce resorption of granulation tissue through an accelerated loss of cells and extra-cellular matrix; however the mechanisms of the tissue loss are unknown (Do-noff and Grillo, 1975). In related studies, Bell et al. (1981) grafted a collagen lattice, containing fibroblasts within the matrix and epidermal cells on the surface, onto the donor of the cells. The graft did not elicit a homograft re-sponse and inhibited wound contraction.

In surgical practice, cryosurgery is known to create relatively little wound contraction (Li et al., 1980a; Shepherd and Dawber, 1984). Freeze injury kills cells but does not completely destroy the connective tissue matrix, which becomes populated by migrating fibroblasts (Ehrlich and Hembry, 1984). To our knowledge, ultrastructural studies have not been done on these fibroblasts to see whether they have features of myofibroblasts. Thus, the reason that cryosurgical wounds do not contract remains uncertain. Billingham and Russel (1956) observed that even frozen dried grafts reduce wound contraction; thus, one wonders whether lack of contraction after a freeze injury is due to mecha-nisms similar to those responsible for inhibition of wound contraction by a skin graft.

The role of myofibroblasts in wound contraction could be further clarified by studies correlating the presence and features of these cells when the rate of wound contraction is modified. Up to now, the ultrastructural, biochemical, and pharmacologic characteristics of myofibroblasts have made them good candidates for the agents responsible for wound contraction. Other candidates are vascular smooth muscle cells and pericytes present in granulation tissue and epidermal cells regenerating over the wound (Baur et al., 1984). However, avascular myofibroblastic tissue introduced in the rat peritoneal cavity exhib-ited contractile properties and drug responses similar to vascularized granula-tion tissue (Ryan et al., 1973). Additional support for the view that vascular smooth muscle cells play a minor role in wound contraction comes from the planimetric observations of Evans et al. (1982). In these studies, the percentage of total tissue area occupied by airways and vascular smooth muscle cells in contractile strips of fibrotic lung did not differ from that of the control lung.

That myofibroblasts by themselves are able to produce forces strong enough to contract wounds is also suggested by a variety of experiments carried out on in vitro fibroblasts, which are structurally similar to in vivo myo-fibroblasts. For instance, serotonin caused contraction of cultured fibroblasts (Majno et al., 1971). Two explants of chicken bone, connected by outgrowths of fibroblasts, draw toward each other as the interconnected fibroblast sheet con-tracts (James and Taylor, 1969). Furthermore, fibroblasts added to polymerized fibrin cause retraction of the fibrin gel in a process similar to platelet-induced clot retraction (Niewiarovski et al., 1972). This phenomenon is inhibited by cytochalasin B and PGE_1 (Niewiarovski and Goldstein, 1973). Bell et al. (1979) showed that fibroblasts incorporated into a collagen lattice cause its contrac-tion, and that the rate of this process is inversely related to the collagen con-centration and directly dependent on cell number. In studies extending the analysis of this in vitro wound-contraction model, fibroblast elongation within the collagen lattice correlated with effective contraction of the lattice (Buttle and Ehrlich, 1983). Furthermore, the collagen lattice contraction is dependent on the tissue origin of the fibroblasts (Bellows et al., 1981). Contraction is suboptimal when SV-40 transformed fibroblasts and fibroblasts from patients with Glanzmann's thrombasthenia (Steinberg et al., 1980) or epidermolysis bullosa dystrophica (Ehrlich and White, 1983) are incorporated into the gel. Interestingly, transformed cells in general have fewer stress fibers than normal cells (Pollack et al., 1975). Tissue repair and fibroblast-induced clot retraction are impaired in Glanzmann's thrombasthenia (Remuzzi et al., 1977; Donati et al., 1977). Fibroblasts of patients with epidermolysis bullosa dystrophica have increased levels of PGE_2 (Ehrlich and White, 1983), known to inhibit the contraction of granulation tissue strips in vitro (Gabbiani et al., 1972a). Cytochalasin B inhibits contraction of collagen lattice by fibroblasts, suggesting a role for microfilaments in the contracting process (Bell et al., 1979). Other reported inhibitors are soluble products of chronic inflammatory cells, which act probably by inducing PGE_2 synthesis by fibroblasts (Ehrlich and Wyler, 1983).

Ultrastructural studies done on fibroblasts incorporated into a collagen lattice showed that they change their phenotype during collagen lattice contraction (Bellows et al., 1982). During the active phase of contraction, fibroblasts exhibited numerous stress fibers and gap junctions. When the collagen gel was fully compacted, however, they changed into a more synthetic phenotype characterized by fewer microfilament bundles and gap junctions and more endoplasmic reticulum. This interesting example of a transition between two cellular isoforms also indicates that stress fibers and intracellular contacts play an important role in fibroblast-induced collagen lattice contraction.

Evidence that stress fibers are probably the force generating element in wound contraction includes (1) glycerol-extracted fibroblasts and stress fibers dissected from rat adenocarcinoma cells contract upon addition of adenosine triphosphatase (ATP) (Hoffmann-Berling, 1954; Isenberg et al., 1976; for review, see Burridge, 1981); and (2) studies of rhodamine-labeled smooth muscle α-actinin microinjected into living fibroblasts, visualized by video-intensified fluorescence microscopy showed that stress fibers are functionally analogous to skeletal muscle fibrils (Kreis and Birchmeier, 1980).

It is conceivable that wound contraction and scar formation involve traction forces rather than true contraction forces. The traction forces exerted by fibroblasts on their substrate are strong enough to distort a sheet of silicon rubber and are weakest in SV-40 transformed cells, leukocytes, and glial cells (Harris et al., 1981). Traction forces have been proposed as responsible for connective tissue morphogenesis and for the formation of tendons and capsule of organs. Traction forces are shearing forces tangential to the cell surface that are exerted by cell spreading and elongation; they should be distinguished from contraction, which involves shortening of the cell (Stopak and Harris, 1982).

Whatever the forces exerted by myofibroblasts, they need to be transmitted to the surrounding connective tissue. Fibronexus (Singer et al., 1984) is probably the key structure in that passive transduction. Gap junctions between myofibroblasts (Gabbiani et al.. 1978) represent the major pathway for the synchronization of contractile and/or retractile activities of these cells.

2.4. Distribution of Myofibroblasts in Normal and Pathologic Tissues

On the basis of ultrastructural studies, myofibroblasts have been observed in tissues during normal and pathologic conditions. In normal conditions, myofibroblasts were found in the external theca of the rat ovarian follicle (O'Shea, 1970); in the human ganglia of the wrist (Ghadially and Mehta, 1971); in the rat duodenal villi (Guldner et al., 1972); in the rat and mouse adrenal gland capsule (Bressler, 1973); in the rat, human, lamb, and monkey pulmonary alveolar septa (Kapanci et al., 1974); in the rat testicular capsule (Gorgas and Böck, 1974); in bovine endometrial caruncle (Tabone et al., 1983) and in the peridontal ligament of rats (Beertsen et al., 1974) and mice (Beertsen, 1975), where they may provide the forces necessary for tooth eruption.

Pathologic conditions in which myofibroblasts are found fall into at least three groups (for review, see Seemayer et al., 1980a, 1981). One group includes situations related to inflammation, wound healing, and tissue remodeling. These include human liver cirrhosis (Bhatal, 1972; Rudolph et al., 1979), experimental liver cirrhosis induced by carbon tetrachloride (Irle et al., 1980), tenosynovitis (Madden, 1973), burn contracture (Larson et al., 1974), kidney fibrosis (Nagle et al., 1973, 1975), pulmonary sarcoidosis (Judd et al., 1975), ischemic contracture of intrinsic muscle of the hand (Madden et al., 1975), hypertrophic scars (Baur et al., 1975), granuloma (El-Labban and Lee, 1983; Roland, 1976), hepatic schistosomial fibrosis (Grimaud and Borojevic, 1977), and pulmonary fibrosis (Adler et al., 1981), regenerating tendon (Postacchini et al., 1977), fibrous capsule around mammary implants (Rudolph et al., 1978; Zimman et al., 1978), liver nodular hyperplasia (Callea et al., 1982), and cataract (Novotny and Pau, 1984). Another group includes fibromatoses, which are fibroblastic proliferative lesions without prominent inflammatory component nor evidence of malignant neoplastic transformation. These include Dupuytren's contracture (Chiu and McFarlane, 1978; Gabbiani and Majno, 1972; Gelberman et al., 1980; Gokel and Hübner, 1977; Hueston et al., 1976; James and Odom, 1980; Meister et al., 1979; Navas-Palacios, 1983), the related La Peyronie's nodule (Ariyan et al., 1978), and plantar fibromatosis or Ledderhose's disease (Gabbiani and Majno, 1972). Some other fibromatoses in which myofibroblasts have been demonstrated are giant cell fibroma of oral mucosa (Weathers and Campbell, 1974), dermatofibroma (Stiller and Katenkamp, 1975), nodular fasciitis (Wirman, 1976), circumscribed fibromatosis (Feiner and Kaye, 1976), mesenchymal hamartoma (Benjamin et al., 1977), uterine plexiform tumor (Fisher et al., 1978), elastofibroma (Ramos et al., 1978), digital fibroma of infancy (Bhawan et al., 1979; Iwasaki et al., 1980), pseudomalignant myositis ossificans (Povysil and Matejovsky, 1979), and cardiac fibromatosis (Turi et al., 1980). The third group involves the stromal response to neoplasia, which is often inflammatory but is sometimes constituted by a vigorous proliferative reaction of myofibroblasts (Seemayer et al., 1980b), known as desmoplasia.

Myofibroblastic desmoplasia was observed in the stroma of invasive carcinoma of breast and pancreas (Martinez-Hernandez et al., 1977; Ohtani and Sasano, 1980; Schürch et al., 1982; Tremblay, 1979), tubular carcinoma of the breast (Harris and Ahmed, 1977), male breast carcinoma (Hassan and Olaizola, 1979), and large bowel carcinoma (Balazs and Kovacs, 1982). A retrospective ultrastructural study of the stroma in a wide variety of carcinomas showed that myofibroblasts are commonly present in the stroma of primary invasive carcinomas and of metastatic carcinomas and are more prominent in neoplasms associated with retraction (Schürch et al., 1981; Seemayer et al., 1979). This raises two important questions: What factor(s) is (are) responsible for the myofibroblastic stromal response? and What is the meaning of this response for tumor progression? According to Seemayer et al. (1980a), epithelial invasion beyond the basal lamina could be one of the factors necessary to evoke myofibroblastic response.

Myofibroblasts have also been described in sarcomas, where they generally constitute a small fraction of the cellular population (Gabbiani et al., 1971b, 1972b; Merkow et al., 1971). In Hodgkin's disease, particularly in the nodular sclerosis type, numerous myofibroblasts were observed, and it was proposed that they may serve to reduce vascular invasion by neoplastic cells (Seemayer et al., 1981). By contrast, no myofibroblasts were described in non-Hodgkin's malignant lymphomas (Levine and Dorfman, 1975).

Finally, there are some reports of malignant myofibroblastic tumors (Blewitt et al., 1983; Churg and Kahn, 1977; D'Andiran and Gabbiani, 1980; Ghadially et al., 1983; Stiller and Katenkamp, 1975; Vasudev and Harris, 1978). However, the existence of true myofibroblastic sarcomas has been questioned since tumoral fibroblasts always exhibit some myofibroblastic features (Seemayer et al., 1980a).

2.5. Cellular Origin

The origin of granulation tissue fibroblasts has been debated for a long time. Cohnheim (1867) introduced the vascular theory proposing that leukocytes become transformed into fibroblasts during the process of repair. Numerous other studies, however, have suggested that blood cells do not have the capacity to transform into fibroblasts and that granulation tissue fibroblasts arise from local connective tissue cells. These antagonist theories were reviewed several times (Allgöwer, 1956; Arey, 1936; Grillo, 1964). Clues for the local origin of granulation tissue fibroblasts came from the sequential autoradiographic experiments of MacDonald (1959) and from the X-irradiation and autoradiographic experiments of Grillo (1963). A convincing refutation of the vascular theory came from Ross et al. (1970), who showed in parabiotic rats that blood cells labeled with [³H]thymidine do not transform into granulation tissue fibroblasts. The question remains open as to whether granulation tissue fibroblasts arise from any mesenchymal cell present in dermis and subcutaneous tissue such as fibroblasts, pericytes, and smooth muscle (Crocker et al., 1970).

The fibroblast origination of the myofibroblast has been a question at least partially clarified by characterizing myofibroblast cytoskeletal proteins such as vimentin (Schürch et al., 1984, Woodcock-Mitchell et al. 1984). Recent studies

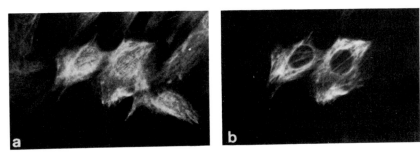

Figure 6. Double immunofluorescent staining of rat medial vascular smooth muscle cell after 4 days of culture. (a) Vimentin. (b) Desmin. All cells are positive for vimentin, but only some also for desmin. Intermediate filaments pattern consists of a perinuclear network of fibers extending to the cell periphery. (×630)

indicate that the cytoskeletal elements desmin, keratin, and vimentin are good markers for determining whether cells are of muscle, epithelial, or mesenchymal lineage, respectively (for review, see Moll et al., 1982; Osborn and Weber. 1982; Rungger-Brändle and Gabbiani, 1983). Neoplastic and fast-growing cells maintain the intermediate filament proteins of the cells from which they derive (for review, see Gabbiani and Kocher, 1983; Gown and Gabbiani, 1984; Osborn and Weber, 1983). Thus, an epidermal tumor metastasis will express cytokeratins, a mesenchymal tumor metastasis will express vimentin, and muscle tissue tumor metastasis will express desmin (Moll et al., 1982; Osborn and Weber, 1983; Rungger-Brändle and Gabbiani, 1983). However, the origin of a mesenchymal cell is more difficult to solve unambiguously by means of intermediate filament analysis, because different cells (e.g., macrophages and fibroblasts) contain the same intermediate filament protein (vimentin). Moreover, cells of the same origin (e.g., smooth muscle cells) may contain two different intermediate filament proteins in different proportions. For instance, vascular smooth muscle cells, although they appear similar ultrastructurally, may express either vimentin alone or vimentin and desmin (Gabbiani et al., 1981; Travo et al., 1982) (Fig. 6). Thus, the fact that myofibroblasts from the stroma of breast carcinoma or from experimental granulation tissue contain only vimentin (Schürch, 1984) (see Section 2.1) unfortunately does not permit unequivocal determination of their origin. In rat granulation tissue, however, desmin-positive cells are found only around the vessels (O. Skalli and G. Gabbiani, unpublished data) (Fig. 3). Because of their location, these desmin-positive cells may be pericytes or smooth muscle cells but certainly are not myofibroblasts.

Actin isoforms have been proposed as useful markers to distinguish between smooth muscle and fibroblastic tissues (Skalli et al., 1987). During evolution, the actin primary sequence was strongly conserved; however, biochemical microheterogeneity has been observed in actins from different tissues (Vandekerckhove and Weber, 1984). These tissue-specific rather than species-specific differences are mainly localized in the 17-amino terminal aminoacids

(Vandekerckhove and Weber, 1981). In mammals, three actin isoforms having different isoelectric points were described by means of two-dimensional gel electrophoresis: α, β, and γ (Garrels and Gibson, 1976; Whalen *et al.*, 1976). Sequencing studies have shown that there are three actin isoforms having an α-electrophoretic mobility, one specific to the striated muscle, one specific to the myocardium, and one specific to smooth muscle (Vanderkerckhove and Weber, 1979). β- and γ-actins correspond to two forms of actin found in every cell, hence are called cytoplasmic actins. In addition, a sixth isoform present in smooth muscle migrates like the γ-cytoplasmic and is referred to as γ-smooth muscle actin (Vandekerckhove and Weber, 1978). Two-dimensional gel electrophoresis of different mesenchymal tissues shows that smooth muscle cells always express the three isoforms although in different proportions, while fibroblastic cells always express only β- and γ-actins in a constant ratio (Skalli *et al.*, 1987). Modulation of the pattern of actin-isoform expression can occur during *in vivo* or *in vitro* conditions (Gabbiani *et al.*, 1984) but even when modulated by pathologic or *in vitro* conditions, smooth muscle cells keep α-, β-, and γ-actins while fibroblasts only show β- and γ-actins. Thus, the presence of α-actin in a tissue or a cell population marks its muscular origin. When applied to rat granulation tissue, two-dimensional gel electrophoresis always shows β- and γ-actins in proportions similar to those found in fibroblastic tissues, a result that strongly indicates the fibroblastic origin of granulation tissue myofibroblastic population (Skalli *et al.*, 1987) (Fig. 7).

The absence of α-smooth muscle actin in myofibroblasts of human and experimental granulation tissue was confirmed by immunofluorescence using a monoclonal antibody specific for α-smooth muscle actin (Skalli *et al.*, 1986a). Surprisingly, stromal cells of breast carcinomas, described as myofibroblasts (see Section 2.4), were stained with this anti-α-actin antibody, unlike stromal cells of the normal breast and typical myofibroblasts of human and experimental granulation tissue (Skalli *et al.*, 1986a). Whether this biochemical heterogeneity among myofibroblasts reflects a separate origin and engagement in different differentiation pathways is unknown (see also Section 2.7).

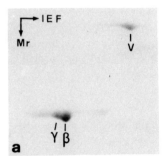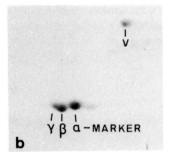

Figure 7. Two-dimensional gel of 15-day-old granulation tissue. (a) Without α-actin marker. (b) With α-actin marker. Granulation tissue contains only β- and γ-actin isoforms, a feature characteristic of fibroblastic tissues compared with smooth muscle tissues. V, vimentin; IEF, direction of the isoelectric gel; M, direction of the SDS-PAGE.

2.6. The Myofibroblast in Culture

There are only a few reports on cells from granulation tissue grown in culture. Ivaska (1973) established a technique to grow cells from experimental rat granuloma by enzymatic digestion. The isolated cells synthesized collagen and glycosaminoglycans and appeared fibroblastic when spread on a petri dish. Unfortunately, no electron microscopic data were provided for these cells. Ultrastructural features and growth dynamics of granulation tissue myofibroblasts and dermal fibroblasts grown from explants were described by Van de Berg et al. (1984). Cultured myofibroblasts have ultrastructural features similar to those found in vivo. Early passage myofibroblasts grow more slowly and possess more microfilament bundles than early passage dermal fibroblasts. However, late passage myofibroblasts and dermal fibroblasts exhibit similar ultrastructure and growth patterns.

When a wound has healed, the granulation tissue is replaced by a scar; interestingly, scar fibroblasts have a shorter in vitro life span, a longer cell population doubling time, and a lower percentage of cells able to incorporate tritiated thymidine than comparable fibroblasts derived from normal dermis (Yamamoto et al., 1982). The diminished proliferative capacity of scar-derived fibroblasts may depend on decreased proliferation capacity acquired during the process of wound repair, as suggested by the fact that early passage myofibroblasts grow more slowly than dermal fibroblasts.

Myofibroblastic cells are also found in fibromatoses such as Dupuytren's disease or La Peyronie's disease (see Section 2.4). When grown from explants, myofibroblasts from Dupuytren's disease exhibit growth properties that are intermediate between those of fibroblasts derived from normal aponeurosis and embryonic or virus transformed fibroblasts (Azzarone et al., 1983) (Table I). In contrast to normal fibroblasts, the cells from Dupuytren's nodules are able to grow in reduced amount of fetal calf serum and produce a high level of the urokinase-like species of plasminogen activator, two characteristics of transformed cells. An enhanced proliferative capacity was also observed when cells grown from explants of La Peyronie's disease were compared to cells grown from explants of normal penile tissue (Somers et al., 1982).

Taken together, these data indicate that when grown in vitro, myofibroblasts from different origins have different growth properties despite their similar ultrastructure. This may be relevant to understanding the biology of the myofibroblast.

2.7. The Myofibroblast Compared with the Fibroblast and the Smooth Muscle Cell

Ultrastructural studies have shown that in vivo myofibroblasts with structural features intermediate between those of fibroblasts and of smooth muscle cells are found in a wide variety of normal and pathologic conditions (Gabbiani et al., 1971a). Tissues in which myofibroblasts are the main cell type exhibit

Table I. Growth Properties of Human Fibroblastic Cell Lines[a]

Cell line	964-S	NMS$_1$	BMS7	DUP-A	DUP-N	DUP-N-SV40	KHOS/NP
Life-span (number of PDs)	45	41	16	30	28	32 up to now	Infinite
Total number of cells produced	NT	NT	NT	27.3×10^6	27.9×10^6	49×10^{6c}	NT
Cells synthesizing DNA at the plateau phase	2.5%	1%	2%	1.5%	2%	54%	42%
Interferon sensitivity (antiviral titer)[b]	>64,000	NT	NT	>64,000	>64,000	600	800
Fibrin clot retraction	100%	100%	100%	100%	100%	<1%	<1%
Formation of spontaneous aggregates in suspension	Negative	Negative	Negative	Negative	Positive	Positive	Positive
Growth in soft agar (number of colonies/Petri dish)	0	0	0	0	80	1600	6000
Colony formation on human epithelial sheet	0	0	0	1%	1%	15%	70%
Number of PDs performed in 2% FCS	1	0	0	2	2	4	3
Response to 1 : 1 split	−3%	−3%	+3%	+59%	+66%	NT	NT
Production of plasminogen activator	Negative	Negative	Negative	Negative	1.2 U×10^6 cells/hr	5.3 U×10^6 cells/hr	1.33 U×10^6 cells/hr

[a]From Azzarone et al. (1983). 964-S, normal embryonic skin; NMS$_1$ and BMS7, normal adult skin; DUP-A, normal aponeurosis; DUP-N, Dupuytren's Nodule; DUP-N-SV40, Dupuytren's Nodule after transformation with SV40; and KHOS/NP, sarcoma.
[b]Reciprocal dilution.
[c]After 28 PDs.

biologic properties similar to smooth muscle tissues in their ability to retract spontaneously *in vivo* and to contract or to relax *in vitro* upon stimulation by certain drugs. We and others (Bellows *et al.*, 1982; Gabbiani *et al.*, 1973) have noted that myofibroblasts possess many ultrastructural characteristics in common with cultured fibroblasts, such as great quantities of rough endoplasmic reticulum and bundles of actin filaments.

The question arises as to whether smooth muscle cells can acquire myofibroblastic features under certain circumstances. Although no systematic study has investigated this possibility, many observations suggest that smooth muscle tissues may contain cells with some ultrastructural characteristics in common with myofibroblasts. *In vitro*, cultured vascular smooth muscle cells develop characteristics corresponding to a morphologic "synthetic" phenotype, as compared to the "contractile" phenotype generally present *in vivo* (Chamley-Campbell *et al.*, 1979). *In vivo*, smooth muscle cells with a phenotype similar to the *in vitro* "synthetic" phenotype were reported in the normal chicken aortic media (Moss and Benditt, 1970), in the human myometrium during pregnancy (Laguens and Lagrutta, 1964), in rat myometrium after estrogen treatment (Ross and Klebanoff, 1967), in the developing rat aortic media (Kocher *et al.*, 1985; Olivetti *et al.*, 1980), and in rat aortic experimental thickening induced by endothelial injury (Kocher *et al.*, 1984; Poole *et al.*, 1971) (Fig. 8).

Thus, it seems that *in vivo*, as well as *in vitro*, fibroblasts or smooth muscle cells can be modulated into cell types having ultrastructural features more or less similar to that of granulation tissue myofibroblasts. These phenotypic modulations may be viewed as isoformic transitions, according to Caplan *et al.* (1983) who defined the transition as "the replacement of individual molecules and cells by molecular and cellular variants called isoforms because they are both similar and distinctly different; these arise and function during embryonic development or later life." Caplan *et al.* (1983) took myosin heavy chains and actin as examples of molecular isoforms, and chondrocytes and osteoclasts as examples of cellular isoforms; they also discussed the question of isoformic transitions during striated muscle development and concluded that transitions involve orderly replacement of discrete cellular or molecular types by the generation of new functioning units, either of cellular or molecular type. Developmental isoformic transitions were then compared to physiologic transitions. During developmental transitions, an external stimulus results in the synthesis of a new set of macromolecules, but when the stimulus is withdrawn the cell does not return to its original phenotype. In contrast, a physiologic transition is reversible (e.g., the action of a hormone can cause synthesis of new molecules, but when the hormone is removed, the target cell will usually shift back to the original pattern of synthesis). Analogous with these concepts, we could define pathologic isoformic transitions as transitions induced by a pathologic stimulus and not reverted by the removal of this stimulus. In evaluating pathologic transitions, it should be kept in mind that pathologic stimuli can persist over a long period of time, leading to situations which may appear irreversible but in actuality are reversible.

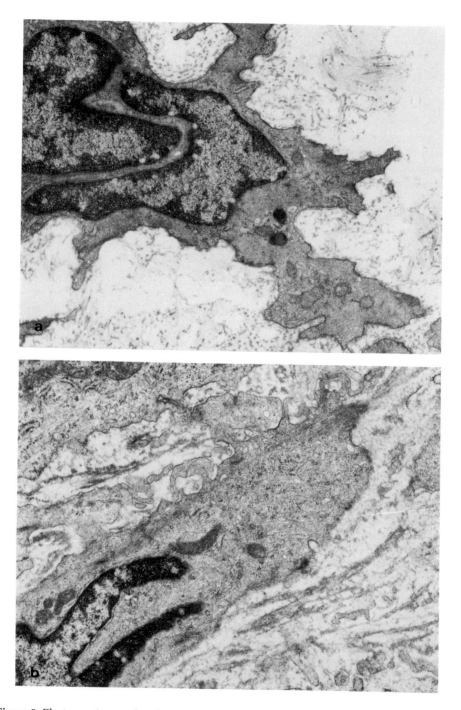

Figure 8. Electron micrographs of (a) rat aortic smooth muscle cell and (b) smooth muscle cells compared with the intima 15 days after endothelial injury. (a) The normal smooth muscle cell shows abundant bundles of microfilaments and only few cisternae of rough endoplasmic reticulum. (b) The intimal smooth muscle cell 15 days after endothelial injury shows an ultrastructure reminiscent of that of the myofibroblast (see Fig. 1b). (×13,000)

Thus, cells having ultrastructural characteristics intermediate between those of fibroblasts and those of smooth muscle cells may be considered cellular isoforms induced by pathologic transitions. During these pathologic transitions, changes in protein isoforms may occur as shown for actin and myosin during the development of experimental and human atheromatosis (Gabbiani et al., 1984; Kocher et al., 1984; Larson et al., 1984a) or during culture of vascular smooth muscle cells (Larson et al., 1984b; Skalli et al., 1986b). Cells having similar ultrastructural features but expressing different protein isoforms can also be considered cellular isoforms. This is the case of vascular smooth muscle cells which may express either vimentin or vimentin and desmin (Gabbiani et al., 1981; Travo et al., 1982) and of myofibroblasts from different lesions which may differ in their actin isoform content (see Section 2.5). These variations in the isoform content may reflect subtle functional differences between cell types of similar ultrastructure. Thus, the study of protein isoforms may be useful for understanding the relationships between different cell types and their respective biology.

Another important point is that fibroblasts and smooth muscle cells grown in culture resemble the myofibroblast counterpart in many respects; this has been shown for vascular smooth muscle cells (Kocher et al., 1984; Kocher et al., 1985; Skalli et al., 1986b) and suggested for fibroblasts (Gabbiani and Rungger-Brändle, 1981; Gabbiani et al., 1973; Guber and Rudolph, 1978) (see Section 2.1). It is tempting to speculate that when placing fibroblasts and smooth muscle cells in culture, one mimics a pathologic transition.

In conclusion, it appears useful to utilize the generic term "myofibroblast" to designate fibroblastic cells having in vivo contractile and synthetic characteristics. A challenging question is whether a myofibroblastic cell represents only an adaptation to pathologic stimuli or whether it also represents an "ancestor" from which fibroblastic and smooth muscle cells develop, and into which normal fibroblasts and smooth muscle cells can dedifferentiate in the adult animal under certain conditions. The last hypothesis may shed new light on the understanding of myofibroblastic pathology.

3. Conclusions

The myofibroblast is a cell with both contractile and synthetic features which generates in vivo forces responsible for wound contraction (Gabbiani et al., 1971a). This is suggested by pharmacologic experiments and by studies done with cultured fibroblasts, which share many structural and biochemical features with in vivo myofibroblasts. Fibroblasts grown in culture exert traction rather than contraction forces on their substrate (Stopak and Harris, 1982). It is likely that myofibroblasts promote granulation tissue contraction also by exerting tractional forces on the surrounding connective tissue, but this remains to be shown in situ.

At the cellular level, stress fibers are presumably the force-generating element, as shown for in vitro fibroblasts (Kreis and Birchmeier, 1980). These forces are probably transduced to the extracellular matrix through the fibronexus, a device linking together stress fibers and collagen via fibronectin (Singer *et al.*, 1984). In addition, myofibroblasts may synchronize their action through gap junctions (Gabbiani *et al.*, 1978) which are classically known to be sites of electrotonic and biochemical coupling. Collagen lattice contraction by fibroblasts may be advantageously investigated as a model for granulation tissue retraction (Bell *et al.*, 1979), since this *in vitro* system is closer to the *in vivo* situation than fibroblasts grown in a petri dish.

Factors producing and regulating granulation tissue contraction *in vivo* are presently unknown. They may be cellular mediators such as serotonin or prostaglandin, or extracellular matrix components or mechanical forces. Studies on the inhibition of wound contraction by skin grafts may help clarify the nature of these factors. In any event, classical and artificial grafts are presently the most useful means to inhibit wound contraction (Bell *et al.*, 1981).

Classical experiments suggest that myofibroblasts originate locally within the affected connective tissue (MacDonald, 1959; Ross *et al.*, 1970). The use of protein markers, such as actin isoforms or intermediate filament proteins, suggests that myofibroblasts arise from fibroblasts (Schürch *et al.*, 1984; Skalli *et al.*, 1986a, 1987). The discovery of the origin of myofibroblasts may be important in understanding their mechanisms of action.

Myofibroblasts have been described in several pathologic situations such as granulation tissue, hypertrophic scars, fibromatosis, and tumor stroma, but they have also been described in some normal conditions where they may play a relevant physiologic role as well. Transition from fibroblast to myofibroblast is probably reversible, at least during normal wound healing, but the factor(s) inducing this transition is still unknown. Platelet-derived growth factor (Vogel *et al.*, 1980; see Chapter 9), fibroblast growth factor (Gospodarowicz, 1975; see Chapter 11), and type β transforming growth factor (Sporn *et al.*, 1983; see Chapter 12) are presently good candidates for the stimulation of myofibroblast production; however, nothing is known about factors which regulate the disappearance of myofibroblasts during scar formation. Further work along these lines may be useful in understanding the mechanism of scar formation, pathologic wound healing, and fibromatosis development.

Ultrastructurally similar myofibroblasts developing in different organs or tissues may have different biologic properties such as different responses to drugs (see Section 2.2), different biochemical markers (see Section 2.5), and different growth activation patterns *in vitro* (see Section 2.6). These cells may be considered "cellular isoforms" of a common cell type. Myofibroblasts are ultrastructurally similar to the "synthetic" smooth muscle cell phenotype found in various conditions (Poole *et al.*, 1971; Chamley-Campbell *et al.*, 1979). However, it should be stressed that myofibroblasts and "synthetic" smooth muscle cells differ from each other in their biochemical phenotype. Presently, we have no substantial information on the developmental relationships between myofibroblasts, "synthetic" smooth muscle cells, fibroblasts, and smooth muscle cells. In any event, it seems that the appearance of a cell type having contractile and synthetic features is common in different responses to injury, such as granulation tissue and atheromatous plaque formation.

In the embryo and the fetus, smooth muscle cells share several features with the fibroblast and vice versa (Greenlee and Ross, 1967; Ross and Greenlee, 1966; Kocher et al., 1985; Olivetti et al., 1980). Thus, it is possible that both in vivo, during pathologic conditions, and in culture, fibroblasts and smooth muscle cells dedifferentiate toward a cellular isotype present during development, thus performing functions which are not normally exerted by these cells in adult animals. Study of the signals stimulating fibroblast and smooth muscle cell differentiation and modulation and of the mechanisms of these phenomena in vitro and in vivo may help elucidate the biological features and functions of myofibroblasts.

References

Abercrombie, M., Flint, M. H., and James, D. W., 1956, Wound contraction in relation to collagen formation in scorbutic guinea pigs, J. Embryol. Exp. Morphol. **4**:167–175.

Adler, K. B., Craighead, J. E., Vallyathan, N. V., and Evans, J. N., 1981, Actin-containing cells in human pulmonary fibrosis, Am. J. Pathol. **102**:427–437.

Allgöwer, M., 1956, The Cellular Basis of Wound Repair, Charles C Thomas, Springfield, Illinois.

Arey, L. B., 1936, Wound healing, Physiol. Rev. **16**:327–406.

Ariyan, S., Enriquez, R., and Krizek, T. J., 1978, Wound contraction and fibrocontractive disorders, Arch. Surg. **113**:1034–1046.

Azzarone, B., Failly-Crepin, C., Daya-Grosjean, L., Chaponnier, C., and Gabbiani, G., 1983, Abnormal behavior of cultured fibroblasts from nodule and nonaffected aponeurosis of Dupuytren's disease, J. Cell Physiol. **117**:353–361.

Balazs, M., and Kovacs, A., 1982, The "transitional" mucosa adjacent to large bowel carcinoma—Electron microscopic features and myofibroblast reaction, Histopathology **6**:617–629.

Baur, P. S., Larson, D. L., and Stacey, T. R., 1975, The observation of myofibroblasts in hypertrophic scars, Surg. Gynecol. Obstet. **141**:22–26.

Baur, P. S., Parks, D. H., and Hudson, J. D., 1984, Epithelial mediated wound contraction in experimental wounds—The purse-string effect, J. Trauma **24**:713–720.

Beertsen, W., 1975, Migration of fibroblasts in the periodontal ligament of the mouse incisor as revealed by autoradiography, Arch. Oral Biol. **20**:659–666.

Beertsen, W., Events, V., and van den Hoof, A., 1974, Fine structure of fibroblasts in the periodontal ligament of the rat incisor and their possible role in tooth eruption, Arch. Oral Biol. **19**:1087–1098.

Bell, E., Ivarsson, B., and Merrill, C., 1979, Production of a tissue-like structure by contraction of collagen lattices by human fibroblasts of different proliferative potential in vitro, Proc. Natl. Acad. Sci. USA **76**:1274–1278.

Bell, E., Ehrlich, H. P., Buttle, D. J., and Nakatsuji, T., 1981, Living tissue formed in vitro and accepted as skin-equivalent tissue of full thickness, Science **211**:1052–1054.

Bellows, C. G., Melcher, A. H., and Aubin, J. E., 1981, Contraction and organization of collagen gels by cells cultured from periodontal ligament, gingiva and bone suggest functional differences between cell types, J. Cell Sci. **50**:299–314.

Bellows, C. G., Melcher, A. H., Bhargava, U., and Aubin, J. E., 1982, Fibroblasts contracting three dimensional collagen gels exhibit ultrastructure consistent with either contraction or protein secretion, J. Ultrastruct. Res. **78**:178–192.

Benjamin, S. P., Mercer, R. D., and Hawk, W. A., 1977, Myofibroblastic contraction in spontaneous regression of multiple congenital mesenchymal hamartomas, Cancer **40**:2343–2352.

Bhatal, P. S., 1972, Presence of modified fibroblasts in cirrhotic livers in man, Pathology **4**:139–144.

Bhawan, J., Bacchetta, C., Joris, I., and Magno, G., 1979, A myofibroblastic tumor. Infantile digital fibroma (recurrent digital fibrous tumor of childhood), Am. J. Pathol. **94**:19–36.

Billingham, R. E., and Russel, P. S., 1956, Studies on wound healing, with special reference to the phenomenon of contracture in experimental wounds in rabbits' skin, *Ann. Surg.* **144**:961–981.

Blewitt, R. W., Aparicio, S. G. R., and Bird, C. C., 1983, Epithelioid sarcoma: A tumor of myofibroblasts, *Histopathology* **7**:573–584.

Block, M., 1960, Wound healing in the new-born opossum (*Didelphis virginianum*), *Nature (Lond.)* **187**:340–341.

Bloom, S., and Cancilla, P. A., 1969, Conformational changes in myocardial nuclei of rats, *Circ. Res.* **24**:189–196.

Bressler, R. S., 1973, Myoid cells in the capsule of the adrenal gland and in monolayers derived from cultured adrenal capsules, *Anat. Rec.* **177**:525–531.

Buckley, I. K., and Porter, K. R., 1967, Cytoplasmic fibrils in living cultured cells. A light and electron microscope study, *Protoplasma* **64**:349–380.

Burridge, K., 1981, Are stress fibers contractile?, *Nature (Lond.)* **294**:691–692.

Burrington, J. D., 1971, Wound healing in the fetal lamb, *J. Pediatr. Surg.* **6**:523–528.

Buttle, D. J., and Ehrlich, H. P., 1983, Comparative studies of collagen lattice contraction utilizing a normal and a transformed cell line, *J. Cell Physiol.* **116**:159–166.

Callea, F., Mebis, J., and Desmet, V. J.. 1982, Myofibroblasts in focal nodular hyperplasia of the liver, *Virchows Arch. [A]* **396**:155–166.

Caplan, A. I., Fiszman, M. Y., and Eppenberger, H. M., 1983, Molecular and cell isoforms during development, *Science* **221**:921–927.

Carrel, A., and Hartmann, A., 1916, Cicatrization of wounds. I. The relation between the size of a wound and the rate of its cicatrization, *J. Exp. Med.* **24**:429–450.

Chamley-Campbell, J., Campbell, G. R., and Ross, R., 1979, The smooth muscle cell in culture, *Physiol. Rev.* **59**:1–61.

Chiu, H. F., and McFarlane, R. M., 1978, Pathogenesis of Dupuytren's contracture: A correlative clinical-pathological study, *J. Hand Surg.* **3**:1–10.

Churg, A. M., and Kahn, L. B., 1977, Myofibroblasts and related cells in malignant fibrous and fibrohistiocytic tumors, *Hum. Pathol.* **8**:205–218.

Cohnheim, J., 1867, Ueber entzündung und Eiterung, *Virchows Arch. [A]* **40**:1–79.

Crocker, D. J., Murad, T. M., and Geer, J. C., 1970, Role of the pericyte in wound healing. An ultrastructural study, *Exp. Mol. Pathol.* **13**:51–65.

D'Andiran, G., and Gabbiani, G., 1980, A metastasizing sarcoma of the pleura composed of myofibroblasts, in: *Progress in Surgical Pathology*, Vol. II (C. M. Fenoglio and M. Wolff, eds.), pp. 31–40, Masson, New York.

Dixon, J. B., 1960, Inflammation in the fetal and neonatal rat: the local reactions to skin burns, *J. Pathol. Bact.* **80**:73–82.

Donati, M. B., Balconi, G., Remuzzi, G., Borgia, R., Morasca, L., and de Gaetano, G., 1977, Skin fibroblasts from a patient with Glanzmann's thrombasthenia do not induce fibrin clot retraction, *Thromb. Res.* **10**:173–174.

Donoff, R. B., and Grillo, H. C., 1975, The effects of skin grafting on healing open wound in rabbits, *J. Surg. Res.* **19**:163–167.

Du Noüy, P. L., 1916a, Cicatrization of wounds. II. Mathematical expression of the curve representing cicatrization, *J. Exp. Med.* **24**:451–460.

Du Noüy, P. L., 1916b, Cicatrization of wounds. III. The relation between the age of the patient, the area of the wound and the index of cicatrization, *J. Exp. Med.* **24**:461–470.

Du Noüy, P. L., 1919, Cicatrization of wounds. X. A general equation for the law of cicatrization of surface wounds, *J. Exp. Med.* **29**:329–350.

Dunphy, J. E., Udapa, K. N., and Edwards, L. C., 1956, Wound healing: A new perspective with particular reference to ascorbic acid deficiency, *Ann. Surg.* **144**:304–317.

Dustin, P., 1978, *Microtubules*, Springer-Verlag, Berlin.

Ehrlich, H. P., and Hembry, R. M., 1984, A comparative study of fibroblasts in healing freeze and burn injuries in rats, *Am. J. Pathol.* **117**:218–224.

Ehrlich, H. P., and White, M. E., 1983, Effects of increased concentrations of prostaglandin E levels with epidermolysis bullosa dystrophica recessive fibroblasts within a populated collagen lattice, *J. Invest. Dermatol.* **81**:572–573.

Ehrlich, H. P., and Wyler, D. J., 1983, Fibroblast contraction of collagen lattices in vitro: Inhibition by chronic inflammatory cell mediators, *J. Cell Physiol.* **116:**345–351.

Ehrlich, H. P., Grislis, G., and Hunt, T. K., 1977, Evidence for the involvement of microtubules in wound contraction, *Am. J. Surg.* **133:**706–709.

El-Labban, N., and Lee, K. W., 1983, Myofibroblasts in central giant cell granuloma of the jaws: An ultrastructural study, *Histopathology* **7:**907–918.

Evans, J. N., Kelley, J., Low, R. B., and Adler, K. B., 1982, Increased contractility of isolated lung parenchyma in an animal model of pulmonary fibrosis induced by bleomycin, *Am. Rev. Respir. Dis.* **125:**89–94.

Feiner, H., and Kaye, G. I., 1976, Ultrastructural evidence of myofibroblasts in circumscribed fibromatosis, *Arch. Pathol. Lab. Med.* **100:**265–268.

Fisher, E. R., Paulson, J. D., and Gregorio, R. M., 1978, The myofibroblastic nature of the uterine plexiform tumor, *Arch. Pathol. Lab. Med.* **102:**477–480.

Franke, W. W., and Schinko, W., 1969, Nuclear shape in muscle cells, *J. Cell Biol.* **42:**326–331.

Fujiwara, K., and Pollard, T. D., 1976, Fluorescent antibody localization of myosin in the cytoplasm, cleavage furrow, and mitotic spindle of human cells, *J. Cell Biol.* **71:**848–875.

Gabbiani, G., and Kocher, O., 1983, Cytocontractile and cytoskeletal elements in pathological processes. Pathogenetic role and diagnostic value, *Arch. Pathol. Lab. Med.* **107:**622–625.

Gabbiani, G., and Majno, G., 1972, Dupuytren's contracture: Fibroblast contraction? An ultrastructural study, *Am. J. Pathol.* **66:**131–146.

Gabbiani, G., and Rungger-Brändle, E., 1981, The fibroblast, in: *Handbook of Inflammation: Tissue Repair and Regeneration*, Vol. 3 (L. E. Glynn, ed.), pp. 1–50, Elsevier/North-Holland Biomedical Press, Amsterdam.

Gabbiani, G., Ryan, G. B., and Majno, G., 1971a, Presence of modified fibroblasts in granulation tissue and their possible role in wound contraction, *Experientia* **27:**549–550.

Gabbiani, G., Kaye, G. I., Lattes, R., and Majno, G., 1971b, Synovial sarcoma. Electron microscopic study of a typical case, *Cancer* **28:**1031–1039.

Gabbiani, G., Hirschel, B. J., Ryan, G. B., Statkov, P. R., and Majno, G., 1972a, Granulation tissue as a contractile organ. A study of structure and function, *J. Exp. Med.* **135:**719–734.

Gabbiani, G., Fu, Y. S., Kaye, G. I., Lattes, R., and Majno, G., 1972b, Epithelioid sarcoma. A light and electron microscopic study suggesting a synovial origin, *Cancer* **30:**486–499.

Gabbiani, G., Majno, G., and Ryan, G. B., 1973, The fibroblast as a contractile cell: The myofibroblast, in: *Biology of the Fibroblast* (J. Pikkarainen and K. Kulonen, eds.), pp. 139–154, Academic, New York.

Gabbiani, G., Chaponnier, C., and Hüttner, I., 1978, Cytoplasmic filaments and gap junctions in epithelial cells and myofibroblasts during wound healing, *J. Cell Biol.* **76:**561–568.

Gabbiani, G., Schmid, E., Winter, S., Chaponnier, C., de Chastonay, C., Vanderkerckhove, J., Weber, K., and Franke, W. W., 1981, Vascular smooth muscle cells differ from other smooth muscle cells: Predominance of vimentin filaments and a specific α-type actin, *Proc. Natl. Acad. Sci. USA* **78:**298–302.

Gabbiani, G., Gabbiani, F., Lombardi, D., and Schwartz, S. M., 1983, Organization of actin cytoskeleton in normal and regenerating arterial endothelial cells, *Proc. Natl. Acad. Sci. USA* **80:**2361–2364.

Gabbiani, G., Kocher, O., Bloom, W. S., Vanderkerckhove, J., and Weber, K., 1984, Actin expression in smooth muscle cells of rat aortic intimal thickening, human atheromatous plaque and cultured rat aortic media, *J. Clin. Invest.* **73:**148–152.

Garrels, J. I., and Gibson, W., 1976, Identification and characterization of multiple forms of actin, *Cell* **9:**793–805.

Gelberman, R. H., Amiel, D., Rudolph, R. M., and Vance, R. M., 1980, Dupuytren's contracture. An electron microscopic, biochemical, and clinical correlative study, *J. Bone Joint Surg.* **62A:**425–432.

Ghadially, F. N., and Mehta, P. N., 1971, Multifunctional mesenchymal cells resembling smooth muscle cells in ganglia of the wrist, *Ann. Rheum. Dis.* **30:**31–42.

Ghadially, F. N., McNaughton, J. D., and Lalonde, J. M. A., 1983, Myofibroblastoma: A tumour of myofibroblasts, *J. Submicrosc. Cytol.* **15:**1055–1063.

Gokel, J. M., and Hübner, G., 1977, Occurrence of myofibroblasts in the different phases of morbus Dupuytren (Dupuytren's contracture), Beitr. Pathol. 161:166–175.

Goldman, R. D., 1975, The use of heavy meromyosin binding as an ultrastructural cytochemical method for localizing and determining the possible functions of actin like microfilaments in nonmuscle cells, J. Histochem. Cytochem. 23:529–542.

Goldman, R. D., Lazarides, E., Pollack, R., and Weber, K., 1975, The distribution of actin in non muscle cells. The use of actin antibody in the localization of actin within the microfilament bundles of mouse 3T3 cells, Exp. Cell Res. 90:333–344.

Gorgas, K., and Böck, P., 1974, Myofibroblasts in the rat testicular capsule, Cell Tissue Res. 154:533–541.

Gospodarowicz, D., 1975, Purification of fibroblast growth factor from bovine pituitary, J. Biol. Chem. 250:2515–2520.

Goss, A. N., 1977, Intra-uterine healing of fetal rat oral mucosal, skin and cartilage wounds, J. Oral Pathol. 6:35–43.

Gown, A. M., and Gabbiani, G., 1984, Intermediate sized (10-nm) filaments in human tumors, in: Advances in Immunohistochemistry (R. A. DeLillis, ed.), pp. 89–109, Masson, New York.

Greenlee, T. K., Jr., and Ross, R., 1967, The development of the rat flexor digital tendon, a fine structure study, J. Ultrastruct. Res. 18:354–376.

Grillo, H. C., 1963, Origin of fibroblasts in wound healing: An autoradiographic study of inhibition of cellular proliferation by local X-irradiation, Ann. Surg. 157:453–467.

Grillo, H. C., 1964, Derivation of fibroblasts in the healing wound, Arch. Surg. 88:218–224.

Grimaud, J. A., and Borojevic, R., 1977, Myofibroblasts in hepatic schistosomal fibrosis, Experientia 33:890–892.

Guber, S., and Rudolph, R., 1978, The myofibroblast, Surg. Gynecol. Obstret. 146:641–649.

Güldner, F. H., Wolff, J. R., and Keyserlingk, D., 1972, Fibroblasts as part of the contractile system in duodenal villi of rat, Z. Zellforsch. 135:349–360.

Harris, A. K., Stopack, D., and Wild, P., 1981, Fibroblast traction as a mechanism for collagen morphogenesis, Nature (Lond.) 290:249–251.

Harris, M., and Ahmed, A., 1977, The ultrastructure of tubular carcinoma of the breast, J. Pathol. 123:79–83.

Hassan, M. O., and Olaizola, M. Y., 1979, Ultrastructural observations on gynecomastia, Arch. Pathol. Lab. Med. 103:624–630.

Heggeness, M. H., Ash, J. F., and Singer, S. J., 1978, Transmembrane linkage of fibronectin in intracellular actin-containing filaments in cultured human fibroblasts, Ann. NY Acad. Sci. 312:414–417.

Herman, I. M., Crisona, N. J., and Pollard, T. D., 1981, Relation between cell activity and the distribution of cytoplasmic actin and myosin, J. Cell Biol. 90:84–91.

Hoffmann-Berling, H., 1954, Adenosintriphosphat als Betriebsstoff von Zellbewegungen, Biochem. Biophys. Acta 14:182–194.

Holund, B., Junker, P., Garbarsch, C., Cristofensen, P., and Lorenzen, I., 1979, Formation of granulation tissue in subcutaneously implanted sponges in rat, Acta Pathol. Microbiol. Scand. Sect. A 87:367–374.

Hueston, J. T., Hurley, J. V., and Whittingham, S., 1976, The contracting fibroblast as a clue to Dupuytren's contracture, Hand 8:10–12.

Hutson, J. M., Niall, M., Evans, D., and Fowler, R., 1979, Effect of salivary glands on wound contraction in mice, Nature (Lond.) 279:793–795.

Hüttner, I., Walker, C., and Gabbiani, G., 1985, The aortic endothelial cell during regeneration: Remodeling of cell junctions, stress fibers, and stress fiber–membrane attachment domains, Lab. Invest. 53:287–302.

Hynes, R. O., Destree, A. T., and Wagner, D. D., 1982, Relationships between microfilaments, cell–substratum adhesion, and fibronectin, Cold Spring Habor Symp. Quant. Biol. 46:659–670.

Irle, C., Kocher, O., and Gabbiani, G., 1980, Contractility of myofibroblasts during experimental liver cirrhosis, J. Submicrosc. Cytol. 12:209–217.

Isenberg, G., Rathke, P. C., Hülsmann, N., Franke, W. W., and Wohlfahrt-Bottermann, K. E., 1976, Cytoplasmic actomyosin fibrils in tissue cultured cells. Direct proof of contractility by visualization of ATP-induced contraction in fibrils isolated by laser microbeam dissection, *Cell Tissue Res.* **166:**427–433.

Ishikawa, H., Bischoff, R., and Holtzer, H., 1969, Formation of arrowhead complexes with heavy meromyosin in a variety of cell types, *J. Cell Biol.* **43:**312–328.

Ivaska, K., 1973, Isolation of viable cells from experimental granulation tissue, *Virchows Arch [B]* **14:**19–30.

Iwasaki, H., Kikuchi, M., Mori, R., Miyazono, J., Enjoji, M., Shinohara, N., and Matsuzaki, A., 1980, Infantile digital fibromatosis. Ultrastructural, histochemical, and tissue culture observations, *Cancer* **46:**2238–2247.

James, D. W., and Taylor, J. F., 1969, The stress developed by sheets of chick fibroblasts *in vitro*, *Exp. Cell Res.* **54:**107–110.

James, W. D., and Odom, R. B., 1980, The role of the myofibroblast in Dupuytren's contracture, *Arch. Dermatol.* **116:**807–811.

Judd, P. A., Finnegan, P., and Curran, R. C., 1975, Pulmonary sarcoidosis: A clinicopathological study, *J. Pathol.* **115:**191–198.

Kapanci, Y., Assimacopoulos, A., Irle, C., Zwahlen, A., and Gabbiani, G., 1974, "Contractile interstitial cells" in pulmonary septa, *J. Cell Biol.* **60:**375–392.

Kocher, O., Skalli, O., Bloom, W. S., and Gabbiani, G., 1984, Cytoskeleton of rat aortic smooth muscle cells. Normal conditions and experimental intimal thickening, *Lab. Invest.* **50:**645–652.

Kocher, O., Skalli, O., Cerutti, D., Gabbiani, F., and Gabbiani, G., 1985, Cytoskeletal features of rat aortic cells during development: An electron microscopic, immunohistochemical and biochemical study, *Circ. Res.* **56:**829–836.

Korn, E. D., 1982, Actin polymerization and its regulation by proteins from nonmuscle cells, *Physiol. Rev.* **62:**672–736.

Kreis, T. E., and Birchmeier, W., 1980, Stress fiber sarcomeres of fibroblasts are contractile, *Cell* **22:**555–561.

Laguens, R., and Lagrutta, J., 1964, Fine structure of human uterine muscle in pregnancy, *Am. J. Obstet, Gynecol.* **89:**1040–1048.

Lane, B. P., 1965, Alterations in the cytologic detail of intestinal smooth muscle in various stages of contraction, *J. Cell Biol.* **27:**199–213.

Larson, D. L., Abston, S., Willis, B., Linares, H., Dobrkovsky, M., Evans, E. B., and Lewis, S. R., 1974, Contracture and scar formation in the burn patient, *Clin. Plast. Surg.* **1:**653–666.

Larson, D. M., Fujiwara, K., Alexander, R. W., and Gimbrone, M. A., Jr., 1984a, Heterogeneity of myosin antigenic expression in vascular smooth muscle *in vivo*, *Lab. Invest.* **50:**401–407.

Larson, D. M., Fujiwara, K., Alexander, R. W., and Gimbrone, M. A., Jr., 1984b, Myosin in cultured vascular smooth muscle cells: Immunofluorescence and immunochemical studies of alterations in antigenic expression, *J. Cell Biol.* **99:**1582–1589.

Lazarides, E., 1975, Tropomyosin antibody: The specific localization of tropomyosin in nonmuscle cells, *J. Cell Biol.* **65:**549–561.

Lazarides, E., and Burrdige, K., 1975, α-actinin: Immunofluorescent localization of a muscle structural protein in nonmuscle cells, *Cell* **6:**289–298.

Le Beux, Y. J., and Willemot, J., 1978, Actin and myosin-like filaments in rat brain pericytes, *Anat. Rec.* **190:**811–826.

Leitzel, K., Cano, C., Marks, J., and Lipton, A., 1982, Failure of nerve growth factor to enhance wound healing in the hamster, *J. Neurosci. Res.* **8:**413–417.

Levine, G. D., and Dorfman, R. F., 1975, Nodular lymphoma: An ultrastructural study of its relationship to germinal centers and a correlation of light and electron microscopic findings, *Cancer* **35:**148–164.

Li, A. K. C., Ehrlich, H. P., Trelstad, R. L., Koroly, M. J., Schattenkerk, M. E., and Malt, R. A., 1980a, Differences in healing of skin wounds caused by burn and freeze injuries, *Ann. Surg.* **191:**244–248.

Li, A. K. C., Koroly, M. J., Schattenkerk, M. E., Malt, R. A., and Young, M., 1980b, Nerve growth factor: Acceleration of the rate of wound healing in mice, *Proc. Natl. Acad. Sci. USA* **77:**4379–4381.

MacDonald, R. A., 1959, Origin of fibroblasts in experimental healing wounds: Autoradiographic studies using tritiated thymidine, Surgery **46**:376–382.

Madden, J. W., 1973, On "the contractile fibroblast," Plat. Reconstr. Surg. **52**:291–292.

Madden, J. W., Morton, D., and Peacock, E. E., 1974, Contraction of experimental wounds. I. Inhibiting wound contraction by using a topical smooth muscle antagonist, Surgery **76**:8–15.

Madden, J. W., Carlson, E. C., and Hines, J., 1975, Presence of modified fibroblasts in ischemic contracture of the intrinsic musculature of the hand, Surg. Gynecol. Obstret. **140**:509–516.

Majno, G., Shea, S. M., and Leventhal, M., 1969, Endothelial contraction induced by histamine-like mediators. An electron microscopic study, J. Cell Biol. **42**:647–672.

Majno, G., Gabbiani, G., Hirschel, B. J., Ryan, G. B., and Statkov, P. R., 1971, Contraction of granulation tissue in vitro: Similarity to smooth muscle, Science **173**:548–550.

Martinez-Hernandez, A., Francis, D. J., and Silverberg, S. G., 1977, Elastosis and other stromal reactions in benign and malignant breast tissue, Cancer **40**:700–706.

Meister, P., Gokel, J. M., and Remberger, K., 1979, Palmar fibromatosis—"Dupuytren's contracture." A comparison of light electron and immunofluorescence microscopic findings, Pathol. Res. Pract. **164**:402–412.

Merkow, L. P., Frich, J. C., Slifkin, M., Kyreages, C. G., and Pardo, M., 1971, Ultrastructure of a fibroxanthosarcoma (malignant fibroxanthoma), Cancer **28**:372–383.

Moll, R., Franke, W. W., Schiller, D. L., Geiger, B., and Krepler, R., 1982, The catalog of human cytokeratins: Patterns of expression in normal epithelia, tumors and cultured cells, Cell **31**:11–24.

Montandon, D., Gabbiani, G., Ryan, G. B., and Majno, G., 1973, The contractile fibroblast. Its relevance in plastic surgery, Plast. Reconstr. Surg. **52**:286–290.

Moss, N. S., and Benditt, E. P., 1970, Spontaneous and experimentally induced arterial lesions. I. An ultrastructural survey of the normal chicken aorta, Lab. Invest. **22**:166–183.

Nagle, R. B., Kneiser, M. R., Bulger, R. E., and Benditt, E. P., 1973, Induction of smooth muscle characteristics in renal interstitial fibroblasts during obstructive nephropathy, Lab. Invest. **29**:422–427.

Nagle, R. B., Evans, L. W., and Reynolds, D. G., 1975, Contractility of renal cortex following complete ureteral obstruction, Proc. Soc. Exp. Biol. Med. **148**:611–614.

Navas-Palacios, J. J., 1983, The fibromatoses. An ultrastructural study of 31 cases, Pathol. Res. Pract. **176**:158–175.

Niewiarowski, S., and Goldstein, S., 1973, Interaction of cultured human fibroblasts with fibrin: modification by drugs and aging in vitro, J. Lab. Clin. Med. **82**:605–610.

Niewiarowski, S., Regoeczi, E., and Fraser Mustard, J., 1972, Adhesion of fibroblasts to polymerizing fibrin and retraction of fibrin induced by fibroblasts, Proc. Soc. Exp. Biol. Med. **140**:199–204.

Novotny, G. E. K., and Pau, H., 1984, Myofibroblast-like cells in human anterior capsular cataract, Virchows Arch. [A] **404**:393–401.

Ohtani, H., and Sasano, N., 1980, Myofibroblasts and myoepithelial cells in human breast carcinoma. An ultrastructural study, Virchows Arch. [A] **385**:247–261.

Olivetti, G., Anversa, P., Melissari, M., and Loud, A. V., 1980, Morphometric study of early postnatal development of the thoracic aorta in the rat, Circ. Res. **47**:417–424.

Osborn, M., and Weber, K., 1982, Intermediate filaments: Cell-type-specific markers in differentiation and pathology, Cell **31**:303–306.

Osborn, M., and Weber, K., 1983, Tumor diagnosis by intermediate filament typing: A novel tool for surgical pathology, Lab. Invest. **48**:372–394.

O'Shea, J. D., 1970, An ultrastructural study of smooth muscle-like cells in the theca externa of the ovarian follicle of the rat, Anat. Rec. **167**:127–131.

Owellen, R. J., Owens, A. H., and Donigian, D. W., 1972, The binding of vincristine, vinblastine and colchicine to tubulin, Biochem. Biophys. Res. Commun. **47**:685–691.

Peacock, E. E., and Van Winkle, W., 1970, Surgery and Biology of Wound Repair, W. B. Saunders, Philadelphia.

Pinto da Silva, P., and Gilula, N. B., 1972, Gap junctions in normal and transformed fibroblasts in culture, Exp. Cell Res. **71**:393–401.

Pollack, R., Osborn, M., and Weber, K., 1975, Patterns of organization of actin and myosin in normal and transformed cultured cells, *Proc. Natl. Acad. Sci. USA* **72**:994–998.

Poole, J. C. F., Cromwell, S. B., and Benditt, E. P., 1971, Behavior of smooth muscle cells and formation of extracellular structures in the reaction of arterial wall to injury, *Am. J. Pathol.* **62**:391–414.

Postacchini, F., Natali, P. G., Accinni, L., Ippolito, E., and De Martino, C., 1977, Contractile filaments in cells of regenerating tendon, *Experientia* **33**:957–959.

Povysil, C., and Matejovsky, Z., 1979, Ultrastructural evidence of myofibroblasts in pseudomalignant myositis ossificans, *Virchows Arch. [A]* **381**:189–203.

Ramos, C. V., Gillespie, W., and Narconis, R. J., 1978, Elastofibroma. A pseudotumor of myofibroblasts, *Arch. Pathol. Lab. Med.* **102**:538–540.

Remuzzi, G., Marchesi, E., de Gaetano, E., and Donati, M., 1977, Abnormal tissue repair in Glanzmann's thrombasthenia, *Lancet* **2**:374–375.

Robbins, S. L., Angell, M., and Kumar, V., 1984, *Basic Pathology*, W. B. Saunders, Philadelphia.

Roberts, P. J., and Häyry, P., 1976, Effector mechanisms in allograft rejection. I. Assembly of "sponge matrix" allografts, *Cell. Immunol.* **26**:160–167.

Roland, J., 1976, Fibroblaste et myofibroblaste dans le processus granulomateux, *Ann. Anat. Pathol.* **21**:37–44.

Ross, M. H., and Reith, E. J., 1969, Perineurium: Evidence for contractile elements, *Science* **165**:604–606.

Ross, R., and Greenlee, T. K., Jr., 1966, Electron microscopy: Attachment sites between connective tissue cells, *Science* **153**:997–999.

Ross, R., and Klebanoff, S. J., 1967, Fine structural changes in uterine smooth muscle and fibroblasts in response to estrogens, *J. Cell Biol.* **32**:155–167.

Ross, R., Everett, N. B., and Tyler, R., 1970, Wound healing and collagen formation. VI. The origin of the wound fibroblast studied in parabiosis, *J. Cell Biol.* **44**:645–654.

Rowlatt, U., 1979, Intrauterine wound healing in a 20 week human fetus, *Virchows Arch. [A]* **381**:353–361.

Rudolph, R., 1976, The effect of skin graft preparation on wound contraction, *Surg. Gynecol. Obstet.* **142**:49–56.

Rudolph, R., and Klein, L., 1973, Healing processes in skin grafts, *Surg. Gynecol. Obstet.* **136**:641–654.

Rudolph, R., and Woodward, M., 1978, Spatial orientation of microtubules in contractile fibroblasts in vivo, *Anat. Rec.* **191**:169–182.

Rudolph, R., Guber, S., Suzuki, M., and Woodward, M., 1977, The life cycle of the myofibroblast, *Surg. Gynecol. Obstet.* **145**:389–394.

Rudolph, R., Abraham, J., Vecchione, T., Guber, S., and Woodward, M., 1978, Myofibroblasts and free silicon around breast implants, *Plast. Reconst. Surg.* **62**:185–196.

Rudolph, R., McLure, W. J., and Woodward, M., 1979, Contractile fibroblasts in chronic alcoholic cirrhosis, *Gastroenterology* **76**:704–709.

Rudolph, R., Kum, I., and Woodward, M., 1981, Use of colchicine to inhibit wound contraction, *Am. J. Surg.* **141**:712–717.

Rungger-Brändle, E., and Gabbiani, G., 1983, The role of cytoskeletal and cytocontractile elements in pathologic processes, *Am. J. Pathol.* **110**:359–392.

Ryan, G. B., Cliff, W. J., Gabbiani, G., Irle, C., Statkov, P. R., and Majno, G., 1973, Myofibroblasts in an avascular fibrous tissue, *Lab. Invest.* **29**:197–206.

Ryan, G. B., Cliff, W. J., Gabbiani, G., Irle, C., Montandon, D., Statkov, P. R., and Majno, G., 1974, Myofibroblasts in human granulation tissue, *Hum. Pathol.* **5**:55–67.

Schürch, W., Seemayer, T. A., and Lagacé, R., 1981, Stromal myofibroblasts in primary invasive and metastatic carcinomas: A combined immunological, light and electron microscopy study, *Virchows Arch. [A]* **391**:125–139.

Schürch, V., Lagacé, R., and Seemayer, T. A., 1982, Myofibroblastic stromal reaction in retracted scirrhous carcinomas of the breast, *Surg. Gynecol. Obstet.* **154**:351–358.

Schürch, W., Seemayer, T. A., Lagacé, R., and Gabbiani, G., 1984, The intermediate filament cytoskeleton of myofibroblasts: An immunofluorescence and ultrastructural study, *Virchows Arch. [A]* **403**:323–336.

Seemayer, T. A., Lagacé, R., Schürch, W., and Tremblay, G., 1979, Myofibroblasts in the stroma of invasive and metastatic carcinoma. A possible host response to neoplasia, Am. J. Surg. Pathol. 3:525–533.

Seemayer, T. A., Lagacé, R., Schürch, W., and Thelmo, W. L., 1980a, The myofibroblast: Biologic, pathologic and theoretical considerations, Pathol. Annual 15(Part I):443–470.

Seemayer, T. A., Lagacé, R., and Schürch, W., 1980b, On the pathogenesis of sclerosis and nodularity in nodular sclerosing Hodgkin's disease, Virchows Arch. [A] 385:283–291.

Seemayer, T. A., Schürch, W., and Lagacé, R., 1981, Myofibroblasts in human pathology, Hum. Pathol. 12:491–492.

Selye, H., 1953, On the mechanism through which hydrocortisone affects the resistance of tissue to injury. An experimental study with the granuloma pouch technique, JAMA 152:1207–1213.

Shepherd, J. P., and Dawber, R. P. R., 1984, Wound healing and scarring after cryosurgery, Cryobiol. 21:157–169.

Shigo, A., 1985, Compartmentalization of decay in trees, Sci. Am. 252:76–83.

Singer, I. I., 1979, The fibronexus: A transmembrane association of fibronectin-containing fibers and bundles of 5 nm microfilaments in hamster and human fibroblasts, Cell 16:675–685.

Singer, I. I., Kawka, D. W., Kazazis, D. M., and Clark, R. A. F., 1984, In vivo co-distribution of fibronectin and actin fibers in granulation tissue: Immunofluorescence and electron microscope studies of the fibronexus at the myofibroblast surface, J. Cell Biol. 98:2091–2106.

Skalli, O., Ropraz, R., Trzeciak, A., Benzonana, G., Gillessen, D., and Gabbiani, G., 1986a, A monoclonal antibody against α-smooth muscle actin: A new probe for smooth muscle differentiation, J. Cell Biol. 103:2787–2796.

Skalli, O., Bloom, W. S., Ropraz, P., Azzarone, B., and Gabbiani, G., 1986b, Cytoskeletal remodeling of rat aortic smooth muscle cells in vitro: Relationships to culture conditions and analogies to in vivo situations, J. Submicrosc. Cytol. 18:481–493.

Skalli, O., Vanderkerckhove, J., and Gabbiani, G., 1987, Actin isoform pattern as marker of normal or pathological smooth muscle and fibroblastic tissues, Differentiation 33:232–238.

Somasundaram, K., and Prathap, K., 1970, Intra uterine healing of skin wounds in rabbit fetuses, J. Pathol. 100:81–86.

Somasundaram, K., and Prathap, K., 1972, The effect of exclusion of amniotic fluid on intra uterine healing of skin wounds in rabbit foetuses, J. Pathol. 107:127–130.

Somers, K. D., Dawson, D. M., Wright, G. L., Leffell, M. S., Rowe, M. J., Bluemink, G. G., Vande Berg, J. S., Gleischman, S. H., Devine, C. J., and Horton, C. E., 1982, Cell culture of Peyronie's disease plaque and normal penile tissue, J. Urol. 127:585–588.

Sporn, M. B., Roberts, A. B., Shull, J. H., Smith, J. M., Ward, J. M., and Sodek, J., 1983, Polypeptide transforming growth factors isolated from bovine sources and used for wound healing in vivo, Science 219:1329–1330.

Steinberg, B. M., Smith, K., Colozzo, M., and Pollack, R., 1980, Establishment and transformation diminish the ability of fibroblasts to contract a native collagen gel, J. Cell Biol. 87:304–308.

Steinert, P. M., Jones, J. C. R., and Goldman, R. D., 1984, Intermediate filaments, J. Cell Biol. 99:22s–27s.

Stiller, D., and Katenkamp, D., 1975, Cellular features in desmoid fibromatosis and well-differentiated fibrosarcomas. An electron microscopic study, Virchows Arch. [A] 369:155–164.

Stopak, D., and Harris, A. K., 1982, Connective tissue morphogenesis by fibroblast traction. I. Tissue culture observations, Dev. Biol. 90:383–398.

Tabone, E., Andujar, M. B., De Barros, S. S., Dos Santos, M. N., Barros, C. L., and Graca, D. L., 1983, Myofibroblast-like cells in non-pathological bovine endometrial caruncle, Cell Biol. Int. Rep. 7:395–400.

Taylor, J. F., 1971, Changes in nuclear dimensions and orientation during contraction of a cultured fibroblast sheet, J. Anat. 108:509–517.

Toyama, Y., 1976, Actin like filaments in the Sertoli cell junctional specializations in the swine and mouse testis, Anat. Rec. 186:477–492.

Toyama, Y., Obinata, T., and Holtzer, H., 1979, Cristalloids of actin like filaments in the Sertoli cell of the swine testis, Anat. Rec. 195:47–62.

Travo, P., Weber, K., and Osborn, M., 1982, Co-existence of vimentin and desmin type intermediate filaments in a subpopulation of adult rat vascular smooth muscle cells growing in primary culture, *Exp. Cell Res.* **139**:87–94.

Tremblay, G., 1979, Stromal aspects of breast carcinoma, *Exp. Mol. Pathol.* **31**:248–260.

Turi, G. K., Albala, A., and Fenoglio, J. J., 1980, Cardiac fibromatosis: An ultrastructural study, *Hum. Pathol.* **11**(Suppl):577–580.

Vande Berg, J. S., Rudolph, R., and Woodward, M., 1984, Comparative growth dynamics and morphology between cultured myofibroblasts from granulating wounds and dermal fibroblasts, *Am. J. Pathol.* **114**:187–200.

Vandekerckhove, J., and Weber, K., 1978, At least six different actins are expressed in higher mammals: An analysis based on the amino acid sequence of the amino terminal tryptic peptide, *J. Mol. Biol.* **126**:783–802.

Vandekerckhove, J., and Weber, K., 1979, The complete amino acid sequence of actins from bovine aorta, bovine heart, bovine fast skeletal muscle and rabbit slow skeletal muscle, *Differentiation* **14**:123–133.

Vandekerckhove, J., and Weber, K., 1981, Actin typing on total cellular extracts. A highly sensitive protein chemical procedure able to distinguish different actins, *Eur. J. Biochem.* **113**:595–603.

Vandekerckhove, J., and Weber, K., 1984, Chordate muscle actins differ distinctly from invertebrate muscle actins. The evolution of the different vertebrate muscle actins, *J. Mol. Biol.* **179**:391–413.

Vasudev, K. S., and Harris, M., 1978, A sarcoma of myofibroblasts. An ultrastructural study, *Arch. Pathol. Lab. Med.* **102**:185–188.

Vogel, A., Ross, R., and Raines, E., 1980, Role of serum components in density dependent inhibition of growth of cells in culture. Platelet derived growth factor is the major serum determinant of saturation density, *J. Cell Biol.* **85**:377–385.

Wang, K., 1977, Filamin, a new high-molecular-weight protein found in smooth muscle and non muscle cells. Purification and properties of chicken gizzard filamin, *Biochemistry* **16**:1857–1865.

Weathers, D. R., and Campbell, W. G., 1974, Ultrastructure of the giant-cell fibroma of the oral mucosa, *Oral Surg.* **38**:550–561.

Weber, K., and Groeschel-Stewart, U., 1974, Antibody to myosin: The specific visualization of myosin-containing filaments in nonmuscle cells. *Proc. Natl. Acad. Sci. USA* **71**:4561–4564.

Wessels, N. K., Spooner, B. S., Ash, J. F., Bradley, M. O., Luduena, M. A., Taylor, E. L., Wrenn, J. T., and Yamada, K. M., 1971, Microfilaments in cellular and developmental processes, *Science* **171**:135–143.

Whalen, R. G., Butler-Browne, G. S., and Gros, F., 1976, Protein synthesis and actin heterogeneity in calf muscle cells in culture, *Proc. Natl. Acad. Sci. USA* **73**:2018–2022.

White, G. E., Gimbrone, M. A., and Fujiwara, K., 1983, Factors influencing the expression of stress fibers in vascular endothelial cells in situ, *J. Cell Biol.* **97**:416–424.

Willingham, M. C., Yamada, S. S., Davies, P. J. A., Rutherford, A. V., Gallo, M. G., and Pastan, I., 1981, Intracellular localization of actin in cultured fibroblasts by electron microscopic immunochemistry, *J. Histochem. Cytochem.* **29**:17–37.

Wirman, J. A., 1976, Nodular fasciitis, a lesion of myofibroblasts. An ultrastructural study, *Cancer* **38**:2378–2389.

Wong, A., Pollard, T. D., and Herman, I. M., 1983, Actin filament stress fibers in vascular endothelial cells in vivo, *Science* **219**:867–869.

Woodcock-Mitchell, J., Adler, K. B., and Low, R. B., 1984, Immunohistochemical identification of cell types in normal and in bleomycin-induced fibrotic rat lung, *Am. Rev. Respir. Dis.* **130**:910–916.

Yamamoto, M., Tsukada, S., and Inoue, M., 1982, Possible age associated change at cellular level in cultured fibroblasts derived from scar tissue, *Chir. Plast.* **7**:51–58.

Zimman, O. A., Robles, J. M., and Lee, J. C., 1978, The fibrous capsule around mammary implants: An investigation, *Aesth. Plast. Surg.* **2**:217–234.

Part III

Extracellular Matrix Production and Remodeling

Chapter 18

Fibronectin

A Primitive Matrix

JOHN A. MCDONALD

1. Introduction

Fibronectins are modular cell-adhesive and matrix-organizing glycoproteins that aid wound healing by stimulating cell attachment and migration and by forming part of the initial connective tissue matrix at wound sites (Hynes, 1986; Hynes and Yamada, 1982; Yamada et al., 1985; Mosher, 1984; Grinnell, 1984; D'Ardenne and McGee, 1984; J. McDonagh, 1985). In vivo, fibronectins occur in soluble form in plasma as well as in basal lamina and loose connective tissue matrices. In culture, so-called cellular fibronectin is produced by many cells, where it is secreted and assembled into an insoluble matrix under and around professional matrix-secreting cells such as fibroblasts, under epithelial cells or largely secreted into the culture medium as is the case for macrophages (Villiger et al., 1981; Alitalo et al., 1980). At wound-healing sites, fibronectin may arise from local synthesis by cells involved in wound healing (macrophages, endothelial cells, fibroblasts, certain epithelial cells) as well as from deposition from plasma (Oh et al., 1981). This chapter reviews recent developments in the fibronectin gene and polypeptide structure, its binding activities, and potential role in extracellular matrix organization and wound healing.

2. Fibronectin Structure

2.1. Protein and Gene Structure

A recent review of the protein and gene structure of the fibronectin molecule is recommended for more detailed information (Hynes, 1985). Fibronectins are complex dimeric glycoproteins composed of two similar but nonidentical subunits of about 250,000 M_r joined near their carboxyl terminal by disulfide bonds. Amino acid sequence analysis of bovine plasma fibronectin by Petersen and co-workers (1983) revealed repeated copies of three distinct

JOHN A. MCDONALD • Respiratory and Critical Care Division, Departments of Biochemistry and Medicine, Washington University School of Medicine, St. Louis, Missouri 63110.

types of polypeptide domains termed types I, II, and III. Each type of domain is partially (25–50%) homologous. Type I and II domains contain 45 to 50 amino acid residues and the type III domains about 90 residues (Fig. 1). The type I and II sequences contain disulfide crosslinks, whereas the type III lack cystine. The type I homology region occurs 12 times: nine times in the amino-terminal fibrin and collagen-binding sequence of fibronectin and three times in the carboxyl terminal fibrin-binding region (see Hynes, 1985). The two type II repeats are confined to the collagen binding domain in the amino-terminal, and the remaining central sequence contains either 15 (plasma fibronectin) or 16 (cellular fibronectin) type III repeats (Fig. 1).

Where analyzed, sequencing of cDNAs has demonstrated that each type I and II homologous sequence is encoded by one exon. Each type III sequence is encoded by two exons, with the exception of the extra domain (ED) region discussed in Section 2.2 (Kornblihtt et al., 1985). Thus, there is a very close association between gene and protein structure in the fibronectins (Odermatt et al., 1985). Because there is considerable (greater than 90%) homology among similar sequences of rat, human, and bovine fibronectins but less between the various homologous repeats or minidomains within one species, it appears that the fibronectins evolved very early in vertebrate evolution and that their structure was subsequently highly conserved (Hynes, 1985). Other proteins possess modules similar to those present in fibronectin (Patthy, 1985; Banyai et al., 1983; Patthy et al., 1984). A type I repeat is found in the fibrin-binding domain of tissue plasminogen activator, whereas urokinase, which lacks fibrin-binding activity, also lacks any type I sequences (Banyai et al., 1983). In addition, members of the serine proteinase or serpine family as well as gelatin-binding proteins found in seminal plasma possess so-called kringle structures homologous to the type II repeats of the collagen-binding domain (Patthy et al., 1984). From these data, one can speculate that functional units present in fibronectin have moved among genes encoding proteins that share similar functions by exon shuffling (Gilbert, 1978).

2.2. Fibronectin Pre-Messenger RNA Splicing

Although cellular and plasma fibronectins differ immunologically and structurally (Yamada and Kennedy, 1979), there is only one functional fibronectin gene located on human chromosome 2 (Kornblihht et al., 1983; Tamkun et al., 1984; Prowse et al., 1986). Hence, post-transcriptional events are responsible for the structural and biologic differences between cellular and plasma fibronectins. The origin of these differences has been elucidated by sequencing complementary DNA (cDNA) clones from rat and human cells, which showed that pre-messenger RNA (mRNA) molecules coding for fibronectin are subjected to a complex scheme of pre-mRNA splicing in at least two regions (Tamkun et al., 1984; Hynes et al., 1984; Schwarzbauer et al., 1983; Kornblihtt et al., 1984a,b, 1985; Hynes, 1985). Figure 2, modified from Sekiguchi et al. (1986), depicts one fibronectin pre-mRNA variably spliced to yield mRNAs coding for the two different subunits of plasma fibronectin. mRNA isolated from cells

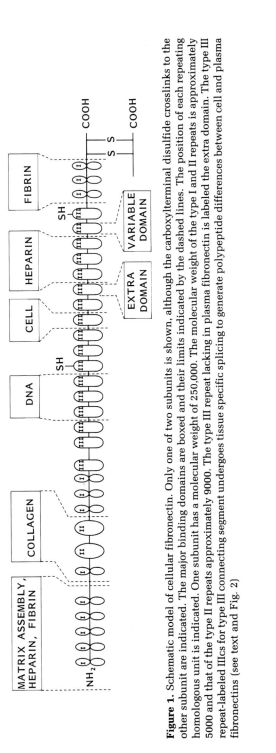

Figure 1. Schematic model of cellular fibronectin. Only one of two subunits is shown, although the carboxylterminal disulfide crosslinks to the other subunit are indicated. The major binding domains are boxed and their limits indicated by the dashed lines. The position of each repeating homologous unit is indicated. One subunit has a molecular weight of 250,000. The molecular weight of the type I and II repeats is approximately 5000 and that of the type III repeats approximately 9000. The type III repeat lacking in plasma fibronectin is labeled the extra domain. The type III repeat-labeled IIIcs for type III connecting segment undergoes tissue specific splicing to generate polypeptide differences between cell and plasma fibronectins (see text and Fig. 2)

Extra Domain   IIIcs

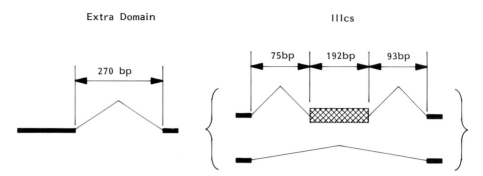

Figure 2. Splicing of plasma fibronectin pre-messenger RNA (mRNA). The pre-mRNA for plasma RNA is spliced at two sites. The extra domain region contains a 270-base pair (bp) nucleotide sequence encoding one type III repeat, which is present in cellular fibronectin messenger RNA (mRNA) and spliced out of plasma fibronectin mRNA. The second region of difference, the variable domain (or IIIcs for type III connecting segment), either contains (hatched box, top) a 192-bp sequence encoding an abbreviated 64-amino acid type III repeat in one subunit of plasma fibronectin or is removed completely (bottom) in the mRNA encoding the other subunit. Cellular fibronectins may contain the extra domain and have additional splicing patterns in the IIIcs or variable region. (See text, Hynes, 1985, and Sekiguchi *et al.*, 1986, for further details. Modified from Sekiguchi *et al.*, 1986.)

synthesizing cellular fibronections either contains or lacks a 270-nucleotide sequence—the ED—encoding one type III repeat of 90 amino acids. This sequence is absent from hepatocyte mRNAs (Sekiguchi *et al.*, 1986), the source of plasma fibronection (Owens and Cimino, 1982; Tamkun and Hynes, 1983). Accordingly, there are 15 type III repeats in plasma fibronectin and 16 in cellular fibronectin (Sekiguchi *et al.*, 1986). A second region of potential sequence difference (the IIIcs or connecting segment region) is located between the last two type III repeats near the carobxyl terminal (Fig. 1). Differential splicing in this region appears to account for the difference in subunit molecular weight of human plasma fibronectin and different proteolytic cleavage patterns of the two plasma fibronectin subunits in the carboxyl terminal domains as well as potential differences amongst cellular fibronectins (Sekiguchi *et al.*, 1986) (Fig. 2). Details of various splicing schemes may be found in Hynes (1985) and Sekiguchi *et al.* (1986).

To summarize, plasma fibronectin is produced by hepatocytes and lacks one type III repeat sequence encoded by the ED region (Fig. 1). In addition, the larger subunit of plasma fibronectin probably contains a 64-amino acid sequence in the IIIcs region, whereas the smaller subunit lacks this sequence (Sekiguchi *et al.*, 1986). It is not yet established whether plasma fibronectin molecules are heterodimers or a mixture of both heterodimers and homodimers. Cellular fibronectins also have polypeptide differences, as mRNAs differing in the IIIcs region have been identified (see Hynes, 1985; Sekiguchi *et al.*, 1986).

Although it is unlikely that this complex scheme of pre-mRNA splicing evolved without purpose, no clear explanation for the structural differences between various forms of fibronectin exists. The biologic differences may be explained by environmentally induced secondary changes, such as multimer formation, or may have been due to other contaminating macromolecules in cellular fibronectin preparations. For example, a distinct macromolecule, termed myotendinous antigen, was responsible for the hemagglutinating activity of cellular fibronectin preparations (Erickson and Inglesias, 1984). Virtually nothing is known about the mechanisms by which splicing of fibronectin pre-mRNAs is regulated in various cells. Plasma fibronectin appears early in wounds at the time of plasma extravasation and clotting, while cellular fibronectin occurs later, at times of tissue regeneration (Clark and Colvin, 1985). It is not known whether these different fibronectins function differently.

2.3. Post-translational Modifications

Fibronectin undergoes a variety of post-translational modifications, including N-linked glycosylation, which protects the collagen-binding domain against proteolysis (Bernard et al., 1982; Fukuda et al., 1982). Polylactosamine units are added to placental fibronectin, altering its collagen-binding avidity (Laine et al., 1984; Yamaguchi et al., 1986). Since tunicamycin, a drug that inhibits N-glycosylation of asparagine residues, does not block fibronectin secretion (Olden et al., 1980), the N-linked carbohydrates do not appear to play a major role in secretion of fibronectin as they do in the secretion of many proteins. [Although monensin inhibits fibronectin secretion, this effect is presumably due to blocking transit through the Golgi rather than by altering glycosylation (Uchida et al., 1980; Ledger et al., 1980).] Fibroblasts cultured with swainsonine, an inhibitor of N-linked oligosaccharide processing, secrete fibronectin with altered glycosylation but with no evidence of functional abnormalities (Ledger et al., 1983; Arumugham and Tanzer, 1983). There is a preliminary report that fibronection from cultured fibroblasts is acylated, raising the potential that fibronectin could have a transmembrane domain (Lange-Mutschler, 1986).

Fibronectin contains phosphoserine (Ledger and Tanzer, 1982); tyrosene-O-sulfate has been identified in sarcoma virus infected rat fibroblast fibronectin (Liu, 1985). Fibronectin contains two sulfhydryl groups (Garcia-Pardo et al., 1985; Vibe-Pedersen et al., 1982; Smith et al., 1982), which are slowly reactive with Ellman's reagent under physiologic conditions (McDonald and Kelly, 1980). There is a plasma transglutaminase (coagulation factor XIIIa) reactive glutamine residue in position 3 (R. P. McDonagh et al., 1981), which can participate in covalent crosslinking of fibronectin to fibrin or collagen or to itself. An additional cryptic transglutaminase crosslinking site is present (Richter et al., 1981).

2.4. Secondary and Tertiary Structure

Plasma fibronectin has considerable β-structure and little α-helical content (Gartner and Bennett, 1985; Odermatt et al., 1982). The type III homologous sequences, the predominant repeating unit of fibronectins, are composed of relatively conserved sequences flanking a more variable central region (Hynes, 1985). Interestingly, computer analysis of the type III sequences in the cell- and heparin-binding regions suggests β-pleated structures with exposed regions located at the center of each type III repeat (Odermatt *et al.*, 1985). When sprayed onto mica and imaged using rotary shadowing, plasma fibronectin molecules are elongated and often V shaped with arms of about 80 nm in length and 2 nm in width, with an angle of about 70% between the arms (Odermatt *et al.*, 1982; Timpl *et al.*, 1981; Erickson and Carrell, 1983; Erickson *et al.*, 1981). This observation fits well with Erickson's estimates for the volume required to contain each minidomain or repeating unit (Erickson and Carrell, 1983).

Hydrodynamic studies based on sedimentation of varying ionic strength demonstrate that plasma fibronectin undergoes a transition to a more compact shape under physiologic conditions (Erickson and Carrell, 1983), suggesting that the fibronectin molecule is opened up during binding to mica. On the basis of this flexibility and charge distribution, models have been proposed in which fibronectin molecules in solution are folded on themselves in such a way as to neutralize charged domains (Homandberg and Erickson, 1986; Homandberg *et al.*, 1985; Markovic *et al.*, 1983; Hormann and Richter, 1986). These models also suggest possible mechanisms for fibronectin assembly into multimers (Hormann and Richter, 1986; Homandberg and Erickson, 1986) by self-association (see Sections 5.4–5.7).

3. Fibronectin-Binding Activities

3.1. Binding Macromolecules

Fibronectins bind many macromolecules, including *Staphylococcus aureus* cell-wall components (Proctor *et al.*, 1982), other bacteria, including *Treponema pallidum* (Thomas *et al.*, 1985), a number of parasites (Ouaossi *et al.*, 1984; Roberts *et al.*, 1985), native and denatured collagens (Engvall *et al.*, 1978; McDonald *et al.*, 1982), actin (Keski-Oja and Yamada, 1981), thrombospondin (Lahav *et al.*, 1984; Bale *et al.*, 1985; Lahav *et al.*, 1982), heparin and heparan sulfate (Gold *et al.*, 1983; Hayashi and Yamada, 1982; Hayashi *et al.*, 1980), hyaluronic acid (Yamada *et al.*, 1980), DNA (Pande *et al.*, 1985; Sieber-Blum, 1984; Hayashi and Yamada, 1982), fibronectins (Ehrismann *et al.*, 1981; Homandberg *et al.*, 1985; Homandberg and Erickson, 1986), fibrin (Garcia-Pardo *et al.*, 1985; Banyai *et al.*, 1983; Sekiguchi and Hakomori, 1980), and cell-surface receptors on fibroblastic cells and myoblasts (Tamkun *et al.*, 1986; Pytela *et al.*, 1985a,b).

3.2. Fibronectin-Binding Domains

Both biophysical and biologic studies (Hynes, 1985; Ingham *et al.*, 1984; McDonald and Kelley, 1980) support the concept of fibronectins as remarkably modular proteins, with protease-resistant macrodomains composed of multiple units of the minidomains or repeated sequences of type I, II, or III (Fig. 1). Hynes (1985) suggested that each repeat of minidomain may possess binding activity and that the larger domains are thus multimeric interactive sites. For example, only one type I repeat is found in plasminogen activator, which binds fibrin (Banyai et al., 1983), whereas fibrin-binding activity in fibronectin is mediated via the amino and carboxyl terminal regions containing several type I repeats. Similarly, type I repeats have been implicated in fibronectin–fibronectin binding; plasminogen activator with its one type I repeat binds to fibronectin as well, although the fibronectin binding site has not been localized (Salonen et al., 1985).

   Although it is not yet known whether each minidomain possesses specific ligand-binding activity, each fibronectin macrodomain clearly displays characteristic binding activities and structure independent of the other macrodomains (Hynes and Yamada, 1982). For example, the major proteolytic fragments of fibronectin comprising virtually the entire sequence have distinctive thermal denaturation characteristics, and the sum of the denaturation curves is very similar to that of the intact molecule (Ingham et al., 1984). The macro- or binding domains are joined with flexible protease-sensitive polypeptide links.

3.3. Isolation of Binding Domains

   Because fibronectin-binding domains are protease resistant, limited proteolysis followed by affinity chromatography of the fibronectin digest on binding macromolecules or on domain specific antibody columns has been useful in probing fibronectin structure and function (McDonald and Kelley, 1980; Zardi et al., 1985). The fibronectin domains binding to Staphylococcus, collagen, cells, heparin, and fibrin have all been isolated, using this strategy. Binding studies using pure components (e.g., denatured collagen and fibronectin) demonstrate that isolated domains retain significant binding activity. As expected, the purified binding domains serve as specific competitive inhibitors of intact fibronectin binding (McDonald and Kelley, 1980; Singer et al., 1985; Johansson, 1985; Akiyama and Yamada, 1985; Akiyama et al., 1985). For example, the purified collagen binding domain of fibronectin competitively inhibits fibronectin binding to collagen but not to cells, whereas sequences containing the cell-adhesive domain inhibit fibronectin binding to cells but have no effect on collagen binding (McDonald and Kelley, 1980; Akiyama and Yamada, 1985).

   An alternative approach to the study of fibronectin structure–function relationships uses recombinant DNA technology to express fibronectin domains as fusion proteins in bacteria. By expressing defined regions, binding ability may be mapped to specific sequences or to certain amino acid residues implicated in binding. Using this approach, Owens and Baralle (1986) determined that a 12,000-M_r region, including the second type II repeat and the initial sequence of a subsequent type I repeat, are important in collagen binding.

3.4. A Molecular Model

These comparisons of structure with function suggest a model of fibronectin as a flexible molecule containing serial binding sites acting more or less independently from one another (Hynes and Yamada, 1982). This union of specific binding sites for macromolecules, a dimeric elongated structure, and a specific site binding to cells suggested that fibronectins could link cells and extracellular matrix molecules (Hynes and Yamada, 1982). In addition to this linking function, fibronectins both self-assemble and form covalent inter- and intramolecular crosslinks. These are properties common to other connective tissue molecules, such as type I collagen, which form extensive matrices.

3.5. The Role of Fibronectin *in Vivo*

Dissociation constants for the binding of fibronectin to hyaluronic acid, heparin (Yamada *et al.*, 1980), collagen α-chains (Forastieri and Ingham, 1983, 1985), and fibroblasts (Akiyama *et al.*, 1985) are indicative of reasonably tight binding, which under certain circumstances may be strengthened considerably by the formation of multivalent complexes (McDonald and Kelley, 1984). The demonstration of fibronectin binding to other macromolecules does not *a priori* indicate that this binding is physiologically significant. For example, the ionic composition in some binding assays has not been physiologic, and binding to both heparin and fibrin is modulated by both divalent cations and ionic strength (Hayashi and Yamada, 1982).

Co-localization of fibronectin with the potential macromolecular or cellular ligand *in vitro* strengthens the case that fibronectin binding *in vitro* is significant. An additional and particularly powerful approach based on new structural information is the use of antibodies or peptides to inhibit fibronectin binding. This approach has been especially helpful in clarifying the role of the fibronectin cell-adhesive receptor. For other fibronectin interactions (e.g., fibronectin binding to collagen, fibrin, proteoglycans, and glycosaminoglycans, *Staphylococcus* cell walls), the physiologic significance is not yet clear. However, the widespread availability of inhibitory peptides and antibodies and possibly the use of antisense RNA should lead rapidly to new insights.

4. The Fibronectin-Receptor Complex

4.1. Identification of the Fibronectin Cell Receptor

A striking activity of fibronectin is its augmentation of fibroblastic cell attachment and spreading on material surfaces, such as collagen-coated and -uncoated plastic culture dishes. This adhesive activity is particularly evident with certain permanent cell lines, such as baby hamster kidney (BHK) and

Chinese Hamster ovary (CHO), which do not secrete endogenous cell-adhesive molecules. Diploid fibroblasts secrete endogenous fibronectin onto the culture substrate and then attach to it and spread (Grinnell and Feld, 1979).

Early studies localizing cell-adhesive activity to specific fibronectin fragments suggested that a specific domain might interact with cells. Pierschbacher et al. (1981) used a monoclonal antibody, which inhibited cell adhesion to fibronectin, in order to immunoaffinity-purify an 11,000-M_r pepsin-resistant cell-adhesive polypeptide. These workers sequenced the peptide and synthesized four nonoverlapping subfragments comprising the entire 11,000-M_r fragment. Only one peptide supported cell-adhesive activity (Pierschbacher et al., 1983). By synthesizing shorter sequences of this peptide, the sequence Arg-Gly-Asp-Ser (RGDS in the single-letter code) was found to possess significant cell-adhesive activity (Pierschbacher and Ruoslahti, 1984). Although this approach could potentially miss other cell-adhesive sites in fibronectin, BHK cell adhesion was inhibited by larger proteolytic fragments or synthetic peptides containing the RGDS sequence, whereas other similar peptides and fragments were noninhibitory. Together, these results demonstrated that there is one principal site in fibronectin interacting with fibroblastic and certain other cells to promote adhesion. Other cell types may recognize more than one site in fibronectin (McCarthy et al., 1986; Humphries et al., 1986).

4.2. Isolation of the Fibronectin Receptor

Initial clues to the identify of specific fibronectin receptors came from the isolation of antibodies inhibiting cell adhesion. Two groups independently obtained monoclonal antibodies inhibiting myoblast and fibroblast adhesion, respectively (Greve and Gottlieb, 1982; Knudsen et al., 1981). These antibodies immunoprecipitated a cell-surface polypeptide complex from cell extracts (Chapman, 1984; Decker et al., 1984). The co-distribution of the cell-surface polypeptide complex with fibronectin is consistent with the possibility that the polypeptide complex is involved in cell recognition of fibronectin (Damsky et al., 1985). A different approach was taken by Ruoslahti's group to isolate potential fibronectin receptors. Using the peptide specificity of fibronectin–cell interaction previously defined, Pytela et al. (1985a) passed extracts of surface-labeled cells over a cell-adhesive fibronectin fragment coupled to a solid support. The column was eluted with a synthetic peptide lacking cell-adhesive activity but similar (one-residue difference) to an active cell-adhesive peptide to remove nonspecifically bound polypeptides. Elution of the column with an active cell-adhesive peptide released two labeled cell-surface glycoproteins of approximately 140,000 M_r. This 140,000-M_r glycoprotein complex bound specifically to liposomes containing fibronectin (Pytela et al., 1985a). A similar receptor complex isolated from chick fibroblasts was demonstrated to bind to fibronectin (Akiyama et al., 1986). In both cases, binding was specifically inhibited by peptides containing the RGDS sequence.

4.3. Isolation of cDNA for the Fibronectin-Receptor Subunits

Using antibodies to the putative fibronectin receptor to probe chick and human cDNA expression libraries, cDNA encoding the carboxyl-terminal of the larger subunit of the human fibronectin receptor (Argraves et al., 1986) and the complete polypeptide sequence for the smallest or band-3 subunit of the chicken fibronectin receptor have been obtained (Tamkun et al., 1986). On the basis of this and unpublished information from the laboratories involved, it is now clear that the subunits of the putative fibronectin receptors from chicken and human fibroblastic cells are closely related on a molecular level.

The fully processed human α-subunit of the fibronectin receptor has a 25,000-M_r light-chain disulfide linked to a 125,000-M_r heavy-chain polypeptide. The deduced amino acid sequence of the carboxyl terminal portion of the α-subunit of the human fibronectin receptor includes a 23–28-amino acid cytoplasmic domain without homology to other known polypeptides, a 34-residue putative transmembrane domain, and an extracellular sequence thought to represent the entire light-chain portion of the α-subunit (Argraves et al., 1986). The deduced polypeptide sequence of the chicken band-3 subunit of the complex has a large extracellular domain with four unique cysteine-rich repeated sequences, a single putative transmembrane hydrophobic domain, and a short intracellular domain homologous to the intracellular portion of the epidermal growth factor (EGF) receptor including a potential tyrosine kinase site. The chicken polypeptide fibronectin-receptor complex has been termed integrin (Tamkun et al., 1986).

4.4. Fibronectin-Receptor Function

On the basis of several areas of evidence, the fibronectin receptor links cytoskeletal components with extracellular fibronectin. In cultured fibroblasts, the receptor is co-localized with extracellular fibronectin and intracellular α-actinin (Damsky et al., 1985; Chen et al., 1985). Both oncogenic transformation and cytoskeletal-disrupting agents alter cytoskeletal organization and cause the loss of organized fibronectin matrices from the cell surface (Tamkun et al., 1986; Chen et al., 1986a; Hirst et al., 1986). Transformation also results in reorganization of the fibronectin receptor to a more diffuse distribution (Chen et al., 1986a; Hirst et al., 1986). Synthetic peptides inhibiting fibronectin-receptor binding also cause loss of matrix fibronectin and a more diffuse appearance of the receptor (Chen et al., 1986a). Interestingly, transformation by viruses associated with tyrosine kinase activity also results in phosphorylation of the fibronectin-receptor complex on tyrosine and serine residues (Hirst et al., 1986). This phosphorylation could alter the binding of the fibronectin receptor to cytoskeletal components and/or fibronectin. Equilibrium gel filtration, a variant of the Hummel-Dreyer (1962) technique, demonstrates that the fibronectin-receptor complex binds talin, a component of cell-surface focal and close contacts and that fibronectin-receptor–talin complexes bind vinculin.

This provides additional support for the proposed role of the fibronectin-receptor complex in coupling matrix to cytoskeleton (Horwitz et al., 1986).

4.5. Related Cell-Adhesive Receptors

The RGDS sequence is also involved in cell adhesion promoted by serum-spreading factor or vitronectin (Pytela et al., 1985b, 1986; Suzuki et al., 1985). An RGDS sequence has been implicated in the interaction of fibronectin, von Willebrand factor, and fibrinogen with the platelet glycoprotein IIb/IIIa complex, an interaction important in hemostasis (Plow et al., 1985, Gardner and Hynes, 1985; Pytela et al., 1986). Thus, the fibronectin-receptor complex appears to be one member of a family of cell-surface-adhesive glycoproteins, including the Mac-1/LFA1 complex of monocytes and neutrophils and glycoproteins IIb/IIIa on platelets and neutrophils (Springer and Anderson, 1986; Burns et al., 1986) that mediate binding to RGDS containing sequences found in fibronectin, fibrin, and vitronectin. Similarly, laminin and vitronectin may both bind to the chicken fibronectin complex (Horwitz et al., 1985).

Identifying an integral membrane protein complex mediating cell adhesion by fibronectin and characterizing the binding helps clarify previously confusing results. Previous difficulty demonstrating binding of soluble fibronectin to cells appears to be explained by the moderate (Kd = 10^6 M) avidity of fibronectin-receptor binding (Akiyama and Yamada, 1985; Akiyama et al., 1985). The binding of fibronectin to the cell-adhesive receptor appears to be largely, if not entirely, responsible for the mediation of initial fibroblast adhesion and spreading by fibronectin (Akiyama and Yamada, 1985). Thus, earlier claims that fibronectin required activation by binding to other substrate-bound macromolecules such as denatured collagen or to synthetic substrates to promote cell adhesion appear less compelling. However, the mechanisms through which the addition of soluble fibronectin partially restores normal receptor distribution and cytoskeletal organization in virally transformed cells (Chen et al., 1986a) remains a mystery. Perhaps oligomers of fibronectin bind and initiate receptor clustering, in turn increasing receptor avidity for cytoplasmic proteins (e.g., talin), linking the receptor to the cytoskeleton.

4.6. Role of Fibronectin and Its Receptor Complex in Wound Healing and Cell Migration

The cell-adhesive domain of fibronectin (and by inference the fibronectin adhesive receptor) has been implicated in chick neural crest cell migration (Bronner-Fraser, 1985; Duband et al., 1986), amphibian gastrulation (Boucaut et al., 1984a,b), and wound re-epithelialization (as discussed in Chapter 14). In addition, evidence implicates the cell-adhesive receptor in the assembly of fibronectin-containing pericellular matrices (see Section 5.7). In the chicken lung, expression of the fibronectin-receptor complex is developmentally regulated, appearing early beneath forming airways and capillaries (Chen et al., 1986b). In adult human lung, the basal lamina of alveolar capillaries and alveolar epithelium contain relatively little fibronectin except during presumed injury and repair accompanying pulmonary fibrosis (Torikata et al., 1985). This is compatible with the use of fibronectin as a temporary adhesive or cell migratory substrate during both development and repair.

Studies of fibronectin in corneal, dermal, and lung alveolar epithelial repair in adults reveal a common theme. Fibronectin appears to play an important role in the initial re-epithelialization by mediating cell adhesion to the fibronectin-rich wound surface via cellular fibronectin receptors. For example, fibronectin augments the movement of corneal epithelial cells over the stromal surface of corneal plugs in vitro and hastens healing of chronic corneal ulcers in vivo (Nishida et al., 1982, 1983a–c, 1984). Both synthetic peptides blocking fibronectin-mediated adhesion and larger proteolytic fragments inhibit corneal re-epithelialization in an in vitro model (M. Berman, personal communication). Similarly, fibronectin has been implicated in keratinocyte adhesion and migration during dermal wound healing (Takashima and Grinnell, 1984, 1985; R. A. F. Clark et al., 1985; Kubo et al., 1984; O'Keefe et al., 1985). Injured lung, similar to the injured dermis and cornea, has increased fibronectin detectable in the basal lamina (Torikata et al., 1985). The cuboidal epithelial cell responsible for re-epithelializing the denuded lung alveolar surface (the type II cell) prefers to attach and spread on fibronectin when presented with several basal lamina and interstitial connective tissue components (R. A. F. Clark et al., 1986). On the basis of this common response to injury, it is likely that expression of the fibronectin receptor is increased during wound healing, although there are currently no available data.

5. The Role of Fibronectin in Matrix Assembly

5.1. Fibronectin and Wound Healing

Fibronectins are thought to play many roles in wound healing, including promotion of re-epithelialization (see Chapters 14 and 23), cell migration (see Chapter 13), wound contraction (see Chapter 17), and matrix deposition. This section comments primarily on the latter role, as the other aspects of the involvement of fibronectin are covered earlier in this volume. Fibronectin is a component of the initial plasma clot in open wounds and is crosslinked both to fibrin and to itself by plasma transglutaminase (coagulation factor XIIIa) (Grinnell et al., 1981; Mosher and Johnson, 1983). The interaction of fibronectin with fibrin appears to be particularly significant. In vitro, fibronectin is required for fibroblast attachment to fibrin; crosslinking of fibronectin to fibrin by factor XIIIa strengthens fibroblast attachment (see Grinnell et al., 1981 and references cited therein). Fibroblasts require factor XIII to proliferate in fibrin clots (Beck et al., 1961; Ueyama and Urayama, 1978), and patients with factor XIII deficiency have impaired wound healing (Alami et al., 1968; Duckert,

1972). Fibrin clots and fibrinopeptides weakly stimulate fibroblast proliferation (Kittlick, 1979). Depletion of fibronectin from plasma clots prevents fibroblast migration (Knox et al., 1986), although the migration of fibroblasts from explanted pieces of lung tissue into fibronectin-depleted plasma clots does occur (Song et al., 1986). Fibronectin and its cell-adhesive fragments are chemotactic for fibroblasts (Postlethwaite et al., 1981) and fibronectin fragments, but surprisingly not the intact molecule, are also chemotactic for monocytes (Clark et al., 1985), which arrive early at wound sites and which also release additional fibroblast attractants such as platelet-derived growth factor (PDGF)-like molecules (Ross et al., 1986).

Wound-invading fibroblasts, presumably under the influence of local polypeptide growth factors, deposit types I and III, and likely other collagens, as well as fibronectin, proteoglycans, and hyaluronic acid (Williams et al., 1984; Barnes et al., 1976). Immunostaining shows early wounds to contain relatively more type III collagen than is found in type I collagen (Williams et al., 1984). Most studies on matrix deposition in vitro use immunostaining, and the thinner type III collagen fibers may be preferentially stained. In addition, biochemical studies demonstrate clearly that dermal and lung fibroblasts in vitro synthesize predominantly type I collagen rather than type III and coordinately regulate synthesis of both (Steinmann et al., 1982; Abe et al., 1979; Liau et al., 1985; Miskulin et al., 1986). However, local influences such as polypeptide growth factors in the wound site may transiently alter the relative proportions of collagens. Similar histologic and biochemical changes appear to occur in other organs and tissues such as lung, where fibrin clots are populated by fibroblasts and a similar sequence of collagen deposition into a fibronectin rich environment occurs (J. G. Clark et al., 1983).

As dermal wounds age, bundles of type I collagen become more evident, and the detectable fibronectin and fibroblasts decrease (Grinnell et al., 1981). Although an important phase in wound healing, nothing is known about the mechanisms responsible for the decreases in fibronectin and fibroblasts in the healing wound.

5.2. Connective Tissue Matrix Organization by Fibronectin

In addition to attracting cells to the wound site and promoting re-epithelialization, fibronectin may also play a direct role in initial matrix deposition or assembly. This speculation follows from both in vitro fibroblast culture experiments and immunohistochemical studies on healing wounds. Preventing the formation of a fibronectin matrix by lung fibroblasts in vitro inhibits deposition of collagen types I and III (McDonald et al., 1982). The fibroblast requirement for a fibronectin matrix to deposit types I and III collagen could be an artifact of tissue culture. However, there are enough similarities between fibroblast culture conditions and those of wound sites to suggest that the fibroblast model is relevant to wound healing.

Light microscopic studies demonstrate that fibroblasts in dermal wound healing are surrounded by a fibronectin-rich matrix during granulation tissue formation (Grinnell *et al.*, 1981; Repesh *et al.*, 1982). Electron microscopic studies of healing experimental dermal wounds demonstrate myofibroblasts with abundant surface fibronectin aligned with intracellular stress fibers (Singer *et al.*, 1984, 1985). This assembly has been termed the fibronexus by Singer (1984). Although double-label immunoelectron microscopy to localize collagen types I or III and fibronectin has not been performed in healing wounds, the normal dermis contains fibers staining with antibodies to both fibronectin and the amino-terminal propeptide of collagen type I (Fleischmajer *et al.*, 1981). The matrix deposited by cultured fibroblasts also contains composite fibrils containing fibronectin, collagen types I, III, VI, and other matrix components. It should not be too surprising that the matrix deposited by fibroblasts grown in culture resembles that found in early wounds, as the serum supplement typically added to fibroblast culture medium contains polypeptide growth factors derived from platelets and fibrinopeptides implicated in wound healing and matrix deposition (Ross *et al.*, 1986).

5.3. Models of Matrix Deposition

Cultured fibroblasts have been used to elucidate many of the features of the deposition of fibronectin in the pericellular matrix. Fibronectin is organized by fibroblastic cells in culture into striking parallel arrays visible using the fluorescent antibody technique (Fig. 3). Immunofluorescence and immunoelectron microscopic observations of smooth muscle (Bornstein and Ash, 1977) and fibroblast cultures (Hedman *et al.*, 1979; McDonald *et al.*, 1982) demonstrate that fibronectin and type I and III (pro)collagen are typically indistinguishably codistributed with fibronectin using the fluorescent antibody technique (Fig. 3).

Fibronectin deposition appears to occur in at least two stages in fibroblast culture. Initially, in the absence of serum, fibronectin secreted within the first 1–2 hr from freshly plated fibroblasts binds to the substrate and permits cell attachment and spreading (Grinnell and Feld, 1979). This fibronectin may be subsequently organized beneath the spreading cells in the form of footprints and linear strands closely associated with the fibronectin receptor (Avnur and Geiger, 1981; Damsky *et al.*, 1985; Chen *et al.*, 1985). Later, following cell proliferation, an extensive three-dimensional pericellular matrix surrounds the fibroblasts (Hedman *et al.*, 1979; Irish and Hasty, 1983; Furcht *et al.*, 1980). It is important to recognize that there may be differences in both the mechanisms of organization of the subcellular material initially deposited by fibroblasts and the material surrounding the cells that Hedman has termed the pericellular matrix (Hedman *et al.*, 1979). Because the pericellular matrix is between and above cells and not simply adherent to a planar surface, it at least topologically more closely resembles the matrix deposited during early wound healing.

The biochemical composition of the pericellular matrix of cultured human fibroblasts has been studied using sodium deoxycholate or other detergents to remove most of the soluble cytoplasmic components and plasma membranes and retain the detergent insoluble matrix. This matrix contains fibronectin, type I and III procollagen, type VI collagen, tenascin or myotendinous antigen, sulfated proteoglycans (including heparan and chondroitin sulfate), and other components (Hedman et al., 1979, 1982, 1984; Wartiovaara et al., 1978; Carter, 1984; Chiquet-Ehrismann et al., 1986). Fibroblast matrix is resistant to digestion by heparitinase and bacterial collagenase yet is disrupted by trypsin, suggesting that once deposited, its structural stability and thus scaffold or core is not dependent on either a heparan sulfate proteoglycan or on collagenous components but is probably glycoprotein in nature (Hedman et al., 1984).

The fibronectin-rich matrix of embryonic chick fibroblasts is insoluble in chaotropic buffers yet is solubilized by dithiothreitol-containing buffers suggesting a disulfide-linked polymer structure (Chen et al., 1978). Indeed, cell-surface fibronectin dimers are disulfide crosslinked to multimeters after secretion from the cell (Choi and Hynes, 1979). Surprisingly, this crosslinking process may involve disulfide interchange within the amino-terminal domains of fibronectin, which lack free cysteine rather than via the two available cysteine residues (McKeown-Longo and Mosher, 1984). Multimer formation requires intimate cell–matrix association. Other components, including type VI collagen, are also present as disulfide-linked multimers in the detergent insoluble matrix but are not disulfide crosslinked to the fibronectin scaffold (Carter, 1984).

The fibronectin matrix deposited by cultured fibroblasts appears to serve as a scaffold for the deposition of type I and III collagen (McDonald et al., 1982) and collagen type VI (Carter, 1984). Human lung fibroblasts cultured with antibodies to the collagen-binding domain of fibronectin (McDonald et al., 1981) were unable to assemble a fibronectin-containing pericellular matrix, even though the antibodies had no effect on cell adhesion, growth, protein synthesis, or cell morphology (McDonald et al., 1982). In the absence of a fibronectin matrix, collagen deposition in the cell layer was strikingly reduced, although its synthesis was unaffected. Although this observation demonstrates that a fibronectin matrix is important for collagen deposition by fibroblasts, processing of type I procollagen, as judged by removal of the carboxyl-terminal propeptides, is deficient in the embryonic lung fibroblast strain used, raising questions about just how faithfully the fibroblast model reproduces *in vivo* conditions (McDonald et al., 1986).

Ultrastructurally, cultured fibroblast fibronectin is found in 10–20-nm fibrils that stain periodically with polyclonal antifibronectin antibodies (Hedman et al., 1978; Hedman, 1980; Livingston et al., 1981; Furcht et al., 1980). Although a study using double-label immunoelectron microscopy has not been published, similar-size fibrils stain with antibodies to procollagen type I (Furcht et al., 1980). As all recognizable fibrils in fibroblast cultures less than 1 week old stained with either fibronectin or procollagen antibodies, it is reasonable to assume that most fibrils formed contain both antigens. However, both the stoichiometry and arrangement of collagenous or fibronectin domains in these fibrils are unknown. Further studies on the immunohistochemical localization of fibronectin and collagen during wound healing and on the effect

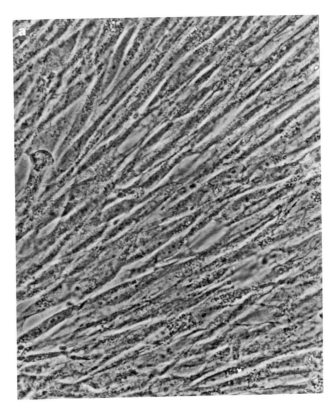

Figure 3. Phase and fluorescent micrographs of IMR-90 embryonic human lung fibroblasts cultured in 5 days in ascorbate supplemented medium. (See McDonald *et al.*, 1987.) (a) Phase microscopy. (b) Procollagen type I. (c) Fibronectin. Note that the matrix parallels the cell alignment and that procollagen and fibronectin are co-distributed in the pericellular matrix. Bar 50 μm.

of specific inhibitors of fibronectin-collagen binding are needed to clarify the possible role of fibronectin in collagen deposition during wound healing.

5.4. Role of Fibroblasts in Matrix Deposition and Organization

Although purified plasma fibronectin forms fibrils under certain non-physiologic conditions *in vitro* (Vuento *et al.*, 1980), an organized pericellular matrix only forms on fibroblasts in culture and never apart from the cells. Although isolated footprints of fibronectin may remain on the substratum where fibroblasts had previously been attached, recognizable matrix is restricted either to the fibroblast surface or to areas between adjacent cells. Thus, fibroblasts must play a critical role in fibronectin matrix assembly. Although cells that do not secrete fibronectin cannot assemble a matrix from exogenous fibronectin, the ability to synthesize and secrete fibronectin is not sufficient for

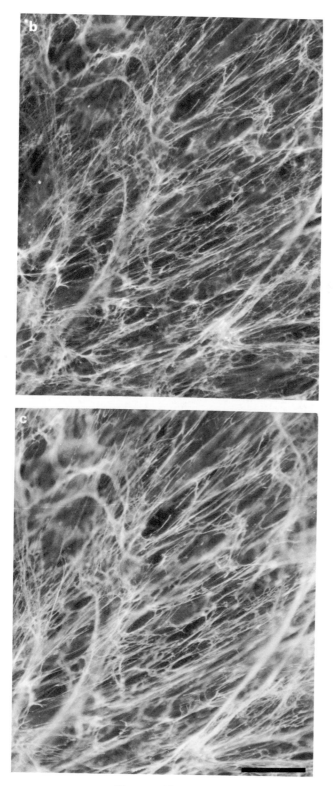

Figure 3. (*Continued*)

matrix assembly. For example, human alveolar macrophages dedicate as much as 70% of their total secreted protein synthesis to fibronectin, yet cannot assemble a pericellular matrix (Villiger *et al.*, 1981).

The fibronectin matrix organized by cultured fibroblasts is related to cell shape and degree of parallel alignment. For example, cultured newborn rat lung fibroblasts are more spread and exhibit less parallel alignment than IMR-90 (see Fig. 3) and lack extensive long matrix fibrils (McDonald and Kelley, 1984). Similarly, F-9 teratocarcinoma cells form more parallel arrays when exposed to retinoic acid and also develop a more organized fibronectin matrix (Dahl and Grabel, 1986). Repesh *et al.* (1982) demonstrated parallel arrays of presumptively migratory fibroblasts and fibronectin matrix at the edge of healing dermal wounds. These observations suggest that the pericellular arrays formed by fibroblasts *in vitro* are created by cell movement, as suggested by Harris and co-workers (Stopak and Harris, 1982; Harris *et al.*, 1981), for the remodeling of preformed collagen gels by fibroblasts. This process, termed traction morphogenesis, results in parallel arrays of collagen fibrils from fibroblasts pulling at opposite poles of an initially disorganized matrix. If this scheme is correct, it implies that cell movement must be taken into account when patterns of matrix assembly are studied. For example, agents perturbing cell movement could alter matrix assembly indirectly without any direct effect on the molecules involved or their cellular receptors.

5.5. Mechanisms of Fibronectin Matrix Assembly

The evidence that fibronectin is pivotal in early matrix assembly makes it important to understand the molecular features of this event. The first clue to a functional domain of fibronectin involved in matrix assembly came from studies performed to probe the role of fibronectin in collagen deposition suggesting that there was a site near the amino-terminal of fibronectin involved in its assembly into fibroblast matrix (McDonald *et al.*, 1981, 1982). McKeown-Longo and Mosher (1983) established that labeled plasma fibronectin binds initially to a detergent soluble pool and is subsequently transferred to a detergent insoluble pool and disulfide crosslinked into multimeric fibronectin. Although immunofluorescence results were stated to suggest that the fibronectin is initially diffusely bound to the cell surface and subsequently transferred into matrix fibrils, simultaneous staining of pre-existing matrix fibronectin using a different fluorochrome was not performed and the published images did not convincingly demonstrate generalized cell-surface staining (McKeown-Longo and Mosher, 1983). Thus, the precise location of this early binding pool of fibronectin remains unclear.

When isolated domains were used as competitive inhibitors, the amino-terminal 70,000- and 25,000-M_r domains of fibronectin were found to inhibit incorporation of plasma fibronectin into matrix. By contrast, a large fingerless 105,000-M_r cell-adhesive fragment from the central portion of the molecule containing only type III repeats had no effect on the incorporation of plasma fibronectin into the matrix (McKeown-Longo and Mosher, 1985). These results confirmed that the amino-terminal domain of fibronectin contained information important for its assemby into matrix and mapped an important region to the first 25,000 M_r. Other studies support the view that the amino-terminal of fibronectin is important in matrix assembly. For example, large fibronectin fragments lacking the amino-terminal are not incorporated into extracellular matrices either in culture or *in vivo* (Millis *et al.*, 1985; Oh *et al.*, 1981), and endogenous fibroblast–fibronectin matrix assembly is effectively inhibited by both antibodies to the amino-terminal 25,000-M_r domain and fragments containing this sequence (McDonald *et al.*, 1987).

5.6. Role of the Amino-Terminal Domain of Fibronectin in Matrix Assembly

McKeown-Longo and Mosher (1983, 1985) suggested that fibroblasts possess a specific matrix assembly receptor that binds to the amino-terminal domain of fibronectin. However, alternative hypotheses have been advanced, and isolation of a receptor with specificity for the amino-terminal domain of fibronectin has not been reported. Plasma membrane-associated heparan sulfate proteoglycans have been suggested as possible alternate fibronectin receptors involved in matrix assembly (Woods *et al.*, 1984, 1985), but high-avidity heparan sulfate binding resides in the carboxyl-terminal heparin-binding domain, not in the amino-terminal (Gold *et al.*, 1983). Alternatively, fibronectin has been shown to bind itself via its amino-terminal and carboxyl-terminal domains containing the type I homology units (Homandberg *et al.*, 1985; Homandberg and Erickson, 1986). Similar results have been obtained by Ehrismann *et al.* (1981, 1982), but the precise origin of the fibronectin–fibronectin-binding site in their studies is unclear. Thus, amino-terminal (or amino-terminal and carboxyl-terminal) domains could be involved in fibril assembly. In this scheme, domains composed of type I repeats would participate in fibril elongation rather than directly mediating the association of fibronectin with the cell (Chernousov *et al.*, 1985; McDonald *et al.*, 1987). An alternate model of intra- and intermolecular interaction of fibronectin based on charge neutralization has been proposed (Hormann and Richter, 1986).

The amino-terminal domain of fibronectin could also mediate matrix assembly by ganglioside binding. The 25,000-M_r amino-terminal domain is a major binding site for oligosaccharides (Thompson *et al.*, 1986), and gangliosides have been implicated in fibronectin matrix assembly (Yamada *et al.*, 1983; Spiegel *et al.*, 1986). If ganglioside binding by the amino-terminal mediates fibronectin matrix assembly, the oligosaccharide moiety of fibronectin-binding gangliosides should inhibit matrix assembly by fibroblasts, similar to the effect of adding a purified amino-terminal domain of fibronectin (Spiegel *et al.*, 1986b; McDonald *et al.*, 1986b). This experiment has not yet been reported.

However, a positive result from this experiment could still be ambiguous, as gangliosides may also play a role in fibronectin binding to its adhesive receptor (Perkins *et al.*, 1982; Cheresh and Klier, 1986). Since the cell-adhesive receptor also mediates matrix assembly, it may be difficult to unambiguously sort out the precise role of gangliosides.

5.7. Role of the Cell-Adhesive Fibronectin Receptor in Matrix Assembly

Several lines of evidence (Tamkun *et al.*, 1986) suggest that the fibronectin cell-adhesive receptor may be involved in organizing the matrix. The fibronectin receptor is co-localized in the fibroblast plasma membrane with both the actin cytoskeleton inside and the fibronectin fibrils outside (Damsky *et al.*, 1985; Chen *et al.*, 1985). Agents disrupting the cytoskeleton of fibroblasts, such as viral transformation or cytochalasins, result in loss or altered organization of the external fibronectin matrix as well as a more diffuse organization of the fibronectin receptor (Hirst *et al.*, 1986; Chen *et al.*, 1986a).

Studies on the role of the fibronectin cell-adhesive site in matrix assembly have yielded seemingly contradictory results. When added to culture medium early during fibroblast growth, both a large proteolytic fragment containing the cell-adhesive receptor-binding site and monoclonal antibodies inhibiting cell adhesion inhibit fibroblast matrix assembly (McDonald *et al.*, 1987). By contrast, McKeown-Longo and Mosher (1985) found that a similar fingerless fragment did not inhibit the binding of exogenous plasma fibronectin to fibroblast cultures. The reason for the discordant results probably relates to differences in the assays used. If the differences in results are real, they undoubtedly give insight into the mechanisms of matrix assembly. The assay used by McKeown-Longo and Mosher uses cells that have already initiated matrix assembly. Because the fibronectin cell-adhesive receptor complex is co-localized with early fibronectin fibrils (Damsky *et al.*, 1985; Chen *et al.*, 1985), it may initiate fibril formation. Thus, in the McKeown-Longo assay, fibronectin could be incorporated via a later step in matrix assembly that is independent of the cell-adhesive receptor. Elongation of fibrils may be a mechanistically separate process involving the amino-terminal and possibly carboxyl-terminal domains (Chernousov *et al.*, 1985; McDonald *et al.*, 1987).

Understanding the molecular and cellular mechanisms of fibronectin's assembly into matrix fibrils and the role played by fibronectin in the deposition of other matrix components *in vivo* may yield valuable pharmacologic agents capable of augmenting or retarding specific events during wound healing. For example, the application of exogenous fibronectin or growth factors stimulating fibronectin synthesis might hasten impaired wound healing, whereas addition of fibronectin-related synthetic peptides or antifibronectin monoclonal antibodies could possibly reduce abnormal increases in connective tissue deposition characterizing keloid formation or other pathologic conditions such as fibrosis.

6. Regulation of Fibronectin Synthesis

6.1. Growth Factors

Capillary endothelium, macrophages, and fibroblasts in wound sites may increase their synthesis of fibronectin (R. A. F. Clark et al., 1982). Polypeptide growth factors (platelet-derived growth factor, brain-derived growth factor, transforming growth factor-β), present in platelets and synthesized by a variety of cells including activated macrophages and lymphocytes, are speculated to play a pivotal role in wound healing by stimulating growth and migration of mesenchymal cells (Ross et al., 1986; Massague, 1985). TGF-β greatly increases the synthesis of connective tissue molecules, particularly fibronectin and procollagen type I by cutured fibroblasts (Ignotz and Massague, 1986; Roberts et al., 1986). This has been dramatically demonstrated by the development of abundant granulation tissue within 24–48 hr after the subcutaneous injection of 800 ng of TGF-β into newborn mice (Roberts et al., 1986). It has been emphasized that TGF-β increases connective tissue synthesis selectively (Ignotz and Massague, 1986; Roberts et al., 1986), a property in keeping with an altered phenotype of wound healing fibroblasts (McDonald et al., 1986). Although there is evidence for coordinate regulation of fibronectin and type I collagen synthesis (Setoyama et al., 1985), it is not yet known whether TGF-β affects connective tissue synthesis at the transcriptional or translational level, nor are its effects on the expression of various matrix receptors known (see also Chapter 12).

6.2. Feedback Regulation

In addition to the stimulatory effect of growth factors on fibronectin synthesis, there is evidence suggesting feedback regulation of this process. For example, smooth muscle cells plated on a fibronectin substrate decrease the synthesis of fibronectin and of type I and III procollagen (Holderbaum and Ehrhart, 1986). Similarly, fibroblasts prevented from assembling a fibronectin pericellular matrix respond by accumulating two- to threefold increases in total fibronectin, perhaps responding to an absent fibronectin matrix by increasing its synthesis (McDonald et al., 1987b). The regulation of fibronectin synthesis by the adjacent matrix, presumably mediated by specific fibronectin receptors, is a potential mechanism of reducing fibronectin synthesis, once wound healing is initiated and the provisional matrix is established. Indeed, if the occupancy of fibronectin receptors were to regulate fibronectin synthesis, increased receptor expression could be a primary event in growth factor-mediated increases in fibronectin synthesis.

Recent advances in the chemistry and cell biology of the fibronectins have yielded a wealth of new information about their structure, function, and interactions with cell receptors and other macromolecules. The application of this information and of reagents such as antibodies, synthetic fragments, and recombinant molecules should rapidly advance our knowledge of the role of fibronectin in wound healing. It is hoped that this knowledge will lead to the development of new diagnostic and therapeutic reagents to modify the wound-healing process selectively.

References

Abe, S., Steinmann, B. U., Wahl, L. M., and Martin, G. R., 1979, High cell density alters the ratio of type III to I collagen synthesis by fibroblasts, *Nature (Lond.)* **279:**442–444.

Akiyama, S. K., and Yamada, K., 1985, Synthetic peptides competitively inhibit both direct binding to fibroblasts and functional biological assays for the purified cell-binding domain of fibronectin, *J. Biol. Chem.* **260:**10402–10405.

Akiyama, S. K., Hasegawa, E., Hasegawa, T., and Yamada, K. M., 1985, The interaction of fibronectin fragments with fibroblastic cells, *J. Biol. Chem.* **260:**13256–13260.

Akiyama, S. K., Yamada, S. S., and Yamada, K. M., 1986, Characterization of a 140-kD avian cell surface antigen as a fibronectin-binding molecule, *J. Cell Biol.* **102:**442–448.

Alami, S. Y., Hampton, J. W., Race, G. J., and Speer, R. J., 1968, Fibrin stabilizing factor (factor XIII), *Am. J. Med.* **44:**1–7.

Alitalo, K., Hovi, T., and Vaheri, A., 1980, Fibronectin is produced by human macrophages, *J. Exp. Med.* **151:**602–613.

Argraves, W. S., Pytela, R., Suzuki, S., Millan, J. L., Pierschbacher, M. D., and Ruoslahti, E., 1986, cDNA sequences from the alpha subunit of the fibronectin receptor predict a transmembrane domain and a short cytoplasmic peptide, *J. Biol. Chem.* **261:**12922–12924.

Arumugham, R. G., and Tanzer, M. L., 1983, Abnormal glycosylation of human cellular fibronectin in the presence of swainsonine, *J. Biol. Chem.* **258:**11883–11889.

Avnur, Z., and Geiger, B., 1981, The removal of extracellular fibronectin from areas of cell–substrate contact, *Cell* **25:**121–132.

Bale, M. D., Westrick, L. G., and Mosher, D. F., 1985, Incorporation of thrombospondin into fibrin clots, *J. Biol. Chem.* **260:**7502–7508.

Banyai, L., Varadi, A., and Patthy, L., 1983, Common evolutionary origin of the fibrin-binding structures of fibronectin and tissue-type plasminogen activator, *FEBS Lett.* **163:**37–41.

Barnes, M. J., Morton, L. F., Bennett, R. C., Bailey, A. J., and Sims, T. J., 1976, Presence of type III collagen in guinea-pig dermal scar, *Biochem. J.* **157:**263–266.

Beck, C., Duckert, F., and Ernst, M., 1961, The influence of fibrin stabilizing factor on the growth of fibroblasts in vitro and wound healing, *Thromb. Haemorr.* **6:**485–491.

Bernard, B. A., Yamada, K. M., and Olden, K., 1982, Carbohydrates selectively protect a specific domain of fibronectin against proteases, *J. Biol. Chem.* **257:**8549–8554.

Bornstein, P., and Ash, J. F., 1977, Cell surface-associated structural proteins in connective tissue cells, *Proc. Natl. Acad. Sci. USA* **74:**2480–2484.

Boucaut, J. C., Darribère, T., Poole, T. J., Aoyama, H., Yamada, K. M., and Thiery, J. P., 1984a, Biologically active synthetic peptides as probes of embryonic development: A competitive peptide inhibitor of fibronectin function inhibits gastrulation in amphibian embryos and neural crest cell migration in avian embryos, *J. Cell Biol.* **99:**1822–1830.

Boucaut, J. C., Darribère, T., Boulekbache, H., and Thiery, J. P., 1984b, Prevention of gastrulation but not neurulation by antibodies to fibronectin in amphibian embryos, *Nature (Lond.)* **307:**364–367.

Bronner-Fraser, M., 1985, Alterations in neural crest migration by a monoclonal antibody that affects cell adhesion, *J. Cell Biol.* **101:**610–617.

Burns, G. F., Cosgrove, L., Triglia, T., Beall, J. A., Lopez, A. F., Werkmeister, J. A., Begley, C. G., Haddad, A. P., d'Apice, A. J., Vadas, M. A., and Cawley, J. C., 1986, The IIb–IIa glycoprotein complex that mediates platelet aggregation is directly implicated in leukocyte adhesion, *Cell* **45:**269–280.

Carter, W. G., 1984, The role of intermolecular disulfide bonding in deposition of GP140 in the extracellular matrix, *J. Cell Biol.* **99:**105–114.

Chapman, A. E., 1984, Characterization of a 140 kD cell surface glycoprotein involved in myoblast adhesion, *J. Cell. Biochem.* **25:**109–121.

Chen, L. B., Murray, A., Segal, R. A., Bushnell, A., and Walsh, M. L., 1978, Studies on intercellular LETS glycoprotein matrices, *Cell* **14:**377–391.

Chen, W. T., Hasegawa, E., Hasegawa, T., Weinstock, C., and Yamada, K. M., 1985, Development of cell surface linkage complexes in cultured fibroblasts, *J. Cell Biol.* **100:**1103–1114.

Chen, W. T., Wang, J., Hasegawa, T., Yamada, S. S., and Yamada, K. M., 1986a, Regulation of fibronectin receptor distribution by transformation, exogenous fibronectin, and synthetic peptides, *J. Cell Biol.* **103:**1649–1661.

Chen, W. T., Chen, J. M., and Mueller, S. C., 1986b, Coupled expression and colocalization of 140K cell adhesion molecules, fibronectin, and laminin during morphogenesis and cytodifferentiation of chick lung cells, *J. Cell Biol.* **103:**1073–1090.

Cheresh, D. A., and Klier, F. G., 1986, Disialoganglioside GD2 distributes preferentially into substrate-associated mocroprocesses on human melanoma cells during their attachment to fibronectin, *J. Cell Biol.* **102:**1887–1897.

Cheresh, D. A., Pierschbacher, M. D., Herzig, M. A., and Mujoo, K., 1986, Disialogangliosides GD2 and GD3 are involved in the attachment of human melanoma and neuroblastoma cells to extracellular matrix proteins, *J. Cell Biol.* **102:**688–696.

Chernousov, M. L., Metsis, M. L., and Koteliansky, V. E., 1985, Studies of extracellular fibronectin matrix formation with fluoresceinated fibronectin and fibronectin fragments, *FEBS Lett.* **183:**365–369.

Chiquet-Ehrismann, R., Mackie, E. J., Pearson, C. A., Sakakura, T. Tenasein—An extracellular matrix protein involved in tissue interactions during fetal development and oncogenesis, *Cell* **47:**131–139.

Choi, M. G., and Hynes, R. O., 1979, Biosynthesis and processing of fibronectin in NIL.8 hamster cells, *J. Biol. Chem.* **254:**12050–12055.

Clark, J. G., Kuhn, C., McDonald, J. A., and Mecham, R. P., 1983, Lung connective tissue, *Int. Rev. Connect. Tissue Res.* **10:**249–331.

Clark, R. A. F., and Colvin, R. B., 1985, Wound repair, in: *Plasma Fibronectin: Structure and Function* (J. McDonagh, ed.), pp. 197–262, Dekker, New York.

Clark, R. A. F., DellaPelle, P., Manseau, E., Lanigan, J. M., Dvorak, H. F., and Colvin, R. B., 1982, Blood vessel fibronectin increases in conjunction with endothelial cell proliferation and capillary ingrowth during wound healing, *J. Invest. Dermatol.* **79:**269–276.

Clark, R. A. F., Folkvord, J. M., and Wertz, R. L., 1985, Fibronectin, as well as other extracellular matrix proteins, mediate human keratinocyte adherence, *J. Invest. Dermatol.* **84:**378–383.

Clark, R. A. F., Mason, R. F., Folkvord, J. M., and McDonald, J. A., 1986, Fibronectin mediates adherence of rat alveolar type II epithelial cells via the fibroblastic cell-attachment domain, *J. Clin. Invest.* **77:**1831–1840.

Cossu, G., and Warren, L., 1983, Lactosaminoglycans and heparan sulfate are covalently bound to fibronectins synthesized by mouse stem teratocarcinoma cells, *J. Biol. Chem.* **258:**5603–5607.

Cossu, G., Andrews, P. W., and Warren, L., 1983, Covalent binding of lactosaminoglycans and heparan sulphate to fibronectin synthesized by a human teratocarcinoma cell line, *Biochem. Biophys. Res. Commun.* **111:**952–957.

Dahl, S. C., and Grabel, L. B., 1986, Retinoic acid induces fibronectin fiber formation in F9 teratocarcinoma stem-cells, *Biol. Bull.* **170:**539.

Damsky, C. H., Knudsen, K. A., Bradley, D., Buck, C. A., and Horwitz, A. F., 1985, Distribution of the cell substratum attachment (CSAT) antigen on myogenic and fibroblastic cells in culture, *J. Cell Biol.* **100:**1528–1539.

D'Ardenne, A. J., and McGee, J. O., 1984, Fibronectin in disease, *J. Pathol.* **142:**235–251.

Decker, C., Greggs, R., Duggan, K., Stubbs, U., and Horwitz, A., 1984, Adhesive multiplicity in the interaction of embryonic fibroblasts and myoblasts with extracellular matrices, *J. Cell Biol.* **99:**1398–1404.

Duband, J. L., Rocher, S., Chen, W. T., Yamada, K. M., and Thiery, J. P., 1986, Cell adhesion and

migration in the early vertebrate embryo: Location and possible role of the putative fibronectin-receptor complex, *J. Cell Biol.* **102**:160–178.

Duckert, F., 1972, Documentation of the plasma factor XIII deficiency in man, *Ann. NY Acad. Sci.*
202:190–198.

Ehrismann, R., Chiquet, M., and Turner, D. C., 1981, Mode of action of fibronectin in promoting
chicken myoblast attachment. M_r = 60,000 gelatin-binding fragment binds native fibronectin,
J. Biol. Chem. **256**:4056–4062.

Ehrismann, R., Roth, D. E., Eppenberger, H. M., and Turner, D. C., 1982, Arrangement of attachment-promoting, self-association, and heparin-binding sites in horse serum fibronectin, *J. Biol.
Chem.* **257**:7381–7387.

Engvall, E., Ruoslahti, E., and Miller, E. J., 1978, Affinitiy of fibronectin to collagens ot different
genetic types and to fibrinogen. *J. Exp. Med.* **147**:1584–1595.

Erickson, H. P., and Carrell, N. A., 1983, Fibronectin in extended and compact conformation.
Electron microscopy and sedimentation analysis, *J. Biol. Chem.* **258**:14539–14544.

Erickson, H. P., and Inglesias, J. L., 1984, A six-armed oligomer isolated from cell surface fibronectin preparations, *Nature (Lond.)* **311**:267–269.

Erickson, H. P., Carrell, N., and McDonagh, J., 1981, Fibronectin molecule visualized in electron
microscopy: A long, thin, flexible strand, *J. Cell Biol.* **91**:673–678.

Fleischmajer, R., Timpl, R., Tuderman, L., Raisher, L., Wiestner, M., Perlish, J. S., and Graves, P. N.,
1981, Ultrastructural identification of extension aminopeptides of type I and III collagens in
human skin, *Proc. Natl. Acad. Sci. USA* **78**:7360–7364.

Forastieri, H., and Ingham, K. C., 1983, Fluid-phase interaction between human plasma fibronectin
and gelatin determined by fluorescence polarization assay, *Arch. Biochem. Biophys.* **227**:358–
366.

Forastieri, H., and Ingham, K. C., 1985, Interaction of gelatin with a fluorescein-labeled 42-kDa
chymotryptic fragment of fibronectin, *J. Biol. Chem.* **260**:10546–10550.

Fukuda, M., Levery, S. B., and Hakomori, S., 1982, Carbohydrate structure of hamster plasma
fibronectin. Evidence for chemical diversity between cellular and plasma fibronectins, *J. Biol.
Chem.* **257**:6856–6860.

Furcht, L. T., Wendelschafer, C., Mosher, D. F., and Foidart, J. M., 1980, An axial periodic fibrillar
arrangement of antigenic determinants for fibronectin and procollagen on ascorbate treated
human fibroblasts, *J. Supramol. Struct.* **13**:15–33.

Garcia-Pardo, A., Pearlstein, E., and Frangione, B., 1985, Primary structure of human plasma
fibronectin. Characterization of a 31,000 dalton fragment from the COOH-terminal region
containing a free sulfhydryl group and a fibrin-binding site, *J. Biol. Chem.* **260**:10320–
10325.

Gardner, J. M., and Hynes, R. O., 1985, Interaction of fibronectin with its receptor on platelets, *Cell*
42:439–448.

Gartner, T. K., and Bennett, J. S., 1985, The tetrapeptide analogue of the cell attachment site of
fibronectin inhibits platelet aggregation and fibrinogen binding to activated platelets, *J. Biol.
Chem.* **260**:11891–11894.

Geerts, A., Geuze, H. L., Slot, J. W., Voss, B., Schuppan, D., Schellinck, P., and Wisse, E., 1986,
Immunogold localization of procollagen III, fibronectin and heparan sulfate proteoglycan on
ultrathin frozen sections of the normal rat liver, *Histochemistry* **84**:355–362.

Gilbert, W., 1978, Why genes in pieces?, *Nature (Lond.)* **271**:501.

Gold, L. I., Frangione, B., and Pearlstein, E., 1983, Biochemical and immunological characterization of three binding sites on human plasma fibronectin with different affinities for heparin,
Biochemistry **22**:4113–4119.

Grinnell, F., 1984, Fibronectin and wound healing, *J. Cell Biochem.* **26**:107–116.

Grinnell, F., and Bennett, M. H., 1981, Fibroblast adhesion on collagen substrata in the presence
and absence of plasma fibronectin, *J. Cell Sci.* **48**:19–34.

Grinnell, F., and Feld, M. K., 1979, Initial adhesion of human fibroblasts in serum-free medium:
Possible role of secreted fibronectin, *Cell* **17**:117–129.

Grinnell, F., Billingham, R. E., and Burgess, L., 1981, Distribution of fibronectin during wound
healing in vivo, *J. Invest. Dermatol.* **76**:181–189.

Harris, A. K., Stopak, D., and Wild, P., 1981, Fibroblast traction as a mechanism for collagen morphogenesis, *Nature (Lond.)* **290**:249–251.

Hayashi, M., and Yamada, K. M., 1982, Divalent cation modulation of fibronectin binding to heparin and to DNA, *J. Biol. Chem.* **257**:5263–5267.

Hayashi, M., Schlesinger, D. H., Kennedy, D. W., and Yamada, K. M., 1980, Isolation and characterization of a heparin-binding domain of cellular fibronectin, *J. Biol. Chem.* **255**:10017–10020.

Hedman, K., 1980, Intracellular localization of fibronectin using immunoperoxidase cytochemistry in light and electron microscopy, *J. Histochem. Cytochem.* **28**:1233–1241.

Hedman, K., Vaheri, A., and Wartiovaara, J., 1978, External fibronectin of cultured human fibroblasts is predominantly a matrix protein, *J. Cell Biol.* **76**:748–760.

Hedman, K., Kurkinen, M., Alitalo, K., Vaheri, A., Johansson, S., and Hook, M., 1979, Isolation of the pericellular matrix of human fibroblast cultures, *J. Cell Biol.* **81**:83–91.

Hedman, K., Johansson, S., Vartio, T., Kjellen, L., Vaheri, A., and Hook, M., 1982, Structure of the pericellular matrix: Association of heparan and chondroitin sulfates with fibronectin–procollagen fibers, *Cell* **28**:663–671.

Hedman, K., Vartio, T., Johansson, S., Kjellen, L., Hook, M., Linker, A., Salonen, E. M., and Vaheri, A., 1984, Integrity of the pericellular fibronectin matrix of fibroblasts is independent of sulfated glycosaminoglycans, *EMBO J.* **3**:581–584.

Hirst, R., Horwitz, A., Buck, C., and Rohrschneider, L., 1986, Phosphorylation of the fibronectin–receptor complex in cells transformed by oncogenes that encode tyrosine kinases, *Proc. Natl. Acad. Sci. USA* **83**:6470–6474.

Holderbaum, D., and Ehrhart, L. A., 1986, Substratum influence on collagen and fibronectin biosynthesis by arterial smooth muscle cells *in vitro*, *J. Cell Physiol.* **126**:216–224.

Homandberg, G. A., and Erickson, J. W., 1986, A model of fibronectin tertiary structure based on studies of interactions between fragments, *Biochemistry* **25**:6917–6925.

Homandberg, G. A., Evans, D. B., Kramer, J., and Erickson, J. W., 1985, Interaction between fluorescence-labeled fibronectin fragments studied by gel high-performance liquid chromatography, *J. Chromatogr.* **327**:434–439.

Hormann, H., and Richter, H., 1986, Models for the subunit arrangement in soluble and aggregated plasma fibronectin, *Biopolymers* **25**:947–958.

Horwitz, A., Duggan, K., Greggs, R., Decker, C., and Buck, C., 1985, The cell substrate attachment CSAT antigen has properties of a receptor for laminin and fibronectin, *J. Cell Biol.* **101**:2134–2144.

Horwitz, A., Duggan, K., Buck, C., Beckerle, M. C., and Burridge, K., 1986, Interaction of plasma membrane fibronectin receptor with talin—A transmembrane linkage, *Nature (Lond.)* **320**:531–533.

Hummel, J. P., and Dreyer, W. J., 1962, Meaurement of protein-binding phenomena by gel filtration, *Biochim. Biophys. Acta* **63**:530–532.

Humphries, M. J., Akiyama, J. K., Komoriya, A., Olden, K., and Yamada, K. M., 1986, Identification of an alternatively spliced site in human plasma fibronectin that mediates cell type-specific adhesion, *J. Cell Biol.* **103**:2637–2647.

Hynes, R. O., 1985, Molecular biology of fibronectin, in: *Annual Review of Cell Biology*, Vol. 1 (G. E. Palade, B. M. Alberts, and J. A. Spudich, eds.), pp. 67–90, Annual Reviews, Palo Alto, California.

Hynes, R. O., 1986, Fibronectins, *Sci. Am.* **254**:42–51.

Hynes, R. O., and Yamada, K. M., 1982, Fibronectins: Multifunctional modular glycoproteins, *J. Cell Biol.* **95**:369–377.

Hynes, R. O., Schwarzbauer, J. E., and Tamkun, J. W., 1984, Fibronectin: A versatile gene for a versatile protein, *Ciba Found. Symp.* **108**:75–92.

Ignotz, R. A., and Massague, J., 1986, Transforming growth factor stimulates the expression of fibronectin and collagen and their incorporation into the extracellular matrix, *J. Biol. Chem.* **261**:4337–4345.

Ingham, K. C., Brew, S. A., Broekelmann, T. J., and McDonald, J. A.. 1984, Thermal stability of human plasma fibronectin and its constituent domains, *J. Biol. Chem.* **259**:11901–11907.

Irish, P. S., and Hasty, D. L., 1983, Immunocytochemical localization of fibronectin in human fibroblast cultures using a cell surface replica technique, *J. Histochem. Cytochem.* **31**:69–77.

Johansson, S., 1985, Demonstration of high affinity fibronectin receptors on rat hepatocytes in suspension, *J. Biol. Chem.* **260**:1557–1561.

Keski-Oja, J., and Yamada, K. M., 1981, Isolation of an actin-binding fragment of fibronectin, *Biochem. J.* **193**:615–620.

Kittlick, P. D., 1979, Fibrin in fibroblast cultures: A metabolic study as a contribution of inflammation and tissue repair, *Exp. Pathol. (Jena)* **17**:312–326.

Knox, P., Crooks, S., and Rimmer, C. S., 1986, Role of fibronectin in the migration of fibroblasts into plasma clots, *J. Cell Biol.* **102**:2318–2323.

Kornblihtt, A. R., Vibe-Pedersen, K., and Baralle, F. E., 1983, Isolation and characterization of cDNA clones for human and bovine fibronectins, *Proc. Natl. Acad. Sci. USA* **80**:3218–3222.

Kornblihtt, A. R., Vibe-Pedersen, K., and Baralle, F. E., 1984a, Human fibronectin: Cell specific alternative mRNA splicing generates polypeptide chains differing in the number of internal repeats, *Nucleic Acids Res.* **12**:5853–5868.

Kornblihtt, A. R., Vibe-Pedersen, K., and Baralle, F. E., 1984b, Human fibronectin: Molecular cloning evidence for two mRNA species differing by an internal segment coding for a structural domain, *EMBO J.* **3**:221–226.

Kornblihtt, A. R., Umezawa, K., Vibe-Pedersen, K., and Baralle, F. E., 1985, Primary structure of human fibronectin—Differential splicing may generate at least 10 polypeptides from a single gene, *EMBO J.* **4**:1755–1759.

Kubo, M., Norris, D. A., Howell, S. E., Ryan, S. R., and Clark, R. A., 1984, Human keratinocytes synthesize, secrete, and deposit fibronectin in the pericellular matrix, *J. Invest. Dermatol.* **82**:580–586.

Lahav, J., Schwartz, M. A., and Hynes, R. O., 1982, Analysis of platelet adhesion with a radioactive chemical crosslinking reagent: Interaction of thrombospondin with fibronectin and collagen, *Cell* **31**:253–262.

Lahav, J., Lawler, J., and Gimbrone, M. A., 1984, Thrombospondin interactions with fibronectin and fibrinogen. Mutual inhibition in binding, *Eur. J. Biochem.* **145**:151–156.

Laine, R. A., Fisher, S. F., Pande, H., Calaycay, J., and Shively, J. E., 1984, Human placental (fetal) fibronectin: Increased glycosylation and higher protease resistance than plasma fibronectin. Presence of polylactosamine glycopeptides and properties of a 44-kilodalton chymotryptic fragment, *J. Biol. Chem.* **259**:3962–3970.

Lange-Mutschler, J., 1986, Acylated fibronectin: A new type of posttranslational modification of cellular fibronectin, *FEBS Lett.* **201**:210–214.

Ledger, P. W., and Tanzer, M. L., 1982, The phosphate content of human fibronectin, *J. Biol. Chem.* **257**:3890–3895.

Ledger, P. W., Uchida, N., and Tanzer, M. L., 1980, Immunocytochemical localization of procollagen and fibronectin in human fibroblasts: Effects of the monovalent ionophore, monensin, *J. Cell Biol.* **87**:663–671.

Ledger, P. W., Nishimoto, S. K., Hayashi, S., and Tanzer, M. L., 1983, Abnormal glycosylation of human fibronectin secreted in the presence of monensin, *J. Biol. Chem.* **258**:547–554.

Liau, G., Yamada, Y., and de-Crombrugghe, B., 1985, Coordinate regulation of the levels of type III and type I collagen mRNA in most but not all mouse fibroblasts, *J. Biol. Chem.* **260**:531–536.

Liu, M. C., and Lipmann, F., 1985, Isolation of tyrosine-O-sulfate by Pronase hydrolysis from fibronectin secreted by Fujinami sarcoma virus-infected rat fibroblasts, *Proc. Natl. Acad. Sci. USA* **82**:34–37.

Livingston, D. C., Smolira, M. A., Hodges, G. M., and Goodman, S. L., 1981, Cell surface distribution of fibronectin in cultures of fibroblasts and bladder derived epithelium: SEM-immunogold localization compared to immunoperoxidase and immunofluorescence, *J. Microsc.* **123**:227–236.

Markovic, Z., Lustig, A., Engel, J., Richter, H., and Hormann, H., 1983, Shape and stability of fibronectin in solutions of different pH and ionic strengths, *Hoppe Seylers Z. Physiol. C* **364**:1795–1804.

Massague, J., 1985, The transforming growth factors, *Trends Biochem. Sci.* **9**:237–240.

McCarthy, J. B., Hagen, S. T., and Furcht, L. T., 1986, Human fibronectin contains distinct adhesion- and motility-promoting domains for metastatic melanoma cells, *J. Cell Biol.* **102**:179–188.

McDonagh, J. (ed.), 1985, *Plasma Fibronectin Structure and Function*, Vol. 5, Dekker, New York.

McDonagh, R. P., McDonagh, J., Petersen, T. E., Thgersen, H. C., Skorstengaard, K., Sottrup-Jensen, L., Magnusson, S., Dell, A., and Morris, H. R., 1981, Amino acid sequence of the factor XIIIa acceptor site in bovine plasma fibronectin, *FEBS Lett.* **127**:174–178.

McDonald, J. A., and Kelley, D. G., 1980, Degradation of fibronectin by human leukocyte elastase. Release of biologically active fragments, *J. Biol. Chem.* **255**:8848–8858.

McDonald, J. A., and Kelley, D. G., 1984, Specific binding of fibronectin–antifibronectin immune complexes to procollagen: A new pitfall in immunostaining, *J. Cell Biol.* **98**:1042–1047.

McDonald, J. A., Broekelmann, T. J., Kelley, D. G., and Villiger, B., 1981, Gelatin-binding domain-specific anti-human plasma fibronectin Fab′ inhibits fibronectin-mediated gelatin binding but not cell spreading, *J. Biol. Chem.* **256**:5583–5587.

McDonald, J. A., Kelley, D. G., and Broekelmann, T. J., 1982, Role of fibronectin in collagen deposition: Fab′ to the gelatin-binding domain of fibronectin inhibits both fibronectin and collagen organization in fibroblast extracellular matrix, *J. Cell Biol.* **92**:485–492.

McDonald, J. A., Broekelmann, T. J., Matheke, M. L., Crouch, E., and Kuhn, C., 1986, Detection of an altered fibroblast phenotype in lung biopsies from patients with active pulmonary fibrosis using a monoclonal antibody to procollagen type I, *J. Clin. Invest.* **78**:1237–1244.

McDonald, J. A., Quade, B. J., Broekelmann, T. J., LaChance, R., Forsman, K., Hasegawa, E., and Akiyama, S., 1987, Both the cell adhesive domain and an aminoterminal matrix assembly domain participate in fibronectin assembly into fibroblast pericellular matrix, *J. Biol. Chem.* **262**:2957–2967.

McKeown-Longo, P., and Mosher, D. F., 1983, Binding of plasma fibronectin to cell layers of human skin fibroblasts, *J. Cell Biol.* **87**:466–472.

McKeown-Longo, P., and Mosher, D. F., 1984, Mechanism of formation of disulfide-bonded multimers of plasma fibronectin in cell layers of cultured human fibroblasts, *J. Biol. Chem.* **259**:12210–12215.

McKeown-Longo, P. J., and Mosher, D. F., 1985, Interaction of the 70,000-mol-wt amino-terminal fragment of fibronectin with the matrix-assembly receptor of fibroblasts, *J. Cell Biol.* **100**:364–374.

Millis, A. J., Hoyle, M., Mann, D. M., and Brennan, M. J., 1985, Incorporation of cellular and plasma (fibronectins) into smooth muscle cell extracellular matrix in vitro, *Proc. Natl. Acad. Sci. USA* **82**:2746–2750.

Miskulin, M., Dalgleish, R., Kluve-Beckerman, B., Rennard, S. I., Tolstoshev, P., Brantly, M., and Crystal, R. G., 1986, Human type III collagen gene expression is coordinately modulated with the type I genes during fibroblast growth, *Biochem.* **25**:1408–1413.

Mosher, D. F., 1984, Physiology of fibronectin, *Annu. Rev. Med.* **35**:561–575.

Mosher, D. F., and Johnson, R. B., 1983, Specificity of fibronectin–fibrin cross-linking, *Ann. NY Acad. Sci.* **408**:583–594.

Nishida, T., Nakagawa, S., Ohashi, Y., Awata, T., and Manabe, R., 1982, Fibronectin in corneal wound healing: Appearance in cultured rabit cornea, *Jpn. J. Ophthalmol.* **26**:410–415.

Nishida, T., Nakagawa, S., Awate, T., Ohashi, Y., Watanabe, K., and Manabe, R., 1983a, Fibronectin promotes epithelial migration of cultured rabbit cornea in situ, *J. Cell Biol.* **97**:1653–1657.

Nishida, T., Nakagawa, S., Awata, T., Tani, Y., and Manabe, R., 1983b, Fibronectin eyedrops for traumatic recurrent corneal lesion. (Letter,) *Lancet* **2**:521–522.

Nishida, T., Ohashi, Y., Awata, T., and Manabe, R., 1983c, Fibronectin. A new therapy for corneal trophic ulcer, *Arch. Ophthalmol.* **101**:1046–1048.

Nishida, T., Nakagawa, S., Nishibayashi, C., Tanaka, H., and Manabe, R., 1984, Fibronectin enhancement of corneal epithelial wound healing of rabbits in vivo, *Arch. Ophthalmol.* **102**:455–456.

Odermatt, E., Engle, J., Richter, H., and Hormann, H., 1982, Shape, conformation and stability of fibronectin fragments determined by electron microscopy, circular dichroism and ultracentrifugation, *J. Mol. Biol.* **159**:109–123.

Odermatt, E., Tamkun, J. W., and Hynes, R. O., 1985, Repeating modular structure of the fibronectin gene: Relationship to protein structure and subunit variation, *Proc. Natl. Acad. Sci. USA* **82:**6571–6575.

Oh, E., Pierschbacher, M., and Ruoslahti, E., 1981, Deposition of plasma fibronectin in tissues, *Proc. Natl. Acad. Sci. USA* **78:**3218–3221.

O'Keefe, E. J., Payne, R. E., Jr., Russell, N., and Woodley, D. T., 1985, Spreading and enhanced motility of human keratinocytes on fibronectin, *J. Invest. Dermatol.* **85:**125–130.

Olden, K., Hunter, V. A., and Yamada, K. M., 1980, Biosynthetic processing of the oligosaccharide chains of cellular fibronectin, *Biochim. Biophys. Acta* **632:**408–416.

Ouaissi, M. A., Afchain, D., Capron, A., and Grimaud, J. A., 1984, Fibronectin receptors on *Trypanosoma cruzi* trypomastigotes and their biological function, *Nature (Lond.)* **308:**380–382.

Owens, J. O., and Baralle, F. E., 1986, Mapping the collagen-binding site of human fibronectin by expression in *Escherichia coli*, *EMBO J.* **5:**2825–2830.

Owens, M. R., and Cimino, C. D., 1982, Synthesis of fibronectin by the isolated perfused rat liver, *Blood* **59:**1305–1309.

Pande, H., Calaycay, J., Hawke, D., Ben-Avram, C. M., and Shively, J. E., 1985, Primary structure of a glycosylated DNA-binding domain in human plasma fibronectin, *J. Biol. Chem.* **260:**2301–2306.

Patthy, L., 1985, Evolution of the proteases of blood coagulation and fibrinolysis by assembly from modules, *Cell* **41:**657–663.

Patthy, L., Trexler, M., Vali, Z., Banyai, L., and Varadi, A., 1984, Kringles: modules specialized for protein binding. Homology of the gelatin-binding region of fibronectin with the kringle structures of proteases, *FEBS Lett.* **171:**131–136.

Perkins, R. M., Kellie, S., Patel, B., and Critchley, D. R., 1982, Gangliosides as receptors for fibronectin? Comparison of cell spreading on a ganglioside-specific ligand with that on fibronectin, *Exp. Cell Res.* **141:**231–243.

Petersen, T. E., Thgersen, H. C., Skorstengaard, K., Vibe-Pedersen, K., Sahl, P., Sottrup-Jensen, L., and Magnusson, S., 1983, Partial primary structure of bovine plasma fibronectin: Three types of internal homology, *Proc. Natl. Acad. Sci. USA* **80:**137–141.

Pierschbacher, M., and Ruoslahti, E., 1984, Variants of the cell recognition site of fibronectin that retain attachment-promoting activity, *Proc. Natl. Acad. Sci. USA* **81:**5985–5988.

Pierschbacher, M., Hayman, E. G., and Ruoslahti, E., 1981, Location of the cell-attachment site in fibronectin with monoclonal antibodies and proteolytic fragments of the molecule, *Cell* **26:**259–267.

Pierschbacher, M., Hayman, E. G., and Ruoslahti, E., 1983, Synthetic peptide with cell attachment activity of fibronectin, *Proc. Natl. Acad. Sci. USA* **80:**1224–1227.

Plow. E. F., Pierschbacher, M. D., Ruoslahti, E., Marguerie, G. A., and Ginsberg, M. H., 1985, The effect of Arg-Gly-Asp-containing peptides on fibrinogen and von Willebrand factor binding to platelets, *Proc. Natl. Acad. Sci. USA* **82:**8057–8061.

Postlethwaite, A., Keski-Oja, J., Balian, G., and Kang, A. H., 1981, Induction of fibroblast chemotaxis by fibronectin. Localization of the chemotactic region to a 140,000 molecular weight nongelatin-binding fragment, *J. Exp. Med.* **153:**494–499.

Proctor, R. A., Mosher, D. F., and Olbrantz, P. J., 1982, Fibronectin binding to Staphylococcus aureus, *J. Biol. Chem.* **257:**14788–14794.

Prowse, K. R., Tricoli, J. V., Klebe, R. J., and Shows, T. B., 1986, Assignment of the human fibronectin structural gene to chromosome-2, *Cytogenet. Cell Genet.* **41:**42–46.

Pytela, R., Pierschbacher, M. D., and Ruoslahti, E., 1985a, Identification and isolation of a 140 kd cell surface glycoprotein with properties expected of a fibronectin receptor, *Cell* **40:**191–198.

Pytela, R., Pierschbacher, M. D., and Ruoslahti, E. A., 1985b, 125/115-kDa cell surface receptor specific for vitronectin interacts with the arginine-glycine-aspartic acid adhesion sequence derived from fibronectin, *Proc. Natl. Acad. Sci. USA* **82:**5766–5770.

Pytela, R., Pierschbacher, M. D., Ginsberg, M. H., Plow, E. F.. and Ruoslahti, E., 1986, Platelet membrane glycoprotein IIb/IIIa: Member of a family of Arg-Gly-Asp—Specific adhesion receptors, *Science* **231:**1559–1562.

Repesh, L. A., Fitzgerald, T. J., and Furcht, L. T., 1982, Fibronectin involvement in granulation tissue and wound healing in rabbits, *J. Histochem. Cytochem.* **30:**351–358.

Richter, H., Seidl, M., and Hormann, H., 1981, Location of heparin-binding sites of fibronectin. Detection of a hitherto unrecognized transaminase sensitive site, *Hoppe Seylers Z. Physiol. C* **362**:399–408.

Roberts, A. B., Sporn, M. B., Assoian, R. K., Smith, J. M., Roche, N. S., Wakefield, L. M., Heine, U. I., Liotta, L. A., Falanga, V., Kehrl, J. H., and Fauci, A. S., 1986, Transforming growth factor type beta: Rapid inducation of fibrosis and angiogenesis in vivo and stimulation of collagen formation in vitro, *Proc. Natl. Acad. Sci. USA* **83**:4167–4171.

Roberts, D. D., Sherwood, J. A., Spitalnik, S. L., Panton, L. J., Howard, R. J., Dixit, V. M., Frazier, W. A., Miller, L. H., and Ginsburg, V., 1985, Thrombospondin binds falciparum malaria parasitized erythrocytes and may mediate cytoadherence, *Nature (Lond.)* **318**:64–66.

Ross, R., Raines, E. W., and Bowen-Pope, D. F., 1986, The biology of platelet-derived growth factor, *Cell* **46**:155–169.

Salonen, E. M., Saksela, O., Vartio, T., Vaheri, A., Nielsen, L. S., and Zeuthen, J., 1985, Plasminogen and tissue-type plasminogen activator bind to immobilized fibronectin, *J. Biol. Chem.* **260**:12302–12307.

Schwarzbauer, J., Tamkun, J. W., Lemischka, I. R., and Hynes, R. O., 1983, Three different fibronectin mRNAs arise by alternative splicing within the coding region, *Cell* **35**:421–431.

Sekiguchi, K., and Hakomori, S., 1980, Identification of two fibrin-binding domains in plasma fibronectin and unequal distribution of these domains in two different subunits: A preliminary note, *Biochem. Biophys. Res. Commun.* **97**:709–715.

Sekiguchi, K., Klos, A. M., Kurachi, K., Yoshitake, S., and Hakomori, S. I., 1986, Human-liver fibronectin complementary DNAs—Identification of 2 different messenger RNAs possibly encoding the alpha-subunit and beta-subunit of plasma fibronectin, *Biochemistry* **25**:4436–4941.

Setoyama, C., Liau, g., and de-Crombrugghe, B., 1985, Pleiotropic mutants of NIH 3T3 cells with altered regulation in the expression of both type I collagen and fibronectin, *Cell* **41**:201–209.

Sieber-Blum, M., 1984, Fibronectin-regulated methionine enkephalin-like and somatostatin-like immunoreactivity in quail neural crest cell cultures, *Neuropeptides* **4**:457–466.

Singer, I. I., Kawka, D. W., Kazazis, D. M., and Clark, R. A. F., 1984, In vivo co-distribution of fibronectin and actin fibers in granulation tissue: Immunofluorescence and electron microscope studies of the fibronexus at the myofibroblast surface, *J. Cell Biol.* **98**:2091–2106.

Singer, I. I., Kazazis, D. M., and Kawka, D. W., 1985, Localization of the fibronexus at the surface of granulation tissue myofibroblasts using double-label immunogold electron microscopy on ultrathin frozen sections, *Eur. J. Cell Biol.* **38**:94–101.

Smith, D. E., Mosher, D. F., Johnson, R. B., and Furcht, L. T., 1982, Immunological identification of two sulfhydryl-containing fragments of human plasma fibronectin, *J. Biol. Chem.* **257**:5831–5838.

Song, J., Broekelmann, T. J., and McDonald, J. A., 1986, Fibrin clot promotes rapid outgrowth of fibroblasts from rat lung explants, *Am. Rev. Respir. Dis.* **133**:259 (abst).

Spiegel, S., Yamada, K. M., Hom, B. E., Moss, J., and Fishman, P. H., 1986, Fibrillar organization of fibronectin is expressed coordinately with cell surface gangliosides in a variant murine fibroblast, *J. Cell Biol.* **102**:1–9.

Springer, T. A., and Anderson, D. C., 1986, The importance of the Mac-1, LFA-1 glycoprotein family in monocyte and granulocyte adherence, chemotaxis, and migration into inflammatory sites: Insights from an experiment of nature, *Ciba Found. Symp.* **118**:102–126.

Steinmann, B. U., Abe, S., and Martin, G. R., 1982, Modulation of type I and type III collagen production in normal and mutant human skin fibroblasts by cell density, prostaglandin E_2 and epidermal growth factor, *Coll. Relat. Res.* **2**:185–195.

Stopak, D., and Harris, A. K., 1982, Connective tissue morphogenesis by fibroblast traction. I. Tissue culture observations, *Dev. Biol.* **90**:383–398.

Suzuki, S., Oldberg, A., Hayman, E. G., Piersbacher, M. D., and Ruoslahti, E., 1985, Complete amino acid sequence of human vitronectin deduced from cDNA. Similarity of cell attachment sites in vitronectin and fibronectin, *EMBO J.* **4**:2519–2524.

Takashima, A., and Grinnell, F., 1984, Human keratinocyte adhesion and phagocytosis promoted by fibroblast, *J. Invest. Dermatol.* **83**:352–358.

Takashima, A., and Grinnell, F., 1985, Fibronectin-mediated keratinocyte migration and initiation of fibronectin receptor function in vitro. *J. Invest. Dermatol.* **85**:304–308.

Tamkun, J. W., and Hynes, R. O., 1983, Plasma fibronectin is synthesized and secreted by hepato-cytes, *J. Biol. Chem.* **258**:4641–4647.

Tamkun, J. W., Schwarzbauer, J., and Hynes, R. O., 1984, A single rat fibronectin gene generates three different mRNAs by alternative splicing of a complex exon, *Proc. Natl. Acad. Sci. USA* **81**:5140–5144.

Tamkun, J. W., DeSimone, D. W., Fonda, D., Patel, R. S., Buck, C., Horwitz, A. F., and Hynes, R. O., 1986, Structure of integrin, a glycoprotein involved in the transmembrane linkage between fibronectin and actin, *Cell* **46**:271–282.

Thomas, D. D., Baseman, J. B., and Alderete, J. F., 1985, Fibronectin mediates *Treponema pallidum* cytoadherence through recognition of fibronectin cell-binding domain, *J. Exp. Med.* **161**:514–525.

Thompson, L. K., Horowitz, P. M., Bentley, K. L., Thomas, D. D., Alderete, J. F., and Klebe, R. J., 1986, Localization of the ganglioside-binding site of fibronectin, *J. Biol. Chem.* **261**:5209–5214.

Timpl, R., Odermatt, E., Engel, A., Madri, J. A., Furthmayr, H., and Rohde, H., 1981, Shapes, domain organizations and flexibility of laminin and fibronectin, two multifunctional proteins of the extracellular matrix, *J. Mol. Biol.* **150**:97–120.

Torikata, C., Villiger, B., Kuhn, C., and McDonald, J. A., 1985, Ultrastructural distribution of fibronectin in normal and fibrotic human lung, *Lab. Invest.* **52**:399–408.

Uchida, N., Smilowitz, H., Ledger, P. W., and Tanzer, M. L., 1980, Kinetic studies of the intra-cellular transport of procollagen and fibronectin in human fibroblasts. Effects of the mono-valent ionophore, monensin, *J. Biol. Chem.* **255**:8638–8644.

Ueyama, M., and Urayama, T., 1978, The role of factor XIII in fibroblast proliferation, *Jpn. J. Exp. Med.* **48**:135–142.

Vibe-Pedersen, K., Sahl, P., Skorstengaard, K., and Petersen, T. E., 1982, Amino acid sequence of a peptide from bovine plasma fibronectin containing a free sulfhydryl group (cysteine), *FEBS Lett.* **142**:27–30.

Villiger, B., Kelley, D. G., Engleman, W., Kuhn, C., and McDonald, J. A., 1981, Human alveolar macrophage fibronectin: Synthesis, secretion, and ultrastructural localization during gelatin-coated latex particle binding, *J. Cell Biol.* **90**:711–720.

Vuento, M., Vartio, T., Saraste, M., von-Bonsdorff, C., and Vaheri, A., 1980, Spontaneous and polyamine-induced formation of filamentous polymers from soluble fibronectin, *Eur. J. Bio-chem.* **105**:33–42.

Wartiovaara, J., Alitalo, K., Hedman, K., Keski-Oja, J., and Kurkinen, M., 1978, Fibronectin and the pericellular matrix of normal and transformed adherent cells, *Ann. NY Acad. Sci.* **312**:434–353.

Williams, E. C., Janmey, P. A., Ferry, J. D., and Mosher, D. F., 1982, Conformational states of fibronectin. Effects of pH, ionic strength, and collagen binding, *J. Biol. Chem.* **257**:14973–14978.

Williams, I. F., McCullagh, K. G., and Silver, I. A., 1984, The distribution of types I and III collagen and fibronectin in the healing equine tendon, *Connect. Tissue Res.* **12**:211–227.

Woods, A., Hook, M., Kjellen, L., Smith, C. G., and Rees, D. A., 1984, Relationship of heparin sulfate proteoglycans to the cytoskeleton and extracellular matrix of cultures fibroblasts, *J. Cell Biol.* **99**:1743–1753.

Woods, A., Couchman, J. R., and Hook, M., 1985, Haparan sulfate proteoglycans of rat embryo fibroblasts. A hydrophobic form may link cytoskeleton and matrix components, *J. Biol. Chem.* **260**:10872–10879.

Wyler, D. J., Sypek, J. P., and McDonald, J. A., 1985, In vitro parasite–monocyte interactions in human leishmaniasis–Possible role of fibronectin in parasite attachment, *Infect. Immun.* **49**:305–311.

Yamada, K. M., and Kennedy, D. W., 1979, Fibroblast cellular and plasma fibroblasts are similar but not identical, *J. Cell Biol.* **80**:492–498.

Yamada, K. M., and Kennedy, D. W., 1984, Dualistic nature of adhesive protein function: Fibronec-tin and its biologically active peptide fragments can autoinhibit fibronectin function, *J. Cell Biol.* **99**:29–36.

Yamada, K. M., Kennedy, D. W., Kimata, K., and Pratt, R. M., 1980, Characterization of fibronectin interactions with glycosaminoglycans and identification of active proteolytic fragments, *J. Biol. Chem.* **255:**6055–6063.

Yamada, K. M., Critchley, D. R., Fishman, P. H., and Moss, J., 1983, Exogenous gangliosides enhance the interaction of fibronectin with ganglioside-deficient cells, *Exp. Cell Res.* **143:**295–302.

Yamada, K. M., Akiyama, S. K., Hasegawa, T., Hasegawa, E., Humphries, M. J., Kennedy, D. W., Nagata, K., Urushihara, H., Olden, K., and Chen, W. T., 1985, Recent advances in research on fibronectin and other cell attachment proteins, *J. Cell Biochem.* **28:**79–97.

Yamaguchi, Y., Isemura, M., Yosizawa, Z., Kan, M., and Sato, A., 1986, A weaker gelatin-binding affinity and increased glycosylation of amniotic fluid fibronectin than plasma fibronectin, *Int. J. Biochem.* **18:**437–443.

Zardi, L., Carnemolla, B., Balza, E., Borsi, L., Castellani, P., Rocco, M., and Siri, A., 1985, Elution of fibronectin proteolytic fragments from a hydroxyapatite chromatography column. A simple procedure for the purification of fibronectin domains, *Eur. J. Biochem.* **146:**571–579.

Chapter 19

Proteoglycans and Wound Repair

JOHN R. COUCHMAN and MAGNUS HÖÖK

1. Introduction

Proteoglycans consist of a protein core to which linear polysaccharides called glycosaminoglycans are covalently linked. This chapter discusses not only proteoglycans, but also hyaluronic acid, which is not covalently bound to protein and therefore does not qualify as a proteoglycan. However, since hyaluronic acid with its repeating disaccharide structure belongs to the family of glycosaminoglycans and has important biologic functions, it is included. The structure of proteoglycans may vary considerably, depending on the size and composition of the core proteins and the size and number of polysaccharide chains. The number of glycosaminoglycan classes is quite small, but some contain a heterodisperse population, in which fine structural variability results in the potential for hundreds of glycosaminoglycan species. It is also becoming clear that each proteoglycan class may contain members with distinctly different core proteins. The net result is the potential for a large variety of proteoglycans within the vertebrate body. Some of these proteoglycans appear to have a general distribution throughout the animal body, whereas others show a high degree of tissue specificity.

All connective tissues contain proteoglycans; in some tissues, such as for example cartilage, proteoglycans are major constituents. In addition, many cells have proteoglycans associated with their surfaces, which may influence many aspects of cellular behavior. It follows that tissue or organ damage will involve the destruction and subsequent regeneration of proteoglycan-rich extracellular matrices. However, wound-repair processes themselves may, in addition, be profoundly influenced by the presence of particular proteoglycan species. An important characteristic of all proteoglycans is their polyanionic nature, which is highly influential in the physicochemical nature of extracellular matrices and cellular responses to them.

In the recent past, there have been several reviews on the structure, biosynthesis, and physicochemical properties of proteoglycans with background

JOHN R. COUCHMAN • Connective Tissue Laboratory, Department of Medicine, B. R. Boshell Diabetes Hospital, University of Alabama in Birmingham, Birmingham, Alabama 35294.
MAGNUS HÖÖK • Department of Biochemistry, Connective Tissue Laboratory, B. R. Boshell Diabetes Hospital, University of Alabama in Birmingham, Birmingham, Alabama 35294.

on their distribution and possible functions (Comper and Laurent, 1978; Lindahl and Höök, 1978; Dorfman, 1981; Hascall and Hascall, 1981; Toole, 1981; Höök et al., 1984, Hascall, 1986; Hassell et al., 1986, Gallagher et al., 1986; Poole, 1986). However, our understanding of the biologic role of these molecules is still in its infancy.

This chapter first summarizes the structures and biosynthesis of the proteoglycans, followed by a discussion of the different types of interactions in which the proteoglycans may participate. Subsequently, the roles of proteoglycans in basic cellular functions, such as adhesion, migration, and proliferation, are discussed. Finally, a section on the possible role of proteoglycans in angiogenesis is included. This is not an in-depth review of the biology of proteoglycans. Rather, we have selected observations, findings, and hypotheses we consider to be of potential importance in wound repair.

Although studies on embryogenesis and *in vitro* experimentation provide valuable basic information on the presence or absence or relative amounts of the various types of glycosaminoglycans and proteoglycans, very little information is available concerning their role in tissue homeostasis. Even less is known about the function of these molecules during the many phases of tissue repair after wounding. Therefore, we do not have a complete picture of the roles of proteoglycans in wound repair. Rather, we point to the possible functions of proteoglycans in cellular reactions that are involved in wound repair.

2. Proteoglycan Structure

2.1. Classification

Proteoglycans varying considerably in overall structure have been isolated and characterized (Fig. 1). Core proteins with molecular weights of $<10,000\ M_r$ to $>300,000\ M_r$ have been reported, and these proteins can carry 1 to more than 100 polysaccharide chains, in turn varying in size from $10,000\ M_r$ to $\sim100,000\ M_r$. Furthermore, in some cases, free glycosaminoglycans without covalently attached protein are present in tissues. Thus, this family of molecules contains members that vary dramatically in terms of structure and presumably function, making the classification of proteoglycans a difficult task. Traditionally, the proteoglycans have been classified according to the structure of the glycosaminoglycan (see Fig. 7). The glycosaminoglycans contain alternating uronic acid (or galactose) and hexosamine residues to form a polymer to which sulfate groups may be coupled in ester or amide linkages. Two major classes of glycosaminoglycans are recognized: the N-acetylgalactosaminoglycans (or chondroitin sulfates), and the N-sulfated glucosaminoglycans, which include heparin and heparan sulfates. In addition, keratan sulfates and hyaluronic acid represent classes of glycosaminoglycans with less structural variation than that found in the two main groups. It is likely that the overall proteoglycan structure is important in determining molecular function, this being a consequence of the number, length, and distribution of polysaccharide chains as well as the

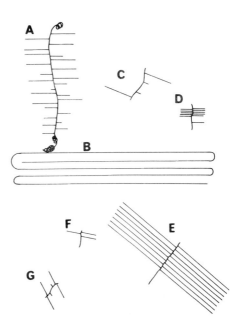

Figure 1. Structural variability of proteoglycans. Schematic models of some proteoglycans and glycosaminoglycans drawn to approximate scale. (A) Large keratan sulfate-bearing cartilage proteoglycan. (B) Hyaluronic acid. (C) Dermatan sulfate proteoglycan of type isolated from loose connective tissues. (D) Dermatan sulfate proteoglycan synthesized by PYS-2 cells in culture. (E) Heparin proteoglycan. (F) Liver cell-surface heparan sulfate proteoglycan. (G) Small heparan sulfate proteoglycan isolated from the EHS tumor. For further explanation, see text.

structure of the core protein. Thus, the usefulness of the traditional classification is somewhat limited. This is highlighted by the recent description of a proteoglycan, which contains both chondroitin and heparan sulfate chains linked to a protein core (Rapraeger *et al.*, 1985; David and van den Berghe, 1985). Once we learn more about core protein structures, these components may provide a basis for a new and more logical classification of proteoglycans (Hassell *et al.*, 1986). Meantime, we must rely on classification based on glycosaminoglycan structures.

2.2. Chondroitin Sulfate Proteoglycans

The chondroitin sulfates contain N-acetylgalactosamine as the hexosamine component. The uronic acid residue is either glucuronic acid or its C-5 epimer, iduronic acid. In the latter case, the galactosaminoglycan is referred to as dermatan sulfate or, in the older literature, chondroitin sulfate B. The glucuronic acid containing chondroitin sulfates are further divided into chondroitin 4-sulfate (chondroitin sulfate A) and chondroitin 6-sulfate (chondroitin sulfate C), depending on which carbon atom of the galactosamine unit carries an ester-linked sulfate group. The nonsulfated polymer composed of glucuronic acid and N-acetylgalactosamine is referred to as chondroitin. Most glycosaminoglycans of this group are hybrids, composed of different disaccharide units in the same polysaccharide chain, although the frequency of the different disaccharides may vary considerably from one proteoglycan to another.

In a chondroitin sulfate proteoglycan, the polysaccharide chains are linked to the core protein via the tetrasaccharide, xylose–galactose–galactose–

glucuronic acid. The xylose unit is joined in a glycosidic linkage to the hydroxyl group of serine residues of the core protein. Proteoglycans may also contain carbohydrates other than glycosaminoglycans. Both N-linked and O-linked oligosaccharides have been demonstrated to be present on the core protein of chondroitin sulfate proteoglycans (Lohmander et al., 1980).

A large hyaluronic acid-binding chondroitin sulfate proteoglycan isolated from cartilage is the most studied proteoglycan (for review see Hascall and Hascall, 1981; Hassell et al., 1986). This proteoglycan consists of a 240,000-M_r core protein to which more than 100 chondroitin sulfate chains are attached. In addition, the proteoglycan is substituted with keratan sulfate chains as well as N- and O-linked oligosaccharides. The hyaluronic acid binding portion of this proteoglycan has been localized to the N-terminal third of the core protein. This region is poorly substituted with carbohydrates. The central region seems to carry most of the keratan sulfate chains, whereas the C-terminal third is rich in chondroitin sulfate chains. Recent results from molecular genetic studies of the core protein have suggested a homology between one domain and the galactose-binding hepatic protein described by Ashwell (Sai et al., 1986). However, an interaction of the core protein with galactose-containing structures has not yet been demonstrated. In vivo, several proteoglycan molecules are bound to a hyaluronic acid molecule forming large complexes that contribute to the structural integrity of cartilage. The interaction between the core protein and hyaluronic acid is stabilized by so-called link proteins. In addition to chondrocytes, other cell types (e.g., smooth muscle cells and fibroblasts) seem to be able to synthesize hyaluronic acid-binding chondroitin sulfate proteoglycans. The structural relationship between these hyaluronic acid binding proteoglycans from different sources is unclear (Hassell et al., 1986; Heinegård et al., 1986).

In addition to the large hyaluronic acid-binding proteoglycan(s), several other proteoglycans of smaller size with galactosaminoglycans as side chains have been isolated and characterized (for reviews, see Hassell et al., 1986; Heinegård et al., 1986). These are abundant in extracellular matrices, although some species have also been found associated with cells (Hedman et al., 1983; Heinegård et al., 1986). The structure of these proteoglycans varies considerably in terms of overall size, length of core protein, number and length of polysaccharide chains, and ratios of 4/6 sulfate and glucuronic/iduronic acid. The structural, functional, and genetic relationship between these proteoglycans is unknown. Thus, chondroitin- and dermatan sulfate-containing proteoglycans appear in many forms and are extremely widespread in all connective tissues, including basement membranes. In cartilage, it is clear that the large chondroitin sulfate- and keratan sulfate-containing proteoglycans have an important structural role in forming a matrix that can withstand the physical stresses to which articular and intervertebral disc cartilages are subjected. In skin, it appears that the interstitial collagens of the dermis have a dermatan sulfate proteoglycan associated with them, which may have a role in collagen fibrillogenesis and bundle formation (Scott and Orford, 1981; Gallagher et al., 1983). Such structural roles may indicate a role for the chondroitin/dermatan sulfate proteoglycans in wound repair.

2.3. Heparin and Heparan Sulfate Proteoglycans

The glycosaminoglycans heparin and heparan sulfate are structurally related. They both contain the same elements (see Fig. 7). The carbohydrate backbone is composed of an alternating sequence of glucosamine and uronic acid (glucuronic acid or iduronic acid) units and is linked to serine residues in the core protein via the same tetrasaccharide as described in Section 2.2 for chondroitin sulfate. To this polysaccharide, sulfate groups may be attached in ester linkages to C-2 of the uronic acid component or C-6 and C-3 of the glucosamine unit. In addition, the amino group of the glucosamine residue may be substituted with sulfate. The presence of N-sulfated hexosamine units in glycosaminoglycans is unique to heparin and heparan sulfate. The glucosamine units that are not N-sulfated usually carry N-acetyl groups.

The classification of the N-sulfated glycosaminoglycans into heparin and heparan sulfate is historically motivated and reflects the early discovery of a highly sulfated polysaccharide with potent anticoagulant activity which was given the name heparin. The term heparan sulfate was given to a polysaccharide described much later, which contained less sulfate and exhibited only minor anticoagulant activity. It has been previously thought that heparin and heparan sulfate could be differentiated by the high anticoagulant activity of the former. However, recent studies have shown that only one-third of heparin molecules are biologically active; the rest of the polymers have low anticoagulant activity despite their high sulfate content. Furthermore, recent studies (Marcum and Rosenberg, 1984; Paulsson et al., 1986; Lane et al., 1986) have shown that some cell types, such as vascular endothelial cells, produce an N-sulfated glycosaminoglycan that, by conventional classification, would be referred to as heparan sulfate but exhibiting powerful anticoagulant activity. In view of these observations, it seems logical to treat these glycosaminoglycans as one group.

Heparan sulfate proteoglycans are preferentially located at the surface of cells. Most adherent cells appear to have a type of cell surface-associated proteoglycan that has its core protein anchored in the plasma membrane. Membrane-associated heparan sulfate proteoglycans from different cell types appear to differ in overall size, length of polysaccharide chains, and size of core proteins (Kjellén et al., 1981; Norling et al., 1981; Fransson et al., 1984; Woods et al., 1985, Rapraeger and Bernfield, 1985; Jalkanen et al., 1985). Heparan sulfate proteoglycans also appear to be present in most, if not all, basement membranes. Different structures of heparan sulfate proteoglycans isolated from this source have been reported (Kanwar and Farquhar, 1979; Hassell et al., 1980; Kobayashi et al., 1983; Parthasarathy and Spiro, 1984; Timpl et al., 1984, Paulsson et al., 1986). Recent studies suggest that the core proteins of the heparan sulfate proteoglycans found in basement membranes and that the cell surfaces are immunologically distinct.

Mast cells produce a highly sulfated N-sulfated glycosaminoglycan exhibiting anticoagulant activity. It seems that this is synthesized as a heparin proteoglycan with 10 or more polysaccharide chains densely packed along a core protein composed mainly of repeating serine and glycine residues. On average,

442

every second serine residue carries a polysaccharide chain. Subsequent to biosynthesis, the heparin proteoglycan may be degraded by an endoglucuronidase releasing large oligosaccharides (7000–20,000 M_r) stored in mast cell granules (Yurt et al., 1977; Robinson et al., 1978; Stevens, 1986).

2.4. Keratan Sulfate Proteoglycans

The known distribution of keratan sulfate is restricted to the cornea, sclera, and cartilage. The polymer is composed of alternating galactose and glucosamine units that may carry sulfate residues attached to C-4 of both residues (Fig. 7). In cartilage, keratan sulfate appears to be linked to the core protein of the large hyaluronic acid-binding chondroitin sulfate proteoglycan via O-glycosidic bonds joining N-acetylglucosamine units to serine residues of the core protein. In the cornea, keratan sulfate occurs as a distinct proteoglycan without chondroitin sulfate chains. The polysaccharide chains are attached to the core protein via N-glycosylamine bonds between N-acetylglucosamine and core protein asparagine residues.

2.5. Hyaluronic Acid

Hyaluronic acid is composed of alternating glucuronic acid and N-acetylglucosamine units. This polysaccharide does not carry sulfate groups, nor does it qualify as a proteoglycan, since it does not appear to contain a covalently attached protein. Hyaluronic acid is synthesized as very large polymers ($\leqslant 10^7$ M_r) by eukaryotic cells and by some bacteria (Stoolmiller and Dorfman, 1969; Sugahara et al., 1979; van de Rijn, 1983; Triscott and van de Rijn, 1986). Hyaluronic acid is a widespread connective tissue component usually associated with other macromolecules, and in such tissues as rooster comb, umbilical cord, and vitreous body hyaluronic acid is a dominant component (Toole, 1981). The large size of this molecule ($\leqslant 10^7$ M_r) and its hydrodynamic properties, however, are probably significant in many connective tissues with respect to cellular behavior, especially in wound repair.

3. Biosynthesis

3.1. Biosynthesis of Proteoglycans

The biosynthesis of the core protein is assumed to follow the pattern demonstrated for other proteins. It is not clear, however, how proteins are selected to be substituted with glycosaminoglycans. Although proteins that normally do not serve as proteoglycan core proteins may occasionally carry one or two glycosaminoglycan chains (Baker et al., 1980; Cossu and Warren, 1983), most proteoglycan core proteins appear to be selected for this role. It is tempting to speculate that protein sequences of proteoglycan cores contain the information needed to direct glycosaminoglycan substitution. Modern molecular genetic techniques will make it possible to determine these primary sequences. So far this approach has resulted in the deduction of the sequence of two dermatan sulfate core proteins (Bourdon *et al.*, 1985, Krusius and Ruoslahti, 1986) as well as partial sequence of the large-cartilage chondroitin sulfate proteoglycan core protein (Sai *et al.*, 1986). In addition, a pre-pro core protein precursor has been identified (Bourdon *et al.*, 1986). In the published sequence analysis, a signal, selecting core protein for glycosaminoglycan substitutions, has been suggested. However, the limited sequence data available so far make it difficult to determine whether such signaling sequences are ubiquitous. This is an area of research in which we can expect rapid progress, and it is likely that several questions regarding core proteins and regulation of proteoglycan biosynthesis will be answered using molecular genetic techniques. Cell-free translation of cartilage messenger RNA (mRNA) suggests that the translation product for the core protein of the large hyaluronic acid-binding chondroitin sulfate is 300,000 M_r (Upholt *et al.*, 1979; Treadwell *et al.*, 1980), whereas newly secreted proteoglycan contains a core protein of 200,000–220,000 M_r. If so, the difference in size conceivably represents segments lost during post-translational modification that could encode information directing chondroitin sulfate and keratan sulfate substitution (Kimura *et al.*, 1981).

The biosynthesis of the glycosaminoglycan chains (except keratan sulfate) is initiated by the transfer of xylose from UDP-xylose to the hydroxyl group of a protein-core serine residue. This reaction is catalyzed by a xylosyl transferase. This step is followed by successive transfers of two galactose units and a glucuronic acid residue, catalyzed by three different enzymes (Dorfman, 1981). The carbohydrate backbone of the glycosaminoglycans is then formed by the alternate transfer of N-acetylhexosamine and glucuronic acid units from corresponding UDP-sugars. The carbohydrate polymers are subsequently subjected to a series of modification reactions. For heparan sulfate, these are initiated by the deacetylation of some N-acetylglucosamine units followed by N-sulfation of exposed amino groups, C-5 conversion of some glucuronic acid units to iduronic acid, and the introduction of ester sulfates. Each of these reactions is catalyzed by distinct enzymes, requiring appropriate cofactors such as phosphoadenylylsulfate as a sulfate donor (Dorfman, 1981). None of these reactions is carried to completion; the extension of polymer modification (hence sulfation) of the heparan sulfate chain seems to depend largely on the extent of the initial N-deacetylation. The corresponding N-deacetylase thus seems to play a key role in regulating the degree of sulfation of heparan sulfate (Riesenfeld *et al.*, 1982; Robinson *et al.*, 1984).

The mechanisms responsible for the regulation of 4/6-sulfation in the biosynthesis of chondroitin sulfate are unknown. However, in general, slower-growing cells seem to make more chondroitin 6-sulfate than do rapidly growing cells (Mathews, 1975). Similarly unknown are the mechanisms responsible for selecting some glucuronic acid residues to become epimerized to iduronic acid. Clearly, in some proteoglycan molecules, a large portion of the uronic acid units are converted to iduronic acid, whereas others contain barely any iduronic acid.

The amounts of proteoglycans produced by a cell seems to be limited by the availability of core protein (discussed in Höök *et al.*, 1984). Some cells (e.g., hepatocytes) that normally do not produce appreciable amounts of chondroitin sulfate proteoglycans still have the complete enzymatic machinery for the biosynthesis of the glycosaminoglycan (L. Kjellén and M. Höök, unpublished observations). This machinery can be activated if a suitable primer for chondroitin sulfate biosynthesis is provided. β-Xylosides can substitute for xylosylated core protein, and the addition of β-xylosides to cells will result in the production of large quantities of chondroitin sulfates, even if protein production has been blocked by addition of inhibitors of protein synthesis. The activity of β-xylosides as primers of heparan sulfate biosynthesis is usually poor and varies for different cell types.

3.2. Biosynthesis of Hyaluronic Acid

Hyaluronic acid is probably not covalently linked to protein and therefore is not a proteoglycan. The mechanisms of hyaluronic acid biosynthesis are incompletely understood. Studies by Prem (1983*a,b*) suggest that this glycosaminoglycan is synthesized on the cytoplasmic side of the plasma membrane. The polymer is believed to grow by the transfer of the next UDP-sugar unit to the reducing end of the nascent chain. In some recent elegant studies, Mian (1986*a,b*) confirmed a plasma membrane location for hyaluronic acid synthesis. He was also able to solubilize and isolate a 450,000-M_r oligomeric protein that catalyzed the formation of hyaluronic acid oligosaccharides. The activity of the hyaluronate synthetase seems to be controlled through phosphorylation of its subunits, one of which displayed tyrosine kinase activity. It is hoped that further studies will demonstrate additional details of this biosynthetic pathway, which resembles those demonstrated for the synthesis of bacterial polysaccharides (Stoolmiller and Dorfman, 1969; Sugahara *et al.*, 1979). Since this glycosaminoglycan seems to have profound effects on cell behavior (i.e., the regulation of hyaluronic acid), size and quantity is of particular interest.

4. Interactions of Glycosaminoglycans

4.1. Interactions with Proteins

Glycosaminoglycans may affect biologic reactions by interacting with proteins. These interactions may serve to (1) anchor specific proteins at certain locations (e.g., heparan sulfate may anchor lipoprotein lipase and its substrate lipoproteins to the same region of the endothelial cell surface); or (2) directly affect the biologic activity of the target protein (e.g., binding of heparin to antithrombin III enhances the activity of this protease inhibitor (for review, see Bjork and Lindahl, 1982). Since glycosaminoglycans are polyanions, interactions involving these molecules would be expected to have a strong ionic character. Any molecule that has a region of net positive charge might bind to the glycosaminoglycans. Undoubtedly, such relatively nonspecific polyanionic–polycationic interactions do occur; for example, polylysine binds strongly to all glycosaminoglycans. However, certain patterns of reactivity have emerged among the different classes of glycosaminoglycans. Most heparan sulfate-binding proteins bind with apparent higher affinity to highly sulfated polymers than to heparan sulfates with low sulfate content. If a protein binds all sulfated glycosaminoglycans, it usually binds more strongly to heparan sulfates than to chondroitin sulfates, even if the two polysaccharides have the same sulfate contents. The content of iduronic acid in a polymer correlates positively with binding strength. These observations remain unexplained.

Some interactions involving the glycosaminoglycans, however, are highly specific and require a specific monosaccharide sequence as well as sulfate substitutions at specific sites; for example, the antithrombin-binding site in heparin has been localized to a pentasaccharide of specific structure. Thus it appears likely that biologically important interactions involving glycosaminoglycans may exhibit different degrees of specificity ranging from relatively nonspecific polyanionic–polycationic interactions to those involving a defined specific structures in the glycosaminoglycans. Unfortunately, our information on specific protein-binding sites in the glycosaminoglycans is limited.

Glycosaminoglycan-binding proteins may sometimes be members of a family of proteins which have similar functions or participate in different steps of a metabolic process. Proteins mediating cell substrate adhesion (e.g., fibronectin, vitronectin, fibrinogen, and laminin) (Yamada, 1983; Suzuki et al., 1984) bind heparin. It is now also apparent that the cell adhesion molecule N-CAM has an aminoterminal heparin-binding domain, which may be important for its adhesion properties (Cole and Glaser, 1986; Cole et al., 1986). Some apolipoproteins (apo-E and apo-B), as well as lipoprotein lipase bind glycosaminoglycans (Shelburne and Quarfordt, 1977; Mahley et al., 1979; Cardin et al., 1984; Olivecrona et al., 1971; Cheng et al., 1981; Weisgraber, et al., 1986). It is tempting to speculate that these interactions have functional implications. An interaction between the adhesive proteins and glycosaminoglycans may facilitate or mediate cell–substrate adhesion (see Section 5.1). In addition a number of growth factors and angiogenic factors have heparin-binding capacity (see Section 5.5). Cell-surface heparan sulfate proteoglycans bind lipoprotein lipase. It is possible that heparan sulfate also binds lipoprotein, and thereby facilitates the interaction between the enzyme and its substrate.

Although the effects of glycosaminoglycan binding are unclear for most proteins, the binding of heparin to antithrombin III has profound effects on blood coagulation (for review, see Bjork and Lindahl, 1982). Antithrombin III is a protease inhibitor capable of reacting with serine proteases of the coagulation

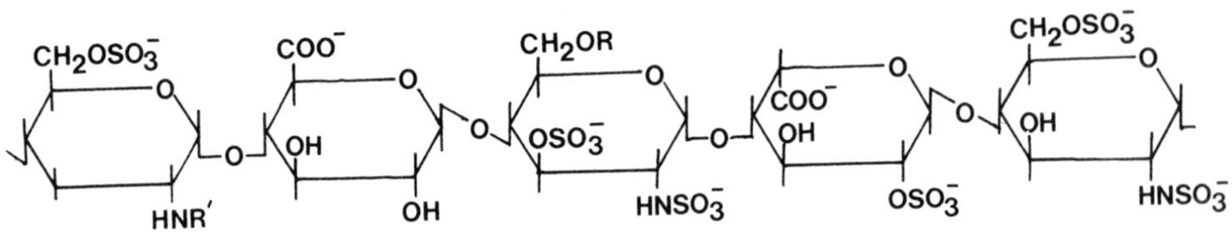

$$R = -H \text{ or } -SO_3^-$$
$$R' = -SO_3^- \text{ or } -COCH_3$$

Figure 2. Structure of the heparin sequence, displaying antithrombin III-binding activity, as reported by Lindahl et al. (1984).

cascade. In the absence of heparin, antithrombin III complexes with and inactivates target proteases; however, this reaction is slow and is greatly enhanced by the addition of heparin. Heparin presumably exerts its effect by binding to and changing the conformation of the protease inhibitor. The antithrombin III binding site in heparin has been localized by Lindahl and co-workers to a pentasaccharide (shown in Fig. 2), which has a specific monosaccharide sequence and sulfate substituents (Thurberg et al., 1982; Lindahl et al., 1984). This pentasaccharide will bind antithrombin III and accelerate the inactivation of some target proteases (e.g., factor Xa) (Choag et al., 1983). However, the observed size of heparin oligosaccharide required to enhance the antiproteinase activity of antithrombin differs depending on the target protease. For some proteases (e.g., thrombin), a longer stretch of heparin is required for optimal antithrombin III activity. In this case, it seems that heparin molecules not only bind to and change the conformation of antithrombin III, but also bind to thrombin (Danielsson et al., 1986). Thus, heparin serves as a template where both the protease and the inhibitor can bind.

Another interaction, studied in some detail, is the binding of hyaluronic acid to large chondroitin sulfate proteoglycans present in cartilage and aortic tissues. A hyaluronic acid binding site is present in the C-terminal globular domain of the core protein of a large-cartilage chondroitin sulfate proteoglycan. The binding of hyaluronic acid to this core protein is specific in that other glycosaminoglycans including heparin, chondroitin sulfates, and chondroitin will not inhibit the binding. Christner et al. (1979) localized the hyaluronic acid binding site to a decasaccharide. In cartilage, the interaction between chondroitin sulfate proteoglycan and hyaluronic acid exhibits a K_d value of 10^{-8} M and is stabilized by a link protein that simultaneously binds both the core protein and hyaluronic acid. Although the binding of hyaluronic acid to link protein has not been studied in great detail, this interaction appears to be similar to the interaction of hyaluronic acid and the core protein. In fact, the link protein and the hyaluronic acid binding region of the core protein appear to share antigenic determinants (Neame et al., 1985) and have an amino acid sequence homology of more than 60% (Neame et al., 1986).

4.2. Glycosaminoglycan–Glycosaminoglycan Interactions

Studies by Fransson et al. (1981, 1982) showed that certain glycosamino-glycans have a strong tendency to self-aggregate. Both galactosaminoglycans and glucosaminoglycans have this ability, although self-aggregation is restricted to certain subspecies. Thus chondroitin sulfates form aggregates with alternating blocks of iduronic and glucuronic acid residues. Certain heparan sulfates will also self-aggregate, but mixed aggregates containing heparan sulfate and chondroitin sulfate are not formed. The molecular basis for the selective specificity of self-aggregating glycosaminoglycans is unclear. Furthermore, although the implication of these interactions is significant and self-aggregation has been a useful tool in the isolation of a iduronic rich chondroitin sulfate proteoglycans from cartilage (Rosenberg et al., 1986), it has not been demonstrated that self-aggregation occurs in vivo.

4.3. Interactions of Proteoglycans and Glycosaminoglycans with Cells

Glycosaminoglycans and proteoglycans are located in close association with the surface of cells as judged by immunohistological and biochemical methods. There are at least three different mechanisms whereby a proteoglycan may be associated with cell membranes (Fig. 3).

Cell-surface-associated proteoglycans that have their protein core anchored in the lipid interior of cell membranes have been demonstrated on several cell types (for review, see Höök et al., 1984; Gallagher et al., 1986). It is conceivable that the core protein may actually span the membrane and be exposed on the cytoplasmic side of the membrane, although evidence proving this mode of membrane association has not yet been presented. In a recent study, Conrad and co-workers showed that a cell-associated proteoglycan could be released from hepatocytes by treatment with phosphatidylinositol-

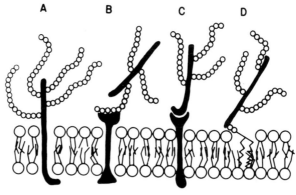

Figure 3. Schematic diagram to represent the various mechanisms by which heparan sulfate proteoglycans may associate with cell surfaces. (A) Core protein intercalated into the cell membrane. (B) Association with a membrane protein binding to a glycosaminoglycan chain of the heparan sulfate proteoglycan. (C) Association with a membrane protein binding to the core protein of the heparan sulfate proteoglycan. (D) Covalent association of the proteoglycan with phosphatidylinositol, which is membrane intercalated.

specific phospholipase C, suggesting that the proteoglycan was covalently linked to membrane lipids (Ishihara et al., 1987). It is possible that the membrane-anchored proteoglycans are ubiquitous in adherent eukaryotic cells, where they may play an important role in substrate adhesion.

Glycosaminoglycans can interact noncovalently with cell membranes. It is clear that some membrane proteins recognize and bind glycosaminoglycans. The function of such proteoglycans and glycosaminoglycans is not fully understood but, since these molecules are widespread and bind specifically to cell surfaces, their interactions with cells are probably biologically significant. Perhaps one of the best examples is heparin binding to smooth muscle cells (Castellot et al., 1985). This interaction may have profound effects on cell growth (see Section 5.3). Endothelial cells can also respond to heparin in terms of angiogenesis (see Section 5.5). Heparin receptors have been identified in hepatocytes, but their function is unclear (Höök et al., 1984). Underhill and Toole (1979, 1980) observed specific binding of [³H]hyaluronic acid to SV-3T3 cells and characterized the putative receptors (Underhill et al., 1983). There is also the possibility of covalent linkage of hyaluronate to a cell-surface protein (Mikuni-Takagaki and Toole, 1981). Binding of hyaluronate to distinct cell-surface molecules was described by Turley (1982) (Fig. 4).

Core proteins of some proteoglycans are noncovalently bound to a membrane component. Information of this type of association is limited. The binding of some chondroitin sulfate proteoglycans to chondrocytes and the binding and endocytosis of a dermatan sulfate proteoglycan to fibroblasts seems to involve the core protein of the proteoglycan (Sommarin and Heinegård, 1983; Glossl et al., 1983).

5. Effects of Proteoglycans on Cellular Behavior in Wound Repair

5.1. Proteoglycans as Modulators of Cell Adhesion

Cellular responses during wound repair involve migration and subsequent proliferation, both of which have particular requirements with respect to organized adhesion. At the outset of repair, epithelial cells at the margin of a skin or corneal wound must develop a new pattern of adhesion whereby a static anchored organization is replaced by one specialized for migration or proliferation. When this phase is complete, a return to a more static adhesion is accompanied by basement membrane synthesis and differentiation. Similar responses must be exhibited by mesenchymal cells. Even leukocytes and macrophages, which are specialized for locomotion and drawn into the wound area by chemotactic signals, exhibit changes in adhesive behavior (see Chapter 6).

Epithelial cells or fibroblasts can adhere to other cells or to macromolecules of the extracellular matrix. Specialized adhesion complexes are commonplace, a number of which are morphologically distinguishable and their molecular constitution is increasingly well understood. These include desmo-

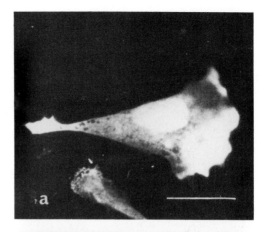

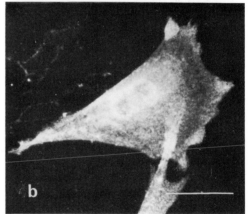

Figure 4. Association of hyaluronate with cell surfaces. Chick heart embryo fibroblasts stained with (a) RITC-hyaluronic acid and (b) a polyclonal antiserum against cell-surface hyaluronate-binding protein. (Courtesy of Dr. E. A. Turley, University of Calgary, Alberta.) Bar = 10 μm.

somes, hemidesmosomes, maculae adherens, or intermediate junctions, and tight junctions. In none of these complexes has a proteoglycan component been identified to date. Response to an injurious event is often accompanied by a loss of these adhesion complexes to facilitate locomotion. It is clear that changes in cytoskeletal organization that facilitate locomotion are coupled with a change in the nature of cell–cell or cell–matrix relationships at the cell surface. Epidermal cells, for example, lose their hemidesmosomes at the onset of cell migration (Krawczyk, 1971). It is therefore apparent that cells require a repertoire of adhesive strategies during wound repair to enable them to respond appropriately to a changing environment.

Although very few studies have been directly concerned with the roles of proteoglycans and glycosaminoglycans in the cellular aspects of wound repair, it is nevertheless possible to draw some parallels from in vitro studies. Proteoglycans are present in all connective tissues but can also be present as cell-surface-associated components (Section 4.3). Not only may they act as a receptor for other matrix molecules, such as fibronectin (Lark and Culp, 1984), but

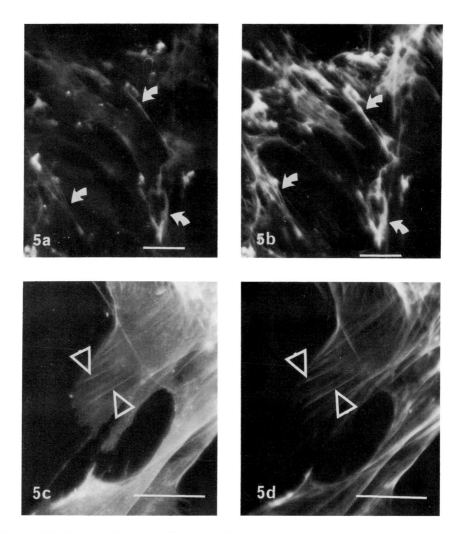

Figure 5. Distribution of heparan sulfate proteoglycans (HSPG) in fibroblast cell layers. Rat embryo fibroblasts stained with antibodies against heparan sulfate proteoglycan (a,c), fibronectin (b), and actin (d). While the matrix form of HSPG codistributes with fibronectin (arrows), that on cell surfaces codistributes with the underlying microfilaments (arrowheads). (Courtesy of A. Woods, University of Alabama at Birmingham.) Bar = 10 μm.

they also may interact directly with the cytoskeleton via their intracellular domain (Rapraeger and Bernfield, 1982). Recent work has shown, for example, that rat embryo fibroblasts possess two populations of heparan sulfate proteoglycans, one codistributing with other matrix molecules such as fibronectin, and the other disposed on the cell surface (Fig. 5), where it coaligns with the underlying microfilament system and is present at focal adhesions (Woods *et al.*, 1984). These proteoglycans probably have distinct core proteins since the cell-surface form is hydrophobic and possibly membrane intercalated while the matrix proteoglycan is not (Woods *et al.*, 1985). Furthermore, when detergent-resistant preparations are made from confluent cultures of rat embryo fibroblasts, up to 30% of the cell-surface heparan sulfate proteoglycan is retained in the detergent-resistant residue along with the microfilaments (Woods *et al.*, 1985).

How does cell-surface heparan sulfate proteoglycan affect cell adhesion? This is not yet entirely clear, but the fact that this molecule can be immunohistochemically localized in focal adhesions and in coalignment with the microfilament bundles of the cytoskeleton (Woods *et al.*, 1984) would, at first sight, implicate it with a role in stable cell adhesion. This is because the presence of large, numerous microfilament bundles is characteristic of nonmotile cells (Couchman and Rees, 1979). In addition, focal adhesions are morphologically and biochemically homologous with maculae adherens, which are characteristic of stable differentiated tissues.

For different reasons, Culp and co-workers have also hypothesized that cell-associated heparan sulfate proteoglycans stabilize adhesion, whereas chondroitin sulfate proteoglycans and hyaluronate destabilize adhesion perhaps to permit locomotion (Laterra *et al.*, 1980). The situation is complex, however, because Woods *et al.* (1984) showed that cell-surface heparan sulfate proteoglycan codistributes with an underlying microfilament meshwork in rat fibroblasts during the early stages of spreading on serum-coated substrata. Cells in these circumstances undergo rapid changes in morphology, contain no microfilament bundles or stress fibers, and lack other peripheral extracellular matrix components such as fibronectin. At later stages of the spreading process, these extracellular matrix proteins appear whereupon the cell-surface heparan sulfate proteoglycan becomes aligned over the submembranous microfilament bundles in a manner similar to fibronectin (Hynes and Destree, 1978). Fibronectin may therefore interact with heparan sulfate proteoglycan and simultaneously establish an extracellular matrix and lock the membrane-intercalated proteoglycan into a transmembrane assembly such as focal adhesions or fibronexus structures (Singer, 1979). Indeed, such structures may be a vital part of wound contraction, as shown by the elegant studies of myofibroblasts by Singer *et al.* (1984) (also see Chapter 17). It would be interesting to know what role proteoglycans have in the assembly or function of these structures. By analogy with focal adhesions, it seems likely that heparan sulfate proteoglycans may be an important component of the fibronexus structure, hence in wound contraction processes.

Recent experiments with cultured fibroblasts have shed some light on the molecular basis of stable adhesion generation in response to matrix molecules; here, proteoglycans may be of central importance. Cells spread on platelet factor 4 (a potent glycosaminoglycan-binding protein) do not assemble stress fibers and focal adhesions (Laterra *et al.*, 1983). In a similar way, we have shown that human fibroblasts that spread on a cell-binding fragment of human plasma fibronectin containing the Arg-Gly-Asp-Ser (RGDS) sequence (Pierschbacher *et al.*, 1982; Pierschbacher and Ruoslahti, 1984) also will not develop focal adhesions. Isolated heparin-binding domains of the fibronectin molecule also promote attachment and partial spreading but not focal adhesion or microfilament bundle formation (Woods *et al.*, 1986). However, a mixture of "cell"- and heparin-binding domains of fibronectin will promote full spreading and focal adhesion formation. Indeed, the heparin- and cell-binding domains of fibronectin have such potent synergism that heparin-binding domain can be added in very small amounts to cells prespread on the "cell"-binding domain and focal adhesions quickly form. Whether the heparin-binding domains of fibronectin can be bound by cell-surface heparan sulfate proteoglycan is not fully established, but preliminary evidence indicates that it can (Lark and Culp, 1984; R. LeBaron, personal communication).

Whether proteoglycans modulate the binding of other matrix molecules such as laminin to cell surfaces is not yet known, but interactions between laminin and glycosaminoglycans have been demonstrated (Sakashita *et al.*, 1980; Del Rosso *et al.*, 1981). A particularly interesting recent finding in this regard has been that neurite outgrowth is promoted by a region of laminin which contains heparin-binding activity (Edgar *et al.*, 1984), but whether this activity is central to its mode of action is unclear. As the authors comment, it is possible that the large laminin fragment tested in these experiments encompasses several biologically active domains. Another cell-adhesion molecule with heparin-binding activity is N-CAM (Cole and Glaser, 1986; Cole *et al.*, 1986). What role this ubiquitous molecule may have in wound healing is unclear. However, this developmentally regulated molecule is thought to be important at least in neuron–neuron, neuron–glial, and neuron–muscle adhesion (reviewed by Edelman, 1986).

Some forms of chondroitin sulfate can also interact with matrix molecules, such as fibronectin and laminin, but in general, the affinity of these interactions is somewhat less than those involving heparan sulfate or heparin (Ruoslahti and Engvall, 1980; Del Rosso *et al.*, 1981; Brennan *et al.*, 1983). This is perhaps consistent with the notion that either through direct interaction, steric hindrance, or the physical nature of the highly hydrated and negatively charged chains, chondroitin sulfate has been shown to decrease adhesion of cells to fibronectin or collagen (Knox and Wells, 1979; Rich *et al.*, 1981; Brennan *et al.*, 1983; Rosenberg *et al.*, 1986). The precise mechanisms are not understood. Studies on normal rat kidney (NRK) cells and human fibroblasts have shown the presence of cell-surface populations of chondroitin sulfate proteoglycan that do not codistribute with other major extracellular matrix components, such as fibronectin and collagen. Whether these are hydrophobic species is unknown, but the chondroitin proteoglycans are apparently excluded from regions of firm adhesion points, such as focal adhesions (Hedman *et al.*, 1983; Avnur and Geiger, 1984). Cell-surface receptors for chondroitin and dermatan sulfate proteoglycans have been demonstrated (Sommarin and Heinegård, 1983; Glossl *et al.*, 1983), and it may be that some of the cell-surface chondroitin sulfate proteoglycans visualized by immunotechniques are in fact involved in exocytosis/endocytosis pathways.

5.2. Proteoglycans and Cell Migration

Cell migration into the wound bed is an integral part of the repair process. Chemotaxis and haptotaxis are almost certainly key physiologic mechanisms by which this cell migration is achieved. In addition, structural cells surrounding the wound area may be responsive to the available space created by wounding events. In any case, the role of extracellular matrices during such migration has received much attention (see Chapter 13). Three major themes have emerged. Firstly, it has been shown, both directly and indirectly, that the locomotion of several cell types is facilitated by fibronectin (Ali and Hynes, 1978; Heasman et al., 1981; Couchman et al., 1982; Nishida et al., 1983; Turner et al., 1983; McCarthy and Furcht, 1984; Boucaut et al., 1984a,b; Takashima and Grinnell, 1985) and that fibronectin peptides can be chemotactic for cells (Postlethwaite et al., 1981; Seppa et al., 1981; Norris et al., 1982). The role of fibronectin in wound healing is discussed in Chapters 13, 18, and 23. Collagen and elastin fragments may also be chemotactic for some cells, but there is now substantial literature supporting a major role for fibronectin in migration both in embryogenesis and in wound healing. Second, it is also clear that migration, both in the embryo and during wound repair, takes place through hyaluronic acid-rich zones. Finally, some chondroitin sulfate proteoglycans may destabilize adhesion, which may in turn allow cell migration to occur. This has been very much the thesis of Culp and co-workers (Culp et al., 1978; Laterra et al., 1980), in which the analysis of fibroblast adhesion areas prepared by ethylene glycol-bis (β-aminoethyl ether) N,N,N′,N′, tetracetic acid (EGTA) detachment indicated that heparan sulfate–fibronectin complexes stabilized adhesion, whereas chondroitin/dermatan sulfate had the opposite effect. More recently, this has been supported by the evidence that a small dermatan sulfate proteoglycan abolished BALB/c3T3 cell attachment to fibronectin (Rosenberg et al., 1986). Brennan et al. (1983) also showed that a chondroitin proteoglycan from a rat yolk sac tumor inhibited cell–fibronectin interactions.

Other evidence from diverse systems has indicated the importance of chondroitin/dermatan sulfate proteoglycans in cell migration (Kinoshita and Saiga, 1979; Solursh et al., 1976; Kinsella and Wight, 1986). One interesting idea to explain persistence in migration is that locomotory cells "condition" collagenous substrata with a chondroitin sulfate proteoglycan, which then renders it unsuitable for adhesion (Funderburg and Markwald, 1986).

The interactions of heparan sulfate proteoglycan and fibronectin at the fibroblast cell surface lead to stable adhesion characterized by focal adhesions at the terminals of microfilament bundle (see Section 5.1). However, such stable adhesion is not consistent with cell migration (Couchman and Rees, 1979; Couchman and Blencowe, 1985). Indeed, neutrophils and macrophages do not assemble such structures either in vivo or in vitro (Abercrombie et al., 1977). The unsolved problem is therefore how fibronectin can promote migration yet also promote stable adhesion or cell–cell junction formation.

A simplistic explanation may lie in the unavailability of cell-surface heparan sulfate proteoglycan, so that cell–fibronectin interactions can only

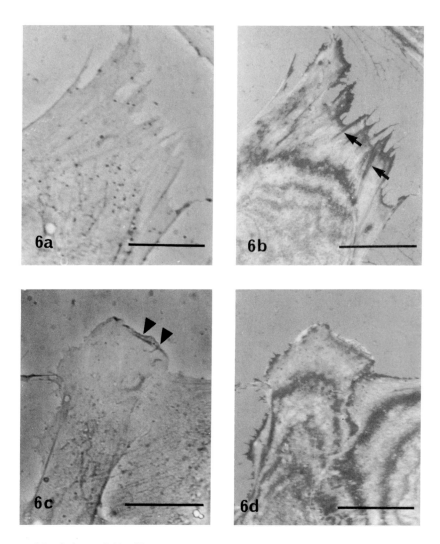

Figure 6. Morphology of fibroblasts in response to fibronectin substrates. Cycloheximide-pre-treated human embryo fibroblasts seeded on intact human plasma fibronectin (a,b) or an 80,000-M_r cell-binding domain of fibronectin (c,d). Note that in contrast to a fibronectin substratum, where spreading is accompanied by focal adhesion formation (arrows), cells on the 80,000-M_r fragment do not develop these structures and retain a motile phenotype with ruffling membrane (arrowheads in c). (a,c) Phase-contrast microscopy. (b,d) Intereference reflection microscopy. Bar = 10 μm.

take place through the fibronectin cell-binding domain (Pierschbacher and Ruoslahti, 1984; Woods *et al.*, 1986). In this case, the resultant adhesion is characterized by the absence of focal adhesions and microfilament bundles (Fig. 6). Such adhesion would then be compatible with migratory responses. Indeed, when tested, it has been documented that the cell-binding domain of plasma fibronectin lacking heparin or gelatin-binding activity is active with respect to locomotion and chemotaxis (Thiery et al., 1985; Donaldson et al., 1985; Seppa et al., 1981; Postlethwaite et al., 1981). Alternative explanations of fibronectin–proteoglycan interactions in cell locomotion are available, however. Chondroitin sulfates and hyaluronic acid have both been reported to bind fibronectin with quite high affinity (Ruoslahti and Engvall, 1980; Yamada, 1983; Brennan et al., 1983; but see also Yamagata et al., 1986), and the latter, particularly, has been put forward as a candidate for promotion of cell migration. Therefore, when fibronectin is bound to either of these ligands, the complex is unable to interact with cell-surface heparan sulfate proteoglycan, and locomotion is facilitated.

There is evidence from a variety of studies that hyaluronic acid is important in wound repair. Alexander and Donoff (1980) reported that in early phases of open wound healing in rabbits, hyaluronic acid is a prominent component of the extracellular matrix at the wound margins, where cell migration is in evidence. Later (after 7 days), hyaluronidase activity is apparent in the granulation tissue, coincident with a phase of proliferation and differentiation. At this time as well, dermatan sulfate is laid down in parallel with collagen fibril formation. In a similar manner, Grimes (1981) reported the presence of hyaluronic acid at the time of cell migration in a study of rabbit ear wounds. This was again followed by elevated hyaluronidase levels, which presumably degraded the hyaluronic acid. In concert with hyaluronic acid removal, the differentiation processes of chondrogenesis and fibrogenesis also occurred.

Ausprunk (1984) studied capillary formation in the chick chorioallantoic membrane and reported that hyaluronate was present during the formation, alignment, or migration of capillary endothelial cells, while sulfated glycosaminoglycans appeared during capillary differentiation. These results may have some bearing on the process of neovascularization, an important event in wound repair. Studies on newt limb regeneration also led Toole and Gross (1971) to conclude that hyaluronic acid levels are high during cell migratory responses. The newt limb-regeneration model is a good example of a repair process that has great similarity to developmental processes.

Much evidence of this sort led Toole (1981) to propose that cell migration, whether it be in wound repair or development, is facilitated by or requires a hydrated hyaluronate-rich environment. Mesenchymal migration in the developing cornea and kidney (Toole and Trelstad, 1971; Toole, 1981), the movement of neural crest cells (Pratt et al., 1975; Pintar, 1978; Thiery et al., 1985), gastrulating ectoderm (Solursh and Morriss, 1977), and the migration of cardiac cushion cells (Markwald et al., 1978) all occur in hyaluranate-rich extracellular matrices. Not all literature supports this view, however. Delauney and Bazin (1964) stated that hyaluronic acid levels are low during the early stages of wound repair and rise later on. This discrepancy is also seen in myocardial infarctions, wherein hyaluronic acid levels are initially low (Shetlar et al., 1978).

Hyaluronic acid has been reported to promote and inhibit neutrophil activity. Hakansson et al. (1980) and Venge et al. (1982) reported that in a range of 10–50 μg/ml, hyaluronic acid enhances neutrophil activities, including adherence, migration, phagocytosis, and oxidative metabolism. They also provide some evidence that hyaluronic acid injections in humans with suppressed neutrophil activity can enhance their activity during wound repair. The *in vitro* effects were, however, potentiated by an uncharacterized serum factor. In contrast, work by Forrester and colleagues showed that hyaluronic acid at concentrations similar to physiologic levels decreased neutrophil adhesiveness and chemotactic responsiveness (Forrester and Lackie, 1981; Forrester and Wilkinson, 1981). In this case, however, serum was not present, and the effects on neutrophil adhesion were not great. In similar assays with chick embryo fibroblasts, Knox and Wells (1979) found no effect of hyaluronic acid or other glycosaminoglycans on fibroblast adhesion to collagen or plastic, although adhesion was inhibited in the presence of a large-cartilage proteoglycan. With respect to diminished chemotactic response by neutrophils in the presence of hyaluronic acid, Forrester and Wilkinson (1981) proposed that hyaluronate interfered with the establishment of a chemotactic gradient and inhibited the binding of the chemotactic agent to the cell surface. It is perhaps likely that hyaluronic acid in solution may sterically hinder the interaction of ligands with their appropriate cell surface receptors. Macrophage migration and phagocytosis may also be suppressed by hyaluronic acid through similar processes (Balazs and Darzynkiewicz, 1973; Forrester and Balazs, 1980). Clearly, the mechanisms by which hyaluronic acid affect cell adhesion and migration are not yet well understood. It does appear, however, that hyaluronate may have considerable impact on many stages of wound healing, not simply by providing a hydrated milieu through which cells may move. No doubt, this whole area of hyaluronate biology will be considerably aided by a more complete understanding of its interactions, as well as more precise methods of localization (Knudsen and Toole, 1985) and quantification.

5.3. Proteoglycans and Cell Proliferation

One aspect of proteoglycan physiology that is currently receiving much attention is control of cell growth. Whether this has a bearing on the proliferative response of cells in wound repair is speculative, but such activity is feasible. Rolin et al. (1975) suggested that heparan sulfate proteoglycans may have a role in density-dependent growth inhibition in cultured 3T3 cells. Furthermore, Kawakami and Terayama (1981) reported that heparan sulfate proteoglycan prepared from liver plasma membranes, a particularly rich source of peripheral and membrane-intercalated species of these proteoglycans (Kjellén et al.. 1981), could exhibit some growth-inhibitory properties when added to hepatoma cells.

Clowes and Karnovsky reported in 1977 that heparin suppresses the growth of vascular smooth muscle. This finding and the discoveries that such molecules can be synthesized by endothelial cells (Castellot et al., 1982) and smooth muscle cells (Fritze and Rosenberg, 1983) and that they are present on cell surfaces in postconfluent rather than proliferative cultures (Fritze et al.,

1985) indicate an important role for heparin-like molecules in tissue home-ostasis. Interestingly it has now been established that anticoagulant activities of heparin are separable from growth suppression. For instance, N-desulfated, re-N-acetylated heparin was found to be antiproliferative, even though it has no anticoagulant properties. However, both activities appear to require 3-O-sul-fated glucosamine (Castellot et al., 1986).

It is possible to envisage these glucosaminoglycans in healthy blood ves-sels acting as a growth suppressor or chalone. When the endothelium is dam-aged, there is perhaps a depletion of growth-suppressing heparan sulfate; under the influence of platelet-derived growth factor (PDGF) (Ross and Glomset, 1976) or similar stimuli, smooth muscle cell migration and proliferation result. Interestingly, the same platelet granules containing PDGF also contain a heparitinase (Oldberg et al., 1980). This pattern of events may be common in all wound-repair responses associated with neovascularization. The situation is clearly complex, however, since a number of growth factors and angiogenic factors have heparin-binding capabilities (see Section 5.5).

While the accumulation of heparan sulfate or similar glycosaminoglycans appears to suppress or decrease growth, proliferating cells often have high levels of hyaluronate associated with them (Tomida et al., 1974; Cohn et al., 1976). Transformation is accompanied by elevated hyaluronate levels (Hop-wood and Dorman, 1977), as is growth stimulation by insulin (Moscathelli and Rubin, 1975) and by epidermal growth factor (EGF) (Lembach, 1976). It would appear that not only does hyaluronate accompany or facilitate cell migration, but it is also synthesized by proliferative cells. This area is becoming particu-larly interesting since E. A. Turley (personal communication) has shown that a cell-surface hyaluronate-binding protein has tyrosine kinase activity, implying that interaction of hyaluronic acid with cell surfaces can stimulate a number of intracelluilar activities, including those of the cytoskeleton.

5.4. Proteoglycans and Cell Differentiation

The restoration of tissue function after damage depends on a succession of cellular events, culminating in the reappearance of the differentiated phe-notype. Such events rely on selective gene expression, accompanied by regu-lated growth, morphology, and secretion of various macromolecules, including those of the extracellular matrix. The profile and organization of the connective tissue components often characterize the mature stabilized tissue (e.g., base-ment membrane beneath epithelia, dermal matrix, cartilage matrix, or bone matrix).

Many reports over the past few years have drawn attention to the important role that extracellular matrix components themselves have on the adhesion, cytoskeletal organization, and subsequent proliferation and differentiation of many cell types. For anchorage-dependent cells, it is clear that a well-organized cellular architecture and cell-surface topography are consistent with differ-entiation, one facet of which is the synthesis of a specific extracellular matrix.

However, few studies have been explicitly directed toward understanding a feedback mechanism exerted directly on cells by exogenously supplied matrix components. Indeed, such studies are difficult to perform, since such molecules affect parameters such as cell shape, proliferation, and migration. During the course of wound repair, however, it is apparent that the extracellular environment undergoes dramatic changes often from a fibrin- and fibronectin-rich provisional matrix accompanied by hyaluronate in the early stages (see Sections 5.2 and 5.3; Chapters 15, 18, and 23) to a later stage where a mature matrix is re-established, often dominated by interstitial collagens (Chapter 20) and sulfated proteoglycans. Studies on chondrocytes have again drawn attention to a cellular sensitivity to hyaluronate-rich environments. Wiebkin and Muir (1973), Solursh et al. (1974), and Handley and Lowther (1976) reported that proteoglycan biosynthesis was reduced by exogenously supplied hyaluronic acid. Studies on myogenesis (Kujawa et al., 1986) showed that the process could be inhibited by plating cells onto surfaces to which hyaluronate had been bonded. All this is consistent with a function of hyaluronate that can be summarized as tending to keep cells in an undifferentiated state (or perhaps dedifferentiated state in a wound healing context) compatible with migration and proliferation. With a decline in hyaluronate levels, differentiation characteristics begin to emerge that include synthesis of a matrix consistent with the differentiated phenotype. Meier and Hay (1974a,b) also showed that extracellular matrix synthesis in the maturing cornea is stimulated by sulfated glycosaminoglycans and collagen.

The extensive studies of Bernfield and co-workers indicated the importance of proteoglycans in the differentiation processes that culminate in the formation of a mature branched salivary gland. The immature basement membranes of this gland have more hyaluronate and chondroitin sulfate proteoglycan associated with them than do mature areas, which have increased levels of heparan sulfate proteoglycans. Moreover, in regions of morphogenetic activity, proteoglycan turnover is elevated, coincident with mitotic activity and basement membrane remodeling (Bernfield and Banerjee, 1982; reviewed by Bernfield et al., 1984).

A recent report has underscored the possible importance in the promotion of differentiation by heparan sulfate proteoglycan. Li et al. (1987) examined the synthesis of mRNA for proteins associated with differentiation of mammary epithelial cells in culture (e.g., caseins). They found that the basement membrane glycoprotein, laminin, in association with a large heparan sulfate proteoglycan (Hassell et al., 1986) could elevate casein mRNA levels (and protein secretion) as well as promote cell shape and organization changes highly reminiscent of the mammary epithelium in vivo. By contrast, cells plated on the proteoglycans alone expressed elevated casein mRNA levels, but remained flatted in culture, did not shape change, nor did they secrete casein. One interpretation is that the interaction of heparan sulfate proteoglycan with cell surfaces can influence transcriptional events or message stability.

The possibility of a role for intracellular heparan sulfate in growth and differentiation has been highlighted by the work of Fedarko and Conrad (1986), which identified populations of nuclear and nuclear membrane heparan sulfate polysaccharides in hepatocytes. Moreover, they contained a high proportion of the unusual disaccharide structure β-D-glucuronosyl (2-SO_4)→D-glycosamine-N,O-(SO_4)$_2$. This structure may be important in the enzymatic processing of the precursor proteoglycan and/or the routing to and function of heparan sulfate in the nucleus. There has been evidence for nuclear glycosaminoglycans previously (Bhavanandan and Davidson, 1975; Furakawa and Terayama, 1977, 1979; Margolis et al., 1976; Stein et al., 1975; Fromme et al., 1976); this, together with effects of heparin on DNA replication and transcription through possible interactions with cationic histones (Kraemer and Coffey, 1970; Arnold et al., 1972; Kovacs et al., 1981; Doneck, 1981; Furakawa and Bhavanandan, 1983), leads to a distinct possibility that glycosaminoglycans can directly influence gene expression. Whether cell-surface or extracellular matrix proteoglycans are the precursors of this pool is unclear. Nevertheless, the possibility exists that glycosaminoglycan uptake, degradation, and transport to the nucleus control cell behavior through selective interactions with other molecules.

5.5. Heparin and Heparan Sulfate in Angiogenesis

The foregoing sections drew attention to some of the potential roles of proteoglycans and glycosaminoglycans in the phases of wound repair. A consideration of angiogenesis, an important component of wound healing, is a potent reminder that such events are not compartmentalized but are contiguous or often parallel in their operation (see Chapter 15). Endothelial cells, once stimulated appropriately, migrate through or perhaps solubilize their subjacent basement membrane, and then by a combination of migration and proliferation (Ausprunk and Folkman, 1977), invade the granulation tissue of the wound. Once established, there must be a series of differentiation events leading to renewal of basement membrane synthesis and deposition (see Chapter 15).

In addition to the role of heparin and related polysaccharides as anticoagulants, they also appear to have wide-ranging effects on the cells of the vascular system that may have some bearing on the process of neovascularization. The situation is probably complex, since members of the heparan sulfate/heparin family, which differ in their fine structure, may have strikingly different effects. For instance, postconfluent vascular smooth muscle cells produce an antiproliferative heparan sulfate species, whereas sparse cells in culture produce species lacking this property (Fritze et al., 1985).

Studies by Taylor and Folkman (1982) show that heparin augments tumor angiogenesis factor in the chick chorioallantoic membrane system and that protamine, a heparin antagonist, severely inhibited the angiogenic process. However, the picture has recently become more complicated, as Folkman et al. (1983) showed that heparin administered with cortisone inhibited capillary proliferation and angiogenesis in several systems, including that in response to inflammation. The biologic action of cortisone here is not yet clear, but the

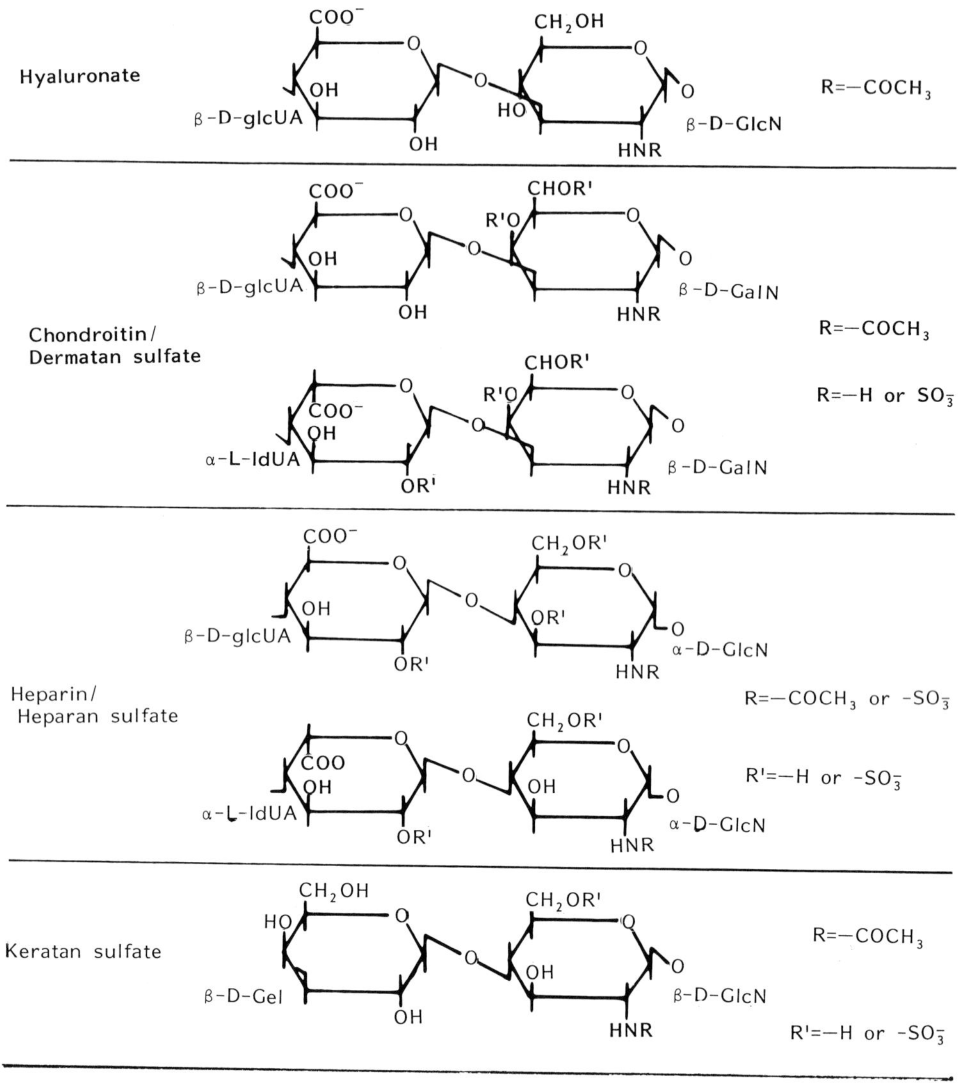

Figure 7. Structure of repeating disaccharide units of the glycosaminoglycans. A large number of structural variants are indicated, especially for heparin/heparan sulfate. It should be pointed out that some of the indicated disaccharide structures may occur at a low frequency due to restrictions in the substrate specifications of the polymer-modifying enzymes.

inhibition of angiogenesis was not derived from anticoagulation effects of heparin, since hexasaccharides lacking anticoagulation activity inhibited angiogenesis.

By contrast, studies by Azizkhan et al. (1980) showed that mast cell heparin promotes capillary endothelial cell migration. This appears to be a highly specific effect, since aortic endothelial cells were unresponsive and heparin-like polysaccharides inhibit vascular smooth muscle cell migration (Majack and Clowes, 1984). Chemically, the effect was also fairly specific as heparan and chondroitin sulfates and hyaluronic acid were inactive. However, dextran sulfate also promoted capillary endothelial cell migration, perhaps indicating the importance of charge density or arrangement. More recently, West *et al.* (1986) confirmed that intact hyaluronic acid was inactive in an angiogenesis assay. Surprisingly, however, degradation products of hyaluronic acid, produced by testicular hyaluronidase, were active in promoting angiogenesis.

Macrophage-derived growth factor(s) (Martin *et al.*, 1981) and endothelial cell growth factor (Schreiber *et al.*, 1985) also stimulate angiogenesis. An interesting property shared by many peptides that stimulate angiogenesis is their ability to bind heparin, in some cases with a high affinity and apparent specificity. For example, a chondrosarcoma-derived angiogenesis promoter required 1.5 M NaCl for elution from a heparin affinity column, whereas PDGF (of similar isoelectric point and also capable of binding heparin) was displaced by one-third of the salt concentration (Shing *et al.*, 1984). A recently described angiogenesis promoter from embryonic kidney is also capable of strong interaction with heparin (Risau and Ekblom, 1986). The factor is apparently mitogenic for endothelial, but not vascular smooth muscle cells. Endothelial cell growth factor also interacts with heparin, and its biologic activity is potentiated by the polysaccharide (Thornton *et al.*, 1983). Many if not all of these angiogenesis factors with high affinity for heparin may be related to acidic or basic fibroblast growth factor (Folkman and Klagsbrun, 1987).

Clearly, the influences of heparin or heparan sulfate in angiogenesis may be multifactorial and may be seen both in terms of capillary endothelial cell proliferation and migration. What are the sources of these glycosaminoglycans? Mast cells that often congregate at sites of chronic inflammation (Dvorak *et al.*, 1976) are a potential source. Endothelial cells themselves also synthesize heparan sulfate proteoglycans (Oohira *et al.*, 1983); some forms of cell-surface heparan sulfate in these cells are anticoagulantly active, possibly partially responsible for the nonthrombogenic properties of the blood vessel luminal surface (Marcum and Rosenberg, 1984).

6. Conclusions

Proteoglycans are ubiquitous components of all connective tissues and can be present on cell surfaces, sometimes as integral membrane components. How widespread cell-associated proteoglycans are has yet to be fully evaluated, but their importance in cellular adhesion and other behavior seems to be increasingly recognized. The involvement of glycosaminoglycans and proteoglycans in the many stages of the complex process of tissue repair has not been well studied; but our conclusion, based on a variety of studies and particularly those on development and embryogenesis, would indicate roles for these molecules at all stages of wound repair.

Heparin may play a role in the control of blood clotting at the site of tissue damage. The cellular environment during the early stages of repair, particularly those involving cell migration, is rich in nonsulfated species such as hyaluronic acid, that, in addition to providing an "open" hydrated milieu through which cells can locomote, can also directly influence cell behavior.

The next stages of tissue repair involve proliferation, differentiation, and synthesis of a mature extracellular matrix. At this time, sulfated proteoglycans are seemingly important; in particular, the appearance of chondroitin and dermatan sulfate proteoglycans is apparent, consistent with previously reported roles for some of these in collagen fibrillogenesis, for example. Heparan sulfate on the cell surface, in matrices such as basement membranes and within the nucleus may also be important at this time.

Clearly, much of the material drawn upon in this chapter was not directly concerned with the molecular events of wound healing, and some of the many gaps in our knowledge have been noted. With the appearance of better tools and methods for the study of proteoglycans, some of these gaps will undoubtedly be filled in the not-too-distant future.

ACKNOWLEDGMENTS The work described in this review, completed in our laboratories, was supported by grants AM27807 and HL34343 (MH) and AR36457 (JRC) from the National Institutes of Health and by grants from the Crippled Children Vitreoretinal Research Foundation (MH, JRC), the Diabetes Research and Training Center, and Diabetes Trust Fund at the University of Alabama (JRC).

References

Abercrombie, M. Dunn, G. A., and Heath, J. P., 1977, Locomotion and contraction in nonmuscle cells, in: *Contractile Systems in Non-Muscle Tissues* (S. V. Perry, A. Margreth, and R. S. Adelstein, eds.), pp. 3–11. North-Holland, Amsterdam.

Alexander, S. A., and Donoff, R. B., 1980, The glycosaminoglycans of open wounds, *J. Surg. Res.* **29**:422–429.

Ali, I. U., and Hynes, R. O., 1978, Effects of LETS glycoprotein on cell motility, *Cell* **14**:439–446.

Arnold, E. A., Yawn, D. H., Brown, D. G., Wyllie, R. C., and Coffey, D. S., 1972, Structural alteration in rat liver nuclei after removal of template restrictions by polyanions, *J. Cell Biol.* **53**:737–757.

Ausprunk, D. H., 1984, Distribution of hyaluronate and sulfated glycosaminoglycans during capillary migration and development in the chick chorioallantoic membrane, *J. Cell Biol.* **99**:168 (abst).

Ausprunk, D. H., and Folkman, J., 1977, Migration and proliferation of endothelial cells in preformed and newly formed blood vessels during tumor angiogenesis, *Microvasc. Res.* **14**:53–65.

Avnur, Z., and Geiger, B., 1984, Immunocytochemical localization of native chondroitin-sulfate in tissues and cultured cells using specific monoclonal antibody, *Cell* **38**:811–822.

Azizkhan, R. G., Azizkhan, J. C., Zetter, B. R., and Folkman, J., 1980, Mast cell heparin stimulates migration of capillary endothelial cells *in vitro*, *J. Exp. Med.* **152**:931–944.

Baker, S. R., Blithe, D. L., Buck, C. A., and Warren, L., 1980, Glycosaminoglycans and other carbohydrate groups bound to proteins of control and transformed cells, *J. Biol. Chem.* **255**:8719–8728.

Balazs, E. A., and Darzynkiewicz, Z., 1973, The effect of hyaluronic acid on fibroblast, mononuclear phagocytes and lymphocytes, in: *The Biology of the Fibroblast* (E. Kulonen and J. Pikkarainen, eds.), pp. 237–252, Academic, London.

Bernfield, M., and Banerjee, S. D., 1982, The turnover of basal lamina glycosaminoglyan correlates with epithelial morphogenesis, *Dev. Biol.* **90**:291–305.

Bernfield, M., Banerjee, S. D., Koda, J. E., and Rapraeger, A. C., 1984, Remodeling of the basement membrane: Morphogenesis and maturation, *Ciba Found. Symp.* **108**:179–196.

Bhavanandan, V. P., and Davidson, E. A., 1975, Mucopolysaccharides associated with nuclei of cultured mammalian cells, *Proc. Natl. Acad. Sci. USA* **72**:2032–2036.

Bjork, I., and Lindahl, U., 1982, Mechanism of the anticoagulant action of heparin. *Mol. Cell. Biochem.* **48**:161–182.

Boucaut, J. C., Darribère, T., Boulekbache, H., and Thiery, J. P., 1984a, Antibodies to fibronectin prevent gastrulation but do not perturb neurulation in gastrulated amphibian embryos, *Nature (London)* **307**:364–367.

Boucaut, J. C., Darribère, T., Poole, T. J., Aoyama, H., Yamada, K. M., and Thiery, J. P., 1984b, Biologically active synthetic peptides as probes of embryonic development: A competitive peptide inhibitor of fibronectin function inhibits gastrulation in amphibian embryos and neural crest cell migration in avian embryo, *J. Cell Biol.* **99**:1822–1830.

Bourdon, M. A., Oldberg, A., Pierschbacher, M., and Ruoslahti, E., 1985, Molecular cloning and sequence analysis of a chondroitin sulfate proteoglycan cDNA, *Proc. Natl. Acad. Sci. USA* **82**:1321–1325.

Bourdon, M. A., Shiga, M., and Ruoslahti, E., 1986, Identification from cDNA of the precursor form of a chondroitin sulfate proteoglycan core protein, *J. Biol. Chem.* **261**:12534–12537.

Brennan, M. J., Oldberg, A., Hayman, E. G., and Ruoslahti, E., 1983, Effect of a proteoglycan produced by rat tumor cells on their adhesion to fibronectin–collagen substrata, *Cancer Res.* **43**:4302–4307.

Cardin, A. D., Witt, K. R., and Jackson, R. L., 1984, Visualization of heparin-binding proteins by ligand blotting with ^{125}I-heparin, *Anal. Biochem.* **137**:368–373.

Castellot, J. J., Favreau, L. V., Karnovsky, M. J., and Rosenberg, R. D., 1982, Inhibition of vascular smooth muscle cell growth by endothelial cell-derived heparin, *J. Biol. Chem.* **257**:11256–11260.

Castellot, J. J., Wong, K., Herman, B., Hoover, R. L., Albertini, D. F., Wright, T. C., Caleb, B. L., and Karnovsky, M. J., 1985, Binding and internalization of heparin by vascular smooth muscle cells, *J. Cell. Physiol.* **124**:13–20.

Castellot, J. J., Choay, J., Lormeau, J.-C., Petitou, M., Sache, E., and Karnovsky, M. J., 1986, Structural determinants of the capacity of heparin to inhibit the proliferation of vascular smooth muscle cells. II. Evidence for a pentasaccharide sequence that contains a 3-O-sulfate group, *J. Cell Biol.* **102**:1979–1984.

Cheng, C.-F., Oosta, G. M., Bensadoun, A., and Rosenberg, R. D., 1981, Binding of lipoprotein lipase to endothelial cells in culture, *J. Biol. Chem.* **256**:12893–12898.

Choay, J., Petitou, M., Lormeau, J. C., Sinay, P., Lasu, B., and Gatti, G., 1983, Structure–activity relationship in heparin: A synthetic pentasaccharide with high affinity for antithrombin III and eliciting high anti-factor Xa activity, *Biochem. Biophys. Res. Commun.* **116**:492–499.

Christner, J. E., Brown, M. L., and Dziewiatkowski, D. D., 1979, Interactions of cartilage proteoglycans with hyaluronate, *J. Biol. Chem.* **254**:4624–4630.

Clowes, A. W., and Karnovsky, M. J., 1977, Suppression by heparin of smooth muscle cell proliferation in injured arteries, *Nature (Lond.)* **265**:625–626.

Cohn, R. H., Cassiman, J. J., and Bernfield, M. R., 1976, Relationship of transformation, cell density and growth control to the cellular distribution of newly synthesized glycosaminoglycan, *J. Cell Biol.* **71**:280–294.

Cole, G. J., and Glaser, L., 1986, A heparin-binding domain from N-CAM is involved in neural cell-substratum adhesion, *J. Cell Biol.* **102**:403–412.

Cole, G. J., Loewy, A., Cross, N. V., Abseson, R., and Glaser, L., 1986, Topographic localization of the heparin-binding domain of the neural cell adhesion molecule N-CAM, *J. Cell Biol.* **103**:1739–1744.

Comper, W. W., and Laurent, T. C., 1978, Physiological function of connective tissue polysaccharides, *Physiol. Rev.* **58:**255–315.

Cossu, G., and Warren, L., 1983, Lactosaminoglycan and heparan sulfate are covalently bound to fibronectins synthesized by mouse stem teratocarcinoma cells, *J. Biol. Chem.* **258:**5603–5607.

Couchman, J. R., and Blencowe, S., 1985, Adhesion and cell surface relationships during fibroblast and epithelial migration *in vitro, Exp. Biol. Med.* **10:**23–38.

Couchman, J. R., and Rees, D. A., 1979, The behavior of fibroblasts migrating from chick heart explants. Changes in adhesion, locomotion, and growth, and in the distribution of actomyosin and fibronectin, *J. Cell Sci.* **39:**149–165.

Couchman, J. R., Rees, D. A., Green, M. R., and Smith, C. G., 1982, Fibronectin has a dual role in locomotion and anchorage of primary chick fibroblasts and can promote entry into the division cycle, *J. Cell Biol.* **93:**402–410.

Danielson, Å., Raub, E., Lindahl, U., and Björk, I., 1986, Role of ternary complexes, in which heparin binds both antithrombin and proteinase, in the acceleration of the reactions between antithrombin and thrombin or factor Xa, *J. Biol. Chem.* **261:**15467–15473.

David, G., and Van den Berghe, H., 1985, Heparan sulfate–chondroitin sulfate hybrid proteoglycan of the cell surface and basement membrane of mouse mammary epithelial cells, *J. Biol. Chem.* **260:**11067–11074.

Delauney, A., and Bazin, S., 1974, Mucopolysaccharides, collagen, and non-fibrillar proteins in inflammation, *Int. Rev. Connective Tissue Res.* **2:**301–325.

Del Rosso, M., Cappelletti, R., Viti, M., Vannucchi, S., and Chiarugi, V., 1981, Binding of the basement-membrane glycoprotein laminin to glycosaminoglycans, *Biochem. J.* **199:**699–704.

Donaldson, D. J., Mahan, J. T., Hasty, D. L., McCarthy, J. B., and Furcht, L. T., 1985, Location of a fibronectin domain involved in newt epidermal cell migration, *J. Cell Biol.* **101:**73–78.

Donecke, D., 1981, Effect of heparin on isolated nuclei, *Biochem. Int.* **3:**73–80.

Dorfman, A., 1981, Proteoglycan biosynthesis, in: *Cell Biology of Extracellular Matrix* (E. D. Hay, ed.), pp. 115–138, Plenum, New York.

Durum, S. K., Schmidt, J. A., and Oppenheim, J. J., 1985, Interleukin 1: An immunological perspective, *Annu. Rev. Immunol.* **3:**263–287.

Dvorak, A. M., Mihm, M. C., and Dvorak, H. F., 1976, Morphology of delayed-type hypersensitivity reactions in man. II. Ultrastructural alterations affecting the microvasculature and the tissue mast cells, *Lab. Invest.* **34:**179–191.

Edelman, G. M., 1986, Cell adhesion molecules in the regulation of animal form and tissue pattern, *Annu. Rev. Cell Biol.* **2:**81–116.

Edgar, D., Timpl, R., and Thoenen, H., 1984, The heparin-binding domain of laminin is responsible for its effects on neurite outgrowth and neuronal survivial, *EMBO J.* **3:**1463–1468.

Fedarko, N. S., and Conrad, H. E., 1986, A unique heparan sulfate in the nuclei of hepatocytes: Structural changes with the growth state of the cell, *J. Cell Biol.* **102:**587–599.

Folkman, J., and Klagsbrun, M., 1987, Angiogenic factors. *Science* **235:**442–447.

Folkman, J., Longer, R., Linhardt, R. J., Hauderschild, C., and Taylor, S., 1983, Angiogenesis inhibition and tumor regression caused by heparin or a heparin fragment in the presence of cortisone, *Science* **221:**719–725.

Forrester, J. V., and Balazs, E. A., 1980, Inhibition of phagocytosis by high molecular weight hyaluronate, *Immunology* **40:**435–446.

Forrester, J. V., and Lackie, J. M., 1981, Effect of hyaluronic acid on neutrophil adhesion, *J. Cell Sci.* **50:**329–344.

Forrester, J. V., and Wilkinson, P. C., 1981, Inhibition of leukocyte locomotion by hyaluronic acid, *J. Cell Sci.* **48:**315–331.

Fransson, L.-Å., Cöster, L., Malmström, A., and Sheehan, J. K., 1982, Self-association of scleral proteodermatan sulfate, *J. Biol. Chem.* **257:**6333–6338.

Fransson, L.-Å., Havsmark, B., and Sheehan, J. K., 1981, Self-association of heparan sulfate, *J. Biol. Chem.* **256:**13039–13043.

Fritze, L. M. S., and Rosenberg, R. D., 1983, Bovine aortic smooth muscle cells produce an inhibitor or smooth muscle cell growth *in vitro, J. Cell Biol.* **97:**90 (abst).

Fritze, L. M. S., Reilly, C. F., and Rosenberg, R. D., 1985, An antiproliferative heparan sulfate species produced by postconfluent smooth muscle cells, *J. Cell Biol.* **100**:1041–1049.

Fromme, H. F., Buddecke, E., von Figura, K., and Kresse, H., 1976, Localization of sulfated glycosaminoglycans within cell nuclei by high resolution autoradiography, *Exp. Cell Res.* **102**:445–449.

Funderburg, F. M., and Markwald, R. R., 1986, Conditioning of native substrates by chondroitin sulfate proteoglycan during cardiac mesenchymal cell migration, *J. Cell Biol.* **103**:2475–2487.

Furakawa, K., and Terayama, H., 1977, Isolation and identification of glycosaminoglycans associated with purified nuclei from rat liver, *Biochim. Biophys. Acta* **499**:278–289.

Furakawa, K., and Terayama, H., 1979, Pattern of glycosaminoglycans and glycoproteins associated with nuclei of regenerating rat liver, *Biochim. Biophys. Acta* **585**:575–588.

Furakawa, K., and Bhavanandan, V. P., 1983, Influences of anionic polysaccharides on DNA synthesis in isolated nuclei and by DNA polymerase alpha: Correlations of observed effects with properties of the polysaccharides, *Biochim. Biophys. Acta* **740**:466–474.

Gallagher, J. T., Gasiunas, N., and Schor, S. L., 1983, Specific association of iduronic acid-rich dermatan sulfate with the extracellular matrix of human skin fibroblasts cultured on collagen gels, *Biochem. J.* **215**:107–116.

Gallagher, J. T., Lyon, M., and Steward, W. P., 1986, Structure and function of heparan sulphate proteoglycans, *Biochem. J.* **236**:313–325.

Glossl, J., Schubert-Prinz, R., Gregory, J. D., Damle, S. P., von Figura, K., and Kresse, H., 1983, Receptor-mediated endocytosis of proteoglycans by human fibroblasts involves recognition of protein core, *Biochem. J.* **215**:295–301.

Grimes, N. L., 1981, The role of hyaluronate and hyaluronidase in cell migration during the rabbit ear regenerative healing response, *Anat. Rec.* **199**:100 (abst).

Håkansson, L., Hallgren, R., and Venge, P., 1980, Regulation of granulocyte function by hyaluronic acid: In vitro and in vivo effects on phagocytosis, locomotion, and metabolism, *J. Clin. Invest.* **66**:298–305.

Handley, C., and Lowther, D. A., 1976, Inhibition of proteoglycan biosynthesis by hyaluronic acid in chondrocytes in cell culture, *Biochem. Biophys. Acta* **444**:69–74.

Hascall, V. C., and Hascall, G. K., 1981, Proteoglycans, in: *Cell Biology of Extracellular Matrix* (E. D. Hay, ed.), pp. 39–63, Plenum, New York.

Hassell, J. R., Kimura, J. H., and Hascall, V. C., 1986, Proteoglycan core protein families, *Annu. Rev. Biochem.* **55**:539–567.

Hassell, J. R., Robey, P. G., Barrach, M.-J., Wilczek, J., Rennard, S. I., and Martin, G. R., 1980, Isolation of a heparan sulfate-containing proteoglycan from basement membrane, *Proc. Natl. Acad. Sci. USA* **77**:4494–4498.

Heasman, J., Hynes, R. O., Swan, A. P., Thomas, V., and Wylie, C. C., 1981, Primordial germ cells of Xenopus embryos: The role of fibronectin in their adhesion during migration, *Cell* **27**:437–447.

Hedman, K., Christner, J., Julkunen, I., and Vaheri, A., 1983, Chondroitin sulfate at the plasma membranes of cultured fibroblasts, *J. Cell Biol.* **97**:1288–1293.

Heinegård, D., Franzén, A., Hedbom, E., and Sommarin, Y., 1986, Common structures of the core proteins of interstitial proteoglycans, in: *Functions of the Proteoglycans*, Ciba Foundation Symposium 124 (D. Evered and J. Whelen, eds.), pp. 65–88, Wiley, New York.

Höök, M., Kjellén, L., Johansson, S., and Robinson, J., 1984, Cell-surface glycosaminoglycans, *Annu. Rev. Biochem.* **53**:847–869.

Hopwood, J. J., and Dorfman, A., 1977, Isolation of lipid glucuronic acid and N-acetylglucosamine from a rat fibrosarcoma, *Biochem. Biophys. Res. Commun.* **75**:472–479.

Hynes, R. O., and Destree, A. T., 1978, Relationships between fibronection (LETS protein) and actin, *Cell* **15**:875–885.

Ishihara, M., Fedarko, N. S., and Conrad, H. E., 1987, Involvement of phosphatidylinositol and insulin in the coordinate regulation of protoheparan sulfate metabolism and hepatocyte growth, *J. Biol. Chem.* **262**:4708–4716.

Jalkanen, M., Nguyen, H., Rapraeger, A., Klein, N., and Bernfield, M., 1985, Heparan sulfate proteoglycan from mouse mammary epithelial cells: Localization on the cell surface with a monoclonal antibody, *J. Cell Biol.* **101**:976–984.

Kanwar, Y. S., and Farquhar, M. G., 1979, Isolation of glycosaminoglycans (heparan sulfate) from glomerular basement membranes, *Proc. Natl. Acad. Sci. USA* **76:**4493–4497.

Kawakami, H., and Terayama, H., 1981, Liver plasma membranes and proteoglycans prepared therefrom inhibit the growth of hepatoma cells *in vitro, Biochim. Biophys. Acta* **646:**161–168.

Kimura, J. H., Thonar, E. J.-M., Hascall, V. C., Reiner, A., and Poole, A. R., 1981, Identification of core protein, an intermediate in proteoglycan biosynthesis in cultured chondrocytes from the Swarm rat chondrosarcoma, *J. Biol. Chem.* **256:**7890–7897.

Kinoshita, S., and Saiga, H., 1979, The role of proteoglycan in the development of sea urchins, *Exp. Cell Res.* **123:**229–236.

Kinsella, M. G., and Wight, T. N., 1986, Modulation of sulfated proteoglycan synthesis by bovine aortic endothelial cells during migration, *J. Cell Biol.* **102:**679–687.

Kjellén, L., Pettersson, I., and Höök, M., 1981, Cell-surface heparan sulfate: An intercalated membrane proteoglycan, *Proc. Natl. Acad. Sci. USA* **78:**5371–5375.

Knox, P., and Wells, P., 1979, Cell adhesion and proteoglycans, *J. Cell Sci.* **40:**77–88.

Knudson, C. B., and Toole, B. P., 1985, Fluorescent morphological probe for hyaluronate, *J. Cell Biol.* **100:**1753–1758.

Kobayashi, S., Oguri, K., Kobayashi, K., and Okayama, M., 1983, Isolation and characterization of proteoheparan sulfate synthesized *in vitro* by rat glomeruli, *J. Biol. Chem.* **258:**12051–12057.

Kovacs, J., Frey, A., and Seifert, K. H., 1981, Activation of transcription complexes of RNA polymerase B by the polyanion heparin, *Biochem. Int.* **3:**645–653.

Kraemer, R. J., and Coffey, D. S., 1970, The interaction of natural and synthetic polyanions with nuclei. I. DNA synthesis, *Biochim. Biophys. Acta* **224:**553–567.

Krawczyk, W. S., 1971, A pattern of epidermal cell migration during wound healing, *J. Cell Biol.* **49:**247–263.

Krusius, T., and Rouslahti, E., 1986, Primary structure of an extracellular matrix proteoglycan core protein deduced from cloned cDNA, *Proc. Natl. Acad. Sci. USA* **83:**7683–7687.

Lane, D. A., Pejler, G., Flynn, A. M., Thompson, E. A., and Lindahl, U., 1986, Neutralization of heparin-related saccharides by histidine-rich glycoprotein and platelet factor 4, *J. Biol. Chem.* **261:**3980–3986.

Lark, M. W., and Culp, L. A., 1984, Multiple classes of heparan sulfate proteoglycans from fibroblast substratum adhesion sites, *J. Biol. Chem.* **259:**6773–6782.

Laterra, J., Ansbacher, R., and Culp, L. A., 1980, Glycosaminoglycans that bind cold-insoluble globulin in cell-substratum adhesion sites of murine fibroblasts, *Proc. Natl. Acad. Sci. USA* **77:**6662–6666.

Laterra, J., Silbert, J. E., and Culp, L. A., 1983, Cell surface heparan sulfate mediated some adhesion responses to glycosaminoglycan-binding matrices, including fibronectin, *J. Cell Biol.* **96:**112–123.

Lembach, K. J., 1976, Enhanced synthesis and extracellular accumulation of hyaluronic acid during stimulation of quiescent human fibroblasts by mouse epidermal growth factor, *J. Cell Physiol.* **89:**277–288.

Lindahl, U., and Höök, M., 1978, Glycosaminoglycans and their binding to biological macromolecules, *Annu. Rev. Biochem.* **47:**385–417.

Lindahl, U., Bäckström, G., Höök, M., Thunberg, L., Fransson, L. Å., and Linker, A., 1979, Structure of the antithrombin-binding site in heparin, *Proc. Natl. Acad. Sci. USA* **76:**3198–3202.

Lindahl, U., Thunberg, L., Bäckström, G., Riesenfeld, J., Nordling, K., and Björk, I., 1984, Extension and structural variability of the antithrombin-binding sequence in heparin, *J. Biol. Chem.* **259:**12368–12376.

Lohmander, L. S., DeLuca, S., Nilsson, B., Hascall, V. C., Caputo, C. B., Kimura, J. H., and Heinegård, D., 1980, Oligosaccharides on proteoglycans from the Swarm rat chondrosarcoma, *J. Biol. Chem.* **255:**6084–6091.

Mahley, R. W., Weisgraber, K. H., and Innerarity, T. L., 1979, Interactions of plasma lipoproteins containing apolipoproteins B and E with heparin and cell surface receptors, *Biochim. Biophys. Acta* **575:**81–91.

Majack, R. A., and Clowes, A. W., 1984, Inhibition of vascular smooth muscle cell migration by heparin-like glycosaminoglycans, *J. Cell Physiol.* **118:**253–256.

Marcum, J. A., and Rosenberg, R. D., 1984, Anticoagulantly active heparin-like molecules from vascular tissue, *Biochemistry* **23**:1730–1737.

Margolis, R. K., Crockett, C. P., Kiang, W. L., and Margolis, R. V., 1976, Glycosaminoglycans and glycoproteins associated with rat brain nuclei, *Biochim. Biophys. Acta* **451**:461–469.

Markwald, R. R., Fitzharris, T. P., Bank, H., and Bernanke, D. H., 1978, Structural analysis on the matrical organization of glycosaminoglycans in developing endocardial cushions, *Dev. Biol.* **62**:292–316.

Martin, B. M., Gimbrone, M. A., Unanue, E. R., Cotran, R. S., 1981, Stimulation of nonlymphoid mesenchymal cell proliferation by a macrophage-derived growth factor, *J. Immunol.* **126**:1510–1515.

Mathews, M. B., 1975, Connective tissues macromolecular structure and evolution, *Mol. Biol. Biochem. Biophys.* **19**:1–318.

McCarthy, J. B., and Furcht, L. T., 1984, Laminin and fibronectin promote the haptotactic migration of B16 mouse melanoma cells *in vitro*, *J. Cell Biol.* **98**:1474–1480.

Meier, S., and Hay, E. D., 1974a, Control of corneal differentiation by extracellular materials. Collagen as a promoter and stabilizer of epithelial stroma production, *Dev. Biol.* **38**:249–270.

Meier, S., and Hay, E. D., 1974b, Stimulation of extracellular matrix synthesis in the developing cornea by glycosaminoglycans, *Proc. Natl. Acad. Sci. USA* **71**:2310–2313.

Mian, N., 1986a, Analysis of cell-growth-phase-related variations in hyaluronate synthase activity of isolated plasma-membrane fractions of cultured human skin fibroblasts, *Biochem. J.* **237**:333–342.

Mian, N., 1986b, Characterization of a high-M_r plasma-membrane-bound protein and assessment of its role as a constituent of hyaluronate synthase complex, *Biochem. J.* **237**:343–357.

Mikuni-Takagaki, Y., and Toole, B. P., 1981, Hyaluronate–protein complex of Rous Sarcoma Virus transformed chick embryo fibroblasts, *J. Biol. Chem.* **256**:8463–8469.

Moscatelli, D., and Rubin, H., 1975, Increased hyaluronic acid production on stimulation of DNA synthesis in chick embryo fibroblasts, *Nature (Lond.)* **254**:65–66.

Neame, P. J., Perin, J.-P., Bonnet, F., Christner, J. E., Jollen, P., and Baker, J. R., 1985, An amino acid sequence common to both cartilage proteoglycans and link protein, *J. Biol. Chem.* **260**:12402–12404.

Neame, P. J., Christner, J. E., and Baker, J. R., 1986, The primary structure of link protein from rat chondrosarcoma proteoglycan aggregate, *J. Biol. Chem.* **261**:3519–3535.

Nishida, T., Nakagawa, S., Awata, T., Ohashi, Y., Watanabe, K., and Mauabe, R., 1983, Fibronectin promotes epithelial migration of cultured rabbit cornea in situ, *J. Cell Biol.* **97**:1653–1657.

Norling, B., Glimelius, B., and Wasteson, Å., 1981, Heparan sulfate proteoglycan of cultured cells: Demonstration of a lipid and a matrix-associated form, *Biochem. Biophys. Res. Commun.* **103**:1265–1272.

Norris, D. A., Clark, R. A. F., Swigart, L. M., Huff, J. C., Weston, W. L., and Howell, S. E., 1982, Fibronectin fragments are chemotactic for human peripheral blood monocytes, *J. Immunol.* **129**:1612–1618.

Oldberg, Å., Heldin, C.-H., Wasteson, Å., Busch, C., and Höök, M., 1980, Characterization of a platelet endoglycosidase degrading heparin-like polysaccharides, *Biochemistry* **19**:5755–5762.

Olivecrona, T., Egelrud, T., Iverius, P.-H., and Lindahl, U., 1971, Evidence for an ionic binding of lipoprotein lipase to heparin, *Biochem. Biophys. Res. Commun.* **43**:524–529.

Oohira, A., Wight, T. N., and Bornstein, P., 1983, Sulfated proteoglycans synthesized by vascular endothelial cells in culture, *J. Biol. Chem.* **258**:2014–2021.

Parthasarathy, N., and Spiro, R. G., 1984, Isolation and characterization of the heparan sulfate proteoglycan of the bovine glomerular basement membrane, *J. Biol. Chem.* **259**:12749–12755.

Paulsson, M., Fujiwara, S., Dziadek, M., Timpl, R., Pejler, G., Bäckström, G., Lindahl, U., and Engel, J., 1986, Structure and function of basement membrane proteoglycans, in: *Functions of the Proteoglycans*, Ciba Foundation Symposium 124 (D. Evered and J. Whelan, eds.), pp. 189–203, Wiley, New York.

Pierschbacher, M. D., and Ruoslahti, E., 1984, Cell attachment activity of fibronectin can be duplicated by small synthetic fragments of the molecule, *Nature (Lond.)* **309**:30–33.

Pierschbacher, M. D., Ruoslahti, E., Sundelin, J., Lind, P., and Peterson, P. A., 1982, The cell attachment domain of fibronectin. Determination of the primary structure, *J. Biol. Chem.* **267**:9593–9597.

Pinter, J. E., 1978, Distribution and synthesis of glycosaminoglycans during quail neural crest morphogenesis, *Dev. Biol.* **67**:444–464.

Poole, A. R., 1986, Proteoglycans in health and disease: Structures and functions, *Biochem. J.* **236**:1–14.

Postlethwaite, A. E., Keski-Oja, J., Bakan, G., Kang, A. H., 1981, Induction of fibroblast chemotaxis by fibronectin, *J. Exp. Med.* **153**:494–499.

Pratt, R. M., Larson, M. A., and Johnston, M. C., 1975, Migration of cranial neural crest cells in a cell-free hyaluronate-rich matrix, *Dev. Biol.* **44**:298–305.

Prehm, P., 1983a, Synthesis of hyaluronate in differentiated teratocarcinoma cells: Characterization of the synthase, *Biochem. J.* **211**:181–189.

Prehm, P., 1983b, Synthesis of hylauronate in differentiated teratocarcinoma cells: Mechanism of chain growth, *Biochem. J.* **211**:191–198.

Rapraeger, A., and Bernfield, M., 1982, An integral membrane proteoglycan is capable of binding components of the cytoskeleton and the extracellular matrix, in: *Extracellular Matrix* (S. P. Hawkes and J. L. Wang, eds.), pp. 265–269, Academic, New York.

Rapraeger, A., and Bernfield, M., 1985, Cell surface proteoglycan of mammary epithelial cells. Proteases release a heparan sulfate-rich ectodomain from a putative membrane-anchored domain, *J. Biol. Chem.* **260**:4103–4109.

Rapraeger, A., Jalkanen, M., Endo, E., Koda, J., and Bernfield, M., 1985, The cell surface proteoglycan from mouse mammary epithelial cells bears chondroitin sulfate and heparan sulfate glycosaminoglycans, *J. Biol. Chem.* **260**:11046–11052.

Rich, A. M., Pearlstein, E., Weissman, G., and Hoffstein, S. T., 1981, Cartilage proteoglycans inhibit fibronectin-mediated adhesion, *Nature (Lond.)* **293**:224–226.

Riesenfeld, J., Höök, M., and Lindahl, U., 1982, Biosynthesis of heparin. Concerted action of early polymer-modification reactions, *J. Biol. Chem.* **257**:421–424.

Risau, W., and Ekblom, P., 1986, Production of a heparin-binding angiogenesis factor by the embryonic kidney, *J. Cell Biol.* **103**:1101–1107.

Robinson, H. C., Horner, A. A., Höök, M., Ögren, S., and Lindahl, U., 1978, A proteoglycan form of heparin and its degradation to single-chain molecules, *J. Biol. Chem.* **253**:6687–6693.

Robinson, J., Viti, M., and Höök, M., 1984, Structure and properties of an under-sulfated heparan sulfate proteoglycan synthesized by a rat hepatoma cell line, *J. Cell Biol.* **98**:946–953.

Rolin, R., Albert, S. O., Gelb, N. A., and Black, D. H., 1975, Cell surface changes correlated with density-dependent growth inhibition. Glycosaminoglycan metabolism in 3T3, SV3T3 and Con A selected revertant cells, *Biochemistry* **14**:347–357.

Rosenberg, L. C., Shoi, H. U., Poole, A. R., Lewandowska, K., and Culp, L. A., 1986, Biological roles of dermatan sulfate proteoglycans, *Ciba Found. Symp.* **124**:47–68.

Ross, R., and Glomset, J. A., 1976, The pathogenesis of atherosclerosis, *N. Engl. J. Med.* **295**:369–377.

Ruoslahti, E., and Engvall, E., 1980, Complexing of fibronectin, glycosaminoglycans and collagen, *Biochim. Biophys. Acta* **631**:350–358.

Sai, S., Tanaka, T., Kosho, R. A., and Tanzer, M. L., 1986, Cloning and sequence analysis of a partial cDNA for chicken cartilage proteoglycan core protein, *Proc. Natl. Acad. Sci. USA* **83**:5081–5085.

Sakashita, S., Engvall, E., and Ruoslahti, E., 1980, Basement membrane glycoprotein laminin binds to heparin, *FEBS Lett.* **116**:243–246.

Schreiber, A. B., Kenney, J., Kowalski, J., Thomas, K. A., Gimenez-Gallego, G., Rios-Candelore, M., DiSalvo J., Barritault, D., Courty, J., Courtois, Y., Moenner, M., Loret, C., Burgess, W. H., Mehlman, T., Friesel, R., Johnson, W., and Maciag, T., 1985, A unique family of endothelial cell polypeptide mitogens: The antigenic and receptor cross-reactivity of bovine endothelial cell growth factor brain-derived acidic fibroblast growth factor, and eye-derived growth factor-II, *J. Cell Biol.* **101**:1623–1626.

Scott, J. E., and Orford, C. R., 1981, Dermatan sulfate-rich proteoglycan associated with rat tail-tendon cartilage at the d band in the gap region, Biochem. J. **197**:213–216.

Seppa, H. E. J., Yamada, K. M., Seppa, S. T., Silver, M. H., Kleinman, H. K., and Schiffman, E., 1981, The cell binding fragment of fibronectin is chemotactic for fibroblasts, Cell Biol. Int. Rep. **5**:813–819.

Shelburne, F. A., and Quarfordt, S. H., 1977, The interaction of heparin with an apoprotein of human very low density lipoprotein, J. Clin. Invest. **60**:944–950.

Shetlar, M. R., Davitt, W. F., Shellar, M. F., Posett, R. L., Cross, M. F., and Lautsch, F. V., 1978, Glycosaminoglycan changes in healing myocardial infarctions, Proc. Soc. Exp. Biol. Med. **158**:210–214.

Shing, Y., Folkman, J., Sullivan, R., Butterfield, C., Murray, J., and Klagsbrun, M., 1984, Heparin affinity: Purification of a tumor derived capillary endothelial cell growth factor, Science **223**:1269–1299.

Singer, I. I., 1979, The fibronexus: A transmembrane association of fibronectin-containing fibers and bundles of Snm microfilaments in hamster and human fibroblasts, Cell **16**:675–685.

Singer, I. I., Kawka, D. W., Kazazis, D. M., and Clark, R. A. F., 1984, In vivo co-distribution of fibronectin and actin fibers in granulation tissue: Immunofluorescence and electron micro-scope studies of the fibronexus at the myofibroblast surface, J. Cell Biol. **98**:2091–2096.

Solursh, M., Mitchell, S. L., and Katow, H., 1986, Inhibition of cell migration in sea urchin embryos by β-D-xyloside, Dev. Biol. **118**:325–332.

Solursh, M., and Morriss, G. M., 1977, Glycosaminoglycan synthesis in rat embryos during the formation of the primary mesenchyme and neural folds, Dev. Biol. **57**:75–86.

Solursh, M., Vaerewyck, S. A., and Reiter, R. S., 1974, Depression by hyaluronic acid of glycos-aminoglycan synthesis by cultured chick embryo chondrocytes, Dev. Biol. **41**:233–244.

Sommarin, Y., and Heinegård, D., 1983, Specific interaction between cartilage proteoglycans and hyaluronic acid at the chondrocyte cell surface, Biochem. J. **214**:777–784.

Stein, G. S., Roberts, R. M., Davis, J. L., Head, W. J., Stein, J. L., Thrall, C. L., van Veen, J., and Welch, D. W., 1975, Are glycoproteins and glycosaminoglycans components of the eukaryotic genome?, Nature (Lond.) **258**:639–641.

Stevens, R. L., 1986, Secretory granule proteoglycans of mast cells on natural killer cells, in: Functions of the Proteoglycans, Ciba Foundation Symposium 125 (D. Evered and J. Whelan, eds.), pp. 272–285, Wiley, New York.

Stoolmiller, A. C., and Dorfman, A., 1969, The biosynthesis of hyaluronic acid by Streptococcus, J. Biol. Chem. **244**:236–246.

Sugahara, K., Schwartz, N., and Dorfman, A., 1979, Biosynthesis of hyaluronic acid by Streptococ-cus, J. Biol. Chem. **254**:6252–6261.

Suzuki, S., Pierschbacher, M. D., Hayman, E. G., Nguyen, K., Öhgren, Y., and Ruoslahti, E., 1984, Domain structure of vitronectin, J. Biol. Chem. **259**:15307–15314.

Takashima, A., and Grinnell, F., 1985, Fibronectin-mediated keratinocyte migration and initiation of fibronectin receptor function in vitro, J. Invest. Dermatol. **85**:304–308.

Taylor, S., and Folkman, J., 1982, Protamine is an inhibitor of angiogenesis, Nature (Lond.) **297**:307–312.

Thiery, J. P., Duband, J. L., and Tucker, G. C., 1985, Cell migration in the vertebrate embryo: Role of cell adhesion and tissue environment in pattern formation, Annu. Rev. Cell Biol. **1**:91–113.

Thornton, S. C., Mueller, S. N., and Levine, E. M., 1983, Human endothelial cells: Use of heparin in cloning and long-term serial cultivation, Science **222**:623–625.

Thunberg, L., Backstrom, G., and Lindahl, U., 1982, Further characterization of the antithrombin binding sequence in heparin, Carbohydrate Res. **100**:393–410.

Timpl, R., Fujiwara, S., Dziadek, M., Aumailley, M., Weber, S., and Engel, J., 1984, Laminin, proteoglycan, nidogen and collagen. IV. Structural models and molecular interactions, Ciba Found. Symp. **108**:25–43.

Tomida, M., Koyama, H., and Ono, T., 1974, Hyaluronic acid synthetase in cultured mammalian cells producing hyaluronic acid. Oscillatory change during the growth phase and suppression by 5-bromodeoxyuridine, Biochim. Biophys. Acta **338**:352–363.

Toole, B. P., 1981, Glycosaminoglycans in morphogenesis, in: *Cell Biology of Extracellular Matrix* (E. D. Hay, ed.), Academic Press, New York, pp. 259–294.

Toole, B. P., and Gross, J., 1971, The extracellular matrix of the regenerating newt limb: Synthesis and removal of hyaluronate prior to differentiation, *Dev. Biol.* **25**:57–77.

Toole, B. P., and Trelstad, R. L., 1971, Hyaluronate production and removal during corneal development in the chick, *Dev. Biol.* **26**:28–35.

Treadwell, B. V., Mankin, D. P., Ho, P. K., and Mankin, H. J., 1980, Cell-free synthesis of cartilage proteins: Partial identification of proteoglycan core and link proteins, *Biochem.* **19**:2269–2275.

Triscott, M. X., and van de Rijn, I., 1986, Solubilization of hyaluronic acid synthetic activity from streptococci and its activation with phospholipids, *J. Biol. Chem.* **261**:6004–6009.

Turley, E. A., 1982, Purification of a hyaluronate-binding protein fraction that modifies cell social behavior, *Biochem. Biophys. Res. Commun.* **108**:1016–1024.

Turner, D. C., Lawton, J., Dollenmeier, P., Ehrismann, R., and Chiquet, M., 1983, Guidance of myogenic cell migration by oriented deposits of fibronectin, *Dev. Biol.* **95**:497–504.

Underhill, C. B., and Toole, B. P., 1979, Binding of hyaluronate to the surface of cultured cells, *J. Cell Biol.* **82**:475–484.

Underhill, C. B., and Toole, B. P., 1980, Physical characteristics of hyaluronate binding to the surface of Simian virus 40-transformed 3T3 cells, *J. Biol. Chem.* **255**:4544–4549.

Underhill, C. B., Chi-Rosso, G., and Toole, B. P., 1983, Effects of detergent solubilization on the hyaluronate-binding protein from membranes of Simian virus 40-transformed 3T3 cells, *J. Biol. Chem.* **258**:8056–8091.

Upholt, W. B., Vertel, B. M., and Dorfman, A., 1979, Translation and characterization of messenger RNAs in differentiating chicken cartilage, *Proc. Natl. Acad. Sci. USA* **76**:4847–4851.

van de Rijn, I., 1983, Streptococcal hyaluronic acid: Proposed mechanisms of degradation and loss of synthesis during stationary phase, *J. Bacteriol.* **156**:1059–1065.

Venge, P., Håkansson, L., and Hallgren, R., 1982, The effect of hyaluronic acid on neutrophil function *in vitro* and *in vivo*, *Adv. Exp. Med. Biol.* **141**:559–565.

Weisgraber, K. H., Rall, S. C., Mahley, R. W., Milne, R. W., Marcely, Y. L., and Sparrow, J. T., 1986, Human apolipoprotein E: Determination of the heparin binding sites of apolipoprotein E3, *J. Biol. Chem.* **261**:2068–2076.

Wiebkin, O. W., and Muir, H., 1973, The inhibition of sulfate incorporation in isolated adult chondrocytes by hyaluronic acid, *FEBS Lett.* **37**:42–46.

Woods, A., Höök, M., Kjellén, L., Smith, C. G., and Rees, D. A., 1984, Relationship of heparan sulfate proteoglycans to the cytoskeleton and extracellular matrix of cultured fibroblasts, *J. Cell Biol.* **99**:1743–1753.

Woods, A., Couchman, J. R., and Höök, M., 1985, Heparan sulfate proteoglycans of rat embryo fibroblasts, *J. Biol. Chem.* **260**:10872–10879.

Woods, A., Couchman, J. R., Johansson, S., and Höök, M., 1986, Adhesion and cytoskeletal organization of fibroblasts in response to fibronectin fragments, *EMBO J.* **5**:665–670.

Yamagata, M., Yamada, K. M., Yaneda, M., Suzuki, S., and Kimata, K., 1986, Chondroitin sulfate proteoglycan (PG-M-like proteoglycan) is involved in the binding of hyaluronic acid to cellular fibronectin, *J. Biol. Chem.* **261**:13526–13535.

Yurt, R. W., Leid, R. W., Austen, K. F., and Silbert, J. E., 1977, Native heparin from rat peritoneal mast cells, *J. Biol. Chem.* **252**:518–521.

Chapter 20

Collagen in Dermal Wound Repair

JOHN M. MCPHERSON and KARL A. PIEZ

1. Introduction

This chapter focuses on collagen, one of the many extracellular matrix mac-romolecules involved in tissue repair. Some of the known interrelationships between collagen and the other biologically active extracellular matrix mac-romolecules and the cells that populate and metabolize it are discussed.

Collagen is a generic term encompassing at least 11 types of molecules, many with two or more subtypes. These are listed in Table I along with some of their properties. All consist largely of the unique collagen triple helix, and in most cases they perform a structural function in aggregate form. More detailed information about the collagen types can be found in recent reviews (Bornstein and Sage, 1980; Miller, 1984; Martin et al., 1985) (see Chapter 22).

Only a few of the collagen types are discussed—I, III, and IV—since the role of these three collagens in wound repair is best defined. Type I collagen is the major structural component of skin, tendon, bone, and many minor struc-tures. Type III collagen is also present in skin in association with type I, al-though that association is not fully understood. How type III collagen fibrils differ in function from type I collagen, and the extent that they do, is unknown. The ratio of I to III varies, a subject to which we return. Type III is usually considered to be in the thin reticular fibrils and type I in the larger fibrils (Martin et al., 1985), but the evidence for this is incomplete. They are similar molecules, and there is some evidence that they may coexist in single fibrils (Henkel and Glanville, 1982).

Type IV collagen, together with other components, including a unique heparan sulfate proteoglycan and the glycoprotein laminin, makes up both the epidermal and endothelial basement membranes. Basement membranes often need to be repaired and replaced in the course of dermal wound healing, as will be discussed later. Type VII collagen deserves mention, as it may form a struc-ture called anchoring fibrils that attach the basement membrane to underlying connective tissue (Bentz et al., 1983), but nothing is known about its role or fate in wound healing. Type V collagen, in fibrillar form, may play a similar role

JOHN M. MCPHERSON and KARL A. PIEZ • Connective Tissue Research Laboratories, Collagen Corporation, Palo Alto, California 94303.

Table I. Collagen Types

Type	Kinds of chains[a]	M_r[b]	Helix length (nm)	Aggregate form	Localization
I	2	300,000	300	67-nm banded fibril	Dermis, tendon, bone
II	1	300,000	300	67-nm banded fibril	Cartilage
III	1	300,000	300	67-nm banded fibril	Dermis
IV	2	550,000	390 (interrupted)	Mat; end interactions	Basement membrane
V	3	400,000	300	Fibril	Dermis
VI	3	550,000	105	100-nm banded fibril	Dermis
VII	1	500,000	450	SLS-like dimer	Anchoring fibrils
VIII	1	500,000	3 × 150 (linked)		
IX	3	210,000	175 (interrupted)		Cartilage
X	1	190,000	140		Cartilage
α1 α2 α3	3	300,000	300		Cartilage

[a]Homo- and heterotrimers may exist, depending on collagen type.
[b]Native trimer.

(Modesti *et al.*, 1984). Types VI and possibly VIII collagen are also present in skin, but their functions are unknown. As more is learned about their functions, a role in wound repair may become manifest. For example, the absence of the minor collagens, or their incorrect utilization, could be a major difference between the highly organized dermis and the fibrotic scar. The other collagen types (II, IX, and X and α1, α2, and α3) are apparently restricted to cartilage.

Types I and III collagen molecules are partially flexible rods about 300 nm in length and 1.5 nm in diameter. Each molecule consists of three polypeptide chains. These chains form an unbroken triple helix except for short nonhelical regions (about 6–26-amino acid residues) at both ends. Molecules associate in staggered array to make the characteristic banded fibrils seen in electron micrographs. The diameters of the fibrils vary from a few tens to a few hundreds of nanometers. Type IV collagen is quite different. It is highly glycosylated (peptidyl glucosylgalactosyl hydroxylysine), has a 400-nm-long helix that is interrupted by several short nonhelical regions, and contains a globular knob at its carboxyl-terminal end. It apparently aggregates at its ends to form a matlike structure associated in an unknown way with other components in the membrane (Timpl *et al.*, 1981). There is considerable structure and organization in the basement membrane that is only evident in electron micrographs of specialized basement membranes such as Reichert's membrane (Farquhar, 1981; Inoue *et al.*, 1983).

It is useful for purposes of discussion to divide the function of collagen in wound repair into four separate categories, which include (1) inflammation; 2) neomatrix formation (synthesis, deposition, and remodeling); (3) wound contraction; and (4) re-epithelialization (Peacock, 1973; Carrico *et al.*, 1984). These processes are not distinct in time but rather overlap during the course of repair;

pre-existing or newly synthesized collagen plays an important role in each of them.

The next section of this chapter illustrates the key role that collagen plays in these four general phases of wound repair. Subsequent sections focus on collagen metabolism during both normal and abnormal wound healing, including naturally occurring factors that regulate collagen synthesis, as well as pharmacologic agents, which have been used in an attempt to control abnormal collagen production. The final section of the chapter is devoted to a discussion of the potential utility of collagen-based biomaterials in various wound-repair applications.

2. Collagen in the Sequence of Events of Wound Repair

2.1. Inflammation

The inflammatory phase of dermal wound repair is initiated almost immediately following tissue injury by either activation of tissue complement or, in the case of associated vascular injury, activation of the coagulation cascade. Activation of both of these pathways leads to the recruitment of inflammatory cells into the area via the generation of C5a or the release of platelet factor 4, fibrin-degradation fragments and perhaps other unidentified factors following platelet aggregation (for review, see Grotendorst et al., 1984). These molecules are chemotactic agents in vitro for specific cell types and may play a critical role in the early events of wound healing. Fibrillar collagens (types I and III) play a pivotal role in the initial stages of wound healing since they are believed to be a key element involved in the promotion of platelet aggregation following vascular injury (for review, see Shoshan, 1981). The binding of platelets to fibrillar collagen in the surrounding connective tissue results in the release of several large glycoproteins such as fibronectin and thrombospondin, the latter of which has been implicated in the subsequent aggregation of platelets to one another (Jaffe et al., 1982). This collagen-induced aggregation of platelets, along with other events in the coagulation cascade, results in the formation of a physical plug that provides hemostasis following vascular injury. Platelet aggregation results in the release of the aforesaid factors, which are chemotactic for inflammatory cells, as well as factors such as platelet-derived growth factor (PDGF) and fibronectin, which have been shown to be chemotactic for fibroblasts and smooth muscle cells (Gauss-Muller et al., 1980; Grotendorst et al., 1981; 1982; Seppa et al., 1982). Other reports in the literature suggest that collagen fragments, which may be generated by collagenases released by granulocytes and macrophages (Woolley, 1984), are chemotactic for fibroblasts (Postlethwaite et al., 1978). Whether this activity is functional in vivo is unknown. PDGF has been shown to be a potent mitogen for fibroblasts (Rutherford and Ross, 1976; Heldin et al., 1981; Bowen-Pope et al., 1982) and thus may serve to mediate repair by promoting connective tissue cell proliferation in wounded areas. Other factors, such as transforming growth factor-β (TGF-β), released by platelets in response to vascular injury, have also been implicated in acceleration of the wound healing response (Sporn et al., 1983). The precise role of these and other platelet-derived factors in the wound healing process is the subject of Chapters 9–12. However, it is clear that fibrillar collagen plays a crucial role in the very earliest stages of wound healing by participating in the early events associated with hemostasis and possibly, as fragments, in the recruitment of connective tissue cells.

2.2. Neomatrix Formation

The migration of fibroblasts into the wounded area and rapid vascularization signal the initiation of another phase in the wound-healing process: synthesis and deposition of collagenous and noncollagenous extracellular matrix proteins in the wound bed. This process of fibroblast invasion and the deposition of a collagen-based extracellular matrix has been termed fibroplasia. If neovascularization also occurs, the process is called granulation tissue formation. This phase is generally considered to begin 3–5 days after wounding and persist for 10–12 days, during which time there is rapid synthesis of type I and III collagen and an associated increase in the tensile strength of the wound (Ross and Benditt, 1986; Madden and Peacock, 1968; Heughan and Hunt, 1975). Cohen et al. (1979) suggested that in rat dermal wounds significant collagen synthesis begins within 24 hr of wounding and is localized in the area of the panniculus carnosis, the muscle layer underlying the dermis. However, inflammation predominates during this period. Remodeling and crosslinking of the collagen follow fibroplasia, continue up to 2 years, and result in generation of fibrillar collagen bundles or fibers. These fibers become oriented according to lines of stress and provide a slow increase in the tensile strength of the healing wound (Heughan and Hunt, 1975). This remodeling phase in the human ultimately results in the formation of a fibrous connective tissue commonly called a scar. The wide degree of variability observed in scar quality will be discussed in detail in Section 4.

2.3. Contraction

The role of type I and III collagen in the contraction process of wound healing remains to be completely elucidated (for review, see Ehrlich, 1984). Current evidence suggests that the surrounding extracellular matrix, not involved in the healing process, as well as the connective tissue deposited in the wound bed play an important role in the contractile process. These matrices provide the anchoring points and connecting cables to which contractile cells, called myofibroblasts (Majno et al., 1971), bind and attempt to reduce the wound volume through an active contraction process (Gabbiani et al., 1972) (see Chapter 17). Several investigators have shown that contraction can be modeled in vitro by placing fibroblasts on or in collagen gels (Bell et al., 1979; Steinberg et al., 1980; Grinnell and Lamke, 1984). At collagen concentrations ranging from 0.5 to 8 mg/ml, these cells can contract the collagen lattices to a fraction of their original volume (Fig. 1). Lattice contraction in these experiments is a function of cell number as well as collagen concentration. It has been proposed that this cellular activity corresponds to the contraction process, which occurs following tissue damage. Using this in vitro experimental approach, it should be possible to identify factors that influence the rate and extent of contraction during wound repair. Although contraction may be desirable in that it presumably reduces healing time, it may not be necessary and it may negatively influence scar quality.

It is important to point out that wound contraction is different from scar contracture. Wound contraction is a relatively early event in the wound healing process which, as stated above, involves an interaction between myofibroblasts and the extracellular matrix, whereas scar contracture is a later event associated primarily with scar remodeling. A primary force in scar contracture may be provided by the underlying musculature and this, in conjunction with reorganization of the collagen matrix, has been proposed as responsible for the distortion of the tissue that may occur in large wounds (Peacock, 1978). This process, at best, is cosmetically unattractive and at worst renders the tissues nonfunctional.

2.4. Re-epithelialization

The type I and III collagenous matrix of early granulation tissue synthesized by fibroblasts in the wound, in conjunction with noncollagenous proteins such as fibronectin and fibrin, provides support for epidermal cell migration and proliferation (hyperplasia) (Clark et al., 1982; Woodley et al., 1985) (Fig. 2). Exposure of a granulating wound to air results in the formation of a scab (eschar) which is composed primarily of dead cells and dehydrated serum and fibrin, which attaches itself to the underlying granulation tissue (Carpenter et al., 1977). Epithelial cells burrow between the eschar and granulation tissue by expressing collagenase and other hydrolases dissolving the collagenous matrix in front of them as they move (Harris and Krane, 1974). Once wound closure is affected the scab is sloughed off. During wound closure the provisional matrix provided by the early granulation tissue and serum-derived components is quite different from the basement membrane, containing type IV collagen, on which these cells normally reside. This results in quite different cellular behavior characterized by lateral cell movement onto the wound bed and cell proliferation rather than the vertical movement and terminal differentiation characteristic of epithelial cells, when they rest on an intact basement membrane (Woodley et al., 1985). Once cell closure of the epidermis is complete, a basement membrane is rapidly synthesized. This signals the end of rapid fibroplasia and the beginning of remodeling and maturation of the wound.

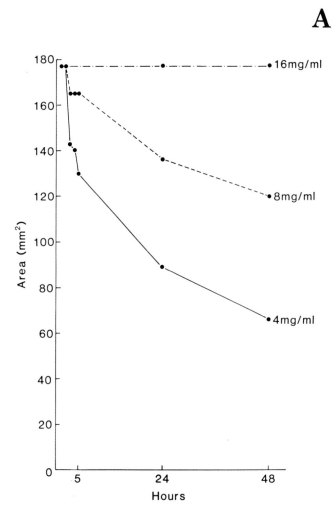

Figure 1. Contraction of fibrillar collagen matrices *in vitro*. (a) Influence of collagen concentration on gel contraction. Pepsin-solubilized, bovine dermal collagen was purified and reconstituted into fibrillar forms at collagen concentrations ranging from 4 to 16 mg/ml (McPherson *et al.*, 1985). Low passage human foreskin fibroblasts (5×10^5 cells) were mixed with 0.5 ml of each of the different fibrillar collagen suspensions, placed in a 24-well tissue culture plate and incubated at 37°C. Surface area measurements were made at various times. (b) Influence of cell number on gel contraction. Low passage human foreskin fibroblasts (5×10^4–1×10^6) were added as described above to fibrillar collagen whose final concentration was 8 mg/ml. Surface area measurements were made at various times. (Data courtesy of Richard Clark, M.D., National Jewish Center, Denver.)

B

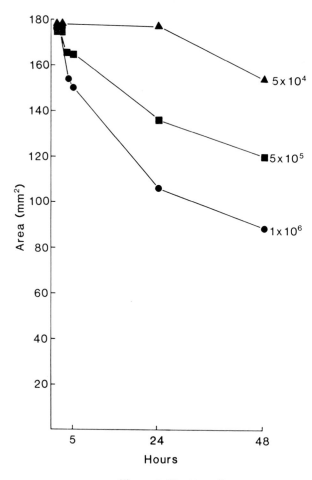

Figure 1. (*Continued*)

Vascularization, like epithelialization, involves cell migration, cell division, and basement membrane formation (see Chapter 15).

3. Collagen Synthesis and Deposition in Normal Wound Repair

3.1. Collagen Types Deposited

The primary collagen types deposited in the wound bed during fibroplasia and associated granulation tissue deposition are interstitial type I and III collagen. Normal mammalian skin contains approximately 80–90% type I col-

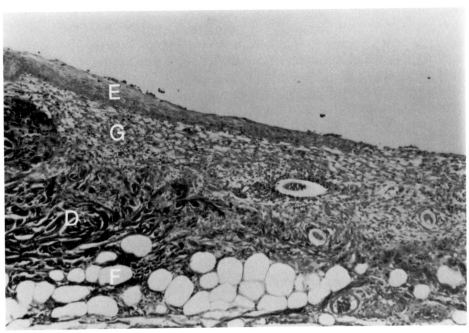

Figure 2. Epidermal cell migration over granulation tissue. Six millimeter partial thickness punch biopsies were made on the shaved backs of guinea pigs to the level of the panniculus carnosis. Wounds were covered with Opsite dressing (Smith and Nephew Inc., Columbia, South Carolina 29205) which was held in place with Elasticon tape (Johnson and Johnson, New Brunswick, New Jersey). Wound sites were surgically removed at 5 days, fixed in formalin embedded in paraffin, sectioned, and treated with Gamori's trichromestain. Components of the skin are identified as follows: E, epidermis; D, dermis; G, granulation tissue; F, fat cells. (Photo courtesy of Philip Ledger, Ph.D., Collagen Corporation, Palo Alto, California.)

lagen and 10–20% type III collagen (Epstein, 1974; Miller, 1976). Bailey and co-workers (1975) reported that during the dermal wound-healing process in rats, the granulation tissue contains significantly higher levels of type III collagen than normally observed in the skin. During the course of the wound-healing process the relative ratio of type III to type I collagen synthesis may change. The work of subsequent investigators has provided evidence that this is indeed the case. Using open skin wounds in the rat as a model, Clore and co-workers (1979) investigated relative rates of collagen synthesis during the wound healing process. Samples were explanted from the wound at various times, placed in tissue culture media containing [³H]proline, and incubated for 2 hrs at 37°C. Following the metabolic labeling period, collagens were isolated by pepsin solubilization and the relative amounts of type I and III determined by molecular sieve chromatography. The results of these experiments suggested that increased type III collagen synthesis (approximately 30% of the total) occurred within the first 10 hr after wounding. However, by 24 hr normal type III collagen levels had returned (approximately 20% of the total). By implanting Cellastic sponges in the wounds of children following surgery and measuring collagen deposition by immunochemical techniques, other investigators demonstrated increased amounts of type III collagen during the first 3–4 days of wound healing, after which time a rapid increase in the amount of type I collagen was noted (Gay et al., 1978). Although the data of these two groups appear to be in some disagreement quantitatively, this may be attributable to differences in experimental design. The elevated rate of type III collagen synthesis at early stages in wound healing is similar to the situation reported for the skin of a developing embryo which has a higher ratio of type III to I collagen than the adult (Epstein, 1974). These data suggest that during the tissue-repair process a key population of cells in the vicinity of the wound follow a program reminiscent of that observed during early development. This behavior is transient, and the physiologic processes that control this type of behavior are not understood.

The relative amount of other collagen types that participate in the wound-healing process are low compared with type I and III collagen. Particularly important in the process of dermal wound healing is type IV collagen synthesis by epidermal cells and the regeneration of the basement membrane. Current evidence suggests that during wound closure epidermal cells migrate on top of a provisional matrix of fibrin/fibrinogen, fibronectin, type I and III collagen, as well as proteoglycans. The synthesis of type V collagen by epidermal cells during this migratory phase has also been reported (Stenn et al., 1979). The production of type IV collagen and regeneration of the basement membrane, including associated glycoproteins such as laminin, is delayed until the wound is covered and the epidermal cells are no longer in a migratory phase.

3.2. Regulation of Collagen Production

The factors regulating collagen production during wound healing can be divided into those that participate in the early, intermediate, and later stages of the process. In the early inflammatory stage of wound repair, platelet factors released during clotting may play a key role in regulating collagen synthesis. One such factor is PDGF (Knighton et al., 1982). This factor could promote collagen synthesis by recruiting connective tissue cells into the wound via its chemotactic activity (Seppa, 1982) and causing them to proliferate via its mitogenic activity (Rutherford and Ross, 1976). Recent work reported by Grotendorst et al. (1985) provides evidence that PDGF can enhance the rate of connective tissue deposition in normal rats and rats whose wound-healing response has been comprised by drug treatment. These investigators treated rats with streptozotocin, a drug that induces diabetes, and subsequently implanted Hunt-Schilling wound chamoers subcutaneously in the experimental animals. The drug-treated animals exhibited a low level of collagen deposition within the chambers that could be significantly enhanced by addition of low levels (50 ng/ml) of PDGF. PDGF in combination with insulin showed a slightly greater effect. PDGF, and PDGF in combination with insulin, also enhanced new collagen synthesis in nontreated control animals. It was concluded that the potent chemotactic and mitogenic activity of PDGF was most likely responsible for its ability to enhance collagen synthesis in this wound model by promoting fibroblast invasion and proliferation in the wound chamber (see also Chapter 9).

Another platelet factor, TGF-β, has been reported to enhance the rate of connective tissue deposition in the rat subcutaneous model (Sporn et al., 1983; Lawrence et al., 1986). Lawrence et al. used Adriamycin to impair wound healing in a rat subcutaneous model similar to that described above. This antineoplastic drug reportedly decreases platelets and white blood cells (Lawrence et al., 1986). These investigators showed that addition of TGF-β (100 ng/ml) to the Hunt-Schilling chambers largely reversed the decreased level of collagen synthesis observed in the drug treated animals. The combination of TGF-β, PDGF, and epidermal growth factor (EGF) showed an even greater effect and restored collagen synthesis to 86% of that observed in control animals. Interestingly, these investigators did not observe an effect of PDGF alone on the wound-healing response in this model.

The increase in new collagen synthesis mediated by TGF-β was not associated with an increase in cell proliferation, suggesting that TGF-β enhances new collagen synthesis by increased collagen production per cell. Support for this hypothesis is provided by recent in vitro experiments that show that addition of very low levels of TGF-β to fibroblasts in culture can significantly increase the rate of new collagen synthesis per cell (Ignotz and Massague, 1986; Roberts et al., 1986) (see also Chapter 12).

It is important to emphasize that the ability to demonstrate a positive effect of growth factors on the wound healing response in animals is not only dependent on the factors chosen but also on the experimental animal models used. Using full-thickness skin wounds in the Syrian hamster Leitzel et al. (1985) were unable to show positive effects of a number of topically applied growth factors, including PDGF, EGF, and fibroblast growth factor (FGF), on the wound-healing response. This may have been due to problems in factor dosage and delivery, or perhaps such factors were not limiting in the wound sites. Alternatively, it is possible that in the more complex full-thickness wounds, where epidermal regeneration as well as granulation tissue deposition is required, a specific combination of factors acting in a concerted fashion will be required to enhance the wound healing response.

Large-scale proliferative response of fibroblasts and associated deposition of connective tissue in the wound bed does not begin until the acute inflammatory phase begins to subside at 3–5 days, when platelets and their factors are presumably gone. The increase in net synthesis of connective tissue is presumably the result not only of more cells but of greater activity per cell. Liebovich and Ross (1975) demonstrated that the initiation of fibroplasia and concomitant deposition of collagen, during the intermediate stages of wound healing, is closely tied to the presence of macrophages. These investigators injected guinea pigs with hydrocortisone systemically to promote monocytopenia and antimacrophage serum in the vicinity of the wound bed, which resulted in the disappearance of macrophages from the wounds. The result was a significant delay in debridement and reduced fibroplasia in surgically induced wounds. Subsequent experiments (Liebovich and Ross, 1976) showed that macrophages, which were cultured *in vitro*, produced and released into the media a factor that caused fibroblast proliferation *in vitro*. This observation has been confirmed in several different laboratories (for review, see Liebovich, 1984). The factor was designated macrophage-derived growth factor (MDGF) (Martin *et al.*, 1981). Recent data provide evidence that MDGF is not a single protein entity but is rather an activity provided by PDGF-like (Shimokado *et al.*, 1985) and FGF-like (Baird *et al.*, 1985) proteins that are synthesized and secreted by macrophages. These factors promote collagen synthesis by increasing the number of connective tissue cells in the wound site.

Several other lines of evidence implicate the macrophage in the control of collagen deposition in wounds. These include studies in which the addition of macrophages to wounds increased collagen synthesis and wound strength (Casey *et al.*, 1976) as well as studies in which injection of macrophages into the corneas of rabbits promoted angiogenesis, fibroplasia, and new collagen synthesis (Clark *et al.*, 1976; Hunt *et al.*, 1984a). Until recently, little information was available regarding whether macrophages produce factors that modulate the amount of collagen produced by a single cell. Limited data from the study of fibroblasts *in vitro* suggested that this was not the case (Diegelmann and Cohen, 1979). However, new studies indicate that macrophages synthesize and secrete a TGF-β-like protein (Assoian *et al.*, 1987), which can increase the rate of collagen synthesis by fibroblasts (Ignotz and Massague, 1986; Roberts *et al.*, 1986).

Thus, it now appears that macrophages play an important role in fibroplasia and associated collagen deposition during the intermediate stages of wound healing by secreting a host of factors that enhance fibroblast proliferation. They promote these cells to synthesize and secrete extracellular matrix proteins (see Chapter 8).

In addition to the requirements for chemoattractants and mitogens to promote new collagen synthesis, some investigators have hypothesized that reduced oxygen tension in the wound, due to the high metabolic activity of cells in the wound bed, also plays an important role in the wound healing process (Hunt *et al.*, 1984b). These investigators suggest that reduced oxygen tension results in local hypoxia and lactate production, which in turn promotes new collagen synthesis (Hunt *et al.*, 1978; Green and Goldberg, 1964; Langness and Udenfriend, 1973; Levene and Bates, 1976). The hypothesis that low oxygen tension promotes wound repair is complicated by the fact that re-epithelialization of the wound is negatively affected by reduced oxygen and positively influenced by increased oxygen levels (Winter, 1978; Silver, 1972). However, Alvarez *et al.* (1983) found no correlation between the oxygen permeability of various wound dressings and the rate of re-epithelialization of these wounds or new collagen synthesis within these wounds. These workers suggested that the blood provides ample oxygen to these wounds. Thus, while there is circumstantial evidence that oxygen tension may play a role in the regulation of new collagen synthesis in wounds, the mechanisms by which this effect may be mediated remains to be determined.

Another regulatory event of collagen production in the healing wound, particularly at the later stages of the process, is the catabolism of newly synthe-

Table II. Potential Points of Regulation in Type I
Collagen Production

Transcriptional control
  mRNA synthesis
  Processing of primary RNA transcript
Translational control
  Feedback regulation by amino-terminal extension peptides
Post-translational control
  Peptidyl hydroxylation
  Peptidyl glycosylation
  Disulfide bond formation and triple-helix formation
Intracellular translocation and secretion
Extracellular processing
  Conversion of procollagen to collagen
  Molecular assembly (fibril formation)
  Oxidative denomination
  Crosslinking

sized collagen. The rate of collagen degradation changes as wound healing proceeds, starting out at a relatively slow rate during the early stages of the process and increasing as wound maturation occurs (Zeitz et al., 1978). Collagenase, which is synthesized by granulocytes and macrophages, as well as fibroblasts and epithelial cells, is a primary mediator of collagen turnover. This protease is secreted as a zymogen that can be activated by certain other proteases such as plasmin (Werb et al., 1977). This activation of the collagenase, as well as inhibition of its enzymatic activity by protease inhibitors such as α_2-macroglobulin, have been proposed to play critical roles in the regulation of expression of collagenolytic activity in vivo (Werb et al., 1974, 1977; Diegelmann et al., 1981). There are probably many other ways in which collagenase activity is regulated during the course of wound healing and beyond but, like so many other aspects of collagen metabolism, these mechanisms are just beginning to be understood (Woolley, 1984).

In addition to the elements for control of collagen synthesis during wound healing that have been briefly described here, there exist transcriptional, translational, and post-translational control mechanisms, which operate during normal collagen metabolism in connective tissues (for review, see Bornstein et al., 1984). Table II summarizes the potential control points for regulation of collagen synthesis.

4. Collagen Synthesis and Deposition in Abnormal Wound Repair

4.1. Definition of Scarring

Deep wounds that penetrate the dermis into the subcutaneous tissue elicit a cascade of events, including inflammation and a fibroproliferative response that results in the deposition of collagen, noncollagenous proteins, and proteoglycans. Scar tissue is the end product of this cascade of events. The proportions of the various components and their organization in scar tissue differ from normal dermis. The differences in connective tissue organization can be easily observed at the light microscopic level. Histologic analysis illustrates that the collagenous matrix of the dermal scar is arranged into thick bundles that are parallel to the epidermis, whereas normal dermis lacks this type of organization (Fig. 3).

The quality of the scar is directly related to the efficiency of the regulation of collagen production during wound healing and, specifically, the balance between new collagen synthesis and collagen degradation during the later stages of the process. It is important to realize that even under optimal conditions the scar is an imperfect substitute for the original tissue, since it has a lower breaking strength, serves as a diffusional barrier to nutrients and oxygen and often results in deformation and reduction of function of the original tissue (Shosan, 1981; Chvapil and Koopmann, 1984). Its advantage apparently is the rapidity by which the structural integrity of the total organism can be re-established.

4.2. Keloid and Hypertrophic Scars

When the equilibrium between collagen synthesis and collagen degradation is not in proper balance, collagen overproduction occurs. In extreme cases, this results in the formation of hypertrophic or keloid scars (Fig. 4). The biologic differences between hypertrophic and keloid scars have not been completely established. They have traditionally been classified on a semiquantitative basis. Exuberant collagen production within the boundaries of the original wound is classified as a hypertrophic scar whereas excessive collagen production beyond the border of the original wound is classified as a keloid scar (Peacock et al., 1970).

4.2.1. Characteristics

Knapp and co-workers (1977) characterized keloid and hypertrophic scars with regard to the ultrastructure of their fibrillar collagen, cell types that inhabited the respective tissues, and the biochemical characteristics of their collagen. Collagen fibers and fiber bundles displayed an inverse correlation between degree of organization and scar abnormality. The collagen in normal skin and mature scar was highly crosslinked, whereas the collagen in hypertrophic and keloid scars demonstrated progressively lower levels of crosslinking. Three morphologically different fibroblastic-like cells were observed in primary cultures of normal mature scars, as well as hypertrophic and keloid scars. These three types seemed to vary in relative amounts among the different scars. These workers concluded that hypertrophic and keloid scars are not distinct pathologic entities but rather represent progressively more aberrant activity in the continuum of the wound healing process.

Other investigators (Kischer et al., 1982) reported that the collagen in

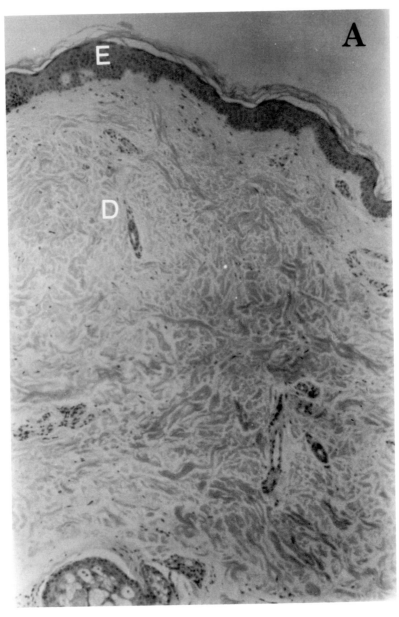

Figure 3. A comparison of normal and scarred human dermis. Normal (A) and scarred tissue (B) were harvested by punch biopsy and fixed in formalin. Samples were imbedded in parafin, sectioned and treated with Gamori's trichrome stain. Components of the skin are identified as follows: E, epidermis; D, dermis. (Photo courtesy of Rosa Armstrong, Ph.D., Collagen Corporation, Palo Alto, California.)

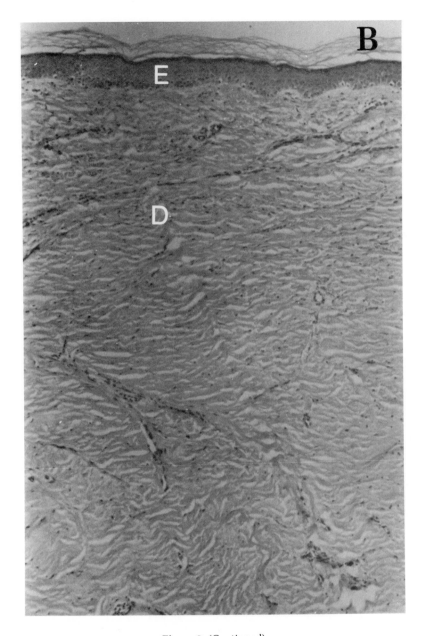

Figure 3. (Continued)

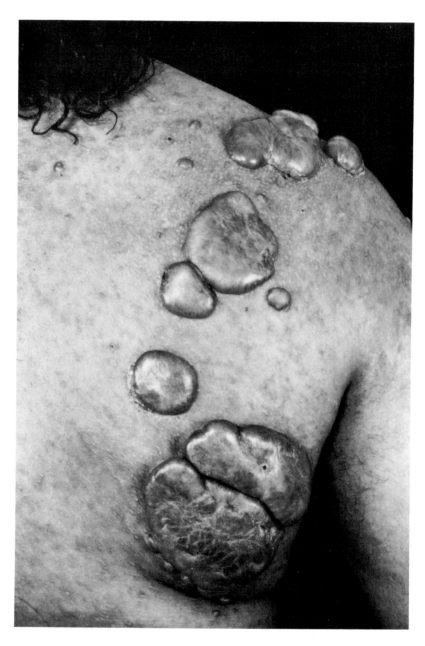

Figure 4. Example of severe keloid scarring on the back of a young black male. (Photo courtesy of David Apfelberg, M.D., Palo Alto Medical Clinic, Palo Alto, California.)

hypertrophic and keloid scars is not less organized than in mature scars or skin, but simply has a different organization with unique structures. These structures, called nodules by Knapp's group, were described as three-dimensional cigar-shaped collagenous bundles that run parallel to the skin surface and tend to flatten as the scar matures.

The fibrillar architecture of the hypertrophic scar, when examined with the electron microscope, also has appeared distinct. Electron-dense links were seen between the collagen bundles within a hypertrophic scar (Kischer, 1974; Kischer and Shetlar, 1974). In addition, the fibrillar bundles were smaller in hypertrophic scars than in mature scar or normal dermis (Kischer et al., 1982). It is clear from the work of these and other investigators that collagen organization in hypertrophic and keloid scars is structurally different from that observed in mature scars and normal skin. The interpretation of these differences is a function of the methods used to analyze them as well as the stage of scar development.

Biochemical analyses of hypertrophic and keloid scars suggest that they have elevated levels of type III collagen relative to mature scar or normal dermis (Bailey et al., 1975a; Chaig et al., 1975). The elevated type III collagen levels observed in these scars is reminiscent of what is observed during rapid granulation tissue deposition. Perhaps hypertrophic and keloid scars are the result of a wound-healing process in which the intermediate collagen synthesis and deposition phase is prolonged.

4.2.2. Basis for Scar Hypertrophy

Diegelmann et al. (1979) reported that fibroblasts derived from keloid scars produce significantly more collagen per cell than do fibroblasts derived from normal skin of normal scar and show no significant differences in collagen-degradation rates. Although these experiments were performed in vitro, extrapolation of these results to the in vivo situation could explain why there is excess deposition of collagen in keloid scars. How this abnormality arises is unknown. Diegelmann et al. (1979) suggested several possible explanations which include (1) keloid fibroblasts are monoclonally derived from mutant cells formed in response to injury; (2) keloid fibroblasts have a unique differentiated capacity to synthesize increased amounts of collagen as a result of injury; and (3) keloid fibroblasts (for some unknown reason) have lost the ability to respond to feedback inhibitory signals that are normally involved in regulation of wound healing.

Kischer and co-workers (1982) proposed that hypertrophic and keloid scar development is related to interruptions of microvasculature regeneration. These investigators suggested that in situations in which microvascular occlusion occurs, low O_2 and high CO_2 levels result, in turn promoting excessive collagen and proteoglycan synthesis. Maturation of this type of scar begins when the scar area becomes so hypoxic that fibroblasts begin to degenerate resulting in the self-limiting resolution of the scar. This hypothesis, although providing an explanation for the basis of excessive connective tissue deposition during the wound-healing process, does not really provide an explanation for why this process is so highly variable from individual to individual.

It has been suggested that the immune system may be involved in the regulation of collagen production in healing wounds (Oluwasanmi et al., 1976). These investigators examined the effect of nonspecific immunization on collagen synthesis in granulomatous tissue (around Ivalon sponges) and showed that in immunostimulated animals the rates of collagen synthesis were significantly higher than in controls. The authors conclude that in certain situations an immune-mediated response may be involved in the excessive collagen synthesis observed in abnormally healing wounds, such as hypertrophic and keloid scars.

An alternative explanation for the excessive connective tissue deposition seen in hypertrophic and keloid scars is that there is variability in the remodeling of the extracellular matrix as the wound-healing process progresses. These temporal differences in the composition of the extracellular matrix could have profound effects on the proliferation or biosynthetic profile of fibroblasts or other cells in the healing wound. Several investigators have shown that the extracellular matrix exerts a powerful effect on the biosynthetic activity of cells *in vitro* and the ability of cells to respond to various factors (Nusgens et al., 1984; Yoshizato et al., 1984). Thus, it seems possible that small differences in the composition of the extracellular matrix during the wound healing process could significantly impact on the final character of the healed wound. Under these circumstances, hypertrophic or keloid scars would develop as a consequence of abnormal turnover of the matrix during the wound healing process. It seems likely that this variability could be modulated by several means including age, disease states, endocrinologic fluctuations, as well as genetic predisposition. All of these parameters have been associated with the etiology of keloid or hypertrophic scars (Murray et al., 1981).

4.2.3. Therapeutic Management of Hypertrophic and Keloid Scars

The traditional treatment of hypertrophic and keloid scars can be classified into five general approaches: (1) surgery, (2) pressure, (3) radiation, (4) corticosteroids, and (5) other drugs (for review, see Murray et al., 1981). These treatments have met with limited success, and it is clear that efficient and predictable management of these conditions awaits scientific breakthroughs that will enable the physician to bring about effective control of collagen production *in vivo*.

Currently, intralesional injection of corticosteroids such as triamcinolone, either alone or in conjunction with surgery, appears to be the most popular means to manage hypertrophic or keloid scars (Maguire, 1965; Minkowitz, 1967; Griffith et al., 1970; Ketchum et al., 1974). The precise mechanism by which corticosteroids influence the characteristics of hypertrophic or keloid scars is unknown. The effects of corticosteroids on inflammation, cell proliferation as well as vasoconstriction are well known, and their effects on mono-cyte/macrophages have been briefly discussed in Section 3.2. However, it seems likely that additional biological activities of these molecules are respon-sible for the effects that are seen in the control of hypertrophic scarring. The studies of corticosteroids on collagen synthesis *in vivo* and *in vitro* has sug-gested that these agents may inhibit collagen synthesis at the transcriptional, translational, or post-translational levels (for review, see Cutroneo *et al.*, 1981). Verification of the mode of control of collagen synthesis in scar tissue either *in vivo* or *in vitro* is unavailable. Several conflicting reports in the literature address the issue of whether these drugs inhibit collagen synthesis or influence wound tensile strength in various experimental modesl (Sandberg, 1964; Vogel, 1970; Stern and Sherman, 1973; Cohen and Keiser, 1973; Cohen *et al.*, 1977; Oxlund *et al.*, 1979). It appears that the conflicts can be attributed to differences in drug doses, methods of introduction, experimental models as well as dif-ferences in the methods of measurement. Thus, it remains to be resolved whether corticosteroids affect scar formation by inhibiting collagen synthesis, by inhibiting fibroblast proliferation, or by some other unrecognized mecha-nism.

An alternative hypothesis to explain the effects of corticosteroids on keloid and hypertrophic scars was presented by Cohen and Diegelmann (1977). These investigators suggested that corticosteroids influence collagen synthesis in scars by enhancing the degradation rate of collagen. They proposed that pro-cess this may be mediated by removing collagenase inhibitors or by promoting the activity of the collagenase present in the scar tissue (Cohen *et al.*, 1977).

Another approach to managing keloid scars following surgical removal has been proposed by Peacock (1981), who used topical applications of β-ami-nopropronitrile (BAPN) in conjunction with colchicine. BAPN is a lathyrogen that inhibits collagen crosslinking by inhibiting the enzyme peptidyl lysine oxidase (Siegel, 1980). Since noncrosslinked fibrillar collagen should be more susceptible to collagenase degradation, the reasoning was that collagen turn-over should be higher in the presence of this compound. Further, colchicine is a drug which disrupts microtubules within cells. Since microtubules are in-volved in collagen secretion from cells (Diegelmann and Peterkofsky, 1972), their disruption should result in reduced collagen production. It has been also reported that colchicine stimulates tissue collagenase (Harris and Krane, 1971; Chvapil *et al.*, 1980). Although a significant reduction in collagen production occurred, a practical treatment for keloids has not resulted.

Clinical investigators have recently begun to investigate the utility of laser therapy in the treatment of keloid scars (Castro *et al.*, 1983; Abergel *et al.*, 1984). The early clinical data from these studies look promising and suggest that laser therapy may provide an effective tool in the management of keloids. The mechanism of action of laser radiation in reducing the keloid scarring seems to be associated with inhibition of keloid fibroblast function, although the potential influence of the laser on the integrity of fibrillar collagen in the scar should not be discounted.

5. Collagen-Based Biomaterials in the Treatment of Dermal Wounds

5.1. Treatment of Burns

One of the most interesting applications of collagen-based biomaterials in the treatment of dermal wounds is the use of the artificial skin developed by Burke et al. (1981) for the treatment of burn victims. This device is composed of two layers, the outer being a Silastic membrane, which serves as a temporary epidermis, and the inner layer composed of a glutaraldehyde-crosslinked fibrillar composite of bovine corium collagen and chrondroitin sulfate, which serves as a template for neodermis regeneration (Yannas and Burke, 1980; Yannas et al., 1980). The artificial skin is designed for temporary use to support dermal regeneration and to control bacterial invasion as well as fluid loss. When donor sites are ready for skin grafting, the Silastic membrane can be removed and epidermal regeneration effected by a split-thickness skin graft. Clinical studies testing the general safety and efficacy of the material continue and, based on preliminary data Burke et al. (1981), suggest that this collagen-based biomaterial and others similar to it may provide a useful tool to physicians who manage patients with severe burns (for review, see Pruitt and Levine, 1984).

It is not unreasonable to expect that this artificial skin might be improved. This may be accomplished through use of a dermal scaffold and the utilization of the technology described by Green et al. (1979), in which epidermal cells from the patient are removed, propagated in cell culture, and then transplanted back to the wound area on the patient (Gallico et al., 1984). The development of an artificial dermis similar to that described by Burke et al. (1981), which could also support epidermal cell proliferation and maturation in vitro, would reduce the complexity of the current epidermal cell transplantation process. A final step will be to use allogeneic epidermal cells already grown in culture, but this will require a solution to the transplant rejection problem. A final problem is that burns vary in size, shape, and degree of tissue involvement and thus require individual treatment.

5.2. Surgical and Traumatic Wounds and Dermal Ulcers

An increasing body of literature provides evidence that collagen-based biomaterials may have clinical value in the treatment of a variety of dermal wounds, particularly those that involve loss of skin and are allowed to heal by secondary intent. Many of these devices are collagen-containing wound dressings that potentially may promote wound healing by enhancing re-epithelialization and accelerating new collagen synthesis (Alvarez et al., 1983; Leipziger et al., 1985). Although these general biologic activities have been observed in noncollagen-containing occlusive and semiocclusive dressings, a particularly advantageous property for certain collagen-containing dressings, may be their ability to reduce wound contraction significantly (Leipyigen *et al.*, 1985; Frank and Bonaldi, 1985).

There is as yet no commercial collagen-based material for the treatment of any type of dermal wound on the market. However, research results have been encouraging enough for trials to continue.

6. Conclusions

The role of collagen in dermal wound repair is clearly an important one. It participates, directly or indirectly, in every phase of wound healing, and its metabolism during the course of the process eventually contributes to the quality of wound repair. Abnormalities in this process can result in scars clinically manifested as cosmetically unattractive lesions that often compromise the functionality of tissues. Scientific progress in understanding this very important biologic problem has been slow in the past, primarily due to the fact that the basic principals which govern collagen production and degradation by cells were poorly understood. The rapid progress made during the past 5 years in developing an understanding of these principles provides hope that a better understanding of scar formation and maturation will be forthcoming in the near future. If this is the case, it may be possible to intervene clinically during the course of the wound repair process to influence the final outcome.

The long-range goals of research programs in this area are to develop biomaterials and biologic control methods that will be useful in regulating the various phases of the wound-healing process (inflammation, collagen synthesis and deposition, wound contraction, and re-epithelialization) and in this way to control the quality of dermal wound healing in a reproducible fashion. It is likely that future strategies will include the use of the various proliferative and chemotactic factors normally involved in the wound-healing process, in conjunction with reconstituted extracellular matrices that will present these factors to cells and perhaps regulate the way in which cells will respond to these signals.

References

Abergel, R. P., Dwyer, R. M., Meeker, C. A., Lask, G., Kelly, A. P., and Uitto, J., 1984, Laser treatment of keloids: A clinical trial and an *in vitro* study with Nd:YAG laser, *Lasers Surg. Med.* **4**:291–295.

Alvarez, O. M., Mertz, P. M., and Eaglstein, W. H., 1983, The effect of occlusive dressings on collagen synthesis and re-epithelialization in superficial wounds, *J. Surg. Res.* **35**:143–148.

Assoian, R. K., Fleurdelys, B. E., Stevenson, H. C., Miller, P. J., Madtes, D. K., Raines, E. W., Ross, R. R., and Sporn, M. B., 1987, Expression and secretion of type-beta transforming growth factor by activated human macrophages, *Proc. Nat. Acad. Sci. USA*, **84**:6020–6024.

Bailey, A. J., Boyin, S., Sims, T. J., Delous, M., Nicoletis, C., and Delaunay, A., 1975a, Characterization of the collagen of human hypertrophic and normal scars, *Biochim. Biophys. Acta* **405**:412–421.

Bailey, A. J., Sims, T. J., LeLous, M., and Bazin, S., 1975b, Collagen polymorphism in experimental granulation tissue, *Biochem. Biophys. Res. Commun.* **66:**1160–1165.

Baird, A., Mormede, P., and Bohlen, P., 1985, Immunoreactive fibroblast growth factor in cells of peritoneal exudate suggests its identity with macrophage-derived growth factor, *Biochem. Biophys. Res. Commun.* **126:**358–364.

Bell, E., Ivarsson, B., and Merril, C., 1979, Production of a tissue-like structure by contraction of collagen lattices by human fibroblasts of different proliferative potential *in vivo, Proc. Natl. Acad. Sci. USA* **76:**1274–1278.

Bentz, H., Morris, N. P., Murray, L. W., Sakai, L. Y., Hollister, D. W., and Burgeson, R. E., 1983, Isolation and partial characterization of a new human collgen with an extended triple-helical structural domain, *Proc. Natl. Acad. Sci. USA* **80:**3168–3172.

Bornstein, P., and Sage, H., 1980, Structurally distinct collagen types. *Annu. Rev. Biochem.* **49:**957–1003.

Bornstein, P., Horlein, D., and McPherson, J., 1984, Regulation of collagen synthesis, in: *Progress in Clinical and Biological Research: Myelofibrosis and the Biology of Connective Tissue* (P. D. Berk, H. Castro-Malaspina, and L. R. Wasserman, eds.), pp. 61–80, Alan R. Liss, New York.

Bowen-Pope, D. F., and Ross, R., 1982, Platelet derived growth factor II. Specific binding to cultured cells, *J. Biol. Chem.* **257:**5161–5171.

Burke, J. F., Yannas, I. V., Quinby, W. C., Bondoc, C. C., and Jung, W. K., 1981, Successful use of a physiologically acceptable artificial skin in the treatment of extensive burn injury, *Ann. Surg.* **194:**413–427.

Carpenter, N. H., Gates, D. J., and Williams, H. T. G., 1977, Normal processes and restraints in wound healing, *Can. J. Surg.* **20:**314–324.

Carrico, T. J., Mehrhof, A. I., and Cohen, I. K., 1984, Biology of wound healing, *Surg. Clin. N. Am.* **64:**721–733.

Casey, W. J., Peacock, E. E., Jr., and Chvapil, M., 1976, Induction of collagen synthesis in rats by transplantation of allogenic macrophages, *Surg. Forum* **27:**53–55.

Castro, D. J., Abergel, R. P., Johnson, K. J., Adomian, G. E., Dwyer, R. M., Uitto, J., and Lesavoy, M. A., 1983, Wound healing: Biological effects of Nd:YAG laser on collagen metabolism in pig skin in comparison to thermal burn, *Ann. Plast. Surg.* **11:**131–140.

Chaig, R. D. P., Scholfield, J. D., and Jackson, D. S., 1975, Collagen biosynthesis in normal and hypertrophic scars and keloid as a function of the duration of the scar, *Br. J. Surg.* **62:**741–744.

Chvapil, M., and Koopman, C. F., 1984, Scar formation: Physiology and pathological states, *Otolaryngol. Clin. North Am.* **17:**265–272.

Chvapil, M., Peacock, E. E., and Carlson, E. G., 1980, Colchicine and wound healing, *J. Surg. Res.* **28:**49–56.

Clark, R. A., Stone, R. D., Leung, P. Y. K., Silver, I., Hohn, D. C., and Hunt, T. K., 1976, Role of macrophages in wound healing, *Surg. Forum* **27:**16–18.

Clark, R. A. F., Lanigan, B. S., Dellapelle, P., Manseau, E., Dvorak, H. F., and Colvin, R. B., 1982, Fibronectin and fibrin provide a provisional matrix for epidermal cell migration during wound reepithelialization, *J. Invest. Dermatol.* **79:**264–269.

Clore, J. N., Cohen, I. K., and Diegelmann, R. F., 1979, Quantitation of collagen types I and III during wound healing in rat skin, *Proc. Soc. Exp. Biol. Med.* **161:**337–340.

Cohen, I. K., and Diegelmann, R. F., 1977, The biology of keloid and hypertrophic scar and the influence of corticosteroids, *Clin. Plast. Surg.* **4:**297–299.

Cohen, I. K., and Keiser, H. R., 1973, Collagen synthesis in keloid and hypertrophic scar following intralesional use of triamcinolone, *Surg. Forum* **24:**521–523.

Cohen, I. K., Diegelmann, R. F., and Johnson, M. L., 1977, Effect of corticosteroids on collagen synthesis, *Surgery* **82:**15–20.

Cohen, I. K., Moore, C. D., and Diegelmann, R. F., 1979, Onset and localization of collagen synthesis during wound healing in open rat skin wounds, *Proc. Soc. Exp. Biol. Med.* **160:**458–462.

Cutroneo, K. R., Rokowski, R., and Counts, D. F., 1981, Glucocorticoids and collagen synthesis: Comparison of *in vivo* and cell culture studies, *Collagen Rel. Res.* **1:**557–568.

Diegelmann, R. F., and Cohen, I. K., 1979, Modulation of fibroblast DNA synthesis by macrophages, *Plast. Surg. Forum* **2:**167–160.

Diegelmann, R. F., and Peterkofsky, B., 1972, Inhibition of collagen secretion from bone and cultured fibroblasts by microtubular disruptive drugs, *Proc. Natl. Acad. Sci. USA* **69**:892–896.

Diegelmann, R. F., Cohen, I. K., and McCoy, B. J., 1979, Growth kinetics and collagen synthesis of normal skin, normal scar and keloid fibroblasts *in vitro, J. Cell Physiol.* **98**:341–346.

Diegelmann, R. F., Cohen, I. K., and Kaplan, A. M., 1981, The role of macrophages in wound repair: A review, *Plast. Reconstr. Surg.* **68**:107–113.

Ehrlich, H. P., 1984, The role of connective tissue matrix in hypertrophic scar contracture, in: *Soft and Hard Tissue Repair* (T. K. Hunt, R. B. Heppenstall, E. Pines, and D. Rovee, eds.), pp. 533–553, Praeger, New York.

Epstein, E. H., 1974, [α1(III)]$_3$ Human skin collagen: Release by pepsin digestion and preponderance in fetal life, *J. Biol. Chem.* **249**:3225–3231.

Farquhar, M. G., 1981, The glomerular basement membrane: A selective macromolecular filter, in: *Cell Biology of Extracellular Matrix* (E. D. Hay, ed.), pp. 335–374, Plenum, New York.

Frank, D. H., and Bonaldi, L. C., 1985, Inhibition of wound contraction: Comparison of full-thickness skin grafts, Biobrane and aspartate membranes, *Ann. Plast. Surg.* **14**:103–110.

Gabbiani, G., Hirschel, B. J., Ryan, G. B., Statkov, P. R., and Majno, G., 1972, Granulation tissue as a contractile organ. A study of structure and function, *J. Exp. Med.* **135**:719–734.

Gallico, G. G., O'Connor, N. E., Compton, C. C., Kehindi, O., and Green, H., 1984, Permanent coverage of large burn wounds with autologous cultured human epithelium, *N. Engl. J. Med.* **311**:448–451.

Gauss-Muller, V., Kleinman, H. K., Martin, G. R., and Schiffman, E., 1980, Role of attachment factors and attractants in fibroblast chemotaxis, *J. Lab. Clin. Med.* **96**:1071–1080.

Gay, S., Viljanto, J., Raekallio, J., and Penttinen, R., 1978, Collagen types in early phases of wound healing in children, *Acta Chir. Scand.* **144**:205–211.

Green, H., and Goldberg, B., 1964, Collagen and cell protein synthesis by an established mammalian fibroblast line, *Nature (Lond.)* **204**:347–349.

Green, H., Kehinde, O., and Thomas, J., 1979, Growth of cultured human epidermal cells into multiple epithelia suitable for grafting, *Proc. Natl. Acad. Sci. USA* **76**:5665–5668.

Griffith, B. H., Monroe, C. W., and McKinney, P., 1970, A follow-up study on the treatment of keloids with triamcinolone acetomide, *Plast. Reconstr. Surg.* **46**:145–150.

Grinnell, F., and Lamke, C. R., 1984, Reorganization of hydrated collagen lattices by human skin fibroblasts, *J. Cell Sci.* **66**:51–63.

Grotendorst, G. R., Seppa, H. E. J., Kleinman, H. K., and Martin, G. R., 1981, Attachment of smooth muscle cells to collagens and their migration toward platelet-derived growth factor, *Proc. Natl. Acad. Sci. USA* **78**:3669–3672.

Grotendorst, G. R., Chang, T., Seppa, H. E. J., Kleinman, H. K., and Martin, G. R., 1982, Platelet derived growth factor is a chemoattractant for vascular smooth muscle cells, *J. Cell Physiol.* **113**:261–266.

Grotendorst, G. R., Pencer, D., Martin, G. R., and Sodek, J., 1984, Molecular mediators of tissue repair, in: *Soft and Hard Tissue Repair* (T. K. Hunt, R. B. Heppenstall, E. Pines, and D. Rovee, eds.), pp. 20–40, Praeger, New York.

Grotendorst, G. R., Martin, G. R., Pencev, D., Sodek, J., and Harvey, A. K., 1985, Stimulation of granulation tissue formation by platelet derived growth factor in normal and diabetic rats, *J. Clin. Invest.* **76**:2323–2329.

Harris, E. D., and Krane, S. M., 1971, Effects of colchicine on collagenase in cultures of rheumatoid synovium, *Arthritis Rheum.* **14**:669–684.

Harris, E. D., and Krane, S. M., 1974, Collagenases, *N. Engl. J. Med.* **291**:652–661.

Heldin, C. H., Westenmark, B., and Wasteson, A., 1981, Specific receptors for platelet-derived growth factor on cells derived from connective tissue and glia, *Proc. Natl. Acad. Sci. USA* **78**:3664–3668.

Henkel, W., and Glanville, R. W., 1982, Covalent crosslinking between molecules of type I and type III collagen, *Eur. J. Biochem.* **122**:205–213.

Heughan, C., and Hunt, T., 1975, Some aspects of wound healing research: A review, *Can. J. Surg.* **18**:118–126.

Hunt, T. K., Conolly, W. B., Aronson, S. B., and Goldstein, P., 1978, Anaerobic metabolism and wound healing: A hypothesis for the initiation and cessation of collagen synthesis in wounds, *Am. J. Surg.* **135:**328–332.

Hunt, T. K., Knighton, D. R., Thakral, K. K., Goodson, W. H., and Andrews, W. S., 1984a, Studies on inflammation and wound healing: Angiogenesis and collagen synthesis stimulated in vivo by resident and activated wound macrophages, *Surgery* **96:**48–54.

Hunt, T. K., Knighton, D. R., Thakral, K. K., Andrews, W., and Michaeli, D., 1984b, Cellular control of repair, in: *Soft and Hard Tissue Repair* (T. K. Hunt, R. B. Heppenstall, E. Pines, and D. Rovee, eds.), pp. 3–19, Praeger, New York.

Ignotz, R. A., and Massague, J., 1986, Transforming growth factor-β stimulates the expression of fibronectin and collagen and their incorporation into extracellular matrix, *J. Biol. Chem.* **261:**4337–4345.

Inoue, S., Leblond, C. P., and Laurie, G. W., 1983, Ultrastructure of Reichert's membrane, a multilayered basement membrane in the parietal wall of the rat yolk sac, *J. Cell Biol.* **97:**1524–1537.

Jaffe, E. A., Leung, L. L. K., Nachman, R. L., Levin, R. I., and Mosher, D. F., 1982, Thrombospondin is the endogenous lectin of human platelets, *Nature (Lond.)* **295:**246–248.

Ketchum, L. D., Cohen, I. K., and Masters, F. W., 1974, Hypertrophic scars and keloids: A collective review, *Plast. Reconstr. Surg.* **53:**140–154.

Kischer, C. W., 1974, Collagen and dermal patterns in the hypertropic scar, *Anat. Rec.* **179:**137–145.

Kischer, C. W., and Shetlar, M. R., 1974, Collagen and myucopolysaccharides in the hypertrophic scar, *Connect. Tissue Res.* **2:**205–213.

Kischer, C. W., Shetlar, M. R., and Chvapil, M., 1982, Hypertrophic scars and keloids: A review and new concept concerning their origin, *Scan. Electron Microsc.* **4:**1699–1713.

Knapp, T. R., Daniels, J. R., and Kaplan, E. N., 1977, Pathologic scar formation, *Am. J. Pathol.* **86:**47–63.

Knighton, D. R., Hunt, T. K., Thakral, K. K., and Goodson, W. H., 1982, Role of platelets and fibrin in the healing sequence: An *in vivo* study of angiogenesis and collagen synthesis, *Ann. Surg.* **196:**379–388.

Langness, U., and Udenfriend, S., 1973, Collagen proline hydroxylases activity and anaerobic metabolism, in: *Biology of Fibroblast* (E. Kulonen and J. Pikkarainen, eds.), pp. 373–378, Academic, New York.

Lawrence, W. T., Norton, J. A., Sporn, M. B., Gorschboth, C., and Grotendorst, E. R., 1986, The reversal of an Adriamycin induced healing impairment with chemottractants and growth factors, *Ann. Surg.* **203:**142–147.

Leipziger, L. S., Glushko, V., DiBernardo, B., Shafaie, F., Noble, J., Nichols, J., and Alvarez, O., 1985, Dermal wound repair: Role of collagen matrix implants and synthetic polymer dressings, *J. Am. Acad. Dermatol.* **12:**409–419.

Leitzel, K., Cano, C., Marks, J. G., and Lipton, A., 1985, Growth factors and wound healing in the hamster, *J. Dermatol. Surg. Oncol.* **11:**617–622.

Levene, C. K., and Bates, C. J., 1976, The effect of hypoxia on collagen synthesis in cultured 3T6 fibroblasts and its relationship to the mode of action of ascorbate, *Biochim. Biophys. Acta* **444:**446–452.

Liebovich, S. J., 1984, Mesenchymal cell proliferation in wound repair: The role of macrophages, in: *Soft and Hard Tissue Repair* (T. K. Hunt, R. B. Heppenstall, E. Pines, and D. Rovee, eds.), pp. 329–351, Praeger, New York.

Liebovich, S. J., and Ross, R., 1975, The role of the macrophage in wound repair: A study with hydrocortisone and antimacrophage serum, *Am. J. Pathol.* **78:**71–91.

Liebovich, S. J., and Ross, R., 1976, A macrophage-dependent factor that stimulates the proliferation of fibroblasts *in vitro, Am. J. Pathol.* **84:**501–513.

Madden, J. W., and Peacock, E. E., 1968, Studies on the biology of collagen during wound healing. I. Rate of collagen synthesis and deposition in cutaneous wounds of the rat, *Surgery* **64:**288–294.

Maguire, H. C., 1965, Treatment of keloids with triamcinolone acetomide injected intralesionally, *JAMA* **192:**325–327.

Majno, G., Gabbiani, G., Hirschel, B. J., Ryan, G. B., and Statkov, P. R., 1971, Contraction of granulation tissue *in vitro*: Similarity to smooth muscle, *Science* **173:**548–550.

Martin, B. M., Gimbrone, M. A., Jr., Unanue, E. R., and Cotran, R. S., 1981, Stimulation of nonlymphoid mesenchymal cell proliferation by a macrophage-derived growth factor, *J. Immunol.* **126**:1510–1515.

Martin, G. R., Timpl, R., Muller, P. K., and Kuhn, K., 1985, The genetically distinct collagens, *Trans. Int. Biol. Soc.* **115**:285–287.

McPherson, J. M., Wallace, D. G., Sawamura, S. J., Conti, A., Condell, R. A., Wade, S., and Piez, K., 1985, Collagen fibrillogenesis *in vitro*: A characterization of fibril quality as a function of assembly conditions, *Collagen Rel. Res.* **5**:119–135.

Miller, E. J., 1976, Biochemical characteristics and biological significance of genetically distinct collagens, *Molec. Cell. Biochem.* **13**:165–189.

Miller, E. J., 1984, Chemistry of collagens and their distribution, in: *Extracellular Matrix Biochemistry* (K. A. Piez and A. H. Reddi, eds.), pp. 41–78, Elsevier, New York.

Minkowitz, F., 1967, Regression of massive keloid following partial excision and postoperative intralesional administration of triamcinolone, *Br. J. Plast. Surg.* **20**:432–435.

Modesti, A., Kalebic, T., Scarpa, S., Togo, S., Grotendorst, G., Liotta, L. A., and Triche, T. J., 1984, Type V collagen in human amnion is a 12 nm component of the pericellular interstitium, *Eur. J. Cell Biol.* **35**:246–255.

Murray, J. C., Pollack, S. V., and Pinnell, S. R., 1981, Keloids: A review, *J. Am. Acad. Dermatol.* **4**:461–470.

Nusgens, B., Merrill, C., LaPierce, C., and Bell, E., 1984, Collagen biosynthesis by cells in a tissue equivalent matrix *in vitro*, *Collagen Rel. Res.* **4**:351–364.

Oluwasanmi, J. O., Lucas, D. O., and Chvapil, M., 1976, Effect of a concurrent immune response on the collagen synthesis around implanted ivalon sponges in rats, *Plast. Reconstr. Surg.* **58**:601–607.

Oxlund, H., Fogdestam, I., and Viidick, A., 1979, The influence of cortisol on wound healing of the skin and distant connective tissue response, *Surg. Gynecol. Obstet.* **148**:876–880.

Peacock, E. E., 1973, Biology of wound repair, *Life Sci.* **13**:1–9.

Peacock, E. E., 1978, Wound contraction and scar contracture. (Letters to the editor), *Plast. Reconstr. Surg.* **62**:600–602.

Peacock, E. E., 1981, Pharmacological control of surface scarring in human beings, *Ann. Surg.* **193**:592–597.

Peacock, E. E., Madden, J. W., and Triea, W. C., 1970, Biologic basis for treatment of keloids and hypertrophic scars, *South. Med. J.* **63**:755–760.

Postlethwaite, E. E., Seyer, J. M., and Kang, A. H., 1978, Chemotactic attraction of human fibroblasts to type I, II and III collagens and collagen derived peptides, *Proc. Natl. Acad. Sci. USA* **75**:871–875.

Pruitt, B. A., and Levine, N. S., 1984, Characteristics and uses of biologic dressings and skin substitutes, *Arch. Surg.* **119**:312–322.

Roberts, A. B., Sporn, M. B., Assoian, R. K., Smith, J. M., Roche, N. S., Heine, U. I., Liotta, L., Falanga, V., Kehrl, J. H., and Fauci, A. S., 1986, Transforming growth factor-beta: Rapid induction of fibrosis and angiogenesis *in vivo* and stimulation of collagen formation *in vitro*, *Proc. Natl. Acad. Sci. USA* **83**:4167–4171.

Ross, R., and Benditt, E. P., 1961, Wound healing and collagen formation. I. Sequential changes in components of guinea pig skin wounds observed in the electron microscope, *J. Biophys. Biochem. Cytol.* **11**:677–700.

Rutherford, R. B., and Ross, R., 1976, Platelet factors stimulate fibroblasts and smooth muscle cells quiescent to plasma serum to proliferate, *J. Cell Biol.* **69**:196–203.

Sandberg, N., 1964, Time relationship between administration of cortisone and wound healing in rats, *Acta Clin. Scand.* **127**:446–455.

Seppa, H. E. J., Grotendorst, G. R., Seppa, S. I., Schiffman, E., and Martin, G. R., 1982, The platelet derived growth factor is a chemoattractant for fibroblasts, *J. Cell. Biol.* **92**:584–588.

Shimokado, K., Raines, E. W., Madtes, D. K., Barrett, T. B., Benditt, E. P., and Ross, R., 1985, A significant part of macrophage-derived growth factor consists of at least two forms of PDGF, *Cell* **43**:277–286.

Shoshan, S., 1981, Wound healing, in *International Review of Connective Tissue Research*, Vol. 9 (D. A. Hall and D. S. Jackson, eds.), pp. 1–26, Academic, New York.

Siegel, R. C., 1980, Lysyl oxidase, *Int. Rev. Connect. Tissue Res.* **8**:73–118.

Silver, I. A., 1972, Oxygen tension and epithelialization, in *Epidermal Wound Healing* (H. I. Maibach and D. T. Rovee, eds.), pp. 291–305, Year Book, Chicago.

Sporn, M. B., Roberts, A. B., Shull, J. H., Smith, J. M., Ward, J. M., and Sodek, J., 1983, Polypeptide transforming growth factors isolated from bovine sources and used for wound healing *in vivo*, *Science* **219**:1329–1330.

Steinberg, B. M., Smith, K., Colozzo, M., and Pollack, R., 1980, Establishment and transformation diminish the ability of fibroblasts to contract a native collagen gel, *J. Cell Biol.* **87**:304–308.

Stenn, K. S., Madri, J. A., and Roll, J. F., 1979, Migrating epidermis produces AB_2 collagen and requires continued collagen synthesis for movement, *Nature (Lond.)* **277**:229–232.

Stern, S. F., and Sherman, A., 1973, Effect of locally administered corticosteroids (soluble and insoluble) on the healing times of surgically induced wounds in guinea pigs, *J. Am. Pod. Assoc.* **63**:374–382.

Timpl, R., Wiedemann, H., von Delden, V., Furthmayr, H., and Kuhn, K., 1981, A network model for the organization of type IV collagen in basement membranes, *Eur. J. Biochem.* **120**:203–211.

Vogel, H. G., 1970, Tensile strength of skin wounds in rats after treatment with corticosteroids, *Acta Endocrinol. (Copenh.)* **64**:295–303.

Werb, Z., 1978, Pathways for the modulation of macrophage collagenase activity, in: *Mechanism of Localized Bone Loss* (J. E. Horton, T. M. Tarpley, and W. F. Davis, eds.), pp. 213–228, Information Retrieval, Washington, D. C.

Werb, Z., Burleigh, M. C., Barrett, A. J., and Starkey, P. M., 1974, The interaction of α-2-macroglobulin with proteinases: Binding and inhibition of mammalian collagenase and other neutral proteases, *Biochem. J.* **139**:359–368.

Werb, Z., Mainardi, C. L., Vater, C. A., and Harris, E. D., 1977, Endogenous activation of latent collgenase by rheumatoid synovial cells: Evidence for a role of plasminogen activator, *N. Engl. J. Med.* **296**:1017–1023.

Winter, G. D., 1978, Oxygen and epidermal wound healing: Oxygen transport to tissue. III. in: *Advances in Experimental Medicine and Biology*, Vol. 94 (I. A. Silver, M. Erecinska, and H. I. Biocher, eds.), pp. 673–678, Plenum, New York.

Woodley, D. T., O'Keefe, E. J., and Prunieras, M., 1985, Cutaneous wound healing: A model for cell–matrix interactions, *J. Am. Acad. Dermatol.* **12**:420–433.

Woolley, D. E., 1984, Mammalian collagenases, in: *Extracellular Matrix Biochemistry* (K. A. Piez and A. H. Reddi, eds.), pp. 119–151, Elsevier, New York.

Yannas, I. V., and Burke, J. R., 1980, Design of an artificial skin. I. Basic design principles, *J. Biomed. Mat. Res.* **14**:65–84.

Yannas, I. V., Burke, J. F., Gordon, P. L., Huang, C., and Rubenstein, R. H., 1980, Design of an artificial skin. II. Control of chemical composition, *J. Biomed. Mat. Res.* **14**:107–132.

Yoshizato, K., Taira, T., and Shioya, N., 1984, Collagen-dependent growth suppression and changes in the shape of human dermal fibroblasts, *Ann. Plast. Surg.* **13**:9–14.

Zeitz, M., Ruiz-Torres, A., and Merker, H. J., 1978, Collagen metabolism in granulating wounds of rat skin, *Arch. Dermatol. Res.* **263**:207–214.

Chapter 21

Role of Degradative Enzymes in Wound Healing

PAOLO MIGNATTI, HOWARD G. WELGUS, and
DANIEL B. RIFKIN

1. Introduction

Several degradative enzymes active on extracellular matrix components play
major roles in the different stages of wound repair. Among the most important
are the plasminogen activators, collagenase, hyaluronidase, and elastase,
which are discussed in this chapter. (See Chapter 8 for a discussion of elastase.)

2. Plasminogen Activators

2.1. Characterization and Properties

Plasminogen activators (PACs) are serine proteinases capable of activating
the inactive zymogen, plasminogen, to plasmin. Originally known as fibrinolysin, because of its role in degrading the fibrin clot, plasmin has a relatively
broad trypsin-like specificity (for review, see Robbins et al., 1981) that can
degrade most proteins, with the notable exceptions of native collagen (Werb et
al., 1977) and elastin. While a number of vertebrate proteins, such as serum
kallikrein and the blood coagulation factors XI and XII (Colman, 1969; Mandle
and Kaplan, 1977; Bouma and Griffin, 1978), and bacterial proteins such as
streptokinase (Christensen, 1945; Summaria et al., 1982) have been shown to
activate plasminogen, the term plasminogen activator is currently restricted to
two enzymes, the urokinase- (u-PA) and the tissue-type (t-PA) plasminogen
activators, which are kinetically extremely efficient activators of plasminogen.
These PAs were purified and characterized and shown to possess structural,
functional, and immunologic differences.

Urokinase, so named because it was originally identified in urine, is a

PAOLO MIGNATTI and DANIEL B. RIFKIN • Department of Cell Biology and Kaplan Cancer
Center, New York University School of Medicine, New York, New York 10016.   HOWARD G.
WELGUS • Department of Medicine, Division of Dermatology, Jewish Hospital at Washington
University Medical Center, St. Louis, Missouri 63110.

50,000-M_r glycoprotein that occurs in one- and two-polypeptide chain forms. The single-polypeptide form is thought to be an inactive proenzyme form of urokinase (pro-u-PA). The two-polypeptide-chain form consists of a 30,000-M_r heavy chain, also termed the β-chain, and a 20,000-M_r light chain (α-chain). The two chains are held together by one disulfide bridge (Sumi and Robbins, 1983; Eaton et al., 1984; Sudol and Reich, 1984). Other enzymatically active forms of u-PA with partially degraded 30,000-M_r α-chains have been reported (Danø and Reich, 1978; Granelli-Piperno and Reich, 1978; Danø et al., 1980). The active site of u-PA has been localized in the β-chain, whose amino acid sequence possesses the structurally conserved regions characteristic of all serine proteinases, with His, Asp, and Ser residues at the active site (Steffens et al., 1982; Strassburger et al., 1983). While some studies have indicated the possible existence of cellular substrates other than plasminogen (Quigley, 1980; Keski-Oja and Vaheri, 1982), the only well-documented protein substrate for u-PA is plasminogen. Urokinase (u-PA) exhibits a high degree of species specificity with respect to plasminogen activation (Wohl et al., 1983), and this is related to the presence of a specific binding pocket in the u-PA molecule (Schoellmann et al., 1982). Urokinase is secreted as the single-chain inactive proenzyme, pro-u-PA, which is converted to the active two-chain form by limited proteolysis (Skriver et al., 1982; Eaton et al., 1984). Trace amounts of plasmin are able to activate pro-u-PA, generating a self-maintained feedback mechanism of pro-u-PA and plasminogen activation. Besides being secreted in human urine in a relatively high concentration, u-PA is present in plasma (Tissot et al., 1982) and in a variety of tissues and body fluids, as well as in the culture medium of several normal and tumor cells (for review, see Danø et al., 1985).

Tissue type-PA, also termed extrinsic plasminogen activator (Collen, 1980), is so named because it was first identified in tissue extracts. It has been purified from various sources, including human uterus, human plasma, blood vessel perfusates, and conditioned cell-culture media (Bachman et al., 1964; Wallen et al., 1983; Heussen et al., 1984). The molecular weight of t-PA is approximately 70,000 (Danø and Reich, 1978; Andreasen et al., 1984). The molecule is glycosylated (McLellan et al., 1980) and, like u-PA, occurs in one- and two-polypeptide-chain forms. The latter consists of two chains (α and β) of approximately equal size, held together by disulfide bonds (Wallen et al., 1983). The proteolytic conversion of the one-chain to the two-chain form is catalyzed by plasmin, tissue kallikrein, and blood coagulation factor Xa, whereas other coagulation factors, such as VIIa, IXa and XIIa, as well as activated protein C, do not catalyze this conversion (Andreasen et al., 1984; Ichinose et al., 1984).

Interesting characteristics are apparent when the amino acid sequences of t-PA and u-PA are compared. Like u-PA, the only known protein substrate for t-PA is plasminogen. The amino acid sequence of the β-chain of t-PA—the one possessing the active site—is similar to that of u-PA and to the corresponding regions of other serine proteinases, with the active site His, Asp, and Ser residues in homologous positions in both activators (Pohl *et al.*, 1984). By contrast, the α-chains of u-PA and t-PA differ significantly in size, even though they show a considerable degree of homology. Unlike u-PA, which contains only one kringle structure, t-PA possesses two such regions in the C-terminal part of the α-chain (Banyai *et al.*, 1983; Pennica *et al.*, 1983). Near the N-terminal end, both activators contain a cysteine-rich region showing homology to blood coagulation factors IX and X, albumin, α-fetoprotein (AFP), and epidermal growth factor (EGF) (Banyai *et al.*, 1983; Pennica *et al.*, 1983; Pohl *et al.*, 1984; Baker, 1985). However, the 43 N-terminal residues of t-PA, have no counterpart in u-PA, and they show a high degree of homology with the finger or type I domains of fibronectin believed to be responsible for its affinity for fibrin (see Chapter 18). This interesting observation may indicate the structural basis of an important characteristic of t-PA, its strong affinity for fibrin (Rijken and Collen, 1981). Plasminogen is also known to bind to fibrin, and fibrin strongly stimulates plasminogen activation by t-PA (Radcliffe, 1983; Suenson *et al.*, 1984). This stimulation results from a lowering of the K_m for plasminogen activation by over 60-fold and is likely explained by a close justaposition of plasminogen and t-PA on the common ligand, fibrin (Hoylaerts *et al.*, 1982; Dunn *et al.*, 1984; Tran-Thang *et al.*, 1984).

The differences in amino acid sequence and in the nucleotide sequence of the corresponding cDNA of u-PA and t-PA afford a definitive demonstration that the two types of activators are probably the products of two independent genes that evolved from a common ancestor gene by duplication and subsequent mutations (Edlund *et al.*, 1983; Pennica *et al.*, 1983).

One of the most important features of the PA–plasmin system is the amplification achieved by the conversion of plasminogen to plasmin by PA and the resultant self-maintained mechanism of pro-PA and plasminogen activation. The amount of circulating plasminogen is relatively high (~70 ng/ml), and in the human approximately 40% of the plasminogen is located in extravascular sites, including the basal layers of epidermis (Isseroff and Rifkin, 1983). The production of even small amounts of PA in a tissue, or at a particular site of a tissue, may therefore result in extremely high levels of local proteolytic activity. Moreover, plasmin is effective in the local activation of procollagenase, the zymogen form of collagenase secreted by most cells (Werb *et al.*, 1977), and in the potentiation of the activity of macrophage elastase, perhaps also by activating a proenzyme (Chapman and Stone, 1984). Thus, the production of a proteinase with restricted specificity, such as PA, can result in the local generation of (at least) three active proteinases: plasmin and elastase, with broad substrate specificities for noncollagen extracellular matrix proteins; and collagenase, which has substrate specificity limited to collagen. Together, these enzymes can degrade most of the protein matrix of connective tissues.

The local high concentration of PA is finely modulated by local and systemic factors acting at each step of its production, for instance, in biosynthesis, release from producer cells, conversion of proenzyme into active enzyme, and enzyme activity. These regulatory factors include hormones (glucocorticoids and polypeptide hormones), cyclic adenosine monophosphate (cAMP) and derivatives (Strickland and Beers, 1976; Vassalli et al., 1976; Granelli-Piperno et al., 1977; Vassalli et al., 1977; Granelli-Piperno and Reich, 1983; Mak et al., 1984; Ny et al., 1985), EGF (Lee and Weinstein, 1978; Eaton and Baker, 1983), colony stimulating factor (Lin and Gordon, 1979), retinoids (Wilson and Reich, 1978), prostaglandins, primarily of the E type (Strickland and Beers, 1976; Conanan and Crutchley, 1983), lymphokines (Vassalli and Reich, 1977), bacterial constituents and toxins (Hamilton et al., 1982; Collen, 1983), ultraviolet (UV) light (Miskin and Reich, 1980; Miskin and Ben-Ishai, 1981), and a number of other natural and synthetic factors (for review, see Danø et al., 1985).

Stimulatory factors and inhibitors appear to be of particular importance in the regulation of PA activity in extracellular matrix degradation. The activity of t-PA is enhanced by fibrin and some fibrin degradation products. The same investigators also demonstrated that fibrinopeptides augment considerably u-PA activation of plasminogen (Suenson et al., 1984). These observations suggest an amplification process whereby local PA activity is triggered by clot formation. The fibrin clot, indeed, can greatly enhance the activity of pre-existing t-PA molecules. The subsequent activation of plasmin and the generation of fibrin degradation products can further stimulate the activity of other t-PA and u-PA molecules. Activated protein C as well as elevated levels of thrombin have also been reported to enhance fibrinolysis by decreasing the levels of a fast-acting inhibitor of t-PA (van Hinsbergh et al., 1985).

By contrast, several specific inhibitors limit, either locally or systemically, the proteolytic activity of these PA enzymes (Thorsen and Philips, 1984; Verheijen et al., 1984). A number of inhibitors specific for PA exist in several tissues and are produced by a variety of cell types, some of which also produce PA, such as fibroblasts, granulocytes, and endothelial cells (Loskutoff and Edgington, 1977; Kopitar et al., 1980; Loskutoff and Edgington, 1981; Collen, 1983; Levin, 1983; Loskutoff et al., 1983; Erickson et al., 1984; Philips et al., 1984; Sprengers et al., 1984; Vassalli et al., 1984; Ny et al., 1985). Protease nexin, a recently discovered proteinase inhibitor produced by cultured human fibroblasts, binds and inhibits u-PA, as well as plasmin and thrombin (Baker et al., 1980; Scott and Baker, 1983). The binding of u-PA by protease nexin may initiate cellular uptake and degradation of u-PA (Baker et al., 1980), pointing to the existence of an additional mechanism of enzyme inactivation.

A rapidly acting inhibitor of u-PA and t-PA produced by cultured endothelial cells and present in platelets and plasma was recently described by Loskutoff and co-workers. The specificity of this inhibitor for PA and its modulation under several different conditions known to affect fibrinolysis indicate that this may be the major physiologic inhibitor of PA (Levin, 1983; Loskutoff et al., 1983).

Urokinase (u-PA) and t-PA have been identified in a variety of body fluids, tissues, and in vitro cell cultures (for review, see Danø et al., 1985). Urokinase is present in a number of cell types, including fibroblasts, endothelial cells, keratinocytes, granulocytes, and macrophages, all of which participate in wound healing. Tissue type-PA has been demonstrated histochemically in virtually all tissues studied, including human skin and the endothelial cells of veins and small vessels that probably represent precapillary sphincters. Both types of activators, but mainly u-PA, are associated with several physiologic and pathologic processes that degrade the extracellular matrix and/or basement membranes. An increased production of PA has been shown to occur in mammary involution following lactation (Ossowski et al., 1979; Larsson et al., 1984), ovulation (Beers, 1975; Strickland and Beers, 1976; Ny et al., 1985; Reich et al., 1985), embryo implantation (Strickland et al., 1976), postpartum uterine involution (Shimada et al., 1985), migration of fibroblasts in vitro (Ossowski et al., 1973), and migration and growth of neuronal cells (Krystosek and Seeds, 1984). These observations point to a role of PA in tissue degradation, cell migration, and tissue remodeling, all of which take place during wound repair. In this context, it is worth mentioning the potential association of PA, along with other proteinases, with the invasive and metastatic capacity of malignant tumors (for review, see Mullins and Rohrlich, 1983).

Other lines of evidence point to the involvement of PA in inflammation. High levels of PA, mainly of the u-PA, are produced by polymorphonuclear leukocytes (Granelli-Piperno and Reich, 1978) and have been associated with macrophage activation (Gordon et al., 1974; Unkeless et al., 1974). More recently, the observation that capillary endothelial cells produce PA and that the synthesis of PA is enhanced by treatment of these cells with angiogenic factors has led to the hypothesis that PA may play a fundamental role in angiogenesis (Gross et al., 1983) (see also Chapter 15). Moreover, PA has been related in vivo to a variety of conditions involving inflammation and/or tissue degradation, such as allergic vasculitis (Toki et al., 1982), xeroderma pigmentosum (Miskin and Ben-Ishai, 1981), pemphigus (Hashimoto et al., 1984), psoriasis (Fraki et al., 1983), corneal ulceration (Berman et al., 1980), and rheumatoid arthritis (Hamilton, 1982).

While all these observations indicate that the primary site of action of PA is at the extracellular level, several lines of evidence suggest that PA may also act at the cell surface or intracellularly. The u-PA produced by macrophages is capable of interacting with surface structures of either producer cells or other cells (Vassalli et al., 1985). The binding to monocytes occurs through the A-chain of u-PA with characteristics similar to the interaction of a hormone with its membrane receptor. Tissue-PA has been shown to bind to cultured human fibroblasts, although more slowly than u-PA binds to monocytes (Hoal et al., 1983). The different cell-binding characteristics of u-PA and t-PA indicate the possible existence of at least two different effects of PA at the cellular level. The presence of cell-surface receptors localizes PA at the cell surface, an optimal site to facilitate parenchymal cell migration (see also Chapter 13). PA production has also been proposed as a mechanism for the infiltration of inflammatory cells into sites of inflammation (see also Chapters 6 and 8). Another possible effect of PA at the cell surface is the degradation of membrane protein components. A 160,000-M_r glycoprotein on the membrane of macrophages has been shown to be very sensitive to plasmin, although the cellular effects of its degradation are not yet fully understood (Remold-O'Donnel and Lewandrowski, 1982).

2.2. Possible Roles of Plasminogen Activators in Wound Repair

Several lines of evidence demonstrate an involvement of PA in those stages of wound healing in which inflammation and tissue remodelling processes are involved. PA may be produced by different cell types in the skin. These can be classified as follows: (1) epidermal cells (keratinocytes); (2) dermal cells (fibroblasts and capillary endothelial cells); and (3) cells that have migrated into the skin and that are active during the different stages of wound repair (granulocytes and macrophages).

2.2.1. Inflammation

During the early and late inflammatory stages of wound healing, several sources may provide the damaged area with high levels of proteolytic activity. From the very moment of tissue injury, blood vessel disruption results in the extravasation of plasma constituents. Plasminogen and PA are therefore released into the open tissue; some of the same factors that take part in the coagulation cascade may also directly activate plasminogen or convert proactivators into active PA. Blood coagulation factors XI and XII, as well as serum kalilkrein, are able to activate plasminogen (Colman, 1969; Mandle and Kaplan, 1977; Bouma and Griffin, 1978), while tissue kallikrein and factor Xa can catalyze the conversion of t-PA from the one-chain zymogen to the two-chain active form of t-PA (Andreasen et al., 1984; Ichinose et al., 1984). Once plasmin is formed, it may activate pro-u-PA molecules, also brought into the wound region with extravasation of blood plasma (Skriver et al., 1982; Eaton et al., 1984). The formation of the fibrin clot provides an early primitive form of extracellular matrix, which potentiates the migration of inflammatory cells into the lesion. Granulocytes and monocytes, the first cells that infiltrate an area of injury and inflammation, secrete high amounts of u-PA (Gordon et al., 1974; Unkeless et al., 1974; Granelli-Piperno et al., 1977; Granelli-Piperno and Reich, 1978; Vassalli et al., 1984). Plasmin, formed by the action of the u-PA produced by these cells, together with the t-PA derived from blood vessel disruption and plasma extravasation, lead to the ultimate dissolution of the fibrin clot. Because of its affinity for fibrin, t-PA is regarded as mainly responsible for clot lysis (Matsuo et al., 1981). The plasmin also degrades glycoprotein components of the extracellular matrix, such as fibronectin and laminin (Werb et al., 1980), and activates other proteinases produced by macrophages in inactive forms, such as procollagenase and proelastase (Werb et al., 1977; Edlund et al., 1983; Chapman and Stone, 1984). Thus, the high level of local proteolytic activity produced by macrophages facilitates debridement of the injured area. While this process constitutes a first step in tissue remodeling, the degradation of the fibrin clot and of the extracellular matrix triggers a mechanism for recruitment of additional monocytes and of parenchymal cells by generating fibrin-, collagen-, elastin-, and fibronectin degradation products (Stecher and Sorkin, 1972; Postlethwaite and Kang, 1976; Fernandez et al., 1978; Senior et al., 1980; Bowersox and Sorgente 1982; Norris et al., 1982).

2.2.2. Granulation Tissue Formation

In granulation tissue formation, fibroblasts and endothelial cells move into the wound space. This migratory phenomenon has been studied in simplified *in vitro* experiments in which a monolayer of cultured fibroblasts is wounded with a razorblade and the movement of cells into the denuded area measured. A serum factor, later identified as plasminogen, is described in several reports as necessary for cell movement into the area (Clarke et al., 1970; Lipton et al., 1971; Burk, 1973; Ossowski et al., 1973). While these *in vitro* experiments oversimplified the *in vivo* situation, they clearly associated plasminogen activation with fibroblast motility. The mechanism of action of PA in cell movement is not yet understood. Besides activating collagenase and directly digesting certain extracellular matrix proteins such as fibronectin, plasmin has the capacity to disrupt actin cables in rat embryo cells (Pollack and Rifkin, 1975), suggesting that PA or plasmin may be capable of modifying intracellular cytoskeletal components as well as extracellular matrix components. Continuous rearrangement of both components is necessary for cell migration (see also Chapter 13).

Other lines of evidence indicate that PA may also play a role in endothelial cell migration and angiogenesis. Vascular endothelial cells have been reported to produce PA both *in vitro* and *in vivo*. Immunohistochemical surveys of tissue sections have shown that human endothelial cells contain t-PA but not u-PA (Kristensen et al., 1984). *In vitro*, human endothelial cells produce t-PA in primary cultures (Philips et al., 1984); at later culture passages, they release both t-PA and u-PA into the culture medium (Levin and Loskutoff, 1982a,b). Preparations containing angiogenic activity, such as bovine retinal extract (D'Amore et al., 1981), mouse adipocyte-conditioned medium (Castellot et al., 1980), a human hepatoma cell line lysate (Zetter, 1980), and, more recently, a human placental extract (Moscatelli et al. 1986), have been shown to promote production of PA and latent collagenase by endothelial cells. This effect appears to be more pronounced with capillary endothelial cells than with large-vessel endothelial cells (Zetter, 1980). The same angiogenic preparations also incude increased cell motility and proliferation at concentrations that correlate reasonably well with those needed to stimulate PA and latent collagenase production (Gross et al., 1983). Mitogens that are not angiogenic, such as insulin, EGF, and PDGF, do not induce increased production of PA and/or collagenase in endothelial cells. It has therefore been postulated that PA as well as collagenase production are essential for angiogenesis to occur, as it may provide high levels of localized proteolytic activity necessary for capillary endothelial cells to degrade the extracellular matrix and penetrate into the tissue to be vascularized (Gross et al., 1983) (see also Chapter 15).

The importance of PA in angiogenesis is also supported by other observations both in vitro and in vivo. Plasma-derived fibrinolytic agents interact with extracellular matrix components and play an important role in the maintenance of vascular integrity. The extracellular matrix, treated with plasmin or trypsin, stimulates rapid organization of human endothelial cells into tubular structures that resemble capillaries (Maciag, 1984); this observation has generated the hypothesis that extracellular matrix degradation initiates a cascade of events that modulate angiogenesis. In this context, it must be considered that in vivo PA, as well as other proteinases, may originate from a variety of cell types, such as granulocytes, macrophages, and fibroblasts, present in the wound area well before angiogenesis actually begins. A sort of cell cooperation, mediated by fibrinolytic enzymes, can therefore be established. Fibronectin and fibronectin fragments have been shown in vitro to be chemotactic for mammalian cells, including endothelial cells (Bowersox and Sorgente, 1982); PA, fibrin, and fibrin degradation products have been demonstrated to be potent stimulators of angiogenesis in vivo (Alessandri et al., 1983). All these factors are actually produced very early after tissue injury. Fibronectin, a major component of the extracellular matrix, is known to be covalently crosslinked to fibrin by activated transglutaminase (factor XIIIa) and to be present in the fibrin clot in a high concentration. Thus, as soon as clot lysis is initiated by the PA in the wound region, fibrin and fibronectin peptides are released in the lesion and may begin to promote angiogenesis by attracting capillary endothelial cells from the damaged vessels and favoring their organization into new capillaries. This view of a cell cooperation in angiogenesis is also supported by a number of reports describing interactions between leukocytes or leukocyte products (interleukins) and microvascular endothelial cells in immune responses (Montesano et al., 1984) (see also Chapter 15).

Indications exist that PA may play a role in the process of re-epithelialization. PA is produced by cultured human epidermal cells (Hashimoto et al., 1983). In cultures of differentiating mouse keratinocytes, the amount of cell-associated PA increases with advanced differentiation. The level of the enzyme then decreases shortly after squame production, and the highest PA levels are found in the squames that have detached from the culture surface. These observations have led to the suggestion that endogenous keratinocyte PA and the subsequent generation of plasmin may facilitate the terminal differentiative events of nuclear dissolution, that characterize keratinocyte differentiation, and be responsible for squame detachment (Risch et al., 1980; Isseroff et al., 1983).

2.2.3. Matrix Formation and Remodeling

In the process of constant remodeling that takes place in the months following the formation of granulation tissue, the elimination of fibronectin from the early extracellular matrix is accomplished by proteinases secreted by the cells present in the wound area. The involvement of the PA–plasmin system in this process is suggested by its similarity with other physiologic processes in which the secretion of PA has been associated with tissue remodeling. Examples are mammary involution following lactation, ovulation, embryo implantation and trophoblast formation, and postpartum uterine involution (Ossowski et al., 1973; 1979; Beers, 1975; Strickland and Beers, 1976; Larsson et al., 1984; Ny et al., 1985; Reich et al., 1985; Shimada et al., 1985). The production of PA by Sertoli cells has also been proposed as a mechanism of tissue remodeling that takes place during spermatogenesis (Fritz et al., 1982; Vihko et al., 1984). Moreover, the ability of plasmin to activate procollagenase may be a key feature in the control of connective tissue turnover (for review, see Senior, 1983).

3. Collagenases

Collagen is the predominant structural protein in all connective tissues of the human organism, including the skin. While as many as 10 distinct genetic types of collagen have been isolated and characterized, all share one feature in common: they are constructed of three polypeptide chains arranged in a ropelike triple-helical conformation. This triple-helical structure, which confers upon collagen its biologic property of high tensile strength, also provides the molecule with an extraordinary degree of resistance to degradation by proteolytic enzymes (see also Chapter 20). Collagenases may be defined as a class of proteinases having the unique ability to cleave the triple helix of collagen at neutral pH under nondenaturing conditions. Thus, common enzymes such as elastase, trypsin, chymotrypsin, and pepsin are unable to cleave most native collagens but readily attack the same substrates when the triple-helical structure is disrupted by thermal denaturation (gelatin). Similarly, the cathepsins are unable to degrade native collagen at neutral pH but have the capacity to cleave the collagen triple helix in an acidic environment, a phenomenon which may be relevant to osteoclast-mediated resorption of the organic matrix of bone (Burleigh et al., 1974).

3.1. Collagenase Specificity

Collagenases may be classified according to the types of collagen they attack. The interstitial collagenases, the designation given the major group of enzymes isolatable from different connective tissue cells and explants of a variety of mammalian organisms, catalyze the cleavage of collagen types I, II, and III (McCroskery et al., 1975; Woolley et al., 1978; Welgus et al., 1981a, 1983). Significantly, basement membrane collagen (type IV) and type V collagen (a pericellular collagen) are resistant to their action. The interstitial collagenase produced by human dermal fibroblasts is the principal collagenolytic enzyme found in skin and is responsible for the turnover of type I and II collagens, the predominant collagens present in this tissue (Welgus *et al.*, 1981a). Type IV-specific collagenases produced by a mouse bone sarcoma (Salo *et al.*, 1983; Fessler *et al.*, 1984) and by human monocytes (Garbisq *et al.*, 1986) have been extensively characterized; these enzymes cleave basement membrane collagen but do not degrade collagen types I, II, III, or V. The secretion of collagenolytic proteinases, which specifically cleave type V collagen, is released by human macrophages (Hibbs *et al.*, 1985) and human sarcoma cell lines (Liotta *et al.*, 1981). However, these enzymes also possess substantial activity against a variety of denatured collagens or gelatins (Mainardi *et al.*, 1985) and have comparatively less activity against native type V collagen; thus, their physiologic significance is unclear. Degradation of the minor collagens, types VI–X, has not been extensively studied, although types VIII and X are reportedly susceptible to interstitial collagenase cleavage (Sage *et al.*, 1983; Schmidt *et al.*, 1986).

The interstitial collagenases degrade susceptible type I, II, and III collagens by a common mechanism: catalyzing the cleavage of a single peptide bond in the three α-chains of each native substrate molecule (Gross and Nagai, 1965; Gross *et al.*, 1974) (Fig. 1). The locus of this proteolytic event is approximately three-fourths the distance from the NH_2-terminal of collagen and involves the scission of either a Gly-Leu (α_2) or Gly-Ile (α_1) bond. The resultant three-quarter-length cleavage product is given the designation TC^A and the one-quarter-length fragment TC^B. At a temperature of 25°C, these digestion products retain their triple-helical conformation and no further catalysis occurs. Physiologic temperature (37°C), however, is significantly above the melting points of both fragments, and TC^A and TC^B spontaneously denature into randomly coiled gelatin peptides (Sakai and Gross, 1967). With the loss of triple-helical structure, these collagenase digestion products are susceptible to further degradation by a wide variety of proteinases (Seltzer *et al.*, 1981; Rantala-Ryhanen *et al.*, 1983).

Since many other Gly-Leu and Gly-Ile bonds are found throughout the type I collagen molecule, the question arises as to why only the single bond at the ¾ : ¼ locus is attacked by collagenase. Renaturation studies performed on collagen peptides following Staph V8 protease digestion indicate that the triple helix of collagen, although intact in this susceptible region, is probably less tightly coiled than in other areas of the molecule, thus permitting enzyme access to this specific substrate site (Highberger *et al.*, 1979). Kinetic studies have demonstrated that the single cleavage in native type I collagen catalyzed by collagenase not only initiates collagen degradation but is also its rate-limiting step (Welgus *et al.*, 1980, 1981a,b, 1982).

3.2. Collagenase Structure and Function

Several common features of the protein structure of interstitial collagenases can be illustrated by examining the prototypic fibroblast collagenase from human skin. This collagenase is a neutral metalloproteinase that exhibits max-

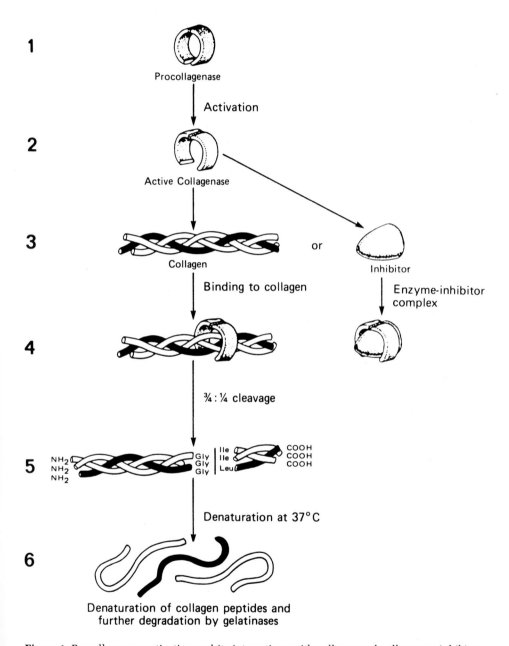

Figure 1. Procollagenase activation and its interactions with collagen and collagenase inhibitor.

imal activity at a neutral pH and contains a zinc atom intrinsically associated with the molecule (Seltzer et al., 1977). Calcium is required as an extrinsic factor for enzyme activity and also provides thermal stability for the proteinase at physiologic temperatures (Seltzer et al., 1976). Perhaps most importantly, collagenases are synthesized and secreted into the extracellular space in zymogen form; human skin procollagenase does not possess catalytic activity and is furthermore unable to bind to the collagen substrate (Stricklin et al., 1977, 1978). Procollagenase can be activated in the laboratory by a proteolytic mechanism involving exposure to trypsin. Trypsin cleaves a 10,000-M_r fragment from the procollagenase molecule, which activates the enzyme (Stricklin et al., 1983a). Plasmin is similarly capable of activating human fibroblast procolleganse (Werb et al., 1977). A specific activator of the procollagenase zymogen has been described in explants of human skin (Tyree et al., 1981), which appears to induce a conformational change in the procollagenase molecule, resulting in catalytic activity without altering the proenzyme's molecular weight. To complicate the situation further, human skin procollagenase is probably capable of activating itself by an autocatalytic mechanism, once a change in its conformation has been induced by heating to 37°C, freeze-thawing, or exposure to chaotropic agents (Stricklin et al., 1977, 1978). Which, if any, of these mechanisms—cleavage by other proteinases, specific activators, or autoactivation—is responsible for the physiologic activation of procollagenase is unknown. Nevertheless, it is crucial to the understanding of human collagen degradation that collagenases are released from both resident fibroblasts and migrating inflammatory cells in an inactive or zymogen form.

Complicating the picture further, human skin fibroblast procollagenase is secreted as a doublet of 55,000 and 60,000 M_r (Stricklin et al., 1977, 1978). In fact, all nonhuman interstitial collagenases as well as rabbit synovial procollagenase occur as doublets (Nagase et al., 1983). Both the 55,000- and 60,000-M_r procollagenase species have been separated chromatographically and they possess equal collagenolytic activity. The preponderance of evidence for both human skin fibroblast and rabbit synovial procollagenases indicate that the protein structure of each doublet species is very similar, if not identical, and that the higher molecular weight form differs only in that it is partially glycosylated (Nagase et al., 1983; Wilhelm et al., 1986). Recently, isolation of a complementary DNA (cDNA) for human skin fibroblast collagenase has permitted determination of the complete primary structure of this molecule (Goldberg et al., 1986).

Interstitial collagenases from other human connective tissues appear to be immunologically and functionally similar, if not identical, to human skin fibroblast collagenase. Thus, the collagenases secreted by human lung fibroblasts, corneal fibroblasts, gingival fibroblasts, uterine smooth muscle cells, and alveolar macrophages in culture react with immunologic identity to antibody prepared from the human skin enzyme, in double immunodiffusion, and in immunoblot assays, and all are catalytically indistinguishable (Welgus et al., 1985a,b; Wilhelm et al., 1985). A notable exception is the collagenase produced by polymorphonuclear leukocytes. Unlike the other human interstitial collagenases, which are not stored intracellularly to a significant extent (Valle and Bauer, 1979), neutrophil collagenase is contained within neutrophil-specific granules. Therefore, its release is governed by factors regulating degranulation of specific granules (Murphy *et al.*, 1982). More importantly, neutrophil collagenase is catalytically different from fibroblast collagenase in its preferential degradation of monomeric type I over type III collagen (Horwitz *et al.*, 1977) (fibroblast collagenase has the opposite specificity) and is readily distinguishable from the fibroblast enzyme by both monoclonal and polyclonal antibody preparations (Hasty *et al.*, 1984, 1986).

3.3. Regulation of Collagenolytic Activity

Regulation of collagen degradation is undoubtedly a complex physiologic process that involves a multitude of biologic events. Control may be achieved by regulating the biosynthesis of procollagenase, its secretion from the cell, zymogen activation in the extracellular space, or via the presence of specific inhibitory proteins. A number of physiologic and pharmacologic modulators of collagenase biosynthesis have been identified.

Perhaps the most extensively studied stimulator of collagenase production in human fibroblasts is mononuclear cell factor (MCF) or interleukin-1 (IL-1). Dayer *et al.* (1977, 1979) demonstrated that monocytes/macrophages isolated from human blood and incubated for one or more days in culture release a soluble factor into culture medium (MCF, IL-1, 15,000–20,000 M_r), which stimulates collagenase production by cultured rheumatoid synovial cells, up to several hundredfold. Similarly, elegant studies of collagenase expression in the rabbit cornea have demonstrated that stromal cells only produce collagenase when co-cultured with epithelial cells from the same tissue (Johnson-Muller and Gross, 1978; Johnson-Wint, 1980). This capacity of epithelial cells to stimulate collagenase biosynthesis by the stromal cells can be reproduced by a soluble factor present in epithelial cell-conditioned medium. The epithelial cell factor is believed to resemble IL-1. Growth factors such as PDGF, EGF, and transforming growth factor-β (TGF-β) have likewise been shown to stimulate selectively the biosynthesis of procollagenase in human dermal fibroblasts and lung fibroblasts (Chua *et al.*, 1985; Bauer *et al.*, 1985). The physiologic roles of soluble mediators such as IL-1 and PDGF in collagen turnover remain to be defined, but these factors are likely to be involved in some capacity during the wound-healing process.

Substances that selectively inhibit collagenase biosynthesis include the glucocorticoids, retinoid compounds, and phenytoin. Low concentrations of dexamethasone or hydrocortisone (10^{-6}–10^{-8} M) have been shown to inhibit the production of collagenase in cultures of human skin, rat uterus (Koob *et al.*, 1974), and mouse macrophages (Werb *et al.*, 1978). The retinoid compounds, including the naturally occurring all-trans-retinoic acid and synthetic analogues such as 13-*cis*-retinoic acid, also inhibit collagenase biosynthesis selectively, i.e. without interfering with general protein synthesis. In cultures of human skin fibroblasts (Bauer *et al.*, 1982) and rheumatoid synovial cells (Brinckerhoff *et al.*, 1980), retinoic acid derivatives decrease collagenase production by approximately 70% at concentrations (10^{-6}–10^{-7} M) that are not toxic to the cells and that are pharmacologically achievable. Of potential importance, an additive effect of glucocorticoids and retinoids on collagenase production *in vitro* has been demonstrated; a 10^{-10} M concentration of either drug alone has no effect on collagenase synthesis, but both drugs added together each at 10^{-0} M inhibit enzyme release by 50% (Brinckerhoff *et al.*, 1981). Another drug, phenytoin, which diminishes collagenase synthesis by 50–60% at concentrations attained clinically, has been used with some success in the long-term treatment of recessive dystrophic epidermolysis bullosa, an hereditary blistering disorder that may be pathogenically related to an excessive release of collagenase from the dermal fibroblasts of afflicted patients (Bauer *et al.*, 1980).

Regulation of collagenase activity can be achieved not only by modulating enzyme biosynthesis but also via the action of collagenase inhibitors. Collagenase inhibitors can be classified according to whether they are found in serum or are produced locally by connective tissues. The principal collagenase inhibitor present in human blood is α_2-macroglobulin, a molecule that irreversibly binds not only collagenase but any active proteinase that gains access to the blood (Eisen *et al.*, 1970). The mechanism of inhibition by α_2-macroglobulin involves hydrolysis by the proteinase of a susceptible bait region in one of the four polypeptide chains of α_2-macroglobulin, with subsequent trapping of the enzyme within this large molecule (Barrett, 1981). The physiologic role of α_2-macroglobulin appears to involve the prevention of proteinase activity within the bloodstream and the restriction of enzyme access to distant tissue sites.

In order to be biologically effective in regulating connective tissue turnover, collagenase inhibitors must be located in the extracellular spaces of specific tissue sites. Such tissue-derived inhibitors of collagenase have been identified in a variety of explants and monolayer cultures of mammalian connective tissue cells (Vater *et al.*, 1979a; Cawston *et al.*, 1981; Stricklin and Welgus, 1983). These inhibitors appear to constitute a distinct biochemical class of glycoproteins that share properties of similar molecular weight (25,000–30,000), resistance to environmental extremes of pH and temperature, and a spectrum of inhibition that includes not only collagenase but also other metalloproteinases of connective tissue origin (Murphy *et al.*, 1981), such as proteoglycanase and gelatinase, hence the designation tissue inhibitors of metalloproteinases (TIMP). TIMP are unable to bind the zymogen forms of such metalloproteinases but complex readily with active collagenase, exhibiting a 1:1 molar stoichiometry of inhibition (1 enzyme molecule–1 inhibitor molecule) (Welgus and Stricklin, 1983) and an extremely high affinity for susceptible proteinases ($K_i \sim 10^{-10}$ M). The TIMP elaborated by human skin fibroblasts has been purified to homogeneity, and its structural stability appears to be explained by a high disulfide bond content, approximately 6% of the molecule (Stricklin and Welgus, 1983; Carmichael *et al.*, 1986). It seems likely that this inhibitory molecule plays a crucial role in regulating matrix turnover throughout the body; glycoproteins immunologically and functionally identical to the skin fibroblast inhibitor are produced by human lung, gingival, tendon, and corneal fibroblasts, by human osteoblasts, by uterine smooth muscle cells, and by alveolar macrophages (Welgus et al., 1985a; Welgus and Stricklin, 1983; Bar-Shavit et al., 1985). Such a molecule has also been identified in human amniotic fluid and in plasma and serum, where it is given the designation β_1-anticollagenase (Woolley et al., 1976). Recently, this same collagenase inhibitor has also been localized to the α-granule of human platelets (Cooper et al., 1985), where its function probably includes a role in the early phases of wound repair. The complete primary structure of human TIMP has been reported using recombinant technology (Docherty et al., 1985; Carmichael et al., 1986).

The catalytic properties of human skin fibroblast collagenase have been extensively studied; several key findings have emerged that may be relevant to understanding collagen degradation in vivo. It is apparent that enzymatic cleavage of the collagen molecule is a very slow process; the calculated value for the turnover number on type I collagen fibrils, the predominant collagen found in skin and the physiologic form of substrate, is only 25 molecules of collagen cleaved per molecule of collagenase per hour at 37°C (Welgus et al., 1980). Therefore, this enzyme catalyzes the proteolytic scission of approximately one α-chain of a collagen molecule every 45 sec. Furthermore, the state of aggregation of the collagen substrate has profound effects on rates of collagenolysis. After individual collagen molecules assemble in the extracellular space into a fibrillar structure, they are covalently crosslinked to one another by the action of the enzyme, lysyl oxidase. Covalent crosslinks not only increase the insolubility of collagen and enhance the tensile strength of the protein but also decrease its susceptibility to proteolytic attack. It has been possible to introduce known amounts of crosslinks into reconstituted collagen fibrils formed in vitro; as few as 0.1 crosslinks per molecule of collagen markedly increase the resistance of this substrate to proteolytic cleavage by human rheumatoid synovial collagenase (Vater et al., 1979b).

Small changes in temperature also affect rates of collagen degradation to a surprising extent. The rate of most enzyme-catalyzed reactions increases two- to threefold for each 10°C change in ambient temperature. By contrast, between the temperatures of 37° and 39°C, human skin fibroblast collagenase increases its cleavage of native type I collagen fibrils by threefold. Over a 5°C temperature change, which could accompany severe inflammation such as within a rheumatoid joint, rates of collagenolysis would be expected to vary by 15-fold. Both the slow rate of collagen degradation by human skin collagenase and the extreme dependence of this reaction process on temperature (energy) are the consequences of the unique triple-helical structure of the collagen molecule and the nature of its aggregation into insoluble fibrils (Welgus et al., 1981b).

3.4. Collagenase in Human Disease

The role of collagenase in disease states can be divided into two major categories: (1) as a mediator of collagen destruction whereby elevated collagenase levels develop secondary to a complex pathologic process; and (2) where a structural and/or expression defect in collagenase itself is directly responsible for the pathogenesis of a particular disease. The first group comprises a large category that includes a variety of destructive inflammatory conditions (e.g., rheumatoid arthritis) and neoplastic processes, whereas only a single clinical entity, called recessive dystrophic epidermolysis bullosa (RDEB), has been identified in the second group. Since collagenases catalyze both the initial and rate-limiting step in collagen degradation, it is not surprising that diseases associated with excessive connective tissue matrix destruction mediate such damage via the presence of overabundant local production of collagenase. Thus, in disorders such as rheumatoid arthritis (Harris *et al.*, 1970), periodontal disease (Birkedal-Hansen, 1980), and alkali burns of the cornea (Brown and Weller, 1971), the severity of connective tissue destruction has been correlated with elevated levels of collagenase that presumably produce such damage.

An increase in the number of fibroblastic cells synthesizing procollagenase, the presence of a variety of inflammatory cells, the release of soluble factors that induce the biosynthesis of new enzymes, the presence of high levels of noncollagenolytic proteinases capable of zymogen activation, and the saturation or inactivation of tissue inhibitors are all factors of potential importance in excessive collagen breakdown in these disease states. Thus, it must be emphasized that such disorders represent extremely complex pathologic processes whereby excessive collagenase activity is one of the final mediators of tissue destruction but that result only after a long series of biologic events that are etiologically more relevant to the intrinsic disease process. Similarly, high levels of collagenase are produced by certain basal cell carcinomas (Bauer *et al.*, 1977), squamous cell carcinomas (Hashimoto *et al.*, 1973), and mammary carcinomas (Bauer and Eisen, 1978). While this increased production of enzyme presumably mediates some of the local destructive and invasive properties of such tumors, it nevertheless reflects the abnormal expression of only one protein in the extremely complex process of neoplasia.

By contrast, RDEB, an hereditary blistering disorder of the skin, may represent a true disease of collagenase. Skin fibroblasts from such patients produce increased amounts of collagenase protein (Bauer and Eisen, 1978), which is correlated with increased translatable collagenase-specific messenger RNA (mRNA) as compared with normal cells or to cells from other genetic variants of epidermolysis bullosa (Kronberger *et al.*, 1982). The collagenase purified from RDEB cells is similar to the enzyme secreted by normal fibroblasts with respect to molecular weight and catalytic properties. However, the RDEB collagenase has a slightly different amino acid composition, a different peptide pattern following cyanogen bromide digestion, and a much lower affinity for the cofactor Ca^{2+} essential for enzymatic activity and stability (Stricklin *et al.*, 1983b). Thus, blister formation in RDEB may be related directly to fibroblast overproduction of a structurally mutant collagenase. It should be mentioned, however, that skin from such patients also contains a greatly diminished number of anchoring fibrils, a finding that may have pathologic relevance to the etiology of this disease process as well.

The role of collagenolytic activity in the wound-healing process is largely speculative. Nevertheless, it seems likely that both the interstitial collagenase and the tissue inhibitor produced by skin fibroblasts must play an active role in dermal repair. Similarly, soluble factors secreted by the overlying regenerating epidermis (e.g., ETAF or IL-I) may be capable of modulating levels of certain proteins (e.g., collagenase) responsible for controlling collagen turnover. Recently, collagenases specific for the degradation of type IV collagen were shown to be released both by migrating epidermal cells (Woodley et al., 1982) and by dermal fibroblasts (Salo et al., 1985). Such proteinases may serve to control the remodeling of the basement membrane zone, the critical area between epidermis and dermis, during the wound-healing process (see also Chapter 23).

4. Hyaluronidase

Studies in several organs during morphogenesis, regeneration, and repair have indicated that a hyaluronate-rich extracellular matrix promotes cell proliferation and migration, whereas a decrease in hyaluronic acid and a parallel increase in sulfated proteoglycans favors the differentiation of the previously migrated or proliferated cells (Reid and Flint, 1974; Bertolami and Donoff, 1978; Toole, 1982; Belsky and Toole, 1983; for review, see Stern, 1984) (see Chapter 19). It has therefore been proposed that hyaluronidase may influence the process of wound repair by affecting the turnover of hyaluronate in the extracellular matrix. Increases in hyaluronidase have been reported in experimental wound healing of skin (Bertolami and Donoff, 1978, 1982). In rabbits, hyaluronidase activity was detected in open granulation tissue subsequent to postwound day 7. The activity increased fivefold between days 7 and 14. No hyaluronidase activity was detectable earlier in the reparative process or in normal rabbit skin. This increase in hyaluronidase activity was paralleled by a 50% decrease in the amount of hyaluronate present in granulation tissue between postwound days 7 and 14, suggesting a functioning degradative system during the second week of healing.

Skin wound hyaluronidase has been partially purified and characterized (Bertolami and Donoff, 1982). Both the crude and purified enzyme appear to have endoglycosidic activity on hyaluronate and chondroitin 4-sulfate, but not on chondroitin 6-sulfate. The optimum pH for enzyme activity is 4.5. The cells responsible for the secretion of this enzyme have not been identified. Since the optimum pH of granulocyte hyaluronidase is 3.7 (Tynelius-Bratthal and Attstrom, 1973) and that of rabbit macrophage hyaluronidase 3.9 (Goggins et al., 1968), it is doubtful that blood leukocytes are the source of skin wound hyaluronidase. Furthermore, wound hyaluronidase activity was at a maximum when inflammatory infiltrates were virtually absent. The characteristics of the hyaluronate degradation products released also appeared to differentiate it from known bacterial hyaluronidases.

The marked drop in hyaluronate during the second week of wound repair was paralleled by increased levels of dermatan sulfate and chondroitin sulfate, products characteristic of differentiated cells. This finding suggests that in wound healing, as in several developmental systems (Toole and Gross, 1971; Toole and Trelstad, 1971; Toole, 1972; Toole *et al.*, 1972; Thet *et al.*, 1983), hyaluronate degradation by hyaluronidase may precede cell differentiation. The presence of an early hyaluronate-rich matrix may favor the infiltration of migratory cells into the injured tissue. On the contrary, its degradation appears to favor or be related to the differentiation of these cells. However, whether hyaluronidase resorption of hyaluronic acid actually initiates cell differentiation during tissue repair, as well as in regeneration and morphogenesis, is merely speculative and still calls for experimental proof.

ACKNOWLEDGMENTS. The authors would like to thank the National Institutes of Health, the American Cancer Society, and the Italian Association for Cancer Research for their support.

References

Alessandri, G., Rajn, K., and Gullino, P. M., 1983, Mobilization of capillary endothelium *in vitro* induced by effectors of angiogenesis *in vivo*, *Cancer Res.* **43**:1790–1797.

Andreasen, P. A., Nielsen, L. S., Grøndahl-Hansen, J., Zenthen, J., Stephens, R., and Danø, K., 1984, Inactive proenzyme to tissue-type plasminogen activator from human melanoma cells identified after affinity purification with a monoclonal antibody, *EMBO J.* **3**:51–56.

Bachman, F., Fletcher, A. P., Alkjaersig, N., and Sherry, S., 1964, Partial purification and properties of the plasminogen activator from pig heart, *Biochemistry* **3**:1578–1585.

Baker, J. B., Low, D. A., Simmer, R. L., and Cunningham, D. D., 1980, Protease nexin: A cellular component that links thrombin and plasminogen activator and mediates their binding to cells, *Cell* **21**:37–45.

Baker, M. E., 1985, Human tissue plasminogen activator is related to albumin and alpha-fetoprotein, *FEBS Lett.* **182**:47–52.

Banyai, L., Varadi, A., and Patthy, L., 1983, Common evolutionary origin of the fibrin-binding structures of fibronectin and tissue-type plasminogen activator, *FEBS Lett.* **163**:37–41.

Bar-Shavit, Z., Teitelbaum, S. L., Stricklin, G. P., Eisen, A. Z., Kahn, A. J., and Welgus, H. G., 1985, Differentiation of a human leukemia cell line and expression of collagenase inhibitor, *Proc. Natl. Acad. Sci. USA* **82**:5380–5384.

Barrett, A. J., 1981, α_2-Macroglobulin, *Methods Enzymol.* **80**:737–754.

Bauer, E. A., and Eisen, A. Z., 1978, Recessive dystrophic epidermolysis bullosa: Evidence for increased collagenase as a genetic characteristic in cell culture, *J. Exp. Med.* **148**:1378–1387.

Bauer, E. A., Gordon, J. M., Reddick, M. E., and Eisen, A. Z., 1977, Quantitation and immunocytochemical localization of human skin collagenase in basal cell carcinoma, *J. Invest. Dermatol.* **69**:363–367.

Bauer, E. A., Cooper, T. W., Tucker, D. R., and Esterly, N. B., 1980, Phenytoin theory of recessive dystrophic epidermolysis bullosa: Clinical trial and proposed mechanism of action on collagenase, *N. Engl. J. Med.* **303**:776–781.

Bauer, E. A., Seltzer, J. L., and Eisen, A. Z., 1982, Inhibition of collagen degradative enzymes by retinoic acid *in vitro*, *J. Am. Acad. Dermatol.* **6**:603–607.

Bauer, E. A., Cooper, T. W., Huang, J. S., Altman, J., and Deuel, T. F., 1985, Stimulation of *in vitro* human skin collagenase expression by platelet-derived growth factor, *Proc. Natl. Acad. Sci. USA* **82**:4132–4135.

Beers, W. H., 1975, Follicular plasminogen and plasminogen activator and the effect of plasmin on ovarian follicle wall, *Cell* **6**:379–386.

Belsky, E., and Toole, B. P., 1983, Hyaluronate and hyaluronidase in the developing chick embryo kidney, *Cell. Diff.* **12**:61–66.

Berman, M., Leary, R., and Gage, J., 1980, Evidence for a role of the plasminogen-plasmin system in corneal ulceration, *Invest. Ophthalmol. Vis. Sci.* **19**:1204–1221.

Bertolami, C. N., and Donoff, R. B., 1978, Hyaluronidase activity during open wound healing in rabbits: A preliminary report, *J. Surg. Res.* **25**:256–259.

Bertolami, C. N., and Donoff, R. B., 1982, Identification, characterization and partial purification of mammalian skin wound hyaluronidase, *J. Invest. Dermatol.* **79**:417–421.

Birkedal-Hansen, H., 1980, Collagenase in periodontal disease, in: *Collagenase in Normal and Pathological Connective Tissues* (D. E. Woolley and J. M. Evanson, eds.), pp. 128–140, Wiley, New York.

Bouma, B. N., and Griffin, J. H., 1978, Deficiency of Factor XII-dependent plasminogen proactivator in prekallikrein-deficient plasma, *J. Lab. Clin. Med.* **91**:148–155.

Bouma, B. N., Miles, L. A., Beretta, G., and Griffin, J. H., 1980, Human plasma prekallikrein. Studies of its activation by activated Factor XII and its inactivation by diisopropylphosphofluoridate, *Biochemistry* **19**:1151–1160.

Bowersox, J. C., and Sorgente, N., 1982, Chemotaxis of aortic endothelial cells in response to fibronectin, *Cancer Res.* **42**:2547–2551.

Brinckherhoff, C. E., McMillan, R. M., Dayer, J. M., and Harris, E. D., Jr., 1980, Inhibition by retinoic acid of collagenase production in rheumatoid synovial cells, *New Engl. J. Med.* **303**:432–436.

Brinckherhoff, C. E., Vater, C. A., and Harris, E. D., Jr., 1981, Effects of retinoids on rabbit synovial fibroblasts and chondrocytes, in: *Cellular Interactions* (J. T. Dingle and J. Gordon, eds.), pp. 215–230, Elsevier/North-Holland, New York.

Brown, S. I., and Weller, C. H., 1971, The pathogenesis and treatment of collagenase-induced diseases of the cornea, *Trans. Am. Acad. Ophthalmol. Otolaryngol.* **74**:375–382.

Burk, R. R., 1973, A factor from a transformed cell line that affects cell migration, *Proc. Natl. Acad. Sci. USA* **70**:369–372.

Burleigh, M. C., Barrett, A. J., and Lazarus, G. S., 1974, A lysosomal enzyme that degrades native collagen, *Biochem. J.* **137**:387–398.

Carmichael, D. F., Sommer, A., Thompson, R. C., Anderson, D. C., Smith, C. G., Welgus, H. G., and Stricklin, G. P., 1986, Primary structure and cDNA cloning of human fibroblast collagenase inhibitor, *Proc. Natl. Acad. Sci. USA* **83**:2407–2411.

Castellot, J. J., Jr., Karnovsky, M. J., and Spiegelman, B. M., 1980, Potent stimulation of vascular endothelial cell growth by differentiated 3T3 adipocytes. *Proc. Natl. Acad. Sci. USA* **77**:6007–6011.

Cawston, T. E., Galloway, W. A., Mercer, E., Murphy, G., and Reynolds, J. J., 1981, Purification of rabbit bone inhibitor of collagenase, *Biochem. J.* **195**:159–165.

Chapman, H. A., and Stone, O. L., Jr., 1984, Cooperation between plasmin and elastase in elastin degradation by intact murine macrophages, *Biochem. J.* **222**:721–728.

Christensen, L. R., 1945, Streptococcal fibrinolysis: A proteolytic reaction due to a serum enzyme activated by streptococcal fibrinolysin, *J. Gen. Physiol.* **23**:363–383.

Chua, C., Geisman, D., Keller, G., and Ladda, R., 1985, Induction of collagenase secretion in human fibroblast cultures by growth promoting factors, *J. Biol. Chem.* **260**:5213–5216.

Clarke, G. D., Stoker, M. G. P., Ludlow, A., and Thorton, M., 1970, Requirement of serum for DNA synthesis in BHK 21 cells: Effects of density, suspension and virus transformation, *Nature (Lond.)* **227**:798–801.

Collen, D., 1980, The regulation and control of fibrinolysis. Edward Kowalski memorial lecture, *Thromb. Haemost.* **43**:77–89.

Collen, D., 1983, Mechanisms of activation of tissue-type plasminogen activator in blood, *Thromb. Haemost.* **50**:678.

Colman, R. W., 1969, Activation of plasminogen by human plasma kallikrein, *Biochem. Biophys. Res. Commun.* **35**:273–279.

Conanan, L. B., and Crutchley, D. J., 1983, Serum-dependent induction of plasminogen activator in human fibroblasts by catecholamines and comparison with the effects of prostaglandin E$_1$, *Biochim. Biophys. Acta* **759**:146–153.

Cooper, T. W., Eisen, A. Z., Stricklin, G. P., and Welgus, H. G., 1985, Platelet-derived collagenase inhibitor: Characterization and subcellular localization, *Proc. Natl. Acad. Sci. USA* **82**:2771–2783.

D'Amore, P. A., Glaser, B. M., Brunson, S. K., and Fenselau, A. H., 1981, Angiogenic activity from bovine retina: Partial purification and characterization, *Proc. Natl. Acad. Sci. USA* **78**:3068–3072.

Danø, K., and Reich, E., 1978, Serine enzymes released by cultured neoplastic cells, *J. Exp. Med.* **147**:745–757.

Danø, K., Andreasen, P. A., Grøndahl-Hansen, J., Kristensen, P., Nielsen, L. S., and Skriver, L., 1985, Plasminogen activators, tissue degradation and cancer, *Adv. Cancer Res.* **44**:139–266.

Danø, K., Nielsen, L. S., Møller, V., and Engelhart, M., 1980, Inhibition of a plasminogen activator from oncogenic virus-transformed cells by rabbit antibodies against the enzyme, *Biochim. Biophys. Acta* **630**:146–151.

Dayer, J. M., Breard, J., Chess, L., and Krane, S. M., 1979, Participation of monocyte–macrophages and lymphocytes in the production of a factor that stimulates collagenase and prostaglandin release by rheumatoid synovium, *J. Clin. Invest.* **64**:1386–1392.

Dayer, J. M., Russell, R. G. G., and Krane, S. M., 1977, Collagenase production by rheumatoid synovial cells: Stimulation by a human lymphocyte factor, *Science* **195**:181–183.

Docherty, A. J., Lyons, A., Smith, B. J., Wright, E. M., Stephens, P. E., Harris, T. J. R., Murphy, G., and Reynolds, J. J., 1985, Sequence of human tissue inhibitor of metalloproteinases and its identity to erythroid-potentiating activity, *Nature (Lond.)* **318**:66–69.

Dunn, F. W., Deguchi, K., Soria, J., Lijnen, H. R., Tobelem, G., and Caen, J., 1984, Importance of the interaction between plasminogen and fibrin for plasminogen activation by tissue-type plasminogen activator, *Thromb. Res.* **36**:345–351.

Eaton, D. L., and Baker, J. B., 1983, Phorbol ester and mitogens stimulate human fibroblast secretion of plasmin-activatable plasminogen activator and protease nexin, an antiactivator/antiplasmin, *J. Cell Biol.* **97**:323–328.

Eaton, D. L., Scott, R. W., and Baker, J. B., 1984, Purification of human fibroblast urokinase proenzyme and analysis of its regulation by proteases and protease nexin, *J. Biol. Chem.* **259**:6241–6247.

Edlund, T., Ny, T., Ranby, M., Heden, L. O., Palm, G., Holmgren, E., and Josephson, S., 1983, Isolation of cDNA sequences coding for a part of human tissue plasminogen activator, *Proc. Natl. Acad. Sci. USA* **80**:349–352.

Eisen, A. Z., Block, K. L., and Sakai, T., 1970, Inhibition of human skin collagenase by human serum, *J. Lab. Clin. Med.* **75**:258–263.

Erickson, L. A., Ginsberg, M. H., and Luskutoff, D. J., 1984, Detection and partial characterization of an inhibitor of plasminogen acivator in human platelets, *J. Clin. Invest.* **74**:1465–1472.

Fernandez, H. N., Henson, P. M., Otani, A., and Hugli, T. E., 1978, Chemotactic response to human C3a and C5a anaphylatoxins. I. Evaluation of C3a and C5a leukotaxis *in vitro* and under simulated *in vivo* conditions, *J. Immunol.* **120**:109–115.

Fessler, L. I., Duncan, K. G., Fessler, J. H., Salo, T., and Tryggvason, K., 1984, Characterization of the procollagen IV cleavage products produced by a specific tumor collagenase, *J. Biol. Chem.* **259**:9783–9789.

Fraki, J. E., Lazarus, G. S., Gilgor, R. S., Marchase, P., and Singer, K. H., 1983, Correlation of epidermal plasminogen activator activity with disease activity in psoriasis, *Br. J. Dermatol.* **108**:39–44.

Fritz, I. B., Parvinen, M., Karmally, K., and Lacroix, M., 1982, Preferential production of testicular plasminogen activator by Sertoli cells in discrete portions (stages VII and VIII) of the seminiferous tubule, *Ann. NY Acad. Sci.* **383**:447–448.

Gallimore, M. J., Farcid, E., and Stormorken, H., 1978, The purification of a human plasma kallikrein with weak plasminogen activator activity, *Thromb. Res.* **12**:409–420.

Garbisq, S., Ballin, M., Gaga-Gordini, D., Fastellio, G., Naturale, M., Negro, A., Semenzato, G., and

Liotta, L. A., 1986, Transient expression of type IV collagenolytic metalloproteinase by human mononuclear phagocytes, *J. Biol. Chem.* **261**:2369–2375.

Goggins, J. F., Lazarus, G. S., and Fullmer, H. M., 1968, Hyaluronidase activity of alveolar macrophages, *J. Histochem. Cytochem.* **16**:688–692.

Goldberg, G. I., Wilhelm, S. M., Kronberger, A., Bauer, E. A., Grant, G. A., and Eisen, A. Z., 1986, Human fibroblast collagenase: complete primary structure and homology to an oncogene transformation-induced rat protein, *J. Biol. Chem.* **261**:6600–6605.

Goldsmith, G. H., Saito, H., and Ratnoff, O. D., 1978, The activation of plasminogen by Hageman Factor (Factor XII) and Hageman Factor fragments, *J. Clin. Invest.* **62**:54–60.

Gordon, S., Unkeless, J. C., and Cohn, Z. A., 1974, Induction of macrophage plasminogen activator by endotoxin stimulation and phagocytosis, *J. Exp. Med.* **140**:995–1010.

Granelli-Piperno, A., and Reich, E., 1983, Plasminogen activators of the pituitary gland: Enzyme characterization and hormonal modulation, *J. Cell Biol.* **97**:1029–1037.

Granelli-Piperno, A., and Reich, E., 1978, A study of proteases and protease-inhibitor complexes in biological fluids, *J. Exp. Med.* **148**:223–234.

Granelli-Piperno, A., Vassalli, J. D., and Reich, E., 1977, Secretion of plasminogen activator by human polymorphonuclear leukocytes. Modulation by glucocorticoids and other effectors, *J. Exp. Med.* **146**:1693–1706.

Gross, J., and Nagai, Y., 1965, Specific degradation of the collagen molecule by tadpole collagenolytic enzyme, *Proc. Natl. Acad. Sci. USA* **54**:1197–1204.

Gross, J., Harper, E., Harris, E. D., Jr., McCroskery, P. A., Highberger, H. H., Corbett, C., and Kang, A. H., 1974, Animal collagenases: Distribution, specificity of action, and structure of the substrate cleavage site. *Biochem. Biophys. Res. Commun.* **61**:605–612.

Gross, J., Moscatelli, D. A., and Rifkin, D. B., 1983, Increased capillary endothelial cell protease activity in response to angiogenic stimuli *in vitro*, *Proc. Natl. Acad. Sci. USA* **80**:2623–2627.

Hamilton, J. A., 1982, Plasminogen activator activity of rheumatoid and non-rheumatoid synovial fibroblasts, *J. Rheumatol.* **9**:834–842.

Hamilton, J. Z., Zabriskie, J. B., Lachman, L. B., and Chen, Y. S., 1982, Streptococcal cell walls and synovial cell activation. Stimulation of synovial fibroblast plasminogen activator activity by monocytes treated with group A streptococcal cell wall sonicates and muramyl dipeptide, *J. Exp. Med.* **155**:1702–1718.

Harris, E. D., Jr., Evanson, J. M., DiBona, D. K., and Krane, S. M., 1970, Collagenase and rheumatoid arthritis, *Arthritis Rheum.* **13**:83–94.

Hashimoto, K., Yamaniski, Y., Maeyens, E., Dabbons, M. K., and Kanzaki, T., 1973, Collagenolytic activities of squamous cell carcinoma of the skin, *Cancer Res.* **33**:2790–2801.

Hashimoto, K., Singer, K., Lide, W. B., Shafran, K., Webber, P., Morioka, S., and Lazarus, G. S., 1983, Plasminogen activator in cultured epidermal cells, *J. Invest. Dermtol.* **81**:424–429.

Hashimoto, K., Singer, K., and Lazarus, G. S., 1984, Penicillamine-induced pemphigus. Immunoglobulin from this patient induces plasminogen activator synthesis by human epidermal cells in culture: Mechanism for acantholysis in pemphigus, *Arch. Dermatol.* **120**:762–764.

Hasty, K. A., Hibbs, M. S., Kang, A. H., and Mainardi, C. L., 1984, Heterogeneity among human collagenases demonstrated by monoclonal antibody that selectively recognizes and inhibits human neutrophil collagense, *J. Exp. Med.* **159**:1455–1463.

Hasty, K. A., Hibbs, M. S., Kang, A. H., and Mainardi, C. L., 1986, Secreted forms of human neutrophil collagenase, *J. Biol. Chem.* **261**:5645–5650.

Heussen, C., Joubert, F., and Dowdle, E. B., 1984, Purification of human tissue plasminogen activator with Erythrina trypsin inhibitor, *J. Biol. Chem.* **259**:11635–11638.

Hibbs, M. S., Hoidal, J. R., and Kang, A. H., 1985, Secretion of a metalloproteinase by human alveolar macrophages which degrades gelatin and native type V collagen, *J. Cell Biol.* **101**:216 (abst).

Highberger, J. H., Corbett, C., and Gross, J., 1979, Isolation and characterization of a peptide containing the site of cleavage of the chick skin collagen α_1 (I) chain by animal collagenase, *Biochem. Biophys. Res. Commun.* **89**:202–208.

Hoal, E. G., Wilson, E. L., and Dowdle, E. B., 1983, The regulation of tissue plasminogen activator activity by human fibroblasts, *Cell* **34**:273–279.

Horwitz, A. L., Hance, A. J., and Crystal, R. G., 1977, Granulocyte collagenase: Selective digestion of type I relative to type III collagen, *Proc. Natl. Acad. Sci. USA* **74**:897–901.

Hoylaerts, M., Rijken, D. C., Lijnen, H. R., and Collen, D., 1982, Kinetics of the activation of plasminogen by human tissue plasminogen activator, *J. Biol. Chem.* **257**:2912–2919.

Ichinose, A., Kisiel, W., and Fjuikawa, K., 1984, Proteolytic activation of tissue plasminogen activator by plasma and tissue enzymes, *FEBS Lett.* **175**:412–418.

Isseroff, R. R., and Rifkin, D. B., 1983, Plasminogen is present in the basal layer of epidermis, *J. Invest. Dermatol.* **80**:297–299.

Isseroff, R. R., Fusenig, N. E., and Rifkin, D. B., 1983, Plasminogen activator in differentiating mouse keratinocytes, *J. Invest. Dermatol.* **80**:217–222.

Johnson-Muller, B., and Gross, J., 1978, Regulation of corneal collagenase production: Epithelial–stromal cell interactions, *Proc. Natl. Acad. Sci. USA* **75**:4417–4421.

Johnson-Wint, B., 1980, Regulation of stromal cell collagenase production in adult rabbit cornea: *In vitro* stimulation and inhibition by epithelial cell products, *Proc. Natl. Acad. Sci. USA* **77**:5331–5335.

Keski-Oja, J., and Vaheri, A., 1982, The cellular target for the plasminogen activator, urokinase, in human fibroblasts—66,000-dalton protein, *Biochim. Biophys. Acta* **720**:141–146.

Koob, T. J., Jeffrey, J. J., and Eisen, A. Z., 1974, Regulation of human skin collagenase activity by hydrocortisone and dexamethasone in organ culture, *Biochem. Biophys. Res. Commun.* **61**:1083–1088.

Kopitar, M., Brzin, J., Babnik, J., Turk, V., and Suhar, A., 1980, Intracellular neutral proteinases and their inhibitors, in: *Enzyme Regulation and Mechanism of Action* (P. Mildner and B. Ries, eds.), pp. 363–375, Pergamon, Oxford.

Kristensen, P., Larsson, L. I., Nielsen, L. S., Grøndal-Hansen, J., Andreasen, P. A., and Danø, K., 1984, Human endothelial cells contain one type of plasminogen activator, *FEBS Lett.* **168**:33–37.

Kronberger, A., Valle, K. J., Eisen, A. Z., and Bauer, E. A., 1982, Enhanced cell-free translation of human skin collagenase in recessive dystrophic epidermolysis bullosa, *J. Invest. Dermatol.* **79**:208–211.

Krystosek, A., and Seeds, N. W., 1984, Peripheral neurons and Schwann cells secrete plasminogen activator, *J. Cell Biol.* **98**:773–776.

Larsson, L. I., Skriver, L., Nielsen, L. S., Grøndahl-Hansen, J., Kristensen, P., and Danø, K., 1984, Distribution of urokinase-type plasminogen activator immunoreactivity in the mouse, *J. Cell Biol.* **98**:894–903.

Lee, L. S., and Weinstein, I. B., 1978, Epidermal growth factor, like phorbol esters, induces plasminogen activator in HeLa cells, *Nature (Lond.)* **274**:696–697.

Levin, E. G., 1983, Latent tissue plasminogen activator produced by human endothelial cells in culture: Evidence for an enzyme-inhibitor complex, *Proc. Natl. Acad. Sci. USA* **80**:6804–6808.

Levin, E. G., and Loskutoff, D. J., 1982a, Cultured bovine endothelial cells produce both urokinase and tissue-type plasminogen activator, *J. Cell Biol.* **94**:631–636.

Levin, E. G., and Loskutoff, D. J., 1982b, Regulation of plasminogen activator production by cultured endothelial cells, *Ann. NY Acad. Sci.* **401**:184–194.

Lin, H. S., and Gordon, S., 1979, Secretion of plasminogen activator by bone marrow-derived mononuclear phagocytes and its enhancement by colony-stimulating factor, *J. Exp. Med.* **150**:231–245.

Liotta, L. A., Lanzer, W. L., and Garbisa, S., 1981, Identification of a type V collagenolytic enzyme, *Biochem. Biophys. Res. Commun.* **98**:184–190.

Lipton, A., Klinger, I., Paul, D., and Holley, R. W., 1971, Migration of mouse 3T3 fibroblasts in response to a serum factor, *Proc. Natl. Acad. Sci. USA* **68**:2799–2801.

Loskutoff, D. J., and Edgington, T. S., 1977, Synthesis of a fibrinolytic activator and inhibitor by endothelial cells, *Proc. Natl. Acad. Sci. USA* **74**:3903–3907.

Loskutoff, D. J., and Edgington, T. S., 1981, An inhibitor of plasminogen activator in rabbit endothelial cells, *J. Biol. Chem.* **256**:4142–4145.

Loskutoff, D. J., van Mourik, J. A., Erickson, L. A., and Lawrence, D., 1983, Detection of an unusually stable fibrinolytic inhibitor produced by bovine endothelial cells, *Proc. Natl. Acad. Sci. USA* **80**:2956–2960.

Maciag, T., 1984, Angiogenesis: The phenomenon, in: *Thrombosis and Haemostasis* (T. H. Spaet, ed.), pp. 167–182, Grune & Stratton, Orlando, Florida.

Mainardi, C. L., Hibbs, M. S., Hasty, K. A., and Seyer, J. M., 1985, Purification of a type V collagen degrading metalloproteinase from rabbit alveolar macrophages, *Collagen Relat. Res.* **4**:479–492.

Mak, W. W. N., Eggo, M. C., and Burrow, G. N., 1984, Thyrotropin regulation of plasminogen activator activity in primary cultures of bovine thyroid cells, *Biochem. Biophys. Res. Commun.* **123**:633–640.

Mandle, R. J., and Kaplan, A. P., 1977, Hageman factor substrates. Human plasma prekallikrein: Mechanism of activation by Hagemen Factor and participation in Hageman factor-dependent fibrinolysis, *J. Biol. Chem.* **252**:6097–6104.

Mandle, R. J., and Kaplan, A. P., 1979, Hageman factor-dependent fibrinolysis: Generation of fibrinolytic activity by the interaction of human activated factor XI and plasminogen, *Blood* **54**:850–862.

Matsuo, O., Rijken, D. C., and Collen, D., 1981, Comparison of the relative fibrinogenolytic, fibrinolytic and thrombolytic properties of tissue plasminogen activator by urokinase *in vitro*, *Thromb. Haemost.* **45**:225–229.

McCroskery, P. A., Richards, J. F., and Harris, E. D., Jr., 1975, Purification and characterization of collagenase extracted from rabbit tumors, *Biochem. J.* **152**:131–142.

McLellan, W. L., Vetterlein, D., and Roblin, R., 1980, The glycoprotein nature of human plasminogen activators, *FEBS Lett.* **115**:181–184.

Miskin, R., and Ben-Ishai, R., 1981, Induction of plasminogen activator by UV light in normal and xeroderma pigmentosum fibroblasts, *Proc. Natl. Acad. Sci. USA* **78**:6236–6240.

Miskin, R., and Reich, E., 1980, Plasminogen activator: Induction of synthesis by DNA damage, *Cell* **19**:217–224.

Montesano, R., Mossaz, A., Ryser, J. E., Orci, L., and Vassalli, P., 1984, Leukocyte interleukins induce cultured endothelial cells to produce a highly organized, glycosaminoglycan-rich pericellular matrix, *J. Cell Biol.* **99**:1706–1715.

Moscatelli, D. A., Presta, M., and Rifkin, D. B., 1986, Purification of a factor from human placenta which stimulates capillary endothelial cell protease production, DNA synthesis and migration, *Proc. Natl. Acad. Sci. USA* **83**:2091–2095.

Mullins, D. E., and Rohrlich, S. T., 1983, The role of proteinases in cellular invasiveness, *Biochim. Biophys. Acta* **695**:177–214.

Murphy, G., McGuire, M. B., Russell, R. G. G., and Reynolds, J. J., 1981, Characterization of collagenase, other metallo-proteinases and an inhibitor (TIMP) produced by human synovium and cartilage in culture, *Clin. Sci.* **61**:711–716.

Murphy, G., Reynolds, J. J., Bretz, V., and Baggiolini, M., 1982, Partial purification of collagenase and gelatinase from human polymorphonuclear leukocytes, *Biochem. J.* **203**:209–221.

Nagase, H., Brinckherhoff, C. L. E., Vater, C. A., and Harris, E. D., Jr., 1983, Biosynthesis and secretion of procollagenase by rabbit synovial fibroblasts. Inhibition of procollagenase secretion by monensin and evidence for glycosylation of procollagenase, *Biochem. J.* **214**:281–288.

Norris, D. A., Clark, R. A. F., Swigart, L. M., Huff, J. C., Weston, W. L., and Howell, S. E., 1982, Fibronectin fragments are chemotactic for human peripheral blood monocytes, *J. Immunol.* **129**:1612–1618.

Ny, T., Bjersing, L., Hsueh, A. J. W., and Loskutoff, D. J., 1985, Cultured granulosa cells produce two plasminogen activators and an anti-activator, each regulated differently by gonadotropins, *Endocrinology* **116**:1666–1668.

Ossowski, L., Biegel, D., and Reich, E., 1979, Mammary plasminogen activator: Correlation with involution, hormonal modulation and comparison between normal and neoplastic tissue, *Cell* **16**:929–940.

Ossowski, L., Quigley, J. P., Kellerman, G. M., and Reich, E., 1973, Fibrinolysis associated with oncogenic transformation. Requirement of plasminogen for correlated changes in cellular morphology, colony formation in agar and cell migration, *J. Exp. Med.* **138**:1056–1064.

Pennica, D., Holmes, W. E., Kohr, W. J., Harkins, R. N., Vehar, G. A., Ward, C. A., Bennet, W. F., Yelverton, E., Seeburg, P. H., Heyneker, H. L., Goeddel, D. V., and Collen, D., 1983, Cloning and expression of human tissue-type plasminogen activator cDNA in E. coli, Nature (Lond.) **301**:214–221.

Philips, M., Juul, A. G., and Thorsen, S., 1984, Human endothelial cells produce a plasminogen activator inhibitor and a tissue-type plasminogen activator–inhibitor complex, Biochim. Biophys. Acta **802**:99–110.

Pohl, G., Kallstrom, M., Bergsdorf, N., Wallen, P., and Jornvall, H., 1984, Tissue plasminogen activator: Peptide analyses confirm an indirectly derived amino acid sequence, identify the active site serine residue, establish glycosylation sites and localize variant differences, Biochemistry **23**:3701–3707.

Pollack, R., and Rifkin, D. B., 1975, Actin-containing cables within anchorage-dependent rat embryo cells are dissociated by plasmin and trypsin, Cell **6**:495–506.

Postlethwaite, A. E., and Kang, A. H., 1976, Collagen and collagen peptide-induced chemotaxis of human blood monocytes, J. Exp. Med. **143**:1299–1307.

Quigley, J. P., Goldfarb, R. H., Scheiner, C., O'Donnel-Tormey, J., and Yeo, T. K., 1980, Plasminogen activator and the membrane of transformed cells, in: Tumor Cell Surfaces and Malignancy (R. O. Hynes and C. F. Fox, eds.), pp. 773–796, Alan R. Liss, New York.

Radcliffe, R., 1983, A critical role of lysine residues in the stimulation of tissue plasminogen activator by denatured proteins and fibrin clots, Biochim. Biophys. Acta **743**:422–430.

Rantala-Ryhanen, S., Ryhanen, L., Nowak, F., and Uitto, J., 1983, Proteinases in human polymorphonuclear leukocytes: Purification and characterization of an enzyme which cleaves denatured collagen and a synthetic peptide with a Gly-Ile sequence, Biochemistry **134**:129–137.

Reich, R., Miskin, R., and Tsafriri, A., 1985, Follicular plasminogen activator: Involvement in ovulation, Endocrinology **116**:516–521.

Reid, T., and Flint, M. H., 1974, Change in glycosaminoglycan content of healing rabbit tendon, J. Embryol. Exp. Morphol. **31**:489–495.

Remold-O'Donnel, E., and Lewandrowski, K., 1982, Macrophage surface component gp160: Sensitivity to plasmin and other proteases, J. Immunol. **128**:1541–1544.

Rijken, D. C., and Collen, D., 1981, Purification and characterization of the plasminogen activator secreted by human melanoma cells in culture, J. Biol. Chem. **256**:7035–7041.

Risch, J., Werb, Z., and Fukuyama, K., 1980, Effect of plasminogen and its activities on nuclear disintegration in newborn mouse skin in culture, J. Invest. Dermatol. **174**:257 (abst)

Robbins, K. C., Summaria, L., and Wohl, R., 1981, Human plasmin, Methods Enzymol. **80**:379–387.

Sage, H., Trueb, B., and Bornstein, P., 1983, Biosynthetic and structural properties of endothelial cell type VIII collagen, J. Biol. Chem. **258**:13391–13401.

Sakai, T., and Gross, J., 1967, Some properties of the products of reaction of tadpole collagenase with collagen, Biochemistry **6**:518–528.

Salo, T., Liotta, L., and Tryggvason, K., 1983, Purification and characterization of a murine basement membrane collagen-degrading enzyme secreted by metastatic tumor cells, J. Biol. Chem. **258**:3058–3063.

Salo, T., Turpeenniemi-Hujanen, T., and Tryggvason, K., 1985, Tumor-promoting phorbol esters and cell proliferation stimulate secretion of basement membrane (type IV) collagen-degrading metalloproteinase by human fibroblasts, J. Biol. Chem. **260**:8526–8531.

Schmidt, T. M., Mayne, R., Jeffrey, J. J., and Linsenmayer, T. F., 1986, Type X collagen contains 2 cleavage sites for a vertebrate collagenase, J. Biol. Chem. **261**:4184–4189.

Scott, R. W., and Baker, J. B., 1983, Purification of protease nexin, J. Biol. Chem. **258**:10439–10444.

Seltzer, J. L., Adams, S. A., Grant, G. A., and Eisen, A. Z., 1981, Purification and properties of a gelatin-specific neutral protease from human skin, J. Biol. Chem. **256**:4662–4668.

Seltzer, J. L., Jeffrey, J. J., and Eisen, A. Z., 1977, Evidence for mammalian collagenases as zinc ion metalloenzymes, Biochim. Biophys. Acta **485**:179–181.

Seltzer, J. L., Welgus, H. G., Jeffrey, J. J., and Eisen, A. Z., 1976, The function of calcium in the action of mammalian collagenases, Arch. Biochem. Biophys. **173**:355–361.

Senior, R. M., 1983, Neutral proteinases from human inflammatory cells. A critical review of their role in extracellular matrix degradation, Clin. Lab. Med. **3**:645–666.

Senior, R. M., Griffin, G. L., and Mecham, R. P., 1980, Chemotactic activity of elastin-derived peptides, *J. Clin Invest.* **66**:859–862.

Shimada, H., Okamura, H., Espey, L. L., and Mori, T., 1985, Increase in plasminogen activator in the involuting uterus of the postpartum rat, *J. Endocr.* **104**:295–298.

Schoellmann, G., Striker, G., and Ong, E. B., 1982, A fluorescent study of urokinase using active site-directed probes, *Biochim. Biophys. Acta* **704**:403–413.

Skriver, L., Nielsen, L. S., Stephens, R., and Dano, K., 1982, Plasminogen activator released as inactive proenzyme from murine cells transformed by sarcoma virus, *Eur. J. Biochem.* **124**:409–414.

Sprengers, E. D., Verheijen, J. H., van Hinsbergh, V. W. M., and Emeis, J. J., 1984, Evidence for the presence of two different fibrinolytic inhibitors in human endothelial cell conditioned medium, *Biochim. Biophys. Acta* **801**:163–170.

Stecher, V. J., and Sorkin, E., 1972, The chemotactic activity of fibrin lysis products, *Int. Arch. Allergy Appl. Immunol.* **43**:879–886.

Steffens, G. J., Gunzler, W. A., Otting, F., Frankus, E., and Flohe, L., 1982, The complete amino acid sequence of low molecular mass urokinase from human urine, *Hoppe Seylers Z. Physiol. Chem.* **363**:1043–1058.

Stern, C. D., 1984, Mini-review: Hyaluronidases in early embryonic development, *Cell Biol. Int. Rep.* **8**:703–717.

Strassburger, W., Wallmer, A., Pitts, J. E., Glover, I. D., Tickle, I. J., Blundell, T. L., Steffens, G. J., Gunzler, W. A., Otting, F., and Flohe, L., 1983, Adaptation of plasminogen activator sequences to known protease structures, *FEBS Lett.* **157**:219–223.

Strickland, S., and Beers, W. H., 1976, Studies on the role of plasminogen activator in ovulation. In vitro response of granulosa cells to gonadotropins, cyclic nucleotides and prostaglandins, *J. Biol. Chem.* **251**:5694–5702.

Strickland, S., and Mahdavi, V., 1978, The induction of differentiation in teratocarcinoma stem cells by retinoic acid, *Cell* **15**:393–403.

Strickland, S., Reich, E., and Sherman, M. I., 1976, Plasminogen activator in early embryogenesis: Enzyme production by trophoblast and parietal endoderm, *Cell* **9**:231–240.

Stricklin, G. P., and Welgus, H. G., 1983, Human skin fibroblast collagenase inhibitor: Purification and biochemical characterization, *J. Biol. Chem.* **258**:12252–12258.

Stricklin, G. P., Bauer, E. A., Jeffrey, J. J., and Eisen, A. Z., 1977, Human skin collagenase: Isolation of precursor and active forms from both fibroblast and organ cultures, *Biochemistry* **16**:1607–1615.

Stricklin, G. P., Eisen, Z. A., Bauer, E. A., and Jeffrey, J. J., 1978, Human skin fibroblast collagenase: Chemical properties of precursor and active forms, *Biochemistry* **17**:2331–2337.

Stricklin, G. P., Jeffrey, J. J., Roswit, W. T., and Eisen, A. Z., 1983a, Human skin procollagenase: Mechanisms of activation by organomercurials and trypsin, *Biochemistry* **22**:61–68.

Stricklin, G. P., Welgus, H. G., and Bauer, E. A., 1983b, Human skin collagenase in recessive dystrophic epidermolysis bullosa: Purification of a mutant enzyme from fibroblast cultures, *J. Clin. Invest.* **69**:1373–1383.

Sudol, M., and Reich, E., 1984, Purification and characterization of a plasminogen activator secreted by a pig kidney cell line, *Biochem. J.* **219**:971–987.

Suenson, E., Lutzen, O., and Thorsen, S., 1984, Initial plasmin-degradation of fibrin as the basis of a positive feed-back mechanism in fibrinolysis, *Eur. J. Biochem.* **140**:513–522.

Sumi, H., and Robbins, K. C., 1983, A functionally active heavy chain derived from human high molecular weight urokinase, *J. Biol. Chem.* **285**:8014–8019.

Summaria, L., Wohl, R. C., Boreisha, I. G., and Robbins, K. C., 1982, A virgin enzyme derived from human plasminogen. Specific cleavage of the arginyl-560-valyl peptide bond in the diisoproxyphosphinyl virgin enzyme by plasminogen activators, *Biochemistry* **21**:2056–2059.

Thet, L. A., Howell, A. C., and Han, G., 1983, Changes in lung hyaluronidase activity associated with lung growth, injury and repair, *Biochem. Biophys. Res. Commun.* **117**:71–77.

Thorsen, S., and Philips, M., 1984, Isolation of tissue-type plasminogen activator–inhibitor complexes from human plasma. Evidence for a rapid plasminogen activator inhibitor, *Biochim. Biophys. Acta* **802**:111–118.

Tissot, J. D., Schneider, P., Hauert, J., Ruegg, M., Kruithof, E. K. O., and Bachman, F., 1982, Isolation from human plasma of a plasminogen activator identical to urinary high molecular weight urokinase, *J. Clin. Invest.* **70**:1320–1323.

Toki, N., Tsushima, H., Yamasaki, M., Yamasaki, R., and Yamura, T., 1982, Isolation of plasminogen activator from skin lesions with allergic vasculitis, *J. Invest. Dermatol.* **78**:18–23.

Toole, B. P., 1971, Hyaluronate production and removal during cornea development in the chick, *Dev. Biol.* **26**:28–35.

Toole, B. P., 1972, Hyaluronate turnover during chondrogenesis in the developing chick limb and axial skeleton, *Dev. Biol.* **29**:321–329.

Toole, B. P., 1982, Transitions in extracellular macromolecules during avian ocular development, *Prog. Clin. Biol. Res.* **28**:17–34.

Toole, B. P., and Gross, J., 1971, The extracellular matrix of the regenerating newt limb: Synthesis and removal of hyaluronate prior to differentiation, *Dev. Biol.* **25**:57–77.

Toole, B. P., and Trelstad, R. L., 1971, Hyaluronate production and removal during cornea development in the chick, *Dev. Biol.* **26**:28–35.

Toole, B. P., Jackson, G., and Gross, J., 1972, Hyaluronate in morphogenesis: Inhibition of chondrogenesis *in vitro*, *Proc. Natl. Acad. Sci. USA* **69**:1384–1386.

Tran-Thang, C., Kruithof, E. K. O., and Bachman, F., 1984, Tissue-type plasminogen activator increases the binding of glu-plasminogen to clots, *J. Clin. Invest.* **74**:2009–2016.

Tynelius-Bratthal, G., and Attstrom, R., 1972, Acid phosphatase, hyaluronidase and protease in crevices of healthy and inflamed gingiva in dogs, *J. Dent. Res.* **51**:279–283.

Tyree, B., Seltzer, J. L., Halme, J., Jeffrey, J. J., and Eisen, A. Z., 1981, The stoichiometric activation of human skin fibroblast procollagenase by factors present in human skin and rat uterus, *Arch. Biochem. Biophys.* **208**:440–443.

Unkeless, J., Gordon, S., and Reich, E., 1974, Secretion of plasminogen activator by stimulated macrophages, *J. Exp. Med.* **139**:834–850.

Valle, K. J., and Bauer, E. A., 1979, Biosynthesis of collagenase by human skin fibroblasts in monolayer culture, *J. Biol. Chem.* **254**:10115–10120.

van Hinsbergh, V. W., Bertina, R. M., van Wijngaarden, A., van Tilburg, N. H., Emeis, J. J., and Haverkate, F., 1985, Activated protein C decreases plasminogen activator–inhibitor activity in endothelial cell-conditioned medium, *Blood* **65**:444–451.

Vassalli, J. D., and Reich, E., 1977, Macrophage plasminogen activator: Induction by products of activated lymphoid cells, *J. Exp. Med.* **145**:429–437.

Vassalli, J. D., Hamilton, J., and Reich, E., 1976, Macrophage plasminogen activator: Modulation of enzyme production by anti-inflammatory steroids, mitotic inhibitors and cyclic nucleotides, *Cell* **8**:271–281.

Vassalli, J. D., Hamilton, J., and Reich, E., 1977, Macrophage plasminogen activator: Induction by concanavalin A and phorbol myristate acetate, *Cell* **11**:695–705.

Vassalli, J. D., Granelli-Piperno, A., and Reich, E., 1978, Secretion of plasminogen activator by macrophages and polymorphonuclear leukocytes, in: *Mechanisms of Localized Bone Loss* (J. E. Horton, T. M. Tarpley, and W. F. Davis, eds.), pp. 201–212, Information Retrieval, Washington, D.C.

Vassalli, J. D., Dayer, J. M., Wohlwend, A., and Belin, D., 1984, Concomitant secretion of pro-urokinase and of a plasminogen activator-specific inhibitor by cultured human monocytes/macrophages, *J. Exp. Med.* **159**:1653–1668.

Vassalli, J. D., Baccino, D., and Belin, D., 1985, A cellular binding site for the M_r 55,000 form of the human plasminogen activator, *J. Cell Biol.* **100**:86–92.

Vater, C. A., Mainardi, C. L., and Harris, E. D., Jr., 1979a, An inhibitor of mammalian collagenases from cultures *in vitro* of human tendon, *J. Biol. Chem.* **254**:3045–3053.

Vater, C. A., Mainardi, C. L., Harris, E. D., Jr., and Siegel, R. C., 1979b, Native cross-links in collagen fibrils induce resistance to human synovial collagenase, *Biochem. J.* **181**:639–645.

Verheijen, J. H., Chang, G. T. G., and Kluft, C., 1984, Evidence for the occurrence of a fast-acting inhibitor for tissue-type plasminogen activator in human plasma, *Thromb. Haemost.* **51**:392–395.

Vihko, K. K., Suominen, J. J. O., and Parvinen, M., 1984, Cellular regulation of plasminogen activator secretion during spermatogenesis, *Biol. Reprod.* **31**:383–389.

Wallen, P., Pohl, G., Bergsdorf, N., Ranby, M., Ny, T., and Jornvall, H., 1983, Purification and characterization of a melanoma cell plasminogen activator, *Eur. J. Biochem.* **132:**681–686.

Welgus, H. G., and Stricklin, G. P., 1983, Human skin fibroblast collagenase inhibitor: Comparative studies in human connective tissues, serum, and amniotic fluid, *J. Biol. Chem.* **258:**12259–12264.

Welgus, H. G., Jeffrey, J. J., Stricklin, G. P., Roswit, W. T., and Eisen, A. Z., 1980, Characteristics of the action of human skin fibroblast collagenase on fibrillar collagen, *J. Biol. Chem.* **255:**6806–6813.

Welgus, H. G., Jeffrey, J. J., and Eisen, A. Z., 1981a, The collagen substrate specificity of human skin fibroblast collagenase, *J. Biol. Chem.* **256:**9511–9515.

Welgus, H. G., Jeffrey, J. J., and Eisen, A. Z., 1981b, Human skin fibroblast collagenase. Assessment of activation energy and deuterium isotope effect with collagenous substrates, *J. Biol. Chem.* **256:**9516–9521.

Welgus, H. G., Jeffrey, J. J., Stricklin, G. P., and Eisen, A. Z., 1982, The gelatinolytic activity of human skin fibroblast collagenase, *J. Biol. Chem.* **257:**11534–11539.

Welgus, H. G., Kobayashi, D. K., and Jeffrey, J. J., 1983, The collagen substrate specificity of rat uterus collagenase, *J. Biol. Chem.* **258:**14162–14165.

Welgus, H. G., Campbell, E. J., Bar-Shavit, Z., Senior, R. M., and Teitelbaum, S. L., 1985a, Human alveolar macrophages produce a fibroblast-like collagenase and collagenase inhibitor, *J. Clin. Invest.* **76:**219–224.

Welgus, H. G., Connolly, N. L., and Senior, R. M., 1985b, TPA-differentiated U937 cells express a macrophage-like profile of neutral proteinases: High levels of secreted collagenase and collagenase inhibitor accompany low levels of intracellular elastase and cathepsin G, *J. Clin. Invest.* **77:**1675–1681.

Werb, Z., Mainardi, C., Vater, C. A., and Harris, E. D., Jr., 1977, Endogenous activation of latent collagenase by rheumatoid synovial cells. Evidence for a role of plasminogen activator, *N. Engl. J. Med.* **296:**1017–1023.

Werb, Z., Foley, R., and Munck, A., 1978, Interaction of glucocorticoids with macrophages. Identification of glucocorticoid receptors in monocytes and macrophages, *J. Exp. Med.* **147:**1684–1694.

Werb, Z., Banda, M. J., and Jones, P. A., 1980, Degradation of connective tissue matrices by macrophages. I. Proteolysis of elastin, glycoproteins and collagen by proteinases isolated from macrophages, *J. Exp. Med.* **152:**1340–1357.

Wilhelm, S. M., Eisen, A. Z., Teter, M., Clark, S. D., Kronberger, A., and Goldberg, G., 1986, Human fibroblast collagenase: Glycosylation and tissue-specific levels of enzyme synthesis, *Proc. Natl. Acad. Sci. USA* **83:**3756–3760.

Wilson, E., and Reich, E., 1978, Plasminogen activator in chick fibroblasts: Induction of synthesis by retinoic acid; synergism with viral transformation and phorbol ester, *Cell* **15:**385–392.

Wohl, R. C., Sinio, L., Summaria, L., and Robbins, K. C., 1983, Comparative activation kinetics of mammalian plasminogen, *Biochim. Biophys. Acta* **745:**20–31.

Woodley, D. T., Liotta, L. A., and Brondage, R., 1982, Adult human epidermal cells migrating on nonviable matrix produce a type IV collagenase, *Clin. Res.* **30:**266A.

Woolley, D. E., Glanville, R. W., Roberts, D. R., and Evanson, J. M., 1978, Purification, characterization and inhibition of human skin collagenase, *Biochem. J.* **169:**265–276.

Woolley, D. E., Roberts, D. R., and Evanson, J. M., 1976, Small molecular weight serum protein which specifically inhibits human collagenases, *Nature (Lond.)* **261:**325–327.

Zetter, B. R., 1980, Migration of capillary endothelial cells is stimulated by tumor-derived factors, *Nature (Lond.)* **285:**41–43.

Chapter 22
Basement Membranes

HEINZ FURTHMAYR

1. Introduction

Tissue repair and wound healing are intimately related to events occurring
outside the cells in the extracellular matrix. Cells respond, in addition to many
other stimuli, to components of the extracellular matrix through direct interaction—adhesion—and use the matrix as a substrate for movement. The extracellular matrix also provides input for the regulation of growth, the phenotypic
expression of cell- and tissue-specific functions, and for the potential restitution of cellular relationships in a fashion typical for a given organ. The final
outcome of the repair process depends on the organ system, the degree of tissue
destruction, and the potential for regeneration of parenchymal cells. In many
ways, the process has to imitate features of development if it is to be successful
in achieving complete restitution of structure and function. Basement membranes are ubiquitous to all organ systems. They are found at the interphase of
epithelial cells, endothelial cells, and even some mesenchymal cells; thus,
tissue repair and proper cell function are closely related to basement membranes.

1.1. What Is a Basement Membrane?

Described originally in the mid-nineteenth century with the help of the
light microscope as a rather homogeneously staining linear region underneath
the epithelial cells in skin and other organs, basement membranes are currently
defined by most investigators using the electron microscope as a thin, amorphous sheetlike structure. The basement membrane varies widely in thickness,
depending on the particular site or species and contains several distinct layers.
Closest to the cells is the lamina lucida, a layer of sparse 10-nm fibrils running
perpendicular to the cell surface. Closest to the connective tissue is the lamina
fibroreticularis, consisting of loose and relatively thin fibrils and with a more
distinct appearance at certain locations. Sandwiched between these two layers

---

HEINZ FURTHMAYR • Department of Pathology, Yale University School of Medicine, New
Haven, Connecticut 06510.

is the lamina densa, mostly amorphous in appearance, but occasionally resolved into thin microfibrils running parallel to the cell layer. In the alveoli of
the lung and the glomeruli of the kidney the basement membrane separates two
distinct cell layers and consists of a lamina densa and an external and internal
lamina lucida. Together the lamina densa and lamina lucida are referred to as
the basal lamina. Frequently this term is used synonymously with basement
membrane.

1.2. What Is the Function of Basement Membranes?

The basal lamina separates certain parenchymal cell types, that is, endothelium and epithelium, from the connective tissue stroma and thus serves as a
boundary between these different tissue elements. The boundary is strictly
respected under normal circumstances by the cells residing on them, yet some
normal migratory cells such as leukocytes can move across it. The second major
function of the basal lamina is to serve as the anchorage matrix of cells. In
epithelial basement membranes, the development of specialized anchorage—
hemidesmosomes and anchoring filaments—is required to withstand extreme
sheer forces. Cells at most other sites presumably interact with basal lamina
components by virtue of plasma membrane receptors. It is likely that this
interaction not only serves to anchor cells but also to maintain polarity of the
cells and possibly to maintain the tissue-specific phenotype. The basal lamina
also serves as a permselective filter restricting the passage of larger molecules.
For instance, this function is particularly important in the kidney to prevent
loss of protein into the urinary space.

During embryogenesis, morphogenesis, and wound repair, the barrier to
movement is altered or destroyed. Either cells leave the boundary and form
new structures (e.g., new blood vessels or new glands), or connective tissue
cells invade the boundary, deposit new matrix, and potentially form new tissue
patterns. The response of cells and tissues to injury depends on the extent of
destruction. It will be different if the basal lamina has been lost together with
the cells and underlying stroma from the response if only the cells lining the
basal lamina are lost. In nerve regeneration, for instance, the basal lamina of the
pre-existing neurolemma serves as a guiding element to establish a new synapse at the same site. If the basal lamina is destroyed, the neuron has no guide
toward the synapse and thus the nerve cannot regenerate.

2. Macromolecular Components of Basement Membranes

Basement membranes represent only a minor portion of most tissues and,
since they are insoluble in general, biochemical analysis is quite difficult.
Fortunately, certain tumor systems have given investigators great quantities of
basement membrane material from which they can isolate and characterize at
least some of the major components present in all or most basement mem-

branes. Various biologic phenomena, however, indicate, that in addition the basal lamina contains organ- or cell-specific components although we know little of their biochemical characteristics, number, or location.

2.1. Background

The bovine lens capsule and renal glomeruli were used in early biochemical studies. Because of the limited amounts of material and solubility problems, it was difficult to define distinct components of the basal lamina in these materials. Pepsin digestion was used by the laboratory of Kefalides (1971) who described a unique collagen consisting of three identical α-chains and suggested it was disulfide linked to noncollagenous glycoproteins (Kefalides et al., 1979). Spiro and collaborators concluded, from studies using denaturing and reducing agents on glomeruli, that the basal lamina was constructed from collagenous and noncollagenous polypeptides of variable size linked together by covalent crosslinks (Sato and Spiro, 1976).

In recent years, most biochemical studies of basement membrane components used either tissue-culture systems [parietal yolk sac (PYS) tumor cells] or transplantable tumors (EHS tumor) (Pierce, 1970; Orkin et al., 1977; Chung et al., 1979). Once enzymatic fragmentation patterns of these compounds were known, it was possible to purify distinct basal lamina protein fragments from the insoluble matrix of human organs such as placenta, kidney, or lung after digestion with proteases. Antibodies to these protein fragments then permitted localization of the macromolecules to the basal lamina by immunohistological methods.

2.2. Molecules Found in All Basement Membranes

Three classes of macromolecules are found in all basement membranes: collagenous proteins, glycoproteins, and proteoglycans. Several of these have been described in sufficient detail to warrant consideration here. Their localization ultrastructurally within the basal lamina or the basement membrane is not well defined.

2.2.1. Collagens

Several distinct types of collagens are contained within the basement membrane (Table I). Interestingly enough, these collagens are organized into structures distinct from typical cross-striated collagen fibrils seen in connective tissue stroma (fibrillar collagens are discussed in Chapter 20). They cannot therefore be defined ultrastructurally without using collagen type-specific antibodies as markers. In general, a collagenous protein is defined by several criteria.

First, a collagenous protein has a primary structure containing repeats of

Table I. Collagens in Basement Membranes

Collagen type	Molecular weight, length, and subunits	Localization
IV	450,000 M_r, 425 nm, twoα1(IV),oneα2(IV)	All basement membranes and organs
V	300,000 M_r, 300 nm, twoα1(V),oneα2(V)	Lamina reticularis in muscle skin; basal lamina in kidney, lung, and other organs
VI	225,000 M_r, 120 nm, twoα1(VI),oneα2(VI)	Lamina reticularis
VII	510,000 M_r, 450 nm, twoα1(VIII),oneα2(VIII)	Anchoring fibrils in skin
VIII	180,000 M_r, ?, twoα1(VII),oneα2(VII)	Endothelial cells, lig. nuchae fibroblasts

the triplet glycine–X–Y, where X and Y are frequently proline and hydroxyproline. However, any amino acid can occupy these X and Y positions. The glycine–X–Y triplets are repeated several hundred times within the so called collagenous domain of the α-chain subunit and are usually uninterrupted by other amino acid sequences (type IV collagen is a notable exception). Second, collagenous proteins contain three α-chains coiled around each other to form the ropelike triple-helical collagen molecule. Variations of this basic and monotonous principle are known and are addressed in Sections 2.2.1a–2.2.1e. Finally, individual collagen molecules interact with each other to form supramolecular assemblies and are usually stabilized by covalent bonds.

2.2.1a. Type IV Collagen. All basement membranes contain this unique collagen type, which presumably provides the structural framework for the basal lamina. Intact type IV collagen can be isolated most readily from the EHS tumor, which can be grown subcutaneously in lathyritic mice (Kleinman et al., 1982; Yurchenco and Furthmayr, 1984). It is also obtained from cells grown in tissue culture: amnionic cells (Crouch and Bornstein, 1979), PF-HR9 endodermal cells (Bächinger et al., 1982b), and other cell types. In addition, by using pepsin under limiting conditions, various fragments of human type IV collagen are obtained from tissues such as placenta, kidney, or lung (Risteli et al., 1980; Kühn et al., 1981). From these and numerous other studies (for reviews, see Timpl and Martin, 1982; Timpl and Dziadek, 1986), it is now clear, that type IV collagen contains two types of α-chains, two α_1- and one α_2-chains with an apparent molecular mass of 185,000 and 175,000 M_r, respectively. In comparison with the so-called interstitial collagens (type I, II, or III), type IV is unusual in several respects: (1) its constituent α-chains are almost twice the size of other collagen α-chains, and the molecular is approximately 425 nm long rather than the 300 nm observed for other collagens; (2) the molecule as found in tissues contains a globular, noncollagenous domain at its carboxy-terminal end (Furthmayr and Madri, 1982; Fessler and Fessler, 1982; Timpl et al., 1981), a domain that is removed from interstitial collagens before complete incorporation of the molecule into the fibril; (3) the regular Gly–X–Y triplet sequence (invariably found in the interstitial collagens) is interrupted a number of times by a variable number of amino acid residues, the so-called nonhelical regions; (4) the molecule does not assemble into fibrils and is more flexible than other collagens (Hoffmann *et al.*, 1984).

Electrophoretic analysis of type IV collagen isolated from tissue culture systems under reducing conditions shows two polypeptides with an apparent molecular mass of 185,000 and 175,000 M_r (Crouch and Bornstein, 1979; Tryggvason *et al.*, 1980; Fessler and Fessler, 1980). It is well established now that the two α-chains are different (Crouch *et al.*, 1980) and that the molecular composition of this collagen is $\alpha1(IV)_2\alpha_2(IV)$, even when isolated from different tissues (Crouch *et al.*, 1980; Gay and Miller, 1979). Since pepsin (usually) and nonspecific tissue proteases (sometimes) were required for solubilization of type IV collagen and its fragments from a variety of tissues, the likely explanations for the earlier reported heterogeneity in fragment size include variations of experimental conditions, tissue source and preparation, and extent of type IV collagen crosslinking. In tissues as well as in solution, the triple helical region of type IV collagen apparently is attacked at multiple sites by enzymes other than type IV specific collagenases. Collagen type-specific collagenases have been described for type I, III, IV, and V collagen and they cleave the respective triple helices at a single site. However, unlike the other collagens, type IV collagen does not require initial cleavage by collagenase before other enzymes will attack its polypeptide chains. Thus, fragments of varying length are released. The sensitivity of this collagen to a variety of proteases presumably is due to intermittent structural differences of the triple helix. This property may be important for rapid turnover during development and organogenesis, for normal turnover, and for rapid reconstruction during inflammatory processes and tumor invasion (Uitto *et al.*, 1980; Mainardi *et al.*, 1980).

The collagenous domains of type IV collagen as well as all the other collagens are readily digested with bacterial collagenases to Gly–X–Y peptides. Timpl *et al.* (1981) took advantage of this sensitivity and isolated the undegraded noncollagenous domains of type IV collagen. One of these fragments, termed noncollagenous region 1 (NC1), is derived from the carboxy-terminal region of the molecule and has a molecular mass of approximately 150,000 M_r. It is composed of six 25,000-M_r subunits that are crosslinked by disulfide and other unknown bonds (Weber *et al.*, 1984). The NC1 fragment thus represents a dimer of the carboxy-terminal domain, indicating a stable interaction of two collagen monomers within this region of the type IV collagen molecule. In fact, when type IV collagen preparations isolated from the EHS tumor or cell-culture matrix are analyzed by the rotary shadowing procedure (Fig. 1), many collagen molecules are dimeric, with an overall length of about 850 nm and contain a globular region at the center of the dimer (Yurchenco and Furthmayr, 1984). By contrast, type IV collagen isolated from the tissue culture medium (Oberbäumer *et al.*, 1982; Bächinger *et al.*, 1982a) is monomeric and contains a globular region at one end of the molecule.

A second unusual fragment, initially termed 7S collagen, was identified in pepsin digests of the EHS tumor, as well as other tissues (Risteli *et al.*, 1980;

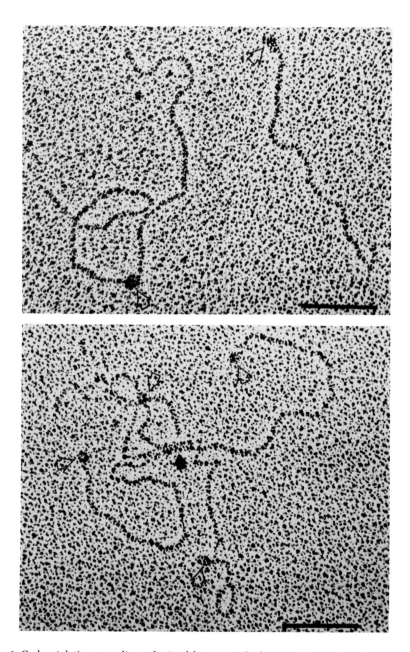

Figure 1. Carbon/platinum replicas obtained by rotary shadowing of type IV collagen monomer (top right) and dimer (top left) and tetramer (bottom) formed from monomers. On the images the carboxy-terminal globular domain is clearly visible (open arrow). The monomeric molecules show the characteristic kink 300 Å away from the amino-terminal end. This region of the molecule is involved in the formation of the tetrameric assembly by parallel–antiparallel alignment (closed arrow). Since most molecules in the tissue or in the matrix of cultured cells exist in the form of stable dimers, the tetramer shown is a relatively rare finding, unless monomers are assembled *in vitro*. Dimeric molecules will assemble, however, in identical fashion to produce octamers and complexes of higher order, as explained in the text. Bar = 1000 Å.

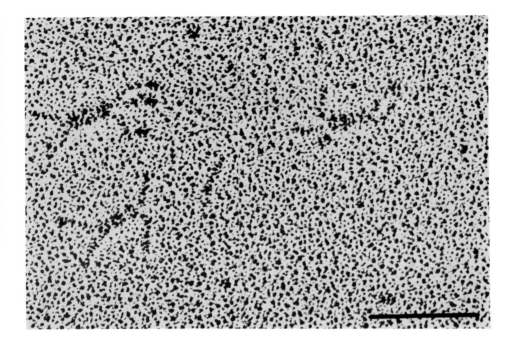

Figure 2. Carbon/platinum replica of the so-called 7S collagen particle obtained by rotary shadowing. The particle can be isolated from tissues by pepsin treatment and it corresponds to the "tetrameric" assembly region of type IV collagen, which in mature tissues is crosslinked by disulfide and other stable bonds. Bar = 500 Å.

Dixit *et al.*, 1981). This 350,000-M_r fragment was resolved into several polypeptides (30,000–160,000 M_r) on polyacrylamide gels after reduction. Images of the fragment obtained by the rotary metal shadow casting technique (Fig. 2) revealed a particle consisting of a central 30-nm rod with two thinner arms extending from each end (Risteli *et al.*, 1980; Furthmayr and Madri, 1982). Kühn *et al.* (1981) isolated a large type IV collagen complex from pepsin digests of human placenta that consisted of four 360-nm-long threadlike structures that overlapped in a central 30-nm region. This finding suggested that a 30-nm region, at the end of the type IV collagen molecule opposite the NC1 globular domain, was capable of parallel–antiparallel interactions with three other molecules to yield tetrameric structures.

The type IV collagen molecule is sensitive to a variety of proteases, probably because the collagen α-chains have discontinuities in the triple-helical Gly–X–Y domains (Schuppan *et al.*, 1980, 1982, 1984; Babel and Glanville, 1984; Glanville *et al.*, 1985; Oberbäumer *et al.*, 1985; Pihlajaniemi *et al.*, 1985). This suggests that the collagen helix in these regions is distorted and vulnerable to proteolytic attack. The discontinuities of the regular helical structure have another consequence; the type IV collagen molecule is considerably more flexible than the interstitial collagens. Images obtained by metal replication show regions of higher flexibility in the amino-terminal and several other regions along the molecule (Hoffmann *et al.*, 1984). A determination of bending angles revealed two types of sites: sites with bending angles distributed narrowly or more widely around the angle zero; and one site with a distinct maximum of 40°. The latter site is frequently observed as a kink on individual molecules and is also observed on tetrameric complexes at a point, at which the collagenous strands emerge from the central rod.

Some of the molecular features of type IV collagen described above are important for assembly, organization, and interactions with other basement membrane macromolecules. These aspects are discussed in Section 3.

2.2.1b. Type V Collagen. A second collagen type, frequently found in association with basement membranes, albeit not necessarily with the basal lamina proper, is type V collagen, initially described by Burgeson et al. (1976). It can best be defined as a family of proteins, since individual molecules have an α-chain composition, which can vary from homotrimers of $\alpha_1(V)_3$, $\alpha_2(V)_3$, $\alpha_3(V)_3$ to the heterotrimer $\alpha_1(V)_2\alpha_2(V)$ (Rhodes and Miller, 1978; Sage and Bornstein, 1979; Haralson et al., 1980; Madri et al., 1982).

Type V collagens have been isolated from a variety of tissues, including blood vessels (Chung et al., 1976), bone (Rhodes and Miller, 1978), skin (Brown and Weiss, 1979), synovium (Brown et al., 1978), skeletal muscle (Bailey et al., 1979), and corneal stroma (Welsh et al., 1980). Endothelial cells and smooth muscle cells (Madri et al., 1980a), tendon and corneal fibroblasts (Fessler et al., 1981), skeletal muscle cells (Bailey et al., 1979), and even some epithelial cells (Stenn et al., 1979) produce type V collagens. The precise ultrastructural location of these collagens in the basement membrane is controversial. Data obtained from immunofluorescence studies on various tissues have shown type V collagen to be present in the interstitium of lung, liver, kidney, and other tissues in addition to basement membranes of blood vessels, skin, eye, kidney tubules, and glomeruli (von der Mark, 1981; Madri et al., 1980a; Madri and Furthmayr, 1980; Roll et al., 1980; Konomi et al., 1984; Modesti et al., 1983; Linsenmayer et al., 1983; von der Mark and Ocalan, 1982). Although in some reports type IV and type V collagens were co-distributed at the ultrastructural level (Roll et al., 1980), implying that type V collagen is present within the basal lamina proper (Fig. 3), several other reports suggested that type V collagen is in fact located in the layer of basement membrane adjacent to the stroma (Martinez-Hernandez et al., 1982; Modesti et al., 1983; Sanes, 1982). In these latter studies, the antibody conjugates to type V collagen labeled non-cross-striated 12-nm fibrils, raising the possibility that type V collagens provide connections between the basal lamina and the stroma. The different techniques used to obtain these data may account for the discrepancies in results; however, the disposition of type V collagen may in fact vary from site to site.

2.2.1c. Type VI Collagen. A 40,000–70,000-M_r disulfide-bonded collagenous protein was originally discovered in limited pepsin digests of aortic intima by Chung et al. (1976) that is referred to as short chain (SC) or intima collagen (Jander et al., 1981, 1983; Furuto and Miller, 1980; Odermatt et al., 1983). However, considerably larger polypeptide chains of 140,000–190,000 M_r were isolated from bovine aorta and nuchal ligaments (Gibson and Cleary, 1982), human placenta and neurofibroma (Heller-Harrison and Carter, 1984;

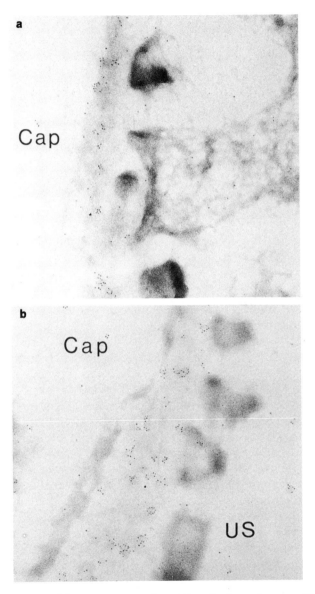

Figure 3. Co-distribution of ferritin anti-IV and anti-V antibody conjugates with type IV (a) and type V (b) collagen, respectively, in the basal lamina of mouse glomeruli on ultrathin frozen sections. (From Roll *et al.*, 1980.)

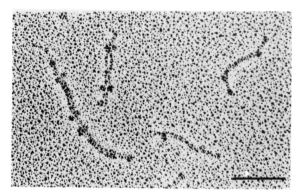

Figure 4. Carbon/platinum replica of pepsin-derived type VI collagen from human placenta. The two particles on the right side of photograph represent dimeric molecules assembled in antiparallel fashion (for details, see Furthmayr *et al.*, 1983), which associate further into tetrameric particles of the same length as the dimer (visualized on the same photograph). This form contains paired and large globular domains separated by collagenous strands and smaller globular domains at the ends. Assembly into microfibrillar structures is suggested by the formation of linear structures such as the one seen on the left side of the photograph. Bar = 1000 Å. (From Furthmayr *et al.*, 1983.)

von der Mark *et al.*, 1984; Hessle and Engvall, 1984), or bovine aorta and uterus (Trüeb and Bornstein, 1984), which apparently constitute the intact α-chains of this protein (Cleary and Gibson, 1983; Engel *et al.*, 1985). Several different cell types produce this protein including: fetal bovine ligamentum nuchae cells (Sear *et al.*, 1981), normal and transformed human lung fibroblasts and skin fibroblasts (Carter, 1982a,b; Bruns, 1984), but apparently not endothelial or epithelial cells (Hessle and Engvall, 1984). On the basis of biochemical data of the pepsin-derived fragment and on images obtained by metal shadow casting and negative staining, a model for this unusual collagen was proposed by Furthmayr *et al.* (1983), and the protein was termed type VI collagen (Fig. 4).

Type VI collagen is a rather unique and unusual collagen. Electron micrographs of the pepsin-derived and partially reduced protein showed rodlike particles 105 nm in length with a large globular domain on one end and a smaller on the other end (Fig. 4). Without reduction, more complex structures are observed, which suggest the presence of side-by-side dimers and tetramers, and the presence of short end-to-end associated filaments (Furthmayr *et al.*, 1983). This overall structure was also found for the intact protein isolated from the tissues or from cells in tissue culture (Jander *et al.*, 1984; von der Mark *et al.*, 1984; Hessle and Engvall, 1984). It has been proposed that the molecule contains three different α-chains (Jander *et al.*, 1983; Trueb and Bornstein, 1984).

A survey of tissues by immunofluorescence revealed that type VI collagen was present predominantly in the interstitial tissue of the papillary and reticular layer of skin, in the aortic media, corneal stroma, around smooth and striated muscle, in the lung and in periportal and perisinusoidal regions of the liver (von der Mark *et al.*, 1984). Basement membranes of renal glomeruli, lung alveoli, and rat diaphragmatic muscle showed weak staining. As judged by immunoelectron microscopy techniques, anti-type VI collagen antibodies appear to react with 5–10-nm-diameter microfibrils, which are quite abundant in the interstitial tissues of the organs mentioned. In muscle, the antibodies react with microfibrils on the stromal side of the basal lamina (Sanes, 1982). Other basement membranes have not been studied in detail as yet. Type VI collagen therefore appears not to be an intrinsic component of the basal lamina. It may, however, serve to connect the basal lamina with stromal elements. Because of its almost ubiquitous presence in the interstitium (Bruns et al., 1986), it is likely that the highly organized and disulfide-bonded molecules will receive further attention in studies on their biologic role.

2.2.1d. Type VII Collagen.   Bentz et al. (1983) isolated a 170-kD collagen from pepsin-digests of human amnion. Because of their large size the molecule has been referred to as long-chain (LC) collagen. Recent studies show that the tissue form of this collagen is arranged as antiparallel dimers (Morris et al., 1986) and that in vitro type VII collagen appears as filaments and fibrils that exhibit a 100-nm axial periodicity (Bruns et al., 1986). Recent evidence indicates that type VII collagen is a major component of the anchoring fibril of skin basement membranes (R. E. Burgeson, personal communication). Segment-long-spacing crystallites prepared from the large pepsin fragments derived from this collagen resemble anchoring fibrils in toad skin (Bruns, 1969). However, the intact molecule contains a large noncollagenous domain at one end, which presumably is utilized to anchor the fibril in the basement membrane.

2.2.1e. Type VIII Collagen.   In addition to types I, III, IV, and V collagen, bovine aortic endothelial cells in culture produce a collagen termed EC or type VIII collagen. It is not found in cultured human endothelial cells or murine hemangioendothelioma, but a human astrocytoma cell line (251 MG) (Alitalo et al., 1983), corneal endothelial cells (Benya, 1986), ligamentum nuchae fibroblasts, and other human tumors (Sage et al., 1980) secrete a collagen with the characteristics of type VIII collagen:polypeptide chains of 125,000 and 100,000, extreme liability to pepsin, and secretion independent of proline hydroxylation. Its location in tissues is unknown, but conceivably it could be associated with basement membranes at certain sites.

2.2.2. Glycoproteins

Noncollagenous glycoproteins are a significant component of basement membranes. The estimated amounts vary widely, and figures between 10 and 50% were given for tissues such as kidney, cornea, or lens capsule (Kefalides et al., 1979). Their content is even higher in the EHS tumor matrix (Timpl et al., 1979). Some of these noncollagenous proteins, such as laminin and entactin/nidogen, have been described in detail and are found associated with virtually all basement membranes. Others such as fibronectin are found in basement membranes probably only under certain conditions. An unknown number of as yet uncharacterized additional proteins are probably present. Such proteins may not exist in all basement membranes but may be associated with the basal lamina at specific sites.

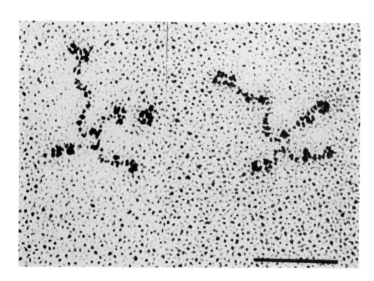

Figure 5. Carbon/platinum replica of laminin obtained by the rotary shadowing technique. The images reveal the cross-shaped organization of the polypeptide chains, the location of distinct globular domains on the short arms, and the complex domain at the end of the long arm. Bar = 500 Å. (From Engel *et al.*, 1981.)

2.2.2a. Laminin. Laminin is a 900,000-M_r glycoprotein originally isolated from the murine EHS tumor (Timpl *et al.*, 1979) and a mouse embryonal carcinoma-derived cell line (Chung *et al.*, 1979). It has also been isolated nearly intact from human placenta (Wewer *et al.*, 1983). The protein is produced by all endothelial and epithelial cells. Endodermal and teratocarcinoma cells are used as model systems to study its biosynthesis and regulation (Cooper *et al.*, 1981; Strickland *et al.*, 1980). Laminin is found in essentially all basement membranes including sites at which a basal lamina cannot be identified by electron microscopy, such as the sinusoids of the liver.

Laminin contains two types of polypeptide chains: one 440,000-M_r α-chain, or heavy chain, and at least two different 200,000-M_r β-chains, or light chains (Cooper *et al.*, 1981; Hogan *et al.*, 1984). Carbon-platinum rotary shadowing images of laminin appeared as an asymmetric cross with three short arms, 36 nm each, and one long arm of 77 nm (Fig. 5). Each short arm contains two small globular regions; the long arm terminates in a large and complex region that may consist of several subdomains (Engel *et al.*, 1981). The same shape and overall features of laminin were found by transmission electron microscopy (TEM) after negative staining and by scanning electron microscopy (SEM) of unstained specimens. Diameters of 5 and 7 nm were measured on negatively stained molecules for the small globular regions of the short arms and the large globular domain of the long arm, respectively. The thin flexible arms have a diameter of about 2.2 nm.

The precise number, localization, and arrangement of the subunits within the intact molecule are not completely understood (Engel and Furthmayr,

1986). The molar ratio of α- to β-chains, as determined by sodium dodecyl sulfate–polyacrylamide gel electrophoresis (SDS-PAGE) was found to vary between 1 : 2 (Howe and Dietzschold, 1983) and 1 : 3 (Engel et al., 1981). Furthermore, studies on the biosynthesis of laminin subunits by endodermal cells and teratocarcinoma cells revealed the synthesis of at least three polypeptide chains with molecular weights of 440,000 (α-chain), 205,000 (β_1-chain), and 185,000 (β_2-chain) (Cooper et al., 1981; Howe and Dietzschold, 1983) rather than the two described initially for laminin from the EHS tumor (Engel et al., 1981). In vitro translation of messenger RNA (mRNA) from parietal endodermal cells has provided evidence for two β_1-chains: β_{1a}, and β_{1b} (Kurkinen et al., 1983; Wang and Gudas, 1983). From these data, it is therefore not clear whether all these polypeptide chains occur in one laminin molecule or whether isoforms are assembled. Recombinant DNA studies of the β_2- and β_{1a},b-chains predict the existence of C-terminal coiled-coil β-helical regions (Barlow et al., 1984). Partial amino acid sequences of a proteolytic fragment derived from the long arm also shows heptad repeats with hydrophobic residues at positions a and d (Paulsson et al., 1985). Such repeats are typical for coiled-coil α-helices found in desmin, myosin, and tropomyosin (two-stranded) and fibrinogen (three-stranded) (Doolittle et al., 1978). Biophysical evidence suggests the α-helices are located in the long arm (Ott et al., 1982; Paulsson et al., 1985). Both α- and β-chains contain this structural feature, but it remains to be seen where in the molecule the individual chains are located. Laminin has unusual properties when studied in vitro (see Section 3).

As far as we know, laminin is the first extracellular matrix protein synthesized in the mouse embryo (Leivo et al., 1980; Wu et al., 1983). In vitro studies show that laminin promotes the attachment and spreading of epithelial cells and hepatocytes (Terranova et al., 1980; Vlodavsky and Gospodarowicz, 1981; Timpl et al., 1983b) and neuronal outgrowth (Baron van Evercooren et al., 1982; Edgar et al., 1984). All of these observations suggest that laminin is a critical matrix molecule during embryonic development and that it mediates the organization of cells into tissues, but how does laminin work?

At the molecular level laminin interacts with itself and other matrix components (Fig. 6), including heparin, heparan sulfate proteoglycan, type IV collagen, and possibly entactin/nidogen. Various domains on the laminin molecule support these interactions (Ott et al., 1982; Edgar et al., 1984; Carlin et al., 1983). It also binds to high-affinity receptors at the surface of the plasma membrane (Rao et al., 1983; Brown et al., 1983; Lesot et al., 1983) at a domain located on the inner parts of the short arms and probably also at the end of the long arm. One can speculate that the protein will be tightly anchored in the basal lamina through certain domains, while others are available for interactions with the cells. It has been argued that the key to the interaction of cells with laminin is not necessarily adhesion or specificity, but rather the recognition of a particular domain or possibly an appropriate spacing of the molecules in the basal lamina (Engvall and Ruoslahti, 1983). This may provide the signals for cellular activity in vivo.

Laminin was localized to essentially all basement membranes by light and

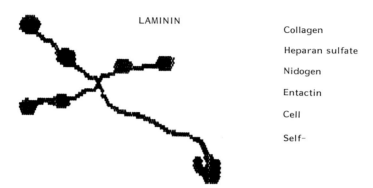

LAMININ

Collagen

Heparan sulfate

Nidogen

Entactin

Cell

Self–

Figure 6. Binding interactions supported by the laminin molecule. See text for description.

electron microscopy (for a recent review, see Martinez-Hernandez and Amenta, 1983). Its precise localization within the basement membrane is controversial, however. Depending on the methods used for preparing the tissue and probably other factors, such as variation in antibody specificity, antibody conjugates localized throughout the entire thickness of the basal lamina, in the lamina lucida only, or in the lamina densa only (Fig. 7). It is also possible that these divergent results reflect either diverse laminin arrays within basement membranes, different laminin isotypes, or organizational differences of the basal lamina that may make certain antigenic sites inaccessible to the antibody probes (Wan et al., 1984).

2.2.2b. Entactin/Nidogen. Entactin, a 150,000-M_r-sulfated protein, was identified in a mouse teratocarcinoma cell line (Carlin et al., 1981; Bender et al., 1981). It has been localized to a number of different basement membranes, but its precise localization within the basal lamina is not clearly established. Entactin or a protein exhibiting similar behavior has also been described in the murine parietal yolk sac basement membrane (Reichert's membrane) and the EHS tumor (Amenta et al., 1983; Kurkinen et al., 1983; Hogan et al., 1984). Nidogen, a glycoprotein of about 100,000 M_r, was isolated from the EHS tumor and named for its ability to aggregate into nestlike structures. Visualization by metal shadow casting revealed a protein consisting of a globule connected to a short rod (Timpl et al., 1983a). However, more recent work from the same group suggests that the nidogen molecule described initially is in fact a proteolytic fragment of a 150,000-M_r protein identical with or related to entactin (Dziadek et al., 1986).

2.2.2c. Fibronectin. This protein (see Chapter 18) has been studied extensively and, despite numerous immunofluorescence studies pointing to the presence of this protein in different basement membranes (Stenman and Vaheri, 1978), its association with the basal lamina is not universally accepted. Based on immunoelectron microscopic findings, the notion was advanced that fibronectin is not found in most basement membranes (Martinez-Hernandez et al., 1981; Roll et al., 1980). The apparently small amounts of fibronectin in basement

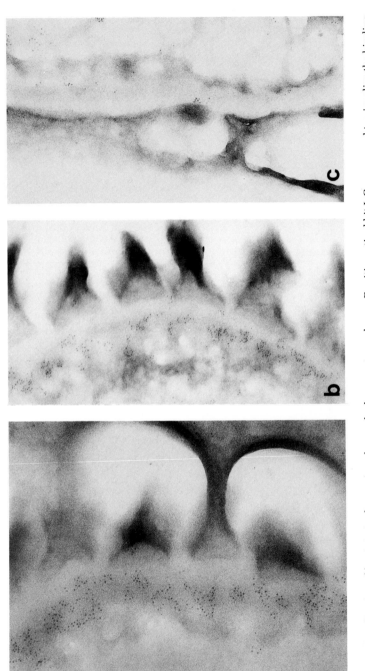

Figure 7. Localization of laminin in the murine glomerular basement membrane. Ferritin-anti rabbit IgGs were used to visualize the binding of rabbit anti-laminin IgG on ultrathin frozen sections. On the segments of the glomerular loop shown in the photograph, laminin apparently is located on the endothelial side of the basal lamina but not on the epithelial side (a,b). By contrast, fibronectin labeling is extremely sparse (c). Magnification: ×60000 (For details see Madri et al., 1980b.)

membranes with high filtering function such as glomerular and Reichert's membranes are possibly due to trapping of serum fibronectin. Under certain circumstances, such as angiogenesis, wound healing, or morphogenesis, fibronectin may be found however in the basal lamina (Clark *et al.*, 1982*a,b*; Wartiovaara *et al.*, 1979; Fujikawa *et al.*, 1981). Endothelial cells *in vitro* are capable of fibronectin production, but it is not clear that endothelial cells of normal, mature blood vessels deposit fibronectin into the basal lamina (Birdwell *et al.*, 1978, Tonnesen *et al.*, 1985).

2.2.3. Heparan Sulfate Proteoglycans

On the basis of studies with cationic probes, numerous histochemical studies have described anionic sites in the basal lamina of many organs (e.g., Kanwar and Farquhar, 1979*a*). Recently more direct evidence was provided that the majority of these highly negative charges in the glomerular basal lamina are sulfate groups linked to the complex macromolecules, heparan sulfate proteoglycans (Kanwar and Farquhar, 1979*b*; Kanwar *et al.*, 1981). Similar molecules have also been isolated from the EHS tumor (Hassell *et al.*, 1980; Fujiwara *et al.*, 1984), and cells in culture (Oohira *et al.*, 1982; Keller and Furthmayr, 1987). These proteoglycans are presumably secreted by all cells attached to basement membranes. At least two distinct molecules have been isolated and presumably are derived from a common precursor molecule (Hassell *et al.*, 1985). For the glomerular basement membrane, it was shown by several techniques that the proteoheparan sulfates are localized ultrastructurally in both the laminae rara interna and externa (Stowe *et al.*, 1985). In addition to the basement membrane form(s) of the proteoheparan sulfate, different heparan sulfate proteoglycans are found on the cell surface of a number of cell types, and these apparently are intercalated into the plasma membrane (Oldberg *et al.*, 1979; Iozzo, 1984). Proteoglycans are discussed at length in Chapter 19.

The large form of the proteoheparan sulfate found in association with basement membranes is tightly linked, since high concentrations of guanidine hydrochloride are required to dissociate the molecules. Some experimental data suggest that proteoheparan sulfate interacts with laminin as well as type IV collagen, which may provide anchoring sites in the basal lamina (Fujiwara *et al.*, 1984; Laurie *et al.*, 1982).

2.3. Molecules Found in Basement Membranes at Distinct Sites

There is ample circumstantial evidence for heterogeneity of basement membranes. Although quantitative data on the content of the different molecules in different basement membranes are difficult to obtain, crude estimates of the collagen content suggest considerably variability from 90% for the bovine lens capsule to 25% for Reichert's membrane. In the EHS tumor the amounts of type IV collagen, laminin, nidogen, and proteoheparan sulfate are about equal in mass (Fujiwara *et al.*, 1984), but it is not likely that a similar relationship will be found for most basement membranes. Equally important are findings suggesting the presence of yet other molecules only at specific sites in certain basement membranes. The following are brief descriptions of some such molecules from various organ systems.

2.3.1. Skin

Stanley et al. (1981b) isolated a 220,000-M_r protein from a spontaneously transformed murine epidermal cell line (PAM 212), which reacted with antisera from human patients with bullous pemphigoid (BP). The BP antibodies stain the basal lamina of skin, urethra, bladder, bronchi, and gallbladder (Beutner et al., 1968). The protein is produced by cultured human epidermal cells (Stanley et al., 1980). Wound-healing experiments show that when epidermal cells leave the basement membrane to re-epithelialize a superficial wound, the BP protein is found beneath the re-epithelializing epidermis prior to laminin and type IV collagen (Stanley et al., 1981a; Hinter et al., 1980; Clark et al., 1982b). Type VII collagen apparently forms the anchoring filaments in skin, but other proteins may be involved as well (Katz, 1984). Chapter 23 presents much additional information about the epidermal–dermal basement membrane.

2.3.2. Muscle

A basal lamina ensheathes each skeletal muscle fiber and passes through the synaptic cleft at the neuromuscular junction. Basal lamina in the synaptic cleft contain considerable amounts of the material thought to play an important role in the formation, function, and maintenance of the synapse. The basal lamina is important for the adhesion of nerve to muscle, contains acetylcholine esterase (AChE), regulates the differentiation of nerve terminals during reinnervation, and has some role in the clustering of post-synaptic acetylcholine receptors (AChR) (Anlister and McMahan, 1984). In addition to the presence of AChE in the synaptic cleft matrix, there are differences in the composition of the basal lamina within or outside the nerve ending, as revealed by immunohistology using antibodies to various matrix molecules (Sanes and Hall, 1979; Sanes, 1982; 1982; Caroni et al., 1985). Specific proteoheparan sulfates appear to be present in the junctional region, although these may be components of the presynaptic plasma membrane rather than of the matrix (Buckley et al., 1983). Matrix material from the electric organ of Torpedo californica also induces clustering of AChR, but the nature of the active principle has yet to be determined (Godfrey et al., 1984).

2.3.3. Glands

During morphogenesis of the mammary gland or salivary gland, marked changes occur in the basement membranes (Bernfield et al., 1984), which presumably involve degradation and reformation of the basal lamina and may control the branching process. Examples of specific molecules found in the basal lamina of glands include Thy-1 antigen beneath the myoepithelial cells in the lactating breast gland (Monaghan *et al.*, 1983).

2.3.4. Neoplastic Tissue

A 200,000-M_r protein has been isolated from a human glioma cell line that reacted with monoclonal antibodies developed against the cell. By peroxidase–antiperoxidase immunohistology, the antibody reacted not only with basement membranes of blood vessels in human tumors, but also with sinusoids in liver, spleen, and with the matrix of renal cortical medullary tubules (Bourdon *et al.*, 1983). The protein apparently is not related to laminin, fibronectin, or other known molecules.

3. Macromolecular Organization of Basement Membranes

How are the many complex macromolecules organized within the basement membrane? Are there differences in organization among different basement membranes? Does the distinction of electron-lucent and electron-dense layers reflect the presence of some molecules only in one or the other layer? These questions can only be partially answered at the present time.

3.1. Topographic Relationships

The modus operandi for localization and distribution of individual components integral to the basement membrane was histochemistry and, more recently, immunohistochemistry. While immunofluorescence light microscopy can screen qualitatively for the presence or absence of a molecule within the basement membrane zone of a tissue (Fig. 8), the electron microscope has been essential in deciphering the ultrastructure of the basement membrane into distinct layers. Considerable effort has been made using different techniques for tissue preparation, labeling, or other manipulations, but these have not always yielded consistent results (for review, see Martinez-Hernandez and Amenta, 1983; Farquhar, 1981). It is therefore not yet possible on the basis of the immunohistochemical work to conclude that various components of the basement membrane are organized into a type IV collagen-rich lamina densa and a laminin and proteoheparan sulfate containing lamina rara, as originally proposed. Likewise, it is not possible to distinguish this model of organization from other models (Furthmayr *et al.*, 1985). Staining of basement membranes with cationic dyes such as ruthenium red most consistently revealed particles in the lamina rara of glomeruli, blood vessels, or alveoli (Vaccaro and Brody, 1981). Antibody staining sometimes confirmed these results, but not invariably. Such discrepancies may reflect properties of antibodies, diffusion of reagents, or other problems of a technical nature.

3.2. *In Vitro* Assemblies

It has long been known that collagen is a fibril-forming protein. Indeed, it was possible to prepare fibrillar structures *in vitro* from soluble type I, II, and III collagens similar to those observed in the tissues as judged by electron microscope examination of cross-striated fibrils. The fibril composed of type I collagen, the collagen quaternary structure which has been most studied and best defined, is produced by parallel alignment of individual molecules in the same direction (C- to N-terminal) and by staggering about one quarter of their length, the D period. Since individual molecules are about 4.4 times the length of this repeat (67 nm), an empty space is created between the C-terminal end of one molecule and the N-terminal of the next. Fibrils with these properties can be produced by incubation of type I, II, or III collagen in aqueous solution at neutral pH. When the process of fibril formation is followed by turbidity measurements, a large increase in turbidity is seen after an initial lag period of about thirty minutes. With the discovery of several additional collagen types it is now clear that different supramolecular structures occur (Fig. 9). Type VI collagen apparently produces a microfibril by end-to-end and precise side-by-side alignment (see Section 2.2.1a). Type VII collagen may be arranged as SLS-crystallites. Similarly, type IV collagen, the major basement membrane constituent, does not form fibrils as defined for the interstitial collagens (type I, II, or III), although 3–5-nm filaments are observed within the lamina densa of the glomerular basement membrane (Farquhar, 1978) or Reichert's membrane (Inoue *et al.*, 1983). The identity of these filament as well as the 10-nm filaments seen in the lamina lucida running perpendicular to the lamina densa is unknown.

Recent studies have revealed some unusual properties of type IV collagen as well as of laminin (Yurchenco and Furthmayr, 1984; Yurchenco *et al.*, 1985; Yurchenco and Furthmayr, 1985). Incubation of dimeric (head–head-associated) type IV collagen, the assembled form found in the matrix of cultured cells and tissue, in a neutral physiologic salt solution caused the protein to further assemble into an organized network. By rotary shadowing, this network appeared as a two-dimensional matrix consisting of polygons with sides varying in length and thickness and that frequently contained a globular domain at the vertices (Fig. 10). These structures apparently are created through side-by-side alignment over variable distances of several (up to three or four) collagenous strands. Pepsin-generated type IV collagen, which lacks the globular domain, or monomeric type IV collagen found in the medium of cells grown in culture do not appear to form this matrix. The so-called lateral association occurs considerably faster than the assembly of the molecules into tetrameric or rather octameric units (Kühn *et al.*, 1981; Yurchenco and Furthmayr, 1984; Yurchenco and Furthmayr, 1985). Three types of associations can thus be described. Presumably, the molecules assemble head–head first, then laterally, and finally the tetrameric interactions occur (Fig. 11). The data have led to a layer model that envisions a two- or three-dimensional array of irregular polygons, which are stabilized by the formation of the N-terminal tetrameric structures.

Laminin also exhibits the property of self-association *in vitro* (Yurchenco

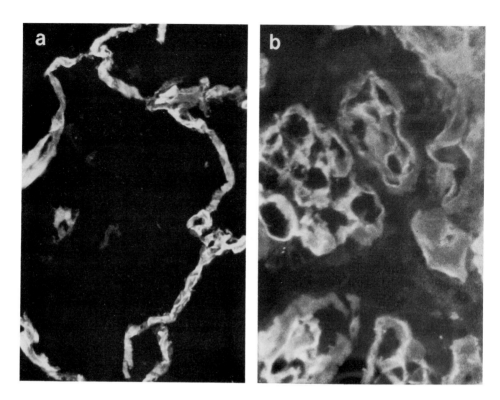

Figure 8. Indirect immunofluorescence of human alveolar (a), placental (b), renal tubular (c), and glomerular (d) basement membranes stained with monoclonal antibodies to human type IV collagen. (From Foellmer *et al.*, 1983.)

et al., 1985). Upon incubation above the critical concentration of about 0.1 mg/ml, at warm temperatures and in the presence of Ca^{2+}, the turbidity of a solution of laminin increases considerably and large aggregates are formed that sediment to the bottom of the tube after ultracentrifugation. In the absence of Ca^{2+}, however, the turbidity increases only slightly and large aggregates do not form. Rotary shadowing of the laminin molecules under these latter conditions revealed that small oligomers are preferentially formed: dimers, trimers, tetramers. These complexes are associated at the globular ends of the molecules with some preference for the tip of the long arm. In the presence of Ca^{2+}, the apparent equilibrium shifts to complexes of larger size by a process akin to nucleation–propagation observed in actin or tubulin assembly (Fig. 12).

Laminin and type IV collagen together can form heterogeneous complexes *in vitro* (Charonis *et al.*, 1985). Mixing experiments demonstrated that laminin interacts with individual collagen molecules at two sites and that this interaction is dependent on the globular regions of laminin, particularly the long-arm globular region. Proteoheparan sulfates and entactin also appear to interact with laminin (Fujiwara *et al.*, 1984; Timpl *et al.*, 1983a). However, the forma-

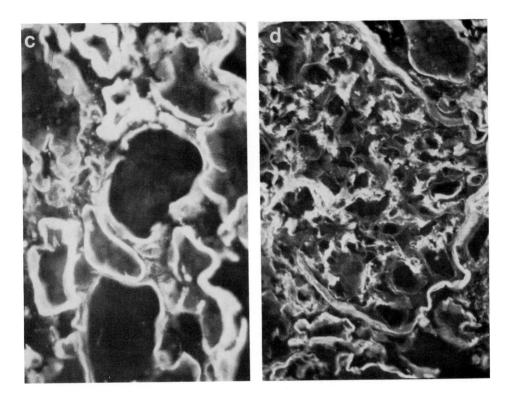

Figure 8. (Continued)

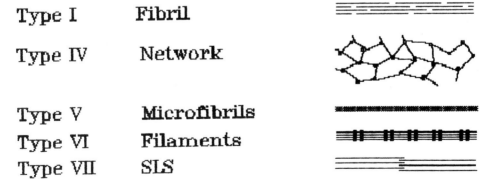

Figure 9. Supramolecular organization of collagen. The various collagen types utilize different ways to assemble structures of higher order.

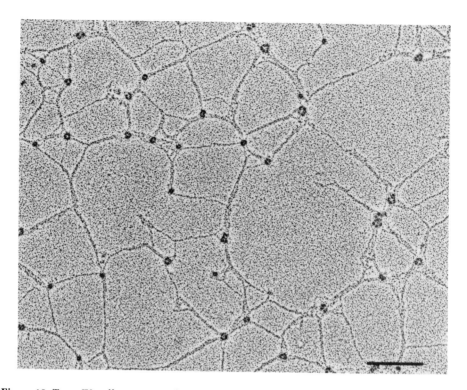

Figure 10. Type IV collagen network assembled *in vitro* from pure collagen. Dimeric type IV collagen molecules associate with segments of their collagenous strands over varying distances with a segment from one or two other molecules and then bend to align with yet other molecules to form a presumably three-dimensional irregular and apparently incomplete polygonal array. The globular particles, located at the center of the dimers in this array, are spaced on the average 170 nm apart. The region of the molecules, which allow for tetrameric assembly, are not clearly seen. However, during the short interval required to form the network, tetrameric stabilization does not occur. Bar = 200 nm. (From Yurchenco and Furthmayr, 1984.)

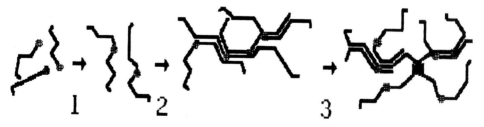

Figure 11. Scheme of the various steps in the *in vitro* assembly of type IV collagen. Monomer to dimer association (step 1) apparently is required to allow for the reversible formation of the lateral assembly (step 2). The exact requirements for step 1 are unknown at this time. Step 3 is relatively slow and may thus represent the last step required for further stabilizing the network *in vivo*.

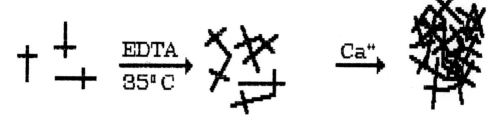

Figure 12. Scheme of the self-assembly of laminin *in vitro*. In the absence of divalent cations laminin forms small oligomers by interactions within the globular end regions, which can be visualized by the rotary shadowing method. In the presence of calcium, the reversible formation of large complexes is observed. (For details, see Yurchenco *et al.*, 1985.)

tion of aggregates of entactin and some of the interactions involving proteoheparan sulfate at low salt concentrations may not occur *in vivo*.

Although we know that the basal lamina proper contains at least type IV collagen, laminin, and proteoheparan sulfate, the precise localization and orientation of these molecules within basement membranes *in situ* are not clearly established. However, given the *in vitro* tendency of these molecules to self-associate and to form multiple interactions with each other, it is possible to construct working models for *in vivo* assembly (Fig. 13).

Several possibilities can be envisioned:

1. *Layer model:* Type IV collagen and laminin form independent assemblies, which are interconnected, and proteoheparan sulfate attaches to either type IV collagen, laminin, or both.
2. *Matrisome model:* The other extreme, proposed by Martin *et al.* (1984), envisions the basement membrane to be assembled from building blocks—the so-called matrisome—consisting of preformed type IV collagen, entactin, laminin, and proteoheparan sulfate complexes.
3. *Assembly polymorphism model:* the various macromolecules are produced and exported by the cell, but not necessarily as prepackaged units; their local concentrations would influence the final assembly.

Model #1, the layer model, suggests that the type IV collagen network is the structural backbone of basement membranes. Laminin forms independent structures that could be space fillers or that could have other functions. Although it is unlikely that large laminin aggregates as formed in test tubes will be found in the basal lamina, it is possible that small complexes may be connected to a type IV lattice. The second model predicts the existence of an essential intermediate—the matrisome—for the assembly process. This intermediate has not been clearly identified. In addition, this model does not address the different biochemical compositions of various basal laminae or the possibility that unique molecular distributions may occur within various basal laminae, or the capability of basement membrane components to self-assemble. Model #3 would allow for variation in the organization of the basal lamina at different

1. LAYER MODEL

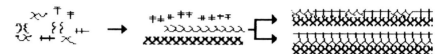

2. MATRISOME MODEL

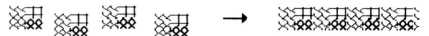

3. ASSEMBLY POLYMORPHISM MODEL

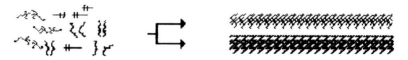

Figure 13. Hypothetical methods for basement membrane assembly. For description, see text.

sites. This would account for the observations that collagen content and laminin localization varies among basement membranes. It certainly addresses the tendency of basement membrane molecules to polymerize. This model predicts that laminin and type IV collagen, and perhaps the proteoheparan sulfates, would influence each other by preventing or modulating the formation of the homopolymers observed *in vitro*. An additional feature of the model would be that the same molecules, albeit in different organizational form (polymorphism of assembly), could support different functional properties of the basal lamina of skin, capillaries in different vascular beds, or other epithelia.

3.3. *In Vivo* Assembly

What is known about the organization of the molecules known to exist within the basal lamina *in situ*? It is not possible to correlate the various filaments seen electron microscopically in the basal lamina with specific molecules by present state-of-the-art immunohistochemistry (see Section 3.1). In considering a general structure for basement membranes, several issues have to be taken into account (Fig. 14): (1) basement membranes vary widely in thickness, (2) they vary in their function as permeability barriers for small molecules, (3) they can be penetrated by cells such as lymphocytes or leukocytes without detectable ultrastructural breaks in their architecture, (4) they support the growth and differentiation of cells, and (5) perhaps they may have biochemical or structural specifities determined by their resident cells.

3.3.1. Developmental Considerations

Laminin is expressed very early in embryogenesis. Although its precise function for the cells at these stages of development is unknown, it may serve as an extracellular matrix for attachment, migration, or other cellular responses. From work on basement membrane development in the kidney, it appears that all the components are seen immunohistologically at the same time, the time of cellular differentiation (Ekblom, 1981; Bonadio et al., 1984). Thus, in organogenesis there does not seem to be a separate time during which laminin or type IV collagen are secreted in newly forming basal lamina.

3.3.2. Ultrastructural Specialization

Reichert's membrane, a thick basement membrane in the parietal wall of rodent yolk sacs, is composed of about 40 distinct dense layers each 25–50 nm in thickness with interspersed lucent spaces of half that thickness (Inoue et al., 1983). The dense layer is composed of 3–8-nm-thick cords, apparently arranged in a three-dimensional network. Immunostaining of these cords with laminin or type IV collagen antibodies before or after plasmin treatment indicates that the cord consists of a core filament of type IV collagen and a sheath of laminin. Scattered among these cords are unbranched straight tubular strucures with a diameter of 7–10 nm, which have been termed basotubules. They appear to consist of a central tubule surrounded by a ribbonlike helical wrapping. The central tubule contains the amyloid P component.

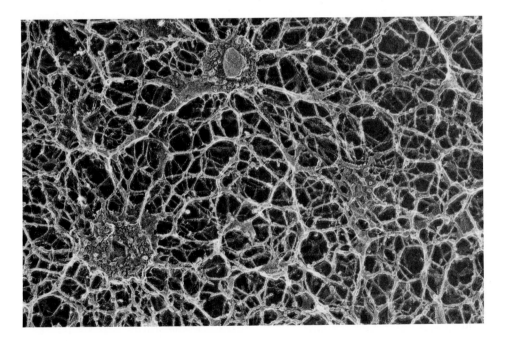

Figure 14. En face view of the bovine amnionic basement membrane prepared by metal replication. The cells were removed to visualize an irregular three-dimensional network of strands that vary in length and thickness. Significantly, the preparation did not allow detection of individual macromolecules, such as type IV collagen or laminin. The larger and rounded structures may represent cell attachment sites. (Courtesy of R. Mecham, Washington University, St. Louis, Missouri.)

Descemet's membrane, another extremely thick basement membrane produced by corneal endothelial cells, has a highly organized appearance in the electron microscope (Sawada, 1982, 1984). In thin sections, the membrane contains stacks of filaments arranged in parallel. Using the freeze-etch replica method, the structures were resolved as a two-dimensional hexagonal lattice consisting of 80-nm-round densities and 120-nm-long rodlike structures connecting these densities. In addition, amorphous material and randomly oriented fine filaments are seen. Similar hexagonal structures appearing as wheels with spokes are demonstrated in the matrix of cultured corneal endothelial cells. The biochemical nature of these structures is unknown. This membrane, as well as Reichert's membrane, contains type IV collagen as well as laminin, but the major collagenous protein in Descemet's membrane may be type VIII collagen (H. Sage, personal communication). In another study, Carlson et al. (1981) visualized densities in renal tubular basement membranes arranged in hexagonal arrays, after proteolytic treatment.

These examples indicate that, at least in some basement membrane, higher order can be observed with some newer technology. It can be anticipated that in the near future replication techniques, antibody labelling studies, and new biochemical information will yield important insight into the complex arrangement of the basal lamina. Interpretation of the image shown in Fig. 13 can be viewed as a challenge. It provides a novel view of organizational features that was hitherto impossible to achieve.

4. The Basement Membrane in Wound Repair

The basal lamina, situated at the interphase between epithelial or endothelial cells and the connective tissue matrix, has been described as a scaffold-facilitating tissue reconstitution after cell injury (Vracko, 1974). Damage to a tissue may be followed by orderly repair and reconstruction; however, to reestablish cellular relationships as they existed prior to repair, several requirements must be met: the reconstituting cell type must be of the same cell type present before injury; the number of replacement cells must be similar to the previous number; and the newly formed cells and the extracellular matrix must be positioned in tissue-specific relationships. There are numerous examples describing the apparent role of the basal lamina in tissue repair. In general, the presence of basal lamina facilitates reconstruction, while its destruction, together with the overlying cells, causes the injury to heal by scar formation. Loss of epithelial cells from the gut lumen, the skin, or renal tubules can be restored completely by re-epithelialization. More extensive damage resulting in deep wounds of the skin or ulcers in the stomach will heal by scar formation (also see Chapter 23). It appears that basal laminae contain information for the cells which facilitates the process of reconstitution perhaps in a site-specific manner. In addition to the events of re-epithelialization, the basal lamina plays an important role during vascularization in the wound-healing process (see Chapters 14 and 19).

Although we have seen an explosion of information on basement membranes and their effects on *in vitro* cell growth, maintenance, and differentiation, we still lack an understanding of the important principles at work. How specific is a basement membrane for its associated cells? What information does the basement membrane contain for its associated cells? Finally, how is the information translated into cellular activity?

References

Alitalo, K., Bornstein, P., Vaheri, A., and Sage, H., 1983, Biosynthesis of an unusual collagen type by human astrocytoma cells *in vitro*, *J. Biol. Chem.* **258**:2653–2661.

Amenta, P. S., Clark, C. C., and Martinez-Hernandez, A., 1983, Deposition of fibronectin and laminin in the basement-membrane of the rat parietal yolk sac. Immunohistochemical and biosynthetic studies, *J. Cell Biol.* **96**:104–111.

Anglister, L., and McMahan, U. J., 1984, Extracellular matrix components involved in neuromuscular transmission and regeneration, *Ciba Found. Symp.* **108**:163–178.

Babel, A., and Glanville, R. W., 1984, Structure of human-basement-membrane (type IV) collagen. Complete amino acid sequence of a 914-residue-long pepsin fragment from the α1 (IV) chain, *Eur. J. Biochem.* **143**:545–556.

Bächinger, H. P., Droege, K. J., Petschek, J. P., Fessler, L. I., and Fessler, J. H., 1982a, Structural implications from an electronmicroscopic comparison of procollagen V with procollagen I, pC-collagen I, procollagen IV and a *Drosophila* procollagen, *J. Biol. Chem.* **257**:14590–14592.

Bachinger, H. P., Fessler, L. I., and Fessler, J. H., 1982b, Mouse procollagen IV: Characterization and supramolecular assembly, *J. Biol. Chem.* **257**:9796–9803.

Bailey, A. J., Shellswell, G. B., and Duance, V. C., 1979, Identity and change of collagen types in differentiating myoblasts and developing chick muscle, *Nature (Lond.)* **278**:67–69.

Barlow, D. P., Green, N. M., Kurkinen, M., and Hogan, B. L. M., 1984, Sequencing of laminin B chain cDNAs reveals C-terminal regions of coiled-coil alpha helix, *EMBO J.* **3**:2355–2362.

Baron van Evercooren, A., Kleinman, H. K., Ohno, S., Marangos, P., Schwartz, J. P., and Dubois-Dalcq, M. E., 1982, Nerve growth factor, laminin and fibronectin promote neurite growth in human fetal sensory ganglia cultures, *J. Neurosci. Res.* **8**:179–193.

Bender, B. L., Jaffe, R., Carlin, B., and Chung, A. E., 1981, Immunolocalization of entactin, a sulfated basement membrane component, in rodent tissues, and comparison with GP-2 (laminin), *Am. J. Pathol.* **103**:419–426.

Bentz, H., Morris, N. P., Murray, L. W., Sakai, L. Y., Hollister, D. W., and Burgeson, R., 1983, Isolation and partial characterization of a new human collagen with an extended triple-helical structural domain, *Proc. Natl. Acad. Sci. USA* **80**:3168–3172.

Benya, P. D., 1986, Isolation and characterization of type VIII collagen synthesis by cultures of rabbit corneal endothelial cells. A conventional structure replaces the interrupted helix model, *J. Biol. Chem.* **261**:4160–4169.

Bernfield, M., Banerjee, S. D., Koda, J. E., and Rapraeger, A. C., 1984, Remodelling of the basement membrane: Morphogenesis and maturation, *Ciba Found. Symp.* **108**:179–192.

Beutner, E. H., Jordon, R. E., and Chorzelski, T. P., 1968, The immunopathology of pemphigus and bullous pemphigoid, *J. Invest. Dermatol.* **51**:63–80.

Birdwell, C. R., Gospodarowicz, D., and Nicolson, G. L., 1978, Localization and role of fibronectin in cultured bovine endothelial cells, *Proc. Natl. Acad. Sci. USA* **75**:3273–3277.

Bonadio, J. F., Sage, H., Cheng, F., Bernstein, J., and Striker, G. E., 1984, Localization of collagen types IV and V, laminin, heparansulfate proteoglycan to the basal lamina of kidney epithelial cells in transfilter metanephric cultures, *Am. J. Pathol.* **116**:289–296.

Bourdon, M. A., Wikstrand, C. J., Furthmayr, H., Matthews, T. J., and Bigner, D. D., 1983, Human glioma–mesenchymal extracellular matrix antigen defined by monoclonal antibody, *Cancer Res.* **43**:2796–2805.

Brown, R. A., and Weiss, J. B., 1979, Possible shared identities of A, B and C chains, *FEBS Lett.* **106:**71–75.

Brown, R. A., Shuttleworth, C. A., and Weiss, J. B., 1978, Three new α-chains from a non-basement membrane source, *Biochem. Biophys. Res. Commun.* **80:**866–872.

Brown, S. S., Malinoff, H. L., and Wicha, M. S., 1983, Connectin–cell surface protein that binds both laminin and actin, *Proc. Natl. Acad. Sci. USA* **80:**5927–5930.

Bruns, R. R., 1969, A symmetrical, extracellular fibril, *J. Cell Biol.* **42:**418–430.

Bruns, R. R., 1984, Beaded filaments and long-spacing fibrils: Relation to type VI collagen, *J. Ultrastruct. Res.* **89:**136–145.

Bruns, R. R., Press, W., Engvall, E., Timpl, R., and Gross, J., 1986, Type VI collagen in extracellular 100 nm periodic filaments and fibrils: Identification by immunoelectron microscopy, *J. Cell Biol.* **103:**393–404.

Buckley, K. M., Schweitzer, E. S., Miljanich, G. P., Clift-O'Grady, L., Kushner, P. D., Reichardt, L. F., and Kelly, R. B., 1983, A synaptic vesicle antigen is restricted to the junctional region of the presynaptic plasma membrane, *Proc. Natl. Acad. Sci. USA* **80:**7342–7346.

Burgeson, R. E., El Adli, F. A., Kaitila, I. I., and Hollister, D. W., 1976, Fetal membrane collagens: Identification of two new collagen α-chains, *Proc. Natl. Acad. Sci. USA* **73:**2579–2583.

Carlin, B. E., Jaffe, R., Bender, B., and Chung, A. E., 1981, Entactin, a novel basal lamina-associated sulfated glycoprotein, *J. Biol. Chem.* **256:**5209–5214.

Carlin, B. E., Durkin, M. E., Bender, B., Jaffe, R., and Chung, A. E., 1983, Synthesis of laminin and entactin by F9 cells induced with retinoic acid and dibutyryl cyclic-AMP, *J. Biol. Chem.* **258:**7729–7737.

Carlson, E. C., Meezan, E., Brendel, K., and Kenney, M. C., 1981, Ultrastructural analyses of control and enzyme treated renal basement membranes, *Anat. Rec.* **200:**421–436.

Caroni, P., Carlson, S. S., Schweitzer, E., and Kelley, R. B., 1985, Presynaptic neurones may contribute a unique glycoprotein to the extracellular matrix at the synapse, *Nature (Lond.)* **314:**441–443.

Carter, W. G., 1982a, The cooperative role of the transformation-sensitive glycoproteins, GP140 and fibronectin, in cell attachment and spreading, *J. Biol. Chem.* **257:**3249–3257.

Carter, W. G., 1982b, Transformation-dependent alterations in glycoproteins of the extracellular matrix of human fibroblasts—characterization of GP250 and the collagen-like GP140, *J. Biol. Chem.* **257:**13805–13815.

Charonis, A. S., Tsilibary, E. C., Yurchenco, P. D., and Furthmayr, H., 1985, Binding of laminin to type IV collagen: A morphological study, *J. Cell Biol.* **100:**1848–1853.

Chung, A. E., Rhodes, R. K., and Miller, E. J., 1976, Isolation of three collagenous components of probable basement membrane origin from several tissues, *Biochem. Biophys. Res. Commun.* **71:**1167–1174.

Chung, A. E., Jaffe, R., Freeman, I. L., Vergnes, J.-P., Braginski, J. E., and Carlin, B., 1979, Properties of a basement membrane-related glycoprotein synthesized in culture by a mouse embryonal carcinoma-derived cell line, *Cell* **16:**277–287.

Clark, R. A. F., Quinn, J. H., Winn, H. J., Lanigan, J. M., Dellapella, P., and Colvin, R. B., 1982a, Fibronectin is produced by blood vessels in response to injury, *J. Exp. Med.* **156:**646–657.

Clark, R. A. F., Lanigan, J. M., DellaPelle, P., Manseau, E., Dvorak, H. F., and Colvin, R. B., 1982b, Fibronectin and fibrin provide a provisional matrix for epidermal cell migration during wound re-epithelialization, *J. Invest. Dermatol.* **79:**264–269.

Cleary, E. G., and Gibson, M. A., 1983, Elastin-associated microfibrils and microfibrillar proteins, *Int. Rev. Connect. Tissue Res.* **10:**97–209.

Cooper, A. R., Kurkinen, M., Taylor, A., and Hogan, B. L. M., 1981, Studies on the biosynthesis of laminin by murine parietal endodermal cells, *Eur. J. Biochem.* **119:**189–197.

Crouch, E., and Bornstein, P., 1979, Characterization of a type IV procollagen synthesized by human amniotic fluid cells in culture, *J. Biol. Chem.* **254:**4197–4204.

Crouch, E., Sage, H., and Bornstein, P., 1980, Structural basis for the apparent heterogeneity of collagens in human basement membranes: Type IV procollagen contains two distinct chains, *Proc. Natl. Acad. Sci. USA* **77:**745–750.

Dixit, S. N., Stuart, J. M., Seyer, J. M., Risteli, J., Timpl, R., and Kang, A. H., 1981, Type IV collagens:

Isolation and characterization of 7S collagen from human kidney, liver and lung, *Collagen Rel. Res.* **1**:549–556.

Doolittle, R. F., Goldbaum, D. M., and Doolittle, L. R., 1978, Designation of sequences involved in the "coiled-coil" interdomain connections in fibrinogen: Construction of an atomic scale model, *J. Mol. Biol.* **120**:311–325.

Dziadek, M., Paulsson, M., and Timpl, R., 1986, Identification and interaction repertoire of large forms of the basement membrane protein nidogen, *EMBO J.* **4**:2513–2518.

Edgar, D., Timpl, R., and Thoenen, H., 1984, The heparin-binding domain of laminin is responsible for its effects on neurite outgrowth and neuronal survival, *EMBO J.* **3**:1463–1468.

Ekblom, P., 1981, Formation of basement membranes in the embryonic kidney: An immunohistological study, *J. Cell Biol.* **91**:1–10.

Engel, J., and Furthmayr, H., 1987, Electronmicroscopy and other physical methods for the characterization of extracellular matrix components: Fibronectin, laminin, collagen IV, collagen VI, and proteoglycans, *Methods Enzymol.* **145**:3–78.

Engel, J., Odermatt, E., Engel, A., Madri, J. A., Furthmayr, H., Rohde, H., and Timpl, R., 1981, Shapes, domain organizations and flexibility of laminin and fibronectin, two multifunctional proteins of the extracellular matrix, *J. Mol. Biol.* **150**:97–120.

Engel, J., Furthmayr, H., Odermatt, E., von der Mark, H., Aumailley, M., Fleischmajer, R., and Timpl, R., 1985, Structure and macromolecular organization of type VI collagen, *Ann. NY Acad. Sci* **460**:25–37.

Engvall, E., and Ruoslahti, E., 1983, Cell adhesive, protein binding, and antigenic properties of laminin, *Collagen Rel. Res.* **3**:359–369.

Farquhar, M. G., 1978, Structure and function in glomerular capillaries. Role of the basement membrane in glomerular filtration, in: *Biology and Chemistry of Basement Membranes* (N. N. Kefalides, ed.), pp. 43–80, Academic, New York.

Farquhar, M. G., 1981, The glomerular basement membrane, a selective macromolecular filter, in: *Cell Biology of the Extracellular Matrix* (E. D. Hay, ed.), pp. 335–378, Plenum, New York.

Fessler, L. I., and Fessler, J. H., 1980, Characterization of basement membrane procollagen made by human endothelial cells, *J. Supramol. Struct.* **4**:178–186.

Fessler, L. I., and Fessler, J. H., 1982, Identification of the carboxyl peptides of mouse procollagen IV and its implications for the assembly and structure of basement membrane procollagen, *J. Biol. Chem.* **257**:9804–9810.

Fessler, L. I., Robinson, W. J., and Fessler, J. H., 1981, Biosynthesis of procollagen ((proα1 (V)2(proα2 V)) by chick tendon fibroblasts and procollagen (proα1 (V)3 by hamster lung cell cultures, *J. Biol. Chem.* **256**:9646–9651.

Foellmer, H. G., Madri, J. A., and Furthmayr, H., 1983, Monoclonal antibodies to type IV collagen: Probes for the study of structure and function of basement membranes, *Lab. Invest.* **48**:639–649.

Fujikawa, L. S., Foster, C. S., Harrist, T. J., Lanigan, J. M., and Colvin, R. B., 1981, Fibronectin in healing rabbit corneal wounds, *Lab. Invest.* **45**:120–128.

Fujiwara, S., Wiedemann, H., Timpl, R., Lustig, A., Engel, J., 1984, Structure and interactions of heparan sulfate proteoglycans from a mouse tumor basement membrane, *Eur. J. Biochem.* **145**:145–157.

Furthmayr, H., and Madri, J. A., 1982, Rotary shadowing of connective tissue macromolecules, *Collagen Rel. Res.* **2**:349–363.

Furthmayr, H., Wiedemann, H., Timpl, R., Odermatt, E., and Engel, J., 1983, Electron-microscopical approach to a structural model of intima collagen, *Biochem. J.* **211**:303–311.

Furthmayr, H., Yurchenco, P. D., Charonis, A. S., and Tsilibary, E. C., 1985, Molecular interactions of type IV collagen and laminin: Models of basement membrane assembly, in: *Basement Membranes* (S. Shibata, ed.), pp. 169–180, Elsevier, Amsterdam.

Furuto, D. K., and Miller, E. J., 1980, Isolation of a unique collagenous fraction from limited pepsin digests of human placental tissues, *J. Biol. Chem.* **255**:290–295.

Gay, S., and Miller, E. J., 1979, Characterization of lens capsule collagen: Evidence for the presence of two unique chains in molecules derived from major basement membrane structures, *Arch. Biochem. Biophys.* **198**:370–378.

Glanville, R. W., Quian, R. Q., Siebold, B., Risteli, J., and Kühn, K., 1985, Amino acid sequence of the N-terminal aggregation and cross-linking (7S domain) of the α1(IV) chain of human basement membrane collagen, *Eur. J. Biochem.* **152**:213–219.

Gibson, M., and Cleary, E., 1982, A collagen-like glycoprotein from elastin-rich tissues, *Biochem. Biophys. Res. Commun.* **105**:1288–1295.

Godfrey, E. W., Nitkin, R. M., Wallace, B. G., Rubin, L. L., and McMahan, J. J., 1984, Components of Torpedo electric organ and muscle that cause aggregation of acetylcholine receptors on cultured muscle cells, *J. Cell Biol.* **99**:615–627.

Haralson, M. A., Mitchell, W. M., Rhodes, R. K., Kresina, T. F., Gay, R., and Miller, E. J., 1980, Chinese hamster lung cells synthesize and confine to the cellular domain a collagen composed solely of B chains, *Proc. Natl. Acad. Sci. USA* **77**:5206–5210.

Hassell, J. R., Gehron Robey, P., Barrach, H. J., Wilczek, J., Rennard, S. I., and Martin, G. R., 1980, Isolation of a heparan sulfate-containing proteoglycan from basement membrane, *Proc. Natl. Acad. Sci. USA* **77**:4494–4498.

Hassell, J. R., Layshon, W. C., Ledbetter, S. R., Tyree, B., Suzuki, S., Kato, M., Kimata, K., and Kleinman, H. K., 1985, Isolation of two forms of basement membrane proteoglycans, *J. Biol. Chem.* **260**:8098–8105.

Heller-Harrison, R. A., and Carter, W. G., 1984, Pepsin-generated type VI collagen is a degradation product of GP 140, *J. Biol. Chem.* **259**:6858–6864.

Hessle, H., and Engvall, E., 1984, Type VI collagen: Studies on its localization, structure, and biosynthetic form with monoclonal antibodies, *J. Biol. Chem.* **259**:3955–3961.

Hinter, H., Fritsch, P. O., Foidart, J. M., Stingl, G., Schuler, G., and Katz, S. I., 1980, Expression of basement membrane zone antigens at the dermo-epidermal junction in organ cultures in human skin, *J. Invest. Dermatol.* **174**:200–204.

Hoffmann, H., Voss, T., Kühn, K., and Engel, J., 1984, Localization of flexible sites in threadlike molecules from electron micrographs: Comparison of interstitial, basement membrane and intima collagens, *J. Mol. Biol.* **172**:325–343.

Hogan, B. L. M., Cooper, A. R., and Kurkinen, M., 1980, Incoporation into Reichert's membrane of laminin-like extracellular proteins synthesized by parietal endoderm cells of the mouse embryo, *Dev. Biol.* **80**:289–300.

Hogan, B. L. M., Taylor, A., Kurkinen, M., and Couchman, J. R., 1982, Synthesis and localization of two sulfated glycoproteins associated with basement membranes and the extracellular matrix, *J. Cell Biol.* **95**:197–204.

Hogan, B. L. M., Barlow, D. P., and Kurkinen, M., 1984, Reichert's membrane as a model for studying the biosynthesis and assembly of basement membrane components, *Ciba Found. Symp.* **108**:60–69.

Howe, C. C., and Dietzschold, B., 1983, Structural analysis of three subunits of laminin from teratocarcinoma-derived parietal endoderm cells, *Dev. Biol.* **98**:385–391.

Inoue, S., Leblond, C. P., and Laurie, G. W., 1983, Ultrastructure of Reichert's membrane, a multilayered basement membrane in the parietal wall of the rat yolk sac, *J. Cell Biol.* **97**:1524–1537.

Iozzo, R. V., 1984, Biosynthesis of heparan sulfate proteoglycan by human colon carcinoma cells and its localization at the cell surface, *J. Cell Biol.* **99**:403–417.

Jander, R., Rauterberg, J., Voss, B., and von Bassewitz, D. B., 1981, A cysteine-rich collagenous protein from bovine placenta. Isolation of its constituent polypeptide chains and some properties of the non-denatured protein, *Eur. J. Biochem.* **114**:17–25.

Jander, R., Rauterberg, J., and Glanville, R. W., 1983, Further characterization of the three polypeptide chains of bovine and human short-chain collagen (intima collagen), *Eur. J. Biochem.* **133**:39–46.

Jander, R., Troyer, D., and Rauterberg, J., 1984, A collagen-like glycoprotein of the extracellular matrix is the undegraded form of type VI collagen, *Biochemistry* **23**:3675–3681.

Kanwar, Y. S., and Farquhar, M. G., 1979a, Anionic sites in the glomerular basement membrane. In vivo and in vitro localization to the laminae rarae by cationic probes, *J. Cell Biol.* **81**:137–153.

Kanwar, Y. S., and Farquhar, M. G., 1979b, Isolation of glycosaminoglycans (heparan sulfate) from the glomerular basement membrane, *Proc. Natl. Acad. Sci. USA* **76**:1303–1307.

Kanwar, Y. S., Hascall, V. C., and Farquhar, M. G., 1981, Partial characterization of newly synthesized proteoglycans isolated from the glomerular basement membrane, *J. Cell Biol.* **90:**527–532.

Katz, S., 1983, The epidermal basement membrane: Structure, ontogeny and role in disease, *Ciba Found. Symp.* **108:**243–259.

Kefalides, N. A., 1971, Isolation of collagen from basement membrane containing three identical α-chains, *Biochem. Biophys. Res. Commun.* **45:**226–234.

Kefalides, N. A., Alper, R., and Clark, C. C., 1979, Biochemistry and metabolism of basement membranes, *Int. Rev. Cytol.* **61:**167–228.

Keller, R., and Furthmayr, H., 1987, Isolation and characterization of basement membrane and cell surface proteoheparan sulfates from HR9 cells, *Eur. J. Biochem.* **161:**707–714.

Kleinman, H. K., McGarvey, M. L., Liotta, L. A., Gehron-Robey, P., Tryggvason, K., and Martin, G. R., 1982, Isolation and characterization of type IV procollagen, laminin and heparan sulfate proteoglycan from the EHS sarcoma, *Biochemistry* **21:**6188–6193.

Kleinman, H. K., McGarvey, M. L., Hassell, J. R., and Martin, G. R., 1983, Formation of a supramolecular complex is involved in the reconstitution of basement membrane components, *Biochemistry* **2:**4969–4974.

Konomi, H., Hayashi, T., Nakayasu, K., and Arima, M., 1984, Localization of type V collagen and type IV collagen in human cornea, lung, and skin, *Am. J. Pathol.* **116:**417–426.

Kühn, K., Wiedemann, H., Timpl, R., Risteli, J., Dieringer, H., Voss, T., and Glanville, R. W., 1981, Macromolecular structure of basement membrane collagens: Identification of 7S collagen as a cross-linking domain of type IV collagen, *FEBS Lett.* **125:**123–128.

Kurkinen, M., Barlow, D. P., Jenkins, J. R., and Hogan, B. L. M., 1983, *In vitro* synthesis of laminin and entactin polypeptides, *J. Biol. Chem.* **258:**6543–6548.

Laurie, G. W., Leblond, C. P., and Martin, G. R., 1982, Localization of type IV collagen, laminin, heparan sulfate proteoglycan, and fibronectin to the basal lamina of basement membranes, *J. Cell Biol.* **95:**340–344.

Leivo, I., Vaheri, A., Timpl, R., and Wartiovaara, J., 1980, Appearance and distribution of collagens and laminin in the early mouse embryo, *Dev. Biol.* **76:**100–114.

Lesot, H., Kühl, U., and von der Mark, K., 1983, Isolation of a laminin-binding protein from muscle cell membranes, *EMBO J.* **2:**861–868.

Linsenmayer, T. F., Fitch, J. M., Schmid, T. M., Zak, N. B., Gibney, E., Sanderson, R. D., and Mayne, R., 1983, Monoclonal antibodies against chicken type V collagen: Production, specificity, and use for immunocytochemical localization in embryonic cornea and other organs, *J. Cell Biol.* **96:**124–132.

Madri, J. A., and Furthmayr, H., 1980, Collagen polymorphism in the lung, *Hum. Pathol.* **11:**353–366.

Madri, J. A., Dreyer, B., Pitlick, F. A., and Furthmayr, H., 1980a, The collagenous components of the subendothelium. Correlation of structure and function, *Lab. Invest.* **43:**303–314.

Madri, J. A., Roll, F. J., Furthmayr, H., and Foidart, J.-M., 1980b, Ultrastructural localization of fibronectin and laminin in the basement membrane of the murine kidney, *J. Cell Biol.* **86:**682–687.

Madri, J. A., Foellmer, H. G., and Furthmayr, H., 1982, Type V collagens of the human placenta: Trimer α-chain composition, ultrastructural morphology and peptide analysis, *Collagen Rel. Res.* **2:**19–29.

Mainardi, C. L., Dixit, S. N., and Kang, A. H., 1980, Degradation of type V (basement membrane) collagen by a proteinase from human polymorphonuclear leucocyte granules, *J. Biol. Chem.* **255:**5435–5441.

Martin, G. R., Kleinman, H. K., Terranova, V. P., Ledbetter, S., and Hassell, J. R., 1984, The regulation of basement membrane formation and cell–matrix interaction by defined supramolecular complexes, *Ciba Found. Symp.* **108:**197–209.

Martinez-Hernandez, A., and Amenta, P. S., 1983, The basement membrane in pathology, *Lab. Invest.* **48:**656–677.

Martinez-Hernandez, A., Marsh, C. A., Clark, C. C., Macarak, E. J., and Brownell, A. G., 1981, Fibronectin: its relationship to basement membranes. II. Ultrastructural studies in rat kidney, *Collagen Rel. Res.* **1:**405–418.

Martinez-Hernandez, A., Gay, S., and Miller, E. J., 1982, Ultrastructural localization of type V collagen in rat kidney, *J. Cell Biol.* **92:**343–349.

Modesti, A., Kalebic, T., Scarpa, S., Togo, S., Liotta, L. A., and Triche, T. J., 1983, Type V collagen in human amnion is a 12 nm fibrillar component of the pericellular interstitium, *Eur. J. Cell Biol.* **35:**246–255.

Monaghan, P., Warburton, M. J., Perusinghe, N., and Rudland, P. S., 1983, Topographical arrangement of basement membrane proteins in lactating rat mammary gland: Comparison of the distribution of type IV collagen, laminin, fibronectin, and thy-1 at the ultrastructural level, *Proc. Natl. Acad. Sci. USA* **80:**3344–3348.

Morris, N. P., Keene, D. R., Glanville, R. W., Bentz, H., and Burgeson, R. E., 1986, The tissue form of type-VII collagen is an antiparallel dimer, *J. Biol. Chem.* **261:**5638–5644.

Oberbäumer, I., Wiedemann, H., Timpl, R., and Kühn, K., 1982, Shape and assembly of type IV procollagen obtained from cell culture, *EMBO J.* **1:**805–810.

Oberbäumer, I., Lautent, M., Schwarz, U., Sakurai, Y., Yamada, Y., Vogeli, G., Voss, T., Siebold, B., Glanville, R. W., and Kuhn, K., 1985, Amino acid sequence of the noncollagenous globular domain (NC1) of the α1 (IV) chain of basement membrane collagen as derived from complementary DNA, *Eur. J. Biochem.* **147:**217–224.

Odermatt, E., Risteli, J., van Delden, V., and Timpl, R., 1983, Structural diversity and domain composition of a unique collagenous fragment (intima collagen) obtained from human placenta, *Biochem. J.* **211:**295–302.

Oldberg, A., Kjellen, L., and Höök, M., 1979, Cell-surface heparansulfate. Isolation and characterization of a proteoglycan from rat liver membranes, *J. Biol. Chem.* **254:**8505–8510.

Oohira, A., Wight, T. N., McPherson, J., and Bornstein, P., 1982, Biochemical and ultrastructural studies of proteoheparansulfates synthesized by PYS-2, a basement membrane-producing cell line, *J. Cell Biol.* **92:**357–367.

Orkin, R. W., Gehron-Robey, P., McGoodwin, E. B., Martin, G. R., Valentine, T., and Swarm, R., 1977, A murine tumor producing a matrix of basement membrane, *J. Exp. Med.* **145:**204–220.

Ott, U., Odermatt, E., Engel, J., Furthmayr, H., and Timpl, R., 1982, Protease resistance and conformation of laminin, *Eur. J. Biochem.* **123:**63–72.

Paulsson, M., Deutzmann, R., Timpl, R., Dalzoppo, D., Odermatt, E., and Engel, J., 1985, Evidence for coiled-coil α-helical regions in the long arm of laminin, *EMBO J.* **4:**309–316.

Pierce, G. B., 1970, Epithelial basement membrane: Origin, development and role in disease, in: *Chemistry and Molecular Biology of the Extracellular Matrix* (E. A. Balazs, ed.), pp. 471–506, Academic, New York.

Pihlajaniemi, T., Tryggvason, K., Myers, J. C., Kurkinen, M., Lebo, R., Cheung, M. C., Prockop, D. J., and Boyd, C. D., 1985, cDNA clones coding for the pro-α1(IV) chain of human type IV procollagen reveal an unusual homology of amino acid sequences in two halves of the carboxy-terminal domain, *J. Biol. Chem.* **260:**7681–7687.

Rao, C. N., Margulies, I. M. K., Tralka, T. S., Terranova, V. P., Madri, J. A., and Liotta, L. A., 1983, Isolation of a subunit of laminin and its role in the molecular structure and tumor cell adhesion, *J. Biol. Chem.* **257:**9740–9744.

Rhodes, R. K., and Miller, E. J., 1978, Physicochemical characterization and molecular organization of the collagen A and B chains, *Biochemistry* **17:**3442–3448.

Risteli, J., Bächinger, H. P., Engel, J., Furthmayr, H., and Timpl, R., 1980, 7S-collagen: Characterization of an unusual basement membrane structure, *Eur. J. Biochem.* **108:**239–250.

Roll, F. J., Madri, J. A., Albert, J., and Furthmayr, H., 1980, Codistribution of collagen types IV and AB2 in basement membranes and mesangium of the kidney: An immunoferritin study of ultrathin frozen sections, *J. Cell Biol.* **85:**597–616.

Sage, H., and Bornstein, P., 1979, Characterization of a novel collagen chain in human placenta and its relation to AB collagen, *Biochemistry* **18:**3815–3822.

Sage, H., Pritzl, P., and Bornstein, P., 1980, A unique, pepsin-sensitive collagen synthesized by aortic endothelial cells in culture, *Biochemistry* **19:**5747–5755.

Sanes, J. R., 1982, Laminin, fibronectin, and collagen in synaptic and extrasynaptic portions of muscle fiber membrane, *J. Cell Biol.* **93:**442–451.

Sanes, J. R., 1983, Roles of the extracellular matrix in neural development, *Annu. Rev. Physiol.* **45**:581–601.

Sanes, J. R., and Hall, Z. W., 1979, Antibodies that bind specifically to synaptic sites on muscle fiber basal lamina, *J. Cell Biol.* **83**:357–370.

Sato, T., and Spiro, R. G., 1976, Studies on the subunit composition of renal glomerular basement membrane, *J. Biol. Chem.* **251**:4062–4070.

Sawada, H., 1982, The fine structure of the bovine Descemet's membrane with special reference to the biochemical nature, *Cell Tissue Res.* **226**:241–255.

Sawada, H., Konomi, H., and Nagai, Y., 1984, The basement membrane of bovine corneal endothelial cells in culture with β-aminoproprionitrile: Biosynthesis of hexagonal lattices of a dumbbell-shaped structure, *Eur. J. Cell Biol.* **35**:226–234.

Schuppan, D., Timpl, R., and Glanville, R. W., 1980, Discontinuities in the triple helical sequence Gly-X-Y of basement membrane (type IV) collagen, *FEBS Lett.* **115**:297–300.

Schuppan, D., Glanville, R. W., and Timpl, R., 1982, Covalent structure of mouse type IV collagen: Isolation, order and partial amino acid sequence of cyanogen and tryptic peptides of pepsin fragment P1 from the α1(IV) chain, *Eur. J. Biochem.* **123**:505–512.

Schuppan, D., Glanville, R. W., and Timpl, R., 1984, Sequence comparison of pepsin resistant segments of basement membrane collagen α1(IV) chain from bovine lens capsule and mouse tumor, *Biochem. J.* **220**:227–233.

Sear, C. H. J., Grant, M. E., and Jackson, D. S., 1981, The nature of the microfibrillar glycoprotein of elastic fibers—A biosynthetic study, *Biochem. J.* **194**:587–598.

Stanley, J. R., Hawley-Nelson, P., Poirier, M., Katz, S. I., and Yuspa, S. H., 1980, Detection of pemphigoid antigen, pemphigus antigen, and keratin filaments by indirect immunofluorescence in cultured human epidermal cells, *J. Invest. Dermatol.* **75**:183–186.

Stanley, J. R., Alvarez, O. M., Bere, E. W., Eaglstein, W. H., and Katz, S. I., 1981a, Detection of basement membrane zone antigens during epidermal wound healing, *J. Invest. Dermatol.* **77**:240–243.

Stanley, J. R., Hawley-Nelson, P., Yuspa, S. H., Shevach, S. M., and Katz, S. I., 1981b, Characterization of bullous pemphigoid antigen: A unique basement membrane protein of stratified squamous epithelia, *Cell* **24**:897–903.

Stenman, J., and Vaheri, A., 1978, Distribution of a major connective tissue protein, fibronectin, in normal human tissues, *J. Exp. Med.* **147**:1054–1064.

Stenn, K. S., Madri, J. A., and Roll, F. J., 1979, Migrating epidermis produces AB₂ collagen and requires continual collagen synthesis for movement, *Nature (Lond.)* **277**:229–232.

Stowe, J. L., Sawada, H., and Farquhar, M. G., 1985, Basement membrane heparansulfate proteoglycans are concentrated in the laminae rare and in podocytes of the rat renal glomerulus, *Proc. Natl. Acad. Sci. USA* **82**:3296–3300.

Strickland, S., Smith, K. K., and Marotti, K. R., 1980, Hormonal induction of differentiation in teratocarcinoma cells: Generation of parietal endoderm by retinoic acid and dibutyryl cAMP, *Cell* **21**:347–355.

Terranova, V. P., Rohrbach, D. H., and Martin, G. R., 1980, Role of laminin in the attachment of PAM 212 (epithelial) cells to basement membrane collagen, *Cell* **22**:719–726.

Timpl, R., and Dziadek, M., 1986, Structure, development and molecular pathology of basement membranes, *Intern. Rev. Exp. Path.* **29**:1–112.

Timpl, R., and Martin, G. R., 1982, Components of basement membranes, in: *Immunochemistry of the Extracellular Matrix*, Vol. 2 (H. Furthmayr, ed.), pp. 119–150, CRC Press, Boca Raton, Florida.

Timpl, R., Rohde, H., Gehron Robey P., Rennard, S. I., Foidart, J. M., and Martin, G. R., 1979, Laminin—A glycoprotein from basement membranes, *J. Biol. Chem.* **254**:9933–9937.

Timpl, R., Wiedemann, H., van Delden, V., Furthmayr, H., and Kühn, K., 1981, A network model for the organization of type IV collagen molecules in basement membranes, *Eur. J. Biochem.* **120**:203–211.

Timpl, R., Dziadek, M., Fujiwara, S., Nowack, H., and Wick, G., 1983a, Nidogen: A new, self-aggregating basement membrane protein, *Eur. J. Biochem.* **137**:455–465.

Timpl, R., Johansson, S., van Delden, V., Oberbäumer, I., and Höök, M., 1983b, Characterization of protease-resistant fragments of laminin mediating attachment and spreading of rat hepatocytes, *J. Biol. Chem.* **258:**8922–8927.

Tonnesen, M. G., Jenkins, Jr., D., Siegal, S. L., Lee, L. A., Huff, J. C., and Clark, R. A. F., 1985, Expression of fibronectin, laminin, and Factor VIII in the human cutaneous microvasculature during development, *J. Invest. Dermatol.* **85:**564–568.

Trueb, B., and Bornstein, P., 1984, Characterization of the precursor form of type VI collagen, *J. Biol. Chem.* **259:**8597–8604.

Tryggvason, K., Gehron Robey, P., and Martin, G. R., 1980, Biosynthesis of type IV procollagen, *Biochemistry* **19:**1284–1289.

Uitto, V.-J., Schwartz, D., and Veiss, A., 1980, Degradation of basement membrane collagen by neutral proteases from human neutrophils, *Eur. J. Biochem.* **105:**409–417.

Vaccaro, C. A., and Brody, J. S., 1981, Structural features of alveolar wall basement membrane in the adult rat lung, *J. Cell Biol.* **91:**427–437.

Vlodavsky, I., and Gospodarowitz, D., 1981, Respective roles of laminin and fibronectin in adhesion of human carcinoma and sarcoma cells, *Nature (Lond.)* **289:**304–306.

von der Mark, K., 1981, Localization of collagen types in tissues, *Int. Rev. Connect. Tissue Res.* **9:**265–324.

von der Mark, K., and Ocalan, M., 1982, Immunofluorescent localization of type V collagen in the chick embryo with monoclonal antibodies, *Collagen Rel. Res.* **2:**541–555.

von der Mark, H., Aumailley, M., Wick, G., Fleischmajer, R., and Timpl, R., 1984, Immunochemistry, genuine size and tissue localization of collagen VI, *Eur. J. Biochem.* **142:**493–502.

Vracko, R., 1974, Basal lamina scaffold—Anatomy and significance for maintenance of orderly tissue structure, *Am. J. Pathol.* **77:**314–346.

Wan, Y.-J., Wu, T.-C., Chung, A. E., and Damjanov, I., 1984, Monoclonal antibodies to laminin reveal the heterogeneity of basement membranes in the developing and adult mouse tissues, *J. Cell Biol.* **98:**971–979.

Wang, S.-Y., and Gudas, L. J., 1983, Isolation of cDNA clones specific for collagen IV and laminin from mouse teratocarcinoma cells, *Proc. Natl. Acad. Sci. USA* **80:**5880–5884.

Wartiovaara, J., Leivo, I., and Vaheri, A., 1979, Expression of the cell surface-associated glycoprotein, fibronectin, in the early mouse embryo, *Dev. Biol.* **69:**247–257.

Weber, S., Engel, J., Wiedemann, H., Glanville, R. W., and Timpl, R., 1984, Subunit structure and assembly of the globular domain of basement membrane collagen type IV, *Eur. J. Biochem.* **139:**401–410.

Welsh, C., Gay, S., Rhodes, R. K., Pfister, R., and Miller, E. J., 1980, Collagen heterogeneity in normal rabbit cornea. I. Isolation and biochemical characterization of the genetically distinct collagens, *Biochim. Biophys. Acta* **625:**77–88.

Wewer, U., Albrechtsen, R., Manthorpe, M., Varon, S., Engvall, E., and Ruoslahti, E., 1983, Human laminin isolated in a nearly intact, biologically active form from placenta by limited proteolysis, *J. Biol. Chem.* **258:**12654–12660.

Wu, T.-C., Wan, Y.-J., Chung, A. E., and Damjanov, I., 1983, Immunohistochemical localization of entactin and laminin in mouse embryos and fetuses, *Dev. Biol.* **100:**496–505.

Yurchenco, P. D., and Furthmayr, H., 1984, Self-assembly of basement membrane collagen, *Biochemistry* **23:**1839–1850.

Yurchenco, P. D., and Furthmayr, H., 1985, Type IV collagen "7S" tetramer formation: Aspects of kinetics and thermodynamics, *Ann. NY Acad. Sci.* **460:**530–533.

Yurchenco, P. D., Tsilibary, E. C., Charonis, A., and Furthmayr, H., 1985, Laminin polymerization in vitro: Evidence for a two step assembly with domain specificity, *J. Biol. Chem.* **260:**7636–7644.

Chapter 23

Re-formation of the Epidermal–Dermal Junction during Wound Healing

DAVID T. WOODLEY and ROBERT A. BRIGGAMAN

1. Introduction

The relationship between keratinocytes and the extracellular matrix upon which they rest is complex and only beginning to be understood. Keratinocytes are capable of synthesizing many of the extracellular matrix molecules that are most closely related to their cell surface, such as the bullous pemphigoid antigen (Woodley and Regnier, 1979; Stanley et al., 1980; Woodley et al., 1980a, 1982) laminin (Stanley et al., 1982c), the epidermolysis bullosa acquisita antigen (Woodley et al., 1985b), and fibronectin (O'Keefe et al., 1984; Kubo et al., 1984). Thus, it is clear that keratinocytes directly influence their extracellular matrix composition. Furthermore, it is becoming apparent that cellular behavior can be modified by contact with a given extracellular matrix molecule. For example, mammary epithelial cells have a decreased requirement for epidermal growth factor when cultured on type IV (basement membrane) collagen as compared with type I (interstitial) collagen (Salomon et al., 1981). The influence on cellular behavior by contact with matrix molecules is often referred to as cell–matrix interactions. The cell–matrix interactions that apply to the keratinocyte may be viewed as a self-contained system, since the keratinocytes synthesize and extracellularly deposit their own matrix components, which in turn directly affects the behavior of cells in contact with the cell plasma membrane.

Matrix molecules that are in direct or near contact with the keratinocyte plasma membrane during wound healing are very different from those of normal epidermis (Table I) (Woodley et al., 1985a). Keratinocytes of normal stratified epidermis that reside on basement membrane eventually move vertically

Abbreviations used in this chapter. BMZ, basement membrane zone; EBA, epidermolysis bullosa acquisita; BP, bullous pemphigoid; IF, immunofluorescence.

DAVID T. WOODLEY and ROBERT A. BRIGGAMAN • Department of Dermatology, University of North Carolina, Chapel Hill, North Carolina 27514.

Table I. Matrices for Keratinocytes

Intact skin	Cutaneous wound
Bullous pemphigoid antigen	Bullous pemphigoid antigen
Laminin	Fibronectin
Heparan sulfate–proteoglycan	Fibrin
Type IV collagen	Fibrinogen
? Type V collagen	Hyaluronic acid
EBA antigen	Sulfated proteoglycans
	Collagen types I and III
	Elastin

leaving the basement membrane, stop dividing, and enter terminal differentiation. At the end of their vertical journey, they become a nonviable anucleated bag of crosslinked keratin in the stratum corneum. These events occur in an epithelium separated from the dermis by a basement membrane composed of the bullous pemphigoid antigen, laminin, heparan sulfate proteoglycan, type IV collagen, perhaps type V collagen, and the epidermolysis bullosa acquisita antigen.

Although there is no direct evidence that components of cutaneous basement membrane have any inductive influence upon the process of keratinization, Prunieras and co-workers (Prunieras *et al.*, 1979, 1983a,b; Regnier *et al.*, 1981) noted that high-molecular-weight keratin bands (67,000 M_r), characteristic of fully differentiated epidermis, are absent from virtually all cultures except when human keratinocytes are cultured on a nonviable human skin basement membrane and kept at an air–fluid interface. Fuchs and Green (1981) found that when vitamin A was removed from cultures by de-lipidizing serum, keratinocytes also synthesized the high-molecular-weight 67,000-M_r keratin band. Thus, it is possible that both extracellular matrix molecules and soluble factors such as retinoic acid may influence keratinization.

During wound healing, keratinocytes adjacent to the wound margin leave their basement membrane matrix and come into contact with a new group of matrix molecules, including fibrinogen, fibrin, fibronectin, elastin, and interstitial collagens (type I and III) (Table I). Keratinocytes migrating on this dermal matrix are in contact with serum (rather than plasma) and with soluble factors that are unfiltered by the basement membrane zone. Under these conditions, the keratinocytes exhibit a different pattern of cell behavior from their steady-state condition; they migrate laterally and continue to proliferate without differentiating until they cover the wound.

Again, there is little direct evidence that this new set of matrix molecules during wound healing has any influence on the observed behavior of the keratinocytes. Nevertheless, it is significant that when keratinocytes are migrating over a wound bed, in addition to covering the wound they reconstitute the cutaneous basement membrane. This chapter reviews the morphology and composition of the epidermal–dermal junction, as well as studies that have examined reconstitution of this structure *in vitro* and *in vivo* wound-healing models.

2. Morphology of the Epidermal–Dermal Junction

The interface between the epidermis and dermis presents an undulating pattern of rete ridges and dermal papillae as viewed by conventional light microscopy. This pattern varies greatly in complexity and configuration in different body regions and is most pronounced on the palms and soles. Special stains, such as periodic acid-Schiff (PAS) and silver (reticulum), show a positive reaction in a zone between the epidermis and dermis that has been termed the basement membrane. The term basement membrane zone (BMZ) in common usage in the immunofluorescence literature refers to the localization of a variety of antibodies including those seen in bullous pemphigoid, lupus erythematosis, and other epidermal–dermal junction diseases. These light and fluorescent microscopic techniques demonstrate a simple-appearing uniform band of reaction between epidermis and dermis.

A greater degree of complexity at epidermal–dermal interface is seen with thin (1-μm) plastic embedded sections than can be appreciated with conventional techniques. The epidermal–dermal interface of the basal cells overlying dermal papillae possess undulating plasma membranes on the basal portion of those cells (Lavker and Sun, 1982). These projections have been termed serrations. By contrast, basal cells in the rete ridge areas have a flat epidermal–dermal interface.

The morphology of the epidermal–dermal junction is best appreciated at the ultrastructural level (Briggaman and Wheeler, 1975; Daroczy et al., 1979). From the epidermal side inward, the junction is composed of the plasma membrane of the basal cell, lamina lucida, lamina densa, and sublamina densa fibrous zone. At intervals along the plasma membrane are studded electron-dense thickenings termed hemidesmosomes. These are structurally similar to the desmosomes present between keratinocytes. Hemidesmosomes are composed of an electron-dense area, the attachment plaque, which is approximately 20–40 nm thick and present on the cytoplasmic surface of the interior leaflet of the plasma membrane. Cytoplasmic tonofilaments radiate toward the attachment plaque and attach to it. Subjacent to the hemidesmosome is an electron-dense line called the subbasal dense plaque (juxtamembrane line), which is situated beneath the outer leaflet of the basal cell plasma membrane.

The lamina lucida is an electron-lucent area between the plasma membrane of the epidermal basal cell and the lamina densa. The lamina lucida is approximately 20–40 nm in thickness. In most areas, the lamina lucida is amorphous. However, fine filaments termed anchoring filaments can be seen in some areas traversing the lamina lucida. They are common in the area of hemidesmosomes.

The lamina densa is a continuous electron-dense layer of fairly uniform thickness (40–50 nm) paralleling the plasma membrane of basal keratinocytes. The lamina densa appears slightly thicker and more dense in the area subjacent to hemidesmosomes. In addition, reduplication of lamina dense is fairly common, even in normal skin, and may result from epidermal–dermal junction remodeling associated with basal cell movement.

Beneath the lamina densa is an array of sublamina densa fibrous components consisting of three morphologically different fiber types. One fibrous element is the anchoring fibril. These have a characteristic morphology consisting of a central asymmetric banded zone that fans at either end into finer filaments. One end fuses with the lamina densa and the other extends into the dermis. The dermal ends frequently connect with adjacent anchoring fibrils producing a network of interconnecting arcades. Bundles of microfibrils (10–12 nm), which appear identical to the microfibrils associated with elastic tissues, constitute a second fibrous element. Their epidermal end fuses directly with the lamina densa frequently at or near the tips of the convolutions of the epidermal–dermal junction previously described as serrations (Lavker and Sun, 1982). This distinctive structural component has been termed the dermal microfibril bundle (Briggaman and Wheeler, 1975) and is identical with the light microscopic oxytylin fiber (Cotta-Pereira et al., 1976, 1979). Dermal microfibril bundles are distributed predominantly in the dermal papillae. The dermal ends of the microfibril bundles have been traced to connections with morphologically distinct dermal elastic fibers (Kobayasi, 1977). The third component, single collagen fibers, or less commonly small bundles of several collagen fibers, is recognized by its characteristic banded periodicity and is distributed beneath the lamina densa in the area corresponding to the papillary dermis on light microscopy. No direct connections occur between the anchoring fibrils and collagen fibers, although collagen fibers are often enmeshed in the network of anchoring fibrils.

It is worth stressing that the epidermal–dermal junction constitutes an integrated structural–functional unit. This unit is composed of cellular (basal cell plasma membrane with its hemidesmosomes) and extracellular (lamina lucida, lamina densa, and sublamina densa fibrous zone) elements.

3. Composition of Basement Membranes—Especially the Epidermal–Dermal Junction

Remarkable advances have been made during the past 10 years in the identification and characterization of basement membrane components, including those of the epidermal–dermal junction (Stanley et al., 1982a; Briggaman, 1983; Katz, 1984) (Tables II and III). Biochemically, these fall into several major categories, including basement membrane collagens; noncollagenous basement membrane proteins, including glycoproteins and proteoglycans; and components known to be in the basement membrane by their reactions with specific antibodies, but whose biochemical characterization is uncertain.

3.1. Basement Membrane Collagens

Type IV collagen is a ubiquitous component of virtually all basement membranes where it is a major structural component of the lamina densa (Foidart and Yaar, 1981; Yaoita et al., 1978). Type IV collagen is composed of two

Table II. Properties of Basement Membrane Components

Macromolecule	Native molecular weight (M_r)	Chain structure	Chain size (M_r)	Role in BMZ	Molecular shape
Bullous pemphigoid	220,000–240,000	An	220,000–240,000	Unknown	Unknown
Laminin	1,000,000	AB$_1$B$_2$	B=200,000 A=400,000	Cell–substrate attachment	
Type IV collagen (BMZ-specific collagen)	540,000	pro 1 (IV)$_3$, pro 2 (IV)$_3$ or heteropolymer	185,000 170,000	Tissue support	
Heparan sulfate proteoglycan	750,000	Central protein core with heparan sulfate glycosaminoglycan (GAG) side chains	GAG side chains of 70,000	Permeability barrier	
Fibronectin	450,000	Disulfide-linked dimers	220,000–225,000	Cell attachment and matrix attachment	
Epidermolysis bullosa acquisita antigen	>800,000	An	290,000	Unkown	Unknown
Entactin	Unknown	?	158,000	Unknown	Unknown

[a]Theoretical shape from known molecular properties.

distinct α-chains (pro-α$_1$ (IV), 185,000 M_r, and proα$_2$ (IV), 170,000 M_r) (Alitalo et al., 1980; Crouch et al., 1980). These α-chains are arranged in a triple-helical macromolecule with an essentially rodlike structure similar to that of other collagens. Type IV collagen differs from the interstitial collagens however in having a more procollagen-like size and frequent nonhelical domains interrupting the triple-helical sequence (Schuppan et al., 1980). In addition, type IV collagen has terminal nonhelical domains. A 7S collagen domain occurs at the N-terminal end, which is resistant to degradation with collagenase (Timpl et al., 1979c; Risteli et al., 1980; Dixit et al., 1983), and a globular carbohydrate-rich domain exists at the C-terminal end (Timple et al., 1981; Fessler and Fessler, 1982). Kuhn et al. (1981) and Timpl et al. (1981) proposed an organization for type IV collagen in basement membranes in which four type IV molecules are connected at their 7S domain, joined with other type IV molecules at the opposite globular ends. Such an arrangement would lead to the formation of the continuous feltwork structure characteristic of basement membrane in distinction from the side-to-side organization of the interstitial collagens, which results in fiber formation.

Table III. Localization of Basement Membrane Components
in the Epidermal–Dermal Junction

Component	Immunohistochemical localization	Ultrastructural localization
Collagenous		
Type IV collagen	+	Lamina densa
Type V collagen	±	Unknown
Type VII collagen	+	Anchoring fibrils
Noncollagenous		
Glycoproteins		
Laminin	+	Lamina lucida
Nidogen	+	Unknown
Entactin	±	Unknown
Bullous pemphigoid antigen	+	Lamina lucida, intracytoplasmic (esp. hemidesmosomes)
Epidermolysis bullosa	+	Sublamina densa and lamina densa
Proteoglycans		
Heparan sulfate proteoglycan	+	Probable lamina densa
Other basement membrane components identified by specific antibodies		
AF-1, AF-2 antigens	+	Anchoring fibrils
KF-1 antigens	+	Lamina densa

Type V collagen is another major collagen class. It is debated whether or not type V collagen is an exclusive basement membrane collagen or even an integral part of basement membranes. Type V collagen is composed of three distinct subunits called α_1 (V), α_2 (V), and α_3 (V), previously called B, A, and C chains, respectively (Burgeson et al., 1976; Chung et al., 1976; Sage and Bornstein, 1979). Type V collagen probably exists as triple helical structures composed of heteropolymers (Rhodes and Miller, 1978) and homopolymers (Bentz et al., 1978). The specific anatomic localization and actual tissue form of type V collagen are unknown. Type V collagen codistributes with type IV collagen within basement membranes according to Madri and Furthmayr (1979), Madri et al. (1980a), and Roll et al. (1980). Other investigators have found type V collagen around the cell surface of a variety of cell types, including smooth muscle (Gay et al., 1981) and endothelial cells (Madri et al., 1980b). The localization of type V at the interface between adjacent connective tissue and cells has justified the term cell-associated or pericellular collagen (Burgeson, 1982). The presence of type V collagen in the epidermal–dermal junction has been disputed (Stenn et al., 1979; Gay et al., 1979).

Type VII collagen was recently isolated and originally termed long-chain (LC) collagen (Bentz et al., 1983). It is distinct from other collagens and unique in the length of its triple-helical domain. Segmental long space crystallites prepared from type VII collagen have a banding pattern identical to previously published electron micrographs of the central banded portion of anchoring fibrils (Bentz et al., 1983). In addition, an antibody specific for type VII collagen localizes to anchoring fibrils in skin by immunoelectron microscopy (Sakai et al., 1986).

3.2. Noncollagenous Basement Membrane Proteins

The noncollagenous glycoproteins represent a diverse group of basement membrane components. Laminin is a well-characterized ubiquitous component of essentially all basement membranes (Timpl et al., 1979a; Chung et al., 1979; Timpl et al., 1983b). It has distinct subunits: two smaller, approximately 220,000-M_r, B chains and a larger 440,000-M_r A chain. The whole laminin molecule is very large (900,000 M_r) and, by rotary shadowing studies, has an asymmetric crosslike configuration. Functionally, laminin binds preferentially to cells (presumably by a cell-surface laminin receptor) Terranova et al., 1980; Malinoff and Wicha, 1983; Terranova et al., 1983), type IV collagen and heparan sulfate (Woodley et al., 1983). Binding domains can be identified in specific portions of the laminin macromolecule (Engel et al., 1981; Rao et al., 1982) (Chapter 22).

Nidogen is another ubiquitous basement membrane component (Timpl et al., 1983a). Nidogen has 100,000–150,000-M_r subunits and readily self-aggregates producing high-molecular-weight forms. Nidogen binds avidly to laminin. Nidogen is present in the epidermal–dermal junction, but its ultrastructural localization is unknown.

Entactin is a highly sulfated glycoprotein that has been shown to promote keratinocyte attachment alone or when mixed with laminin (Carlin et al., 1981; Bender et al., 1981; Alstadt et al., 1985). Immunolocalization studies have associated entactin with a variety of basement membranes, although its presence in skin is uncertain. In addition, other related sulfated glycoproteins have been found, so this group may be recognized as more diverse with further investigation.

Fibronectin is a large noncollagenous glycoprotein widely distributed in most tissues, especially at cell surfaces and in connective tissue matrices (Yamada and Olden, 1978; Pearlstein et al., 1980; Ruoslahti et al., 1981; Mosher and Furcht, 1981). Fibronectin has been extensively studied and is known to be a dimer composed of two similar disulfide-linked subunits (220,000 M_r). Fibronectin undergoes molecular interactions with a diverse group of other materials, including all types of collagen, C1q component of complement, cells, glycoaminoglycans, fibrinogen, and fibrin. Fibronectin is organized functionally, into segregated binding domains (see Chapter 18). Interesting analogies can be drawn between fibronectin and laminin concerning their overall molecular organization and binding functions. Its presence in basement membranes has been reported (Stenman and Vaheri, 1978; Couchman et al., 1979; Fyrand, 1979) and localized to the epidermal cell surface and the lamina lucida in the epidermal–dermal junction (Couchman et al., 1979). However, its role as a specific basement membrane component has been denied by others (Boselli et al., 1981; Martinez-Hernandez et al., 1981; Laurie et al., 1982). Fibronectin is more consistently found within fetal basement membranes. Recent studies have indicated that fibronectin is synthesized and laid down by migrating epidermal cells in culture (O'Keefe et al., 1984; Kubo et al., 1984).

Bullous pemphigoid antigen is a noncollagenous basement membrane glycoprotein recognized by its reactivity with sera from patients with the disease, bullous pemphigoid. Very low- (Diaz et al., 1977; Diaz and Marcelo, 1978) and high-molecular-weight peptides (Stanley et al., 1981b) have been isolated and react with bullous pemphigoid sera. However, the recent isolation of a high-molecular-weight bullous pemphigoid antigen (200,000 M_r) from cultured mouse and human epidermal cells represents the major subunit chain for the bullous pemphigoid antigen (Stanley et al., 1982c). Bullous pemphigoid antigen was initially localized ultrastructurally to the lamina lucida (Schaumburg-Lever, 1975; Holubar et al., 1975). Recently, however, evidence indicates that bullous pemphigoid antigen is closely associated with the epidermal cell surface. Moreover, a major intraepidermal pool of bullous pemphigoid antigen has been identified in association with hemidesmosomes (Yamasaki and Nishikawa, 1983; Mutasim et al., 1985; Westgate et al., 1985; Regnier et al., 1985). Bullous pemphigoid antigen is limited in its distribution to the basement membrane of stratified squamous epithelia and is not a ubiquitous component of all basement membranes.

Epidermolysis bullosa acquisita (EBA) antigen has been identified in basement membrane-rich dermal extracts by immunoblot analysis using the sera of patients with epidermolysis bullosa acquisita (Woodley et al., 1984). Two components have been identified, a major 290,000-M_r band and a minor 145,000-M_r band. Current evidence indicates that these proteins are biochemically different. EBA antigen is limited in distribution to mammalian basement membranes of stratified squamous epithelia. Ultrastructurally, EBA antigen is localized to the area immediately below the lamina densa and the lower portion of the lamina densa (Nieboer et al., 1980; Yaoita et al., 1981).

Heparan sulfate proteoglycans are ubiquitous components of nearly all basement membranes. Several heparan sulfate-containing proteoglycans have been identified. These proteoglycans consist of a central core protein surrounded by heparan sulfate side chains (see Chapter 19). Although heparan sulfate has been identified in a wide variety of tissues, the core proteins associated with the basement membrane proteoglycans appear to be basement membrane specific. The basement membrane heparan sulfate proteoglycans are biochemically heterogeneous and vary in their overall molecular size, central core protein size, and composition of the heparan sulfate side chains (Hassell et al., 1980; Kanwar and Farquhar, 1979; Kanwar et al., 1981; Oohira et al., 1982). The qualitative heterogeneity in the specific heparan sulfate proteoglycan content of different tissues could influence the biologic function of different basement membranes. At least one heparan sulfate proteoglycan is known to be a component of the epidermal–dermal junction, although its ultrastructural localization is uncertain (Hassell et al., 1980). Indirect evidence using polyanionic probes suggests that a high concentration of polyanions, presumably heparan sulfate proteoglycans, exists on either side of the lamina densa (Manabe and Ogawa, 1985).

3.3. Antibodies to Uncharacterized Basement Membrane Zone Antigens

Both bullous pemphigoid antigen and EBA antigen represent two cutaneous basement membrane antigens that were originally recognized by their reactivity with naturally occurring antibodies. Recently, several other antibodies have been developed to as yet uncharacterized antigens present in the dermal–epidermal junction. Goldsmith and Briggaman (1982, 1983) reported two mouse monoclonal antibodies (AF-1 and AF-2) that reacted exclusively with primate basement membrane zone. Ultrastructurally, these antibodies were localized to the anchoring fibrils. Bacterial collagenase, which destroys the anchoring fibrils and the lamina densa, abolishes AF-1 and AF-2 binding to epidermal–dermal junction, whereas human leukocyte elastase, which removes lamina densa but not anchoring fibrils, does not eliminate the binding by these antibodies (Briggaman et al., 1984). In addition, AF-1 and AF-2 binding is absent in the skin of patients with severe dystrophic epidermolysis bullosa recessive, where anchoring fibrils are known to be absent but not from types of epidermolysis bullosa with retained fibrils (Goldsmith and Briggaman, 1983). We believe that these antibodies represent anchoring fibril-associated antigens.

Breathnach et al. (1983) raised a mouse monoclonal antibody (KF-1) that localized to the epidermal–dermal junction in primate skin but not vascular basement membrane. On immunoelectron microscopy, KF-1 bound to the lamina densa of human skin. Bacterial collagenase treatment of skin did not abolish KF-1 binding, indicating that the antigen is a noncollagenous protein.

4. Events in Early Wound Healing

Clark et al. (1982b) focused on early events in skin wound healing and the provisional extracellular matrix upon which the first migrating cells must contact. While this is not reconstitution of the BMZ per se, the provisional matrix may be important not only in initiating cell migration but in directing the migrating cells to orchestrate the reconstitution of the BMZ as well. The initial wound bed is extremely rich in fibronectin, which derives predominantly from serum, but is also produced locally by fibroblasts. Recently, O'Keefe et al. (1984) and Kubo et al. (1984) showed that fibronectin is synthesized and deposited extracellularly by human epidermal cells in culture without the presence of mesenchymal cells or fibronectin containing medium. Furthermore, O'Keefe et al. (1984) observed that fibronectin tracks are deposited on the floor of Petri dishes as the keratinocytes migrate. In a follow-up study, O'Keefe et al. (1985)

demonstrated fibronectin-mediated cell spreading in keratinocyte cultures grown in both high (1.1-mM) and low (0.1-mM) calcium concentrations. In addition, fibronectin enhanced the motility of keratinocytes when added to the cultures. These studies are in accordance with earlier studies that demonstrated that human keratinocytes attach and grow on fibronectin-coated Petri dishes (Gilchrist et al., 1980, 1982; Maciag et al., 1981). Taken as a whole, these studies show that human keratinocytes respond to fibronectin and that fibronectin can act as a matrix factor for keratinocytes in vitro. Earlier studies had suggested that fibronectin is a matrix molecule for fibroblasts and mesenchymal cells (Kleinman et al., 1981; Yamada, 1982) but is not biologically active for epithelial cells. This incorrect notion was perhaps encouraged by the observation that fibronectin was often not found in adult cutaneous basement membranes and was consistently absent from the epidermis of skin sections stained with antifibronectin antibodies. However, during wound healing, the migrating epidermis comes into intimate contact with fibronectin and other dermal and serum molecules. Perhaps it is during wound healing that fibronectin–keratinocyte interactions become important in vivo. In studies of guinea pig wounds, Clark et al. (1982b) found that the regenerating epidermis migrated over a provisional matrix rich in fibronectin and fibrin but lacked laminin and type IV collagen, two major components of the intact junction. Thus, the advancing edge of migrating epidermis does not have a normal junction beneath it but rests on a homogeneous dense fibrillar zone that is thick, irregular, and rich in fibronectin and fibrin (Clark et al., 1982b). As healing progresses and the epidermis becomes more stationary, marked remodeling of this transient matrix occurs. Around day 7 of the wound, the BMZ began to appear more normal with a thinner, more regular histology. Further, antifibronectin no longer stained the new junction and antifibrinogen was markedly weaker and more focal. This suggested that these two early matrix components were markedly decreased in maturing wounds. Simultaneously with the decrease in fibronectin and fibrinogen, laminin and type IV collagen began to appear in the reconstituted BMZ beneath the wound epithelium (Clark et al., 1982b). It is not known whether fibronectin induces lamina and type IV collagen formation in the newly formed basement membrane. It is known that fibronectin binds to most types of collagen except Ascaris cuticle collagen (Kleinman et al., 1981; Yamada, 1982; Woodley et al., 1983). Furthermore, fibronectin binds to proteoglycans (Yamada, 1982; Hynes, 1982; Hynes and Yamada, 1982) and cells. Fibroblasts align along the same axis as the extracellular fibronectin that they produce and deposit (Clemmons et al., 1980; Clark et al., 1982b; Repesh et al., 1982). Collagen deposition then appears to occur along the fibronectin–fibroblast axis. It is possible that fibronectin serves as a scaffolding for the deposition of collagen and other matrix molecules during wound healing (see Chapter 18). In fibroblast cultures, both collagen fibrils and a fibronectin matrix are seen (McDonald et al., 1982). When the cultures are grown without ascorbate, a necessary requirement for collagen synthesis, the fibroblasts do not produce collagen but only produce a dense fibronectin matrix (Chen et al., 1978). In the presence of ascorbate both fibronectin and collagen are formed. However, if an antifibronectin antibody that blocks fibronectin binding to collagen is added to the system, collagen deposition in the extracellular matrix is diminished as well as fibronectin accumulation (McDonald et al., 1982). These studies suggest that an interaction with fibronectin may be necessary before collagen fibrils are formed and that new collagen is formed on a matrix of fibronectin (Clark, 1985).

Similar observations have also been made in an in vivo wound-healing model (Kurkinen et al., 1980). Cellulose sponge implants were placed in rats and the sequential appearance of connective tissue components observed. First, fibroblasts migrated into the sponges and fibronectin was deposited. Small amounts of new collagen were deposited behind the leading edge of fibroblasts and fibronectin. Mature type I collagen formed later at a time when fibronectin deposits were less, probably due to degradation from cellular proteinases (Kurkinen et al., 1980; Clark, 1985). Thus, both in vitro and in vivo studies would support the notion that fibronectin deposition occurs before collagen formation. At least in fibroblast cell cultures fibronectin appears to invoke collagen deposition and fibril formation (see Chapter 18). Whether fibronectin and collagen deposition are causatively related events in vivo is not known.

There is some evidence that fibronectin might play a role in the formation of basement membrane. First, there is the general observation that fibronectin is frequently detected in fetal basement membrane and is much more difficult to detect in adult basement membranes. Second, Brownell et al. (1981) showed that fibronectin may induce isolated epithelium to form a lamina densa containing laminin and type IV collagen. These investigators isolated epithelial and mesenchymal elements from mouse molar tooth organs. Isolated epithelium cultured in chemically defined medium without serum or embryonic extracts did not reconstitute a lamina densa. However, in the presence of fibronectin or mesenchyme-preconditioned medium containing fibronectin as a major component, the epithelium was capable of producing a lamina densa. These studies suggested that lamina densa formation resulted from super-molecular interactions between epithelium-derived macromolecules (e.g., type IV collagen, laminin, proteoglycans) and mesenchymal-derived fibronectin (Brownell et al., 1981). In vitro studies with human skin cultures have shown that cultured epidermal cells in contact with living dermis form an ultrastructural lamina densa and type IV collagen at this interface while identical cells in contact with dead dermis do not have a lamina densa or type IV collagen formed at the cell–matrix junction (Woodley et al., 1980b). In other systems, it has been clearly shown that the character and composition of matrix or basement membrane can influence cellular behavior (Dodson and Hay, 1971; Hay, 1982; Salomon et al., 1981; Gospodarowicz, 1983; Grinnell, 1983; Woodley et al., 1984) and induce the cells to produce structural components. For example, basement membrane-containing anchoring fibrils will induce epithelial cells to produce hemidesmosomes while basement membranes without anchoring fibrils will not (Gipson et al., 1983).

Glycosaminoglycans (GAGs) are high-molecular-weight polymers composed of repeating amino sugars and uronic acids (see Chapter 19). GAGs and GAGs bound to a protein core (proteoglycans) may also play a role in the biology of an early wound matrix. Bernfield and co-workers (1978; Bernfield and Banerjee, 1973) have shown the presence of acidic GAG molecules at the junction between epithelium and mesenchyme in developing salivary glands (Wessells, 1977a; Toole, 1983). A lamina densa is formed at this interface. However, if the GAG molecules are removed from the epithelial surface by enzymatic treatment, the lamina densa disappears and the epithelial cells round up and lose their polarity and clefted morphology. It appears that GAGs are required for maintenance of epithelial shape and morphogenesis. Hyaluronic acid (HA), one type of GAG that is nonsulfated, may be present in early granulation tissue of wounds (Balazs, 1950) and play a role in morphogenesis during development and wound healing (Clark, 1985). In developing cornea, an inner layer of endothelial cells secretes large amounts of HA into the stroma inducing tissue swelling and the subsequent migration of mesenchymal cells into the stroma (Toole and Trelstad, 1971; Toole, 1983; Wessells, 1977a). Later, these migrating cells secrete hyaluronidase and degrade the HA, after which the cells stop migrating. This has led to the general notion that cells migrate on swollen HA-rich connective tissue stroma and stop migrating at the time that hyaluronidase appears and HA content in the tissue decreases (Wessells, 1977b). Furthermore, these observations suggest that the extracellular matrix can influence cell migration and that this function is not the exclusive domain of the intracellular cytoskeleton. It is interesting that HA content is very high in the granulation tissue of early wounds at a time when lateral keratinocyte migration must be induced (Clark, 1985; Bentley, 1967).

It is interesting that both GAGs and fibronectin are abundant in the provisional matrix of early wound beds and that fibronectin has a specific binding domain for the sulfated GAGs, heparin, and heparan sulfate. It has been suggested that cell-surface associated heparan sulfate and fibronectin interact to attach the cells to their connective tissue matrix (Culp et al., 1979). Furthermore, HA is thought to abrogate cell–matrix adherence. Therefore, it is possible that the mechanisms of cell migration include an alternating sequence of cell–substrate adhesive forces mediated by molecules such as fibronectin and heparan, and cell–substrate releasing forces, such as HA (Culp et al., 1979).

Proteoglycans such as chondroitin 4-sulfate can accelerate collagen fibrillogenesis (Wood, 1960). This mechanism may play a role in the ultimate healing of dermal wounds and the processing of newly synthesized and aligned interstitial collagens. However, it may not play a role in the induction of type IV collagen since the latter is nonfibrillar in nature. Studies to examine type IV collagen induction by proteoglycan have not been done. It is known, however, that type IV collagen and BMZ heparan sulfate proteoglycan bind together by domains that are not in common with the laminin binding sites on each molecule (Woodley et al., 1983; Terranova et al., 1983). Thus, it may be possible that heparan sulfate proteoglycan in the BMZ region promotes BMZ regeneration by aligning other essential matrix molecules as type IV collagen and laminin.

Hay and co-workers (Hay, 1982; Sugrue and Hay, 1981; Dodson and Hay,

1971, 1974) have shown that the plasma membrane of corneal epithelium undergoes blebbing when isolated from underlying connective tissue stroma (side that would be apposed to matrix in intact tissue) surface, but not on their lateral or apical sides. The "blebbed" side has the appearance of small fingers or pseudopodia. When the investigators placed the epithelium on nonviable collagen, the epithelium stopped blebbing and produced a new stroma consisting of interstitial collagens (Dodson and Hay, 1971; Linsenmayer et al., 1977), a lamina densa (Hay and Dodson, 1973) and GAGs (Meier and Hay, 1973). When the same epithelium is placed on a Millipore filter, it continued to bleb and did not produce a stroma. If isolated epithelium is placed on a Millipore filter saturated with collagens (I, II, or IV), laminin or fibronectin, the blebs retract in 2 hr and completely disappear in 6 hr. This does not occur when the filters are saturated with IgG, albumin, GAGs, or proteoglycan (Sugrue and Hay, 1981). Soluble collagen did not stimulate stromal production to the same degree as an insoluble collagen gel (Meier and Hay, 1974). Type I collagen worked as well as type IV (basement membrane) collagen.

The epithelial blebs have actin filaments inside them and when they retract the actin filaments condense and merge with other cytoskeletal microfilaments to form the inner corona of the cytoskeleton (Sugrue and Hay, 1981; Hay, 1982). If the blebs are viewed as pseudopodia reaching out to initiate directional migration, the high levels of GAGs and relative low concentration of collagen in early wound beds would promote and perhaps initiate migration. Later, with lower levels of HA and higher levels of fibronectin and collagen, the cell cytoskeleton would be more stabilized by interactions with these molecules and cellular energy directed more toward an anchoring junction, and eventually differentiation. While this is speculative, the experiments of Hay and co-workers clearly show that extracellular matrix molecules can exert a response at the cell surface and in the cytoskeleton of the cell. Cell shape and morphology may be affected by extracellular matrix and also direct the metabolism of the cell overall and the cellular responses to soluble growth factors in its environment (Gospodarowicz et al., 1978). We are just beginning to understand how these events are orchestrated, but studying the biology of wound healing should continue to provide clues as to how extracellular matrices influence keratinocytes to cover the wound, regenerate a basement membrane, and return to a pattern of normal differentiation.

5. Basement Membrane Reconstruction

5.1. *In Vivo* Studies

The epidermal–dermal junction is completely restored following skin wounding in vivo. All ultrastructural elements of the junction and at least certain of the biochemical components are re-formed after injury (Tables IV and V). Some variation in these studies results from use of different animal species and different skin-wounding techniques. Nevertheless, serious disagreement

Table IV. Basement Membrane Reformation During Skin Wound Healing *In Vivo*

System/Subject	Ultrastructural studies	Immunohistochemical studies	Investigators
Partial-thickness incision wound—human	Junction re-formed	—	Odland and Ross (1968)
Full-thickness incision wound—mouse	Junction re-formed	—	Croft and Tarin (1970)
Subepidermal blister suction induced—mice	Rapid re-formation of hemidesmosomes	—	Krawczyk and Wilgram (1973)
Subepidermal blister, suction induced—human	Rapid re-formation of hemidesmosomes	—	Beerens *et al.* (1975)
Split thickness wound—pig	—	BP antigen, followed by type IV collagen and laminin	Stanley *et al.* (1981a)
Full-thickness incision wound—guinea pig	—	BP fibronectin, followed by type IV collagen and laminin	Clark *et al.* (1982b)
Split-thickness incision wound—non-human primate	—	Laminin, fibronectin and type IV collagen followed by BP, EBA, and CP antigens; later KF-1 antigen	Fine *et al.* (1985)

exists in the sequence of the restoration of basement membrane components in certain of the studies.

Incision wounds, into or through the dermis, heal with the formation of granulation tissue in the dermal portion of the wound over which epidermis migrates from the wound margin to cover the wound gap. Ultrastructurally, the epidermal–dermal junction of the stationary epidermis at the periphery of the wound is intact, but junctional structures are absent beneath the migrating epidermis (Odland and Ross, 1968; Croft and Tarin, 1970). The basal surface of the migrating epidermal cells rests directly on the granulation tissue wound base, frequently associated with fibrin deposits but rarely directly opposed to collagen fibers, fibroblasts, or inflammatory cells. Restoration of the epidermal–dermal junction proceeds from the margin of the wound with all structures of the junction including lamina densa, lamina lucida, and hemidesmosomes formed more or less simultaneously. The latter point has not been specifically addressed, and sequential formation of junctional structures might occur. Complete restoration of the junction lags well behind reepithelialization of the wound. Several studies have examined the reformation of basement membrane components during skin wound healing. Stanley *et al.* (1981a) evaluated basement membrane components beneath the regenerating epidermis in split-thickness wounds on the Yorkshire pigs by immunofluorescence using antibodies to laminin, type IV collagen, and BP antigen. As expected, laminin and type IV collagen were present at the intact epidermal–dermal junction at the wound margin but were absent initially under the regenerating epidermis. Gradually, laminin and type IV collagen were found extending from the margins of the wound but never extended as far as the distal tip of the migrating epidermis. After completion of re-epithelialization, laminin and type IV collagen appeared at the newly formed epidermal–dermal junction throughout the length of the wound. By contrast, BP antigen was expressed beneath the entire length of the migrating epidermis, including the most distal tip during all stages of wound healing. In similar *in vivo* studies on incisional wounds in guinea pigs, Clark *et al.* (1982a,b) noted the early appearance of BP antigen beneath the migrating epidermis and a marked delay in the appearance of laminin and type IV collagen. Fibrin and fibronectin were present closely opposed to the migrating epidermis and formed a provisional matrix during early wound healing. Later, fibrin and fibronectin gradually disappear with the reappearance of laminin and type IV collagen at the basement membrane zone.

Table V. Basement Membrane Formation by Skin Models In Vitro[a]

System	Junctional ultrastructures formed	BM component by immunohistochemical studies	Investigators
Human skin organ culture, epiboly	HD, continuous LD	—	Sarkany and Gaylarde (1970)
Human skin recombinant grafts on CAM	Focal to continuous LD, AF	—	Briggaman *et al.* (1971)
Human skin organ culture, epiboly	Limited, focal LD	BP ag	Marks *et al.* (1975)
Guinea pig epidermal cell culture on coll gel	HD focal LD	—	Mann and Constable (1977)
Human newborn foreskin organ culture	Junction re-formed	BP ag	Brickman *et al.* (1977)
Mouse skin organ culture, epiboly	—	Type V coll—Type IV coll absent	Stenn *et al.* (1979)
Human skin organ culture, epiboly and outgrowth on Millipore filter	—	BP ag	Woodley *et al.* (1979)
Human epidermal cell culture on coll gel	HD, focal LD	Type IV coll	Hirone and Taniguchi (1979, 1982)
Human skin organ culture, epiboly	HD, LD, AF	B ag early, type IV coll, later laminin	Hintner *et al.* (1980)
Human epidermal outgrowth on nonviable dermis	No LD	BP ag—type IV coll absent	Woodley *et al.* (1980)

[a]Abbreviations: BP ag, bullous pemphigoid antigen; LD, lamina densa; AF, anchoring fibril; CAM, chorioallantoic membrane; coll, collagen.

The sequence of reappearance of basement membrane components during wound healing, namely BP antigen followed by a laminin and type IV collagen, differs from the sequence found during gestational development where laminin, type IV collagen, and fibronectin are the first detectable basement membrane antigens followed by EBA antigen, BP antigen, and KF-1 antigen (Fine *et al.*, 1984). This has led to the belief that the formation of the epidermal–dermal junction during wound healing is fundamentally different from that during fetal development.

In a recent abstract by Fine *et al.* (1985), it was reported that in split thickness skin wounds on monkeys, BP antigen was expressed in the newly reconstituted basement membrane zone 48 hr after laminin and type IV collagen, a sequence of basement membrane formation in accordance with the gestational studies. Fine *et al.* (1985) raised the question whether previous *in vivo* wound-healing studies performed on pigs may not reflect the sequence of events that occurs when primates are wounded.

No study has examined the ultrastructural and biochemical events concomitantly during the healing of cutaneous wounds *in vivo*. Moreover, the only *in vivo* human skin study was the early ultrastructural study by Odland and Ross (1968). A study of human skin wound healing with correlation of ultrastructural and biochemical events during basement membrane re-formation might help resolve the conflicting reports.

In closed suction-induced subepidermal blisters, re-epithelialization occurred by migration of epidermal cells over residual, intact lamina densa at the base of the blister. This type of skin wound offers the opportunity to examine the reattachment of epidermal cells onto lamina densa (Krawczyk and Wilgram, 1973; Beerens *et al.*, 1975). The restoration of hemidesmosomes and cell–lamina densa attachment proceeds rapidly in a matter of 8–12 hr after separation. The sequence of events is the bridging of the plasma membrane to lamina densa with anchoring filaments, formation of sub-basal dense plaque (juxtamembrane line) beneath the membrane, followed by the formation of an attachment plaque on the cytoplasmic surface of the plasma membrane and finally the attachment of tonofilaments to the plaque (Krawczyk and Wilgram, 1973). Studies in a corneal epithelium system indicate that hemidesmosome formation is calcium dependent and probably mediated by calmodulin (Trinkaus-Randall and Gipson, 1984). Little is known about the composition of hemidesmosomes, although desmoplakins I and II may be components of hemidesmosomes as well as desmosomes (Mueller and Franke, 1983). Bullous pemphigoid antigen has also been associated with hemidesmosomes (Mutasim *et al.*, 1985; Westgate *et al.*, 1985; Regnier *et al.*, 1985). These proteins have not been examined in relation to hemidesmosome reformation.

5.2. *In Vitro* Studies

Several *in vitro* studies employing cultured skin or skin components have been used to study basement membrane formation (Table V). Although these *in vitro* systems are not skin wound healing per se, they are analogous and have yielded valuable insights into the process. Basement membrane formation has been demonstrated by ultrastructural observation, by immunohistochemical identification of basement membrane components or, in several studies, by a combination of these two approaches.

In explant cultures of small pieces of split-thickness skin, epidermal cells migrate off the cut edge of the cutaneous basement membrane onto the dermis and eventually surround the sides and inferior aspect of the explant. This is termed epiboly, and the new junction between the migrating cells and the dermis of the explant is called the epibolic–dermal junction. Using such cultures as an *in vitro* wound healing model, Sarkany and Gaylarde (1970) demonstrated new lamina densa formation beneath migrating epibolic epidermis in adult human skin organ cultures maintained for 3 days. In studies by Marks *et al.* (1975) using human skin organ cultures, no new junctional structures were noted beneath the migrating epidermis until after the second day when hemidesmosomes and focal areas of lamina densa formed in limited areas near the original edge of the explant. By indirect immunofluorescence with sera from bullous pemphigoid (BP) patients, these authors observed a small amount of fragmented fluorescent material between the epibolized cells and the explant dermal surface in some of the explants. This suggested that the BP antigen could be synthesized in culture, but it was unclear if its cell of origin was the migrating epidermal cells, the cells in the dermis, or both. If the epidermal cells produced the bullous pemphigoid antigen, these studies did not address the question of whether cells or other factors from the dermis (e.g., metabolic factors secreted by resident dermal fibroblasts, endothelial cells, mast cells) were required to induce the epidermal cells to produce it.

Using short-term (7-day) organ cultures of neonatal foreskin, Brickman *et al.* (1977) found that BP antigen was present on the first day of culture, but then degenerated and was completely absent by the fourth day. This loss of BP antigen staining was paralleled by degeneration of the lamina densa within the junction when examined ultrastructurally. However, these events were slightly out of synchrony; the lamina densa was maximally degenerated by 72 hr of culture while the degeneration of the BP antigen was not complete until the fourth day of culture. As the cultures continued, the investigators noted regeneration of both BP antigen and the ultrastructural lamina densa. The lamina densa began to regenerate by day 4 of culture and was complete on day 5. The BP antigen, which was negative at day 4 (the same time point as when the lamina densa began to regenerate), did not completely regenerate until day 6 of culture. These studies showed a disappearance and reappearance of the BP antigen and ultrastructural lamina densa. The reappearance sequence was similar to that described in early gestational studies of the BMZ in which the lamina densa formed first followed by the lamina lucida (Breathnach and Robins, 1969; Muller *et al.*, 1973). However, this finding may have been a function of the later occurring BP antigen degradation (day 4) compared with that of the lamina densa (day 3). Again, these organ culture studies did not clarify which cell produced the BP antigen since both the epidermis and dermis are viable in routine organ cultures.

Using human skin explants in culture, Hintner *et al.* (1980) examined the epibolic–dermal junction created by newly migrated cells growing around the explant dermis. In this model of BMZ neogenesis, these workers found that type IV collagen, bullous pemphigoid antigen, and laminin were detected within the epibolic–dermal junction by IF with antibodies to junctional components. BP antigen was found at the epibolic–dermal junction from the first 24 hr throughout day 7 and extended the full length of the newly formed junction. By contrast, the appearance of laminin did not occur until day 4 of culture. Moreover, laminin was always confined to the most proximal areas of the epiboly and absent from the advancing edge. Likewise, the expression of type IV collagen was delayed at the newly formed BMZ but appeared earlier (days 2–3 of culture) than laminin. From day 4 of culture until day 7, an increasing portion of the epibolic-dermal junction expressed type IV collagen as the migrating epidermis extended over the dermal surface of the explant. However, type IV collagen and laminin were always absent beneath the advancing tip of the migrating cells. In vivo studies by Clark et al. (1982b) confirmed this time sequence of bullous pemphigoid antigen, type IV collagen, and laminin.

Ultrastructurally Hintner et al. (1980) noted that between day 0 and day 2, there was no lamina densa in the epibolic–dermal junction. By contrast, hemidesmosomes and anchoring filaments were plentiful. Then from days 4 through 7, a lamina densa was formed at the junction but always lagged far behind the advancing tip of the migrating epidermis. These studies showed that (1) lamina densa was not required for the cells to migrate; (2) BP antigen was the first BMZ component reconstituted, while there was a delay in the expression of laminin and type IV collagen; and (3) the sequence of BMZ component reformation in an in vitro wound-healing model was different from that during gestation and the organ-culture studies of Brickman et al. (1977). These studies did not address the cell of origin of any of the BMZ components, since both the epidermis and dermis were viable in these cultures.

Stenn et al. (1979) examined collagen production in organ culture of mouse skin in which the epidermal cells from the original explant migrate off of the explant and across a Millipore filter. They found that the migrating epidermal cells did not produce interstitial collagens (types I and III) or basement membrane collagen (type IV). However, they did find that the migrating cells produced type V (AB$_2$) collagen and that its synthesis was required for cell migration.

In the human explants and epiboly experiments of Hintner et al. (1980), small amounts of type IV collagen were expressed at the newly reconstituted junction while in the experiments by Stenn and colleagues (1979) no type IV collagen was synthesized. However, these experiments cannot be directly compared for several reasons: (1) mouse and human skin may behave differently; (2) the cultures by Stenn et al. (1979) were for 48 hr only, while those of Hintner et al. (1980) were for 7 days, and type IV collagen production was not noted until day 4; and (3) the migrating epidermal cells in the Stenn cultures were apposed to a nonviable Millipore filter, while those in the Hintner system were apposed to a living dermis that could potentially influence the migrating cells.

Using a human explant system similar to that of Hintner et al. (1980) but modified such that the cultures were placed on Millipore filters, permitting epibolized epidermal cells simultaneous contact with both a viable dermis and a nonviable nitrocellulose substrate, Woodley and Regnier (1979) demonstrated that newly synthesized BP antigen was expressed at both the epibolic–dermal junction and the junction between the epibolized cells and the Millipore filter. This finding suggests that human keratinocytes can synthesize and extracellularly deposit BP antigen in culture without contact with living dermis or mesenchymal tissue. In a similar in vitro system in which human keratinocytes migrate across nonviable reticular dermis, it was shown that BP antigen was synthesized by the migrating cells and deposited within the junction formed by the living culture cells and the nonviable dermal substrate (Woodley et al., 1980a). BP antigen expression occurred from day 4 of culture throughout day 50, when the cultures were terminated. In addition to extracellular deposition of the BP antigen within the junction, in early cultures BP antigen was also detected within the migrating cells. When these cultures were examined ultrastructurally for lamina densa formation and by IF for type IV collagen expression, neither a lamina densa or type IV collagen could be demonstrated (Woodley et al., 1980a,b). These studies showed that BP antigen could by synthesized by human keratinocytes without the contact or influence of viable dermal cells, and that BP antigen expression was independent from, and did not require the synthesis of an ultrastructural lamina densa or type IV collagen.

In later studies (Woodley et al., 1982), human keratinocytes were cultured on nonviable human skin basement membrane or tissue culture plastic and evaluated for BP antigen expression. Again, the BP antigen formed at the junction between the cultured cells and the nonviable basement membrane in a linear extracellular distribution akin to that seen when normal human skin substrate is stained by IF with BP sera. When cultured on polystyrene dishes, the interface between cultured cells and tissue culture plastic could not be assessed. Furthermore, when in situ cultures were stained with BP antibodies by IF, it was difficult to observe BP antigen expression clearly. However, when the cultured cells were removed from the cultures and resuspended by trypsinization, air-dried on slides, and examined for BP antigen, it was easily demonstrated that the cultured cells synthesized BP antigen and that the percentage of BP-positive cells correlated with percentage of basal cells in culture. Moreover, in both primary and secondary cultures, there was a dramatic increase in the number of BP positive cells in culture over time. These studies showed that BP antigen could be synthesized by human keratinocytes cultured on nonviable dermis, basement membrane or plastic, that the basal cells in the cultures were the synthesizing cells, that BP antigen synthesis over time was due to the greater percentage of basal cells in the cultures, and that BP antigen was localized both intracellularly and extracellularly in keratinocytes.

Briggaman and Wheeler (1971) studied the formation of lamina densa and anchoring fibrils in adult human skin using a recombinant graft procedure in which the skin recombinants were grown on chorioallantoic membrane or embryonated chicken eggs. After recombination of trypsin-separated epidermis and dermis, the epidermal–dermal interface of the graft contained no lamina densa or anchoring fibrils, although hemidesmosomes and tonofilaments were intact on the freshly trypsinized epidermal cell surface. Three days after grafting, lamina densa began to form subjacent to hemidesmosomes of the epidermal basal cells. Lamina densa was not seen in the absence of hemidesmosomes which seemed to act as organizing centers for lamina densa formation. From the fifth to the seventh day after grafting, lamina densa became progressively more dense and extended in many areas to become continuous at the epidermal–dermal interface of the graft. On the fifth day after grafting, anchoring fibrils first appeared in the graft and became progressively more numerous thereafter. No immunohistochemical studies were done. In order to determine the origin of lamina densa and anchoring fibrils in this system, the dermal portion of the graft was rendered nonviable by repeated freezing and thawing, after which it was recombined with viable epidermis. Lamina densa formed as rapidly in these recombinants of viable epidermis with freeze-thaw-killed dermis as with recombinants with viable dermis, indicating that dermal viability was not essential for the formation of lamina densa and supporting the epidermal origin for this structure. By contrast, anchoring fibrils did not re-form in the recombinants containing nonviable dermis, indicating that dermal viability was required for anchoring fibril formation and suggesting that the anchoring fibrils were of dermal origin.

Basement membrane formation was also studied in epidermal cell cultures grown on collagen substrates. Mann and Constable (1977) grew guinea pig epidermal cell suspensions on both collagen gel and hydrated collagen lattice. During the first week of cultivation, hemidesmosomes formed along the plasma membrane of epidermal cells at the interface with collagen gel, usually at sites where collagen fibers were abundant. Lamina densa-like material was first detected subjacent to the hemidesmosomes and never by itself. Lamina densa remained focal at these locations and did not become continuous even though the cultures were maintained for 2 weeks. Recently, the formation of lamina densa in human skin epidermal cell cultures was demonstrated on collagen gel (Hirone and Taniguchi, 1979; Taniguchi and Hirone, 1982). No lamina densa formation was found when the same cells were grown on a plastic surface. Hemidesmosomes formed at about the fifth day of cultivation on collagen gel. Beneath some of the hemidesmosomes, lamina densa appeared focally on the surface of the collagen. Hemidesmosomes became more numerous and lamina densa progressively extended to become continuous in many areas of the culture.

It is noteworthy that in all three studies, hemidesmosomes appeared to act as an organizing site for the deposition of new lamina densa (Briggaman and Wheeler, 1971; Mann and Constable, 1977; Hirone and Taniguchi, 1979). In addition, the presence of abundant collagen in the dermis appeared to act as a site for hemidesmosome formation (Mann and Constable, 1977; Taniguchi and Hirone, 1982). Similar observations were made during hemidesmosome formation in a corneal epithelial system in which hemidesmosomes formed preferentially over areas of pre-existing lamina densa, especially at sites of anchoring fibril attachment to the lamina densa (Gipson et al., 1983). It would appear then that the presence of one element of the junction may act as a site for initiating re-formation of the complete junction by the deposition of other junctional components.

The formation of lamina densa in both guinea pig and human epidermal cell cultures grown in vitro on collagen gel provides persuasive evidence for the epidermal origin of lamina densa. This is further supported by the variety of epithelial cell lines that have been demonstrated to produce type IV collagen in vitro.

6. Summary

The dermal–epidermal junction is completely reconstituted in a healed wound to the limits of our observation by light and electron microscopy and immunohistochemical techniques. The epidermal cells migrating over the wound contribute many of the components in the newly formed junction zone. Most of the in vitro and in vivo studies suggest that there is an orderly sequence of reappearance of the junctional components. The BP antigen has been the junctional component that appears first and most consistently beneath migrating epidermis with a delay in the appearance of type IV collagen and laminin. However, a definitive in vivo study of human skin wounds has not been performed and designed to examine specifically the sequence of events in the re-formation of the dermal–epidermal junction as they are defined today.

ACKNOWLEDGMENT. This work was supported by grants AM33625 (D. T. W.) and AM10546 (R. A. B.) from the National Institutes of Health.

References

Alitalo, K., Vaheri, A., Kreig, T., and Timpl, R., 1980, Biosynthesis of two subunits of type IV procollagen and of other basement membrane proteins by a human tumor cell line, Eur. J. Biochem. **109**:247–255.

Alstadt, S. P., Hebda, P., Chung, A., and Eaglstein, W., 1985, The enhancement of epidermal cell attachment by basement membrane entactin, J. Invest. Dermatol. **84**:353 (abst).

Balazs, A., and Holmgren, H. J., 1950, The basic dye-uptake and the presence of growth inhibiting substance in the healing tissue of skin wounds, Exp. Cell Res. **1**:206–216.

Beerens, E., Slot, J., and Van der Leun, J., 1975, Rapid regeneration of the dermal-epidermal junction after partial separation by vacuum: An electron microscopic study, J. Invest. Dermatol. **65**:513–521.

Bender, B. L., Jaffe, R., Carlin, B., and Chung, A., 1981, Immunolocalization of entactin, a sulfated basement membrane component in rodent tissues and comparison with GP-2 (laminin), Am. J. Pathol. **103**:419–426.

Bentley, J. P., 1967, Fate of chondroitin sulfate formation in wound healing, Ann. Surg. **165**:186–191.

Bentz, H., Bachinger, H., Granville, R., and Kuhn, K., 1978, Physical evidence for the assembly of A and B chains of human placental collagen in a single triple helix, *Eur. J. Biochem.* **92**:563–567.

Bentz, H., Morris, N., Murray, L., Sakai, L., Hollister, D., and Burgeson, R., 1983, Isolation and partial characterization of a new human collagen with an extended triple-helical structural domain, *Proc. Natl. Acad. Sci. USA* **80**:3168–3172.

Bernfield, M. R., and Banerjee, S. D., 1978, The basal lamina in epithelial–mesenchymal morphogenetic interactions, in: *Biology and Chemistry of Basement Membranes* (N. A. Kefalides, eds.), pp. 137–148, Academic, New York.

Bernfield, M. R., Cohn, R. N., and Banerjee, S. D., 1973, Glycosaminoglycans and epithelial organ formation, *Am. Zool.* **13**:1067–1083.

Boselli, J., Macarale, E., Clark, C., Brownell, A., and Martinex-Hernandez, A., 1981, Fibronectin: Its relationship to basement membranes. I. Light microscopic studies, *Collagen Relat. Res.* **1**:391–404.

Breathnach, A. S., and Robins, J., 1969, Ultrastructural features of epidermis of a 14 MM. (6 weeks) human embryo, *Br. J. Dermatol.* **81**:504–516.

Breathnach, S. M., Fox, P. A., Neises, G. R., Stanley, J. R., and Katz, S. I., 1983, A unique epithelial basement membrane antigen defined by a monoclonal antibody (KF-1), *J. Invest. Dermatol.* **80**:392–395.

Brickman, F., Soltani, K., Medenica, M., and Taylor, M. E. M., 1977, Antigenic and morphologic regeneration of epidermal basement membrane in short term organ culture of human skin, *Lab. Invest.* **36**:296–302.

Briggaman, R., 1983, Biochemical composition of the epidermal–dermal junction and other basement membrane, *J. Invest. Dermatol.* **81**:74s–81s.

Briggaman, R. A., and Wheeler, C. E., Jr., 1971, Formation and origin of basal lamina and anchoring fibrils in adult human skin, *J. Cell Biol.* **51**:384–395.

Briggaman, R., and Wheeler, C. E., Jr., 1975, The epidermal–dermal junction, *J. Invest. Dermatol.* **65**:71–84.

Briggaman, R. A., Schechter, N., Fraki, J., and Lazarus, G. S., 1984, Degradation of the epidermal–dermal junction by proteolytic enzymes from human skin and human polymorphonuclear leukocytes, *J. Exp. Med.* **160**:1027–1042.

Brownell, A. G., Bessen, C. C., and Slavkin, H. C., 1981, Possible functions of mesenchyme cell-derived fibronectin on the formation of basal lamina, *Proc. Natl. Acad. Sci. USA* **178**:3711–3725.

Burgeson, R., 1982, Genetic heterogeneity of collagens, *J. Invest. Dermatol.* **79**:25s–30s.

Burgeson, R., Adli, F., Kaitila, I., and Hollister, D., 1976, Fetal membrane collagens: Identification of two new collagen alpha chains, *Proc. Natl. Acad. Sci. USA* **73**:2579–2583.

Carlin, B. R., Jaffe, R., Bender, B., and Chung, A., 1981, Entactin, a novel basal lamina associated sulfated glycoprotein, *J. Biol. Chem.* **256**:5209–5214.

Chen, L. B., Murray, A., Segal, R. A., Bushnell, A., and Walsh, M., 1978, Studies on intracellular LETS glycoprotein matrices, *Cell* **14**:377–391.

Chung, A. E., Rhodes, K., and Miller, E., 1976, Isolation of three collagenous components of probable basement membrane origin from several tissues, *Biochem. Biophys. Res. Commun.* **71**:1167–1174.

Chung, A. E., Jaffe, R., Freeman, I. L., Vergnes, J.-P., Braguiski, J. E., and Carlin, B., 1979, Properties of a basement membrane related glycoprotein synthesized in culture by a mouse embryonal carcinoma-derived line, *Cell* **16**:277–287.

Clark, R. A. F., 1985, Cutaneous tissue repair: Basic biological considerations, *J. Am. Acad. Dermatol.* **13**:701–725.

Clark, R. A. F., Dellapelle, P., Manseau, E., Lanigan, J., Dvorak, H., and Colvin, R., 1982a, Blood vessel fibronectin increases in conjunction with endothelial cell proliferation and capillary ingrowth during wound healing, *J. Invest. Dermatol.* **79**:269–276.

Clark, R. A. F., Lanigan, J. M., Dellapelle, P., Manseau, E., Dvorak, H., and Colvin, R., 1982b, Fibronectin and fibrin provide a provisional matrix for epidermal–dermal cell migration during wound re-epithelialization, *J. Invest. Dermatol.* **79**:264–269.

Clemmons, D. R., Van Wyk, J. J., and Pledger, W. J., 1980, Sequential addition of plotted factor and plasma to BALB/c 373 fibroblast cultures stimulates somatomedin-C binding in early cell cycle, *Proc. Natl. Acad. Sci. USA* **77**:6644–6648.

Cotta-Pereira, G., Rodrigo, F., and Bittencourt-Sampaio, S., 1976, Oxytalan, elaunin and elastic fibers in the human skin, *J. Invest. Dermatol.* **66**:143–148.

Cotta-Pereira, G., Kattenback, W., and Guerra-Rodrigo, F., 1979, Elastic-related fibers in basement membrane, *Front. Matrix Biol.* **7**:90–100.

Couchman, J., Gibson, W., Thom, D., Weaver, A., Dees, D., and Parish, W., 1979, Fibronectin distribution in epithelial and associated tissues in the rat, *Arch. Dermatol. Res.* **266**:295–310.

Croft, C. B., and Tarin, D., 1970, Ultrastructural studies of wound healing in mouse skin. I. Epithelial behavior, *J. Anat.* **106**:63–77.

Crouch, E., Sage, H., and Bornstein, P., 1980, Structural basis for apparent heterogeneity of collagens in human basement membranes: Type IV procollagen contains two distinct chains, *Proc. Natl. Acad. Sci. USA* **77**:745–749.

Culp, L. A., Murray, B. A., and Rollins, B. J., 1979, Fibronectin and proteoglycans as determinants of cell–substratum adhesion, *J. Supramol. Struct.* **11**:401–427.

Daroczy, J., Feldman, J., and Kiraly, K., 1979, Human epidermal basal lamina: Its structure, connections and functions, *Front. Matrix Biol.* **7**:208–234.

Diaz, L. A., and Marcelo, C. L., 1978, Pemphigoid and pemphigus antigens in cultured epidermal cells, *Br. J. Dermatol.* **98**:631–637.

Diaz, L., Calvanico, N., Tomasi, T., and Jordan, R., 1977, Bullous pemphigoid antigen: Isolation from normal human skin, *J. Immunol.* **118**:455–460.

Dixit, S., Mainarda, D., Beachey, E., and Kang, A., 1983, 7S domains constitutes the amino terminal end of type IV collagen: An immunochemical study, *Collagen Relat. Res.* **3**:263–269.

Dodson, J. W., and Hay, E. D., 1971, Secretion of collagenous stroma by isolated epithelium grown, in vitro, *Exp. Cell Res.* **65**:215–220.

Dodson, J. W., and Hay, E. D., 1974, Secretion of collagen by corneal epithelium. II. Effect of the underlying substratum on secretion and polymerizations of epithelial products, *J. Exp. Zool.* **189**:51–72.

Engel, J., Odermatt, E., Engel, A., Madri, J., Furthmayr, H., Rohde, H., and Timpl, R., 1981, Shapes, domain organization and flexibility of lamini and fibronectin two multifunctional proteins of the extracellular matrix, *J. Mol. Biol.* **150**:97–120.

Fessler, L. I., and Fessler, J. H., 1982, Identification of the carboxyl peptides of mouse procollagen IV and its implications for the assembly and structure of basement membrane procollagen, *J. Biol. Chem.* **257**:9804–9810.

Fine, J. D., Smith, L. T., Holbrook, K. A., and Katz, S. I., 1984, The appearance of four basement membrane zone antigens in developing human fetal skin, *J. Invest. Dermatol.* **83**:66–69.

Fine, J. D., Redmer, D. A., and Goodman, A. L., 1985, Reappearance of seven basement membrane antigens in primate skin following split-thickness wound induction, *J. Invest. Dermatol.* **84**:353 (abst).

Fleischmajer, R., and Timpl, R., 1984, Ultrastructural localization of fibronectin to different anatomic structures of human skin, *J. Histochem. Cytochem.* **32**:315–321.

Foidart, J., and Yaar, M., 1981, Type IV collagen, laminin and fibronectin at the dermoepidemal junction, *Front. Matrix Biol.* **9**:175–188.

Foidart, J. M., Bere, E. W., Yaar, M., Rennard, S. I., Qullino, M., Martin, G. R., and Katz, S. I., 1980, Distribution and immunoelectron microscopic localization of laminin, a non-collagenous basement membrane glycoprotein, *Lab. Invest.* **42**:336–342.

Fuchs, E., and Green, H., 1981, Regulation of terminal differentiation of cultured human keratinocytes by vitamin A, *Cell* **25**:617–625.

Fyrand, O., 1979, Studies on fibronectin in the skin, *Br. J. Dermatol.* **101**:263–270.

Gay, S., Kresina, T., Gay, R., Miller, E., and Montes, L., 1979, Immunohistochemical demonstration of basement membrane collagen in normal skin and in psoriasis, *J. Cutan. Pathol.* **6**:91–95.

Gay, S., Martinez-Hernandez, A., Rhodes, R. K., and Miller, E. J., 1981, The collagenous exocytoskeleton of smooth muscle cells, *Collagen Relat. Res.* **1**:377–384.

Gilchrest, B. A., Nemore, R. E., and Maciag, T., 1980, Growth of human keratinocytes on fibronectin coated plates, *Cell Biol. Int. Rep.* **4**:1009–1016.

Gilchrest, B. A., Alhoun, J. K., and Maciag, T., 1982, Attachment and growth of human keratinocytes in a serum-free environment, *J. Cell Physiol.* **112**:197–206.

Gipson, I. K., Grill, S. M., Spurr, S. J., and Brennan, S. J., 1983, Hemidesmosome formation *in vitro*, *J. Cell Biol.* **97**:849–857.

Goldsmith, L. A., and Briggaman, R. A., 1982, Monoclonal antibodies to normal and abnormal epithelial antigens, in: *Normal and Abnormal Epidermal Differentiation* (M. Seiji and I. Bernstein, eds.), pp. 1–23, University of Tokyo Press, Tokyo.

Goldsmith, L. A., and Briggaman, R. A., 1983, Monoclonal antibodies to anchoring fibrils for the diagnosis of epidermolysis bullosa, *J. Invest. Dermatol.* **81**:464–466.

Gospodarowicz, D., 1983, The control of mammalian cell proliferation by growth factors, basement lamina and lipoproteins, *J. Invest. Dermatol.* **81**:40s–49s.

Gospodarowicz, D., Greenburg, G., and Birdwell, C. R., 1978, Determination of cellular shape by extracellular matrix and its correlation with the control of cellular growth, *Cancer Res.* **38**:4155–4171.

Grinnell, F., 1983, The role of fibronectin in the bioreactivity of material surfaces, in: *Biocompatible Polymers, Metals and Composites*, (M. Szycher, ed.), pp. 673–699, Technomic Publishing Co., Lancaster, Pennsylvania.

Hassell, R. J., Gehron-Robey, P., Barrach, H. J., Wilczek, J., Rennard, S. I., and Martin, G. R., 1980, Isolation of a heparan sulfate containing proteoglycan from basement membrane, *Proc. Natl. Acad. Sci. USA* **77**:4494–4498.

Hay, E. D., 1982, Collagen and embryonic development, in: *Cell Biology of the Extracellular Matrix* (E. D. Hay, ed.), pp. 379–409, Plenum, New York.

Hay, E. D., and Dobson, J. W., 1973, Secretion of collagen by corneal epithelium. I. Morphology of the collagenous products produced by isolated epithelia grown on frozen-killed lens, *J. Cell Biol.* **57**:190–213.

Hintner, H., Fritsch, P. O., Foidart, J. M., Stingl, G., Schuler, G., and Katz, S., 1980, Expression of basement membrane zone antigens at the dermo-epibolic junction in organ culture of human skin, *J. Invest. Dermatol.* **74**:200–205.

Hirone, T., and Taniguchi, S., 1979, Basal lamina formation by epidermal cells in culture, in: *Biochemistry of Normal and Abnormal Epidermal Differentiation* (I. Bernstein and M. Seiji, eds.), pp. 159–169, University of Tokyo Press, Tokyo.

Holubar, K., Wolff, K., Konrad, K., and Beutner, E. H., 1975, Ultrastructure localization of immunoglobulins in bullous pemphigoid skin, *J. Invest. Dermatol.* **64**:220–227.

Hynes, R. O., 1982, Fibronectin and its relation to cellular structure and behavior, in: *Cell Biology of the Extracellular Matrix* (E. D. Hay, ed.), pp. 295–334, Plenum, New York.

Hynes, R. O., and Yamada, K. M., 1982, Fibronectins: Multifunctional modular glycoproteins, *J. Cell Biol.* **95**:369–377.

Kanwar, Y. S., and Farquhar, M. D., 1979, Isolation of glycosaminoglycans (heparan sulfate) from glomerular basement membranes, *Proc. Natl. Acad. Sci. USA* **76**:4493–4497.

Kanwar, Y. S., Hascall, V. C., and Farquhar, M. G., 1981, Partial characterization of newly synthesized proteoglycans isolated from the glomerular basement membrane, *J. Cell Biol.* **90**:527–533.

Katz, S. I., 1984, The epidermal basement membrane zone—Structure, ontogeny, and role in disease. *J. Am. Acad. Dermatol.* **11**:1025–1037.

Kleinman, H. K., Klebe, R. J., and Martin, G. R., 1981, Role of collagenous matrices in the adhesion and growth of cells, *J. Cell Biol.* **88**:473–485.

Kobayasi, T., 1977, Anchoring of basal lamina to elastic fibers by elastic fibrils, *J. Invest. Dermatol.* **68**:389–390.

Krawczyk, W. S., and Wilgram, G., 1973, Hemidesmosome and desmosome morphogenesis during epidermal wound healing, *J. Ultrastruct. Res.* **45**:93–101.

Kubo, M., Norris, D. A., Howell, S. E., Ryan, S. R., and Clark, R. A. F., 1984, Human keratinocytes synthesize, secrete and deposit fibronectin in the pericellular matrix, *J. Invest. Dermatol.* **82**:580–586.

Kuhn, K., Weidemann, H., Timpl, R., Risteli, J., Dieringer, H., Voss, T., and Glanville, R. W., 1981, Macromolecular structure of basement membrane collagens identification of 7S collagen as a crosslinking domain of type V collagen, *FEBS Lett.* **125**:123–238.

Kurkinen, M., Vaheri, A., Roberts, P. J., and Stenman, S., 1980, Sequential appearance of fibronectin and collagen in experimental granulation tissue, *Lab. Invest.* **43**:47–51.

Laurie, G. W., LeBlond, C., and Martin, G., 1982, Localization of type IV collagen, laminin, heparan sulfate proteoglycan and fibronectin to the basal lamina of basement membrane, *J. Cell Biol.* **95**:340–344.

Lavker, R., and Sun, T.-T., 1982, Heterogeneity in epidermal basal keratinocytes: Morphological and functional correlations, *Science* **215**:1239–1241.

Linsenmayer, T. F., Smith, G. N., and Hay, E. D., 1977, Synthesis of two collagen types by embryonic chick corneal epithelium *in vitro*, *Proc. Natl. Acad. Sci. USA* **74**:39–43.

Maciag, T., Nemore, R. E., Weinstein, R., and Gilchrest, B. A., 1981, An endocrine approach to control of epidermal growth: Serum free cultivation of human keratinocytes, *Science* **211**:1452–1454.

Madri, J. A., and Furthmayr, H., 1979, Isolation and tissue localization of type B_2 collagen from normal lung parenchyma, *Am. J. Pathol.* **94**:323–330.

Madri, J. A., Roll, J., Furthmayr, H., and Foidart, J. M., 1980a, Ultrastructural localization of fibronectin and laminin in the basement membrane of the murine kidney, *J. Cell Biol.* **86**:682–687.

Madri, J. A., Dreyer, B., Pitlick, F. A., and Furthmayr, H., 1980b, The collagenous components of the subendothelium, *Lab Invest.* **43**:303–315.

Malinoff, H., and Wicha, M. S., 1983, Isolation of a cell surface receptor protein for laminin from murine fibrosarcoma cells, *J. Cell Biol.* **96**:1475–1479.

Manabe, M., and Ogawa, H., 1985, Ultrastructural demonstration of anionic sites in basement membrane zone by cationic probes, *J. Invest. Dermatol.* **84**:19–21.

Mann, P., and Constable, H., 1977, Induction of basal lamina formation in epidermal cell cultures *in vitro*, *Br. J. Dermatol.* **96**:421–426.

Marks, R., Abell, E., and Nishikawa, T., 1975, The junctional zone beneath migrating epidermis, *Br. J. Dermatol.* **92**:311–319.

Martinez-Hernandez, A., Marsh, C., Clark, C., Macarak, E., and Brownell, A., 1981, Fibronectin: Its relationship to basement membranes. II. Ultrastructural studies in rat kidney, *Collagen Relat. Res.* **1**:405–418.

McDonald, J. A., Kelley, D. G., and Broekelmann, T. J., 1982, Role of fibronectin in collagen deposition: Fab¹ antibodies to the gelatin-binding domain of fibronectin inhibits both fibronectin and collagen organization in fibroblast extracellular matrix, *J. Cell Biol.* **92**:485–492.

Meier, S., and Hay, E. D., 1973, Synthesis of sulfated glycosaminoglycans by embryonic corneal epithelium, *Dev. Biol.* **35**:318–331.

Meier, S., and Hay, E. D., 1974, Stimulation of extracellular matrix synthesis in developing cornea by glycosaminoglycans, *Proc. Natl. Acad. Sci. USA* **71**:2310–2313.

Mosher, D. F., and Furcht, L., 1981, Fibronectin: Review of its structure and possible functions, *J. Invest. Determatol.* **77**:175–180.

Mueller, H., and Franke, W. W., 1983, Biochemical and immunological characterization of desmoplakins I and II, the major polypeptides of the desmosomal plaque, *J. Mol. Biol.* **163**:645–671.

Muller, H. K., Kalnins, R., and Sutherland, R., 1973, Ontogeny of pemphigus and bullous pemphigoid antigens in human skin, *Br. J. Dermatol.* **88**:443–446.

Mutasim, D. F., Takahashi, Y., Labib, R. S., Anhalb, G. J., Patel, H. P., and Diaz, L. A., 1985, A pool of bullous pemphigoid antigen(s) is intracellular and associated with the basal cell cytoskeleton–hemidesmosome complex, *J. Invest. Dermatol.* **84**:47–53.

Nieboer, C., Boorsma, D. M., Woerdeman, M. J., and Kalsbeek, G. L., 1980, Epidermolysis bullosa acquisita: Immunofluorescence, electron microscopic and immunoelectron microscopic studies in four patients, *Br. J. Dermatol.* **102**:383–392.

Odland, G., and Ross, R., 1968, Human wound repair. I. Epidermal regeneration, *J. Cell Biol.* **39**:135–151.

O'Keefe, E. J., Woodley, D. T., Castillo, G., Russell, N., and Payne, R., 1984, Production of soluble and cell-associated fibronectin in cultured keratinocytes, *J. Invest. Dermatol.* **82**:150–155.

O'Keefe, E. J., Payne, R. E., Russell, N., and Woodley, D. T., 1985, Spreading and enhanced motility of human keratinocytes on fibronectin, *J. Invest. Dermatol.* **85**:125–130.

Oohira, A., Wight, T., McPherson, J., and Bornstein, P., 1982, Biochemical and ultrastructural studies of proteoheparan sulfates synthesized by PYS-Z, a basement membrane producing cell line, *J. Cell Biol.* **92:**357–367.

Pearlstein, E., Gold, L., and Garcia-Pardo, A., 1980, Fibronectin: A review of its structure and biological activity, *Mol. Cell Biochem.* **29:**103–128.

Prunieras, M., Regnier, M., and Schlotterer, M., 1979, Nouveau procédé de culture des cellules épidermiques humaine sur derme homologue ou hétérologue: Préparation de greflons recombinés, *Ann. Chir. Plast. Esthet.* **24:**357–362.

Prunieras, M., Regnier, M., Fougere, S., and Woodley, D., 1983a, Keratinocytes synthesize basal lamina proteins in culture, *J. Invest. Dermatol.* **81:**74s–81s.

Prunieras, M., Regnier, M., and Woodley, D., 1983b, Methods for cultivation of keratinocytes with air–liquid interface, *J. Invest. Dermatol.* **81:**28s–33s.

Rao, C. N., Margulies, I., Tralka, T., Terranova, V., Madri, J., and Liotta, L., 1982, Isolation of a subunit of laminin and its role in molecular structure and tumor cell attachment, *J. Biol. Chem.* **257:**9740–9744.

Regnier, M., Prunieras, M., and Woodley, D., 1981, Growth and differentiation of adult human epidermal cells on dermal substrates, *Front. Matrix Biol.* **9:**4–35.

Regnier, M., Voigot, P., Michel, S., Prunieras, M., 1985, Localization of bullous pemphigoid antigen in isolated human keratinocytes, *J. Invest. Dermatol.* **85:**187–190.

Repesh, L. A., Fitzgerla, T. J., and Furcht, L. T., 1982, Fibronectin involvement in granulation tissue and wound healing in rabbits, *J. Histochem. Cytochem.* **30:**351–358.

Rhodes, R., and Miller, E., 1978, Physiochemical characterization and molecular organization of collagen A and B chains, *Biochemistry* **17:**3442–3448.

Risteli, J., Bachinger, H., Engel, J., Furthmayr, H., and Timpl, R., 1980, 7S collagen characterization of an unusual basement membrane structure, *Eur. J. Biochem.* **108:**239–250.

Roll, J., Madri, J. A., Albert, J., and Furthmayr, H., 1980, Codistribution of collagen types IV and AB_2 in basement membranes and mesangium of the kidney, *J. Cell Biol.* **85:**597–616.

Ruoslahti, E., Engvall, E., and Hayman, E. G., 1981, Fibronectin: Current concepts of its structure and function, *Collagen Relat. Res.* **1:**95–128.

Sage, H., and Bornstein, P., 1979, Characterization of a novel collagen chain in human placenta and its relation to AB collagen, *Biochemistry* **18:**3815–3822.

Salomon, D. S., Liotta, L. A., and Kidwell, W. R., 1981, Differential growth factor responsiveness of rat mammary epithelial plate on different collagen substrate in serum-free medium, *Proc. Natl. Acad. Sci. USA* **176:**382–386.

Sakai, L., Keene, D. R., Morris, N. P., and Burgeson, R. F., 1986, Type VII collagen is a major structural component of anchoring fibrils, *J. Cell Biol.* **103:**1577–1586.

Sarkany, I., and Gaylarde, P., 1970, Ultrastructural changes in human skin maintained in organ culture, *Br. J. Dermatol.* **83:**572–581.

Schaumburg-Lever, G., Rule, R. A., Schmidt-Ullrich, B., and Lever, W. F., 1975, Ultrastructural localization of *in vivo* bound immunoglobulins in bullous pemphigoid: A preliminary report, *J. Invest. Dermatol.* **64:**47–49.

Schuppan, D., Timpl, R., and Granville, R., 1980, Discontinuities in the triple helical sequences Gly–X–Y of basement membrane (type IV) collagen, *FEBS Lett.* **115:**297–300.

Stanley, J. R., Foidart, J. M., Murray, J. C., Martin, G. R., and Katz, S. I., 1980, The epidermal cell which selectively adheres to a collagen substrate is the basal cell, *J. Invest. Dermatol.* **74:**54–58.

Stanley, J. R., Alvarez, O. M., Bere, E. W., Eaglstein, W., and Katz, S., 1981a, Detection of basement membrane antigens during epidermal wound healing, *J. Invest. Dermatol.* **77:**240–243.

Stanley, J. R., Hawley-Nelson, P., Yuspa, S. H., Shevach, E., and Katz, S., 1981b, Characterization of bullous pemphigoid antigen: A unique basement membrane protein of stratified squamous epithelia, *Cell* **24:**897–903.

Stanley, J., Woodley, D., Katz, S., and Martin, G., 1982a, Structure and function of basement membrane, *J. Invest. Dermatol.* (Suppl.) **79:**69s–72s.

Stanley, J. R., Beckwith, J. B., Fuller, R. P., and Katz, S. I., 1982b, A specific antigenic defect of the basement membrane is found in basal cell carcinoma but not in other epidermal tumors, *Cancer* **50:**1486–1490.

Stanley, J. R., Hawley-Nelson, P., Yaar, M., Martin, G. R., and Katz, S. I., 1982c, Laminin and bullous pemphigoid antigen are distinct basement membrane proteins synthesized by epidermal cells, J. Invest. Dermatol. **78:**456–459.

Stenman, S., and Vaheri, A., 1978, Distribution of a major connective tissue protein, fibronectin in normal tissue, J. Exp. Med. **147:**1054–1064.

Stenn, K. S., Madri, J. A., and Roll, F. J., 1979, Migrating epidermis produces AB$_2$ collagen and requires continued collagen synthesis for movement, Nature (Lond.) **277:**229–232.

Sugrue, S. P., and Hay, E. D., 1981, Response of basal epithelial cell surface and cytoskeleton to solubilize extracellular matrix molecules, J. Cell Biol. **91:**45–54.

Taniguchi, S., and Hirone, T., 1982, Synthesis of basal lamina by epidermal cells in vitro, in: Normal and Abnormal Epidermal Differentiation (M. Seiji and I. Bernstein, eds.), pp. 127–133, University of Tokyo Press, Tokyo.

Terranova, V. P., Rohrbach, D. H., and Martin, G. R., 1980, Role of laminin in the attachment of PAM 212 (epithelial) cells to basement membrane collagen, Cell **22:**719–729.

Terranova, V., Rao, C., Kalebic, T., Margulies, I., and Liotta, L., 1983, Laminin receptor on human breast carcinoma cells, Proc. Natl. Acad. Sci. USA **80:**444–448.

Timpl, R., Rhode, H., Gehron Robey, P., Rennard, S. I., Foidart, J. M., and Martin, G. R., 1979a, Laminin—A glycoprotein from basement membranes, J. Biol. Chem. **254:**9933–9937.

Timpl, R., Risteli, J., and Bachinger, H., 1979b, Identification of a new basement membrane collagen by the aid of a large fragment resistant to bacterial collagenase, FEBS Lett. **101:**265–268.

Timpl, R., Granville, R., Wick, G., and Martin, G., 1979c, Immunochemical study on basement membrane (type IV) collagen, Immunology **38:**109–116.

Timpl, R., Wiedemann, H., van Delden, V., Furthmayr, H., and Kuhn, K., 1981, A network model for the organization of type IV collagen molecules in basement membranes, Eur. J. Biochem. **120:**203–211.

Timpl, R., Dziadek, M., Fujiwara, S., Nowack, H., and Wick, G., 1983a, Nidogen: A new self-aggregating basement membrane protein, Eur. J. Biochem. **139:**401–410.

Timpl, R., Engel, J., and Martin, G., 1983b, Laminin—A multifunctional protein of basement membranes, Trends Biol. Sci. **8:**207–209.

Toole, B. P., 1983, Glycosaminoglycans in morphogenesis, in: Cell Biology of Extracellular Matrix (E. D. Hay, ed.), pp. 259–294, Plenum, New York.

Toole, B. P., and Trelstad, R. L., 1971, Hyaluronate production and removal during corneal development in the chick, Dev. Biol. **26:**28–35.

Trinkaus-Randall, V., and Gipson, I., 1984, Role of calcium and calmodulin in hemidesmosome formation in vitro, J. Cell Biol. **98:**1565–1571.

Wessells, N. K., 1977a, Extracellular materials and tissue interactions, in: Tissue Interactions and Development (N. K. Wessells, ed.), pp. 213–229, Benjamin-Cummings, Menlo Park, California.

Wessells, N. K., 1977b, Cell surface and development, in: Tissue Interactions and Development (N. K. Wessells, ed.), pp. 181–196, Benjamin-Cummings, Menlo Park, California.

Westgate, G. E., Weaver, A. C., and Couchman, J. R., 1985, Bullous pemphigoid antigen localization suggests an intracellular association with hemidesmosomes, J. Invest. Dermatol. **84:**218–224.

Wood, G. C., 1960, The formation of fibrils from collagen solutions. Effect of chondroitin sulfate and other naturally occurring polyanions on the rate of formation, Biochem. J. **75:**605–612.

Woodley, D. T., and Regnier, M., 1979, Bullous pemphigoid antigen deposited on a millipore filter, Arch. Dermatol. Res. **266:**319–322.

Woodley, D., Didierjean, L., Regnier, M., Saurat, J., and Prunieras, M., 1980a, Bullous pemphigoid antigen synthesized in vitro by human epidermal cells, J. Invest. Dermatol. **75:**148–151.

Woodley, D., Regnier, M., and Prunieras, M., 1980b, In vitro basal lamina formation may require non-epidermal cell living substrate, Br. J. Dermatol. **103:**397–404.

Woodley, D. T., Saurat, J. H., Prunieras, M., and Regnier, M., 1982, Pemphigoid, pemphigus and Pr antigens in adult human keratinocytes grown on nonviable substrates, J. Invest. Dermatol. **79:**23–29.

Woodley, D. T., Rao, D. N., Hassell, J. R., Liotta, L., Martin, G., and Kleinman, H., 1983, Interactions of basement membrane components, Biochim. Biophys. Acta **761:**278–283.

Woodley, D. T., Briggaman, R., O'Keefe, E., Inman, A., Queen, L., and Gammon, W. R., 1984,

Identifications of epidermolysis bullosa acquisita antigen—A normal component of human skin basement membrane, *N. Engl. J. Med.* **310:**1007–1013.

Woodley, D. T., O'Keefe, E. J., and Prunieras, M., 1985a, Cutaneous wound healing: A model for cell–matrix interactions, *J. Am. Acad. Dermatol.* **12:**420–433.

Woodley, D. T., Briggaman, R. A., Gammon, W. R., and O'Keefe, E. J., 1985b, Epidermolysis bullosa acquisita antigen is synthesized by human keratinocytes cultured in serum-free medium, *Biochem. Biophys. Res. Commun.* **130:**1267–1272.

Yamada, K. M., 1982, Fibronectin and other structural proteins, in: *Cell Biology of the Extracellular Matrix* (E. D. Hay, ed.), pp. 95–115, Plenum, New York.

Yamada, K., and Olden, K., 1978, Fibronectins—Adhesive glycoproteins of cell surface and blood, *Nature (Lond.)* **275:**179–184.

Yamasaki, Y., and Nishikawa, T., 1983, Ultrastructural localization of *in vitro* binding sites of circulating antibasement membrane zone antibodies in bullous pemphigoid, *Acta Derm. Venereol. (Stockh.)* **63:**501–596.

Yaoita, H., Foidart, J. M., and Katz, S. I., 1978, Localization of the collagenous component in skin basement membrane, *J. Invest. Dermatol.* **70:**191–193.

Yaoita, H., Briggaman, R. A., Lawley, T. J., Provost, T. T., and Katz, S. I., 1981, Epidermolysis bullosa acquisita: Ultrastructural and immunological studies, *J. Invest. Dermatol.* **76:**288–292.

Index

Italicized numbers indicate pages where entry is discussed in detail.